Cultural Diversity
in Health and Illness

CULTURALCARE

There is something that transcends all of this
I am I . . . You are you
Yet. I and you
Do connect
Somehow, sometime.

To understand the "cultural" needs
Samenesses and differences of people
Needs an open being
See—Hear—Feel
With no judgment or interpretation
Reach out
Maybe with that physical touch
Or eyes, or aura
You exhibit your openness and willingness to
Listen and learn
And, you tell and share
In so doing—you share humanness
It is acknowledged and shared
Something happens—
Mutual understanding

—Rachel E. Spector

Cultural Diversity in Health and Illness

SEVENTH EDITION

Rachel E. Spector, PhD, RN, CTN, FAAN

CULTURALCARE Consultant,
Needham, MA 02494

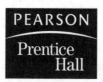

PEARSON
Prentice
Hall

Upper Saddle River, New Jersey 07458

Library of Congress Cataloging-in-Publication Data
Spector, Rachel E.
   Cultural diversity in health and illness / Rachel E. Spector.—7th ed.
     p. ; cm.
   Rev. ed. of: Cultural diversity in health & illness / Rachel E. Spector. 6th ed. c2004.
   Includes bibliographical references and index.
   ISBN-13: 978-0-13-503589-4
   ISBN-10: 0-13-503589-9
   1. Transcultural medical care—United States.
   2. Health attitudes—United States.
   3. Transcultural nursing—United States.
   I. Spector, Rachel E., 1940-Cultural diversity in health & illness. II. Title.
   [DNLM: 1. Cultural Diversity—United States.
   2. Attitude to Health—ethnology—United States.
   3. Cultural Competency—United States.
   4. Delivery of Health Care—United States.
   5. Ethnic Groups—United States.
   6. Health Status—United States. WA 31 S741c 2009]
   RA418.5.T73S64 2009
   362.1'0425-dc22   2008020984

I would like to dedicate this text to

My husband, Manny;
Sam, Hilary, Julia, and Emma;
Becky, Perry, Naomi, Rose, and Miriam;
the memory of my parents, Joseph J. and Freda F. Needleman,
and my in-laws, Sam and Margaret Spector;
and the memory of my beloved mentor, Irving Kenneth Zola.

Contents

Preface

Every book, every volume you see here, has a soul. The soul of the person who wrote it and of those who read it and lived and dreamed with it.

—Carlos Ruiz Zafon,
The Shadow of the Wind, 2001

In 1977—more than 30 years ago—I prepared the first edition of *Cultural Diversity in Health and Illness*. Now, as I begin the seventh edition of this book—the sixth revision—I realize that this is an opportunity to reflect on an endeavor that has filled a good deal of my life for the past 30 years. I believe this book has a soul and it, in turn, has become an integral part of my soul. I have lived—through practice, teaching, and research—this material since 1974 and have developed many ways of presenting this content. In addition, I have tracked for 30 years

1. The United States Census
2. Immigration—numbers and policies
3. Poverty—figures and policies
4. Health care—costs and policies
5. Morbidity and mortality rates
6. Nursing and other health care manpower issues

My metaphors are *HEALTH*, defined as "the balance of the person, both within one's being—physical, mental, and spiritual—and in the outside world—natural, communal, and metaphysical"; *ILLNESS*, the imbalance of the person, both within one's being—physical, mental, and spiritual—and in the outside world—natural, communal, and metaphysical; and *HEALING*, the restoration of balance, both within one's being—physical, mental, and spiritual—and in the outside world—natural, communal, and metaphysical." I have learned over these years that within many traditional heritages (defined as "old," not contemporary or modern) people tend to define HEALTH, ILLNESS, and HEALING in this manner. Imagine a kaleidoscope—the tube can represent HEALTH. The objects reflected within the kaleidoscope reflect the traditional tools used to care for a given person's HEALTH. If you love kaleidoscopes, you know what I am describing and that the patterns that emerge are infinite.

In addition, I have had the unique opportunity to travel to countless places in the United States and abroad. I make it a practice to visit the traditional markets, pharmacies, and shrines and dialogue with the people who work in or patronize the settings and have gathered invaluable knowledge and unique items and images. My tourist dollars are invested in amulets and remedies and my collection is large. Digital photography has changed my eyes; I may be a "digital immigrant," rather than a "digital native," but the camera has proven to be my most treasured companion. I have been able to use the images of sacred objects and sacred places to create HEALTH Traditions Imagery. The opening images for each chapter and countless images within the chapters are the results of these explorations. Given that there are times when we do not completely understand a concept or an image, several images are slightly blurred or dark to represent this wonderment.

The first edition of this book was the outcome of a *promesa*—a promise— I once made. The promise was made to a group of Asian, Black, and Hispanic students I taught in a medical sociology course in 1973. In this course, the students wound up being the teachers, and they taught me to see the world of health care delivery through the eyes of the health care consumer rather than through my own well-intentioned eyes. What I came to see I did not always like. I did not realize how much I did not know; I believed I knew a lot. I promised the students that I would take that which they taught me regarding HEALTH and teach it to students and colleagues. I have held on to the *promesa*, and my experiences over the years have been incredible. I have met people and traveled. At all times I have held on to the idea and goal of attempting to help nurses and other health care providers be aware of and sensitive to the HEALTH, ILLNESS, and HEALING beliefs and needs of their patients.

I know that looking inside closed doors carries with it a risk. I know that people prefer to think that our society is a melting pot and that the traditional beliefs and practices have vanished with the expected acculturation and assimilation into mainstream North American modern life. Many people, however, have continued to carry on the traditional customs and culture from their native lands and heritage, and HEALTH, ILLNESS, and HEALING beliefs are deeply entwined within the cultural and social beliefs that people have. To understand HEALTH and ILLNESS beliefs and practices, it is necessary to see each person in his or her unique sociocultural world. The theoretical knowledge that has evolved for the development of this text is cumulative and much of the "old" material is relevant today as many HEALTH, ILLNESS, and HEALING beliefs do not change. However, many beliefs and practices do go underground.

The purpose of each edition has been to increase awareness of the dimensions and complexities involved in caring for people from diverse cultural backgrounds. I wished to share my personal experiences and thoughts concerning the introduction of cultural concepts into the education of health care professionals. The books represented my answers to the questions:

- ■ "How does one effectively expose a student to cultural diversity?"
- ■ "How does one examine health care issues and perceptions from a broad social viewpoint?"

As I have done in the classroom, I attempt to bring you, the reader, into direct contact with the interaction between providers of care within the North American health care system and the consumers of health care. The staggering issues of health care delivery are explored and contrasted with the choices that people may make in attempting to deal with health care issues.

It is now imperative, according to the most recent policies of the Joint Commission of Hospital Accreditation and the Centers for Medicare & Medicaid Services, that all health care providers be "culturally competent." In this context, cultural competency implies that within the delivery of care the health care provider understands and attends to the total context of the patient's situation; it is a complex combination of knowledge, attitudes, and skills, yet

■ How do you *really* inspire people to hear the content?
■ How do you *motivate* providers to see the worldview and lived experience of the patient?
■ How do you assist providers to *really* bear witness to the living conditions and life ways of patients?
■ How do you liberate providers from the burdens of prejudice, xenophobia, the "isms"—racism, ethnocentrism—and the "antis"?

It can be argued that the development of CULTURALCOMPETENCY does not occur in a short encounter with cultural diversity but that it takes time to develop the skills, knowledge, and attitudes to safely and satisfactorily deliver CULTURALCARE. Indeed, the reality of becoming "CULTURALCOMPETENT" is a complex process—it is time consuming, difficult, frustrating, and extremely interesting. CULTURALCOMPETENCY embraces the premise that all things are connected. Imagine a dandelion that has gone to seed. Each seed is a discrete entity, yet each is linked to the other (Figure P–1). Each facet discussed in this text—heritage, culture, ethnicity, religion, socialization, and identity—is connected to diversity—demographic change—population, immigration, and poverty. These facets are connected to health/HEALTH, illness/ILLNESS, curing/HEALING, and beliefs and practices, modern and traditional. All of these facets are connected to the health care delivery system—the culture, costs, and politics of health care, the internal and external political issues, public health issues, and housing and other infrastructure issues. In order to fully understand a person's health/HEALTH beliefs and practices, each of these topics must be in the background of a provider's mind.

I have had the opportunity to live and teach in Spain and to explore many areas, including Cadiz and the surrounding small villages. There was a fake door within the walls of a small village, *Vejer de la Frontera* (Figure P–2), that appeared to be bolted shut. The door was placed there during the early 14th century to fool the Barbary pirates. The people were able to vanquish them while they tried to pry the door open. It reminded me of the attempt to keep other ideas and people away from us and to not open ourselves up to new and different ideas. Another door (Figure P–3), found in Avila, Spain, was made of a translucent glass. Here, the person has a choice—you could peer through the door and view the garden behind it or open it and actually go into the garden

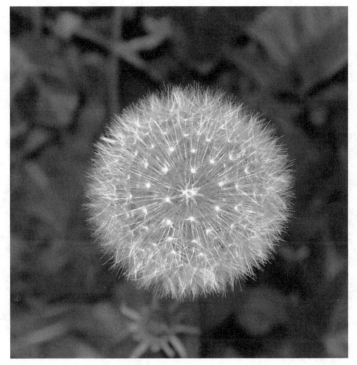

Figure P-1 A dandelion in seed.

for a finite walk. This reminded me of people who are able to understand the needs of others and return to their own life and heritage when work is completed. This polarity represents the challenges of "CULTURALCOMPETENCY."

The way to CULTURALCOMPETENCY is complex, but I have learned over the years that there are five steps (Figure P–4) to climb to begin to achieve this goal:

1. Personal heritage—Who are *you*?? What is *your* heritage? What are your health/HEALTH beliefs?
2. Heritage of others—demographics—Who is the patient? Family? Community?
3. Health and HEALTH beliefs and practices—competing philosophies
4. Health care culture and system—all the issues and problems
5. Traditional HEALTH Care Systems—The way HEALTH was for most and the way HEALTH still is for many

Once you have reached the sixth step, CULTURALCOMPETENCY, you are ready to open the door to CULTURALCARE.

Each step represents a discrete unit of study. The steps are composed of "bricks" and these provide the ingredients for the content. The "bricks" are

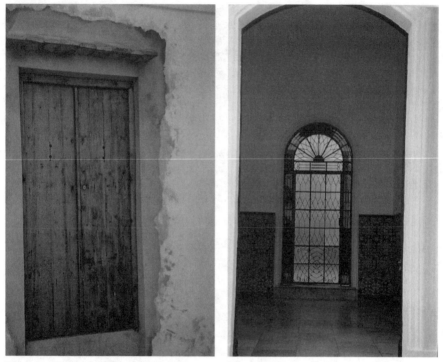

Figure P–2   Solidly closed door.   **Figure P–3   Transparent door.**

defined in the glossary, Appendix A and are the language of CULTURALCARE. The side rails represent responsibility and resiliency—for it is the responsibility of health care providers to be CULTURALLYCOMPETENT and, if this is not met, the consequences will be dire. The resiliency of providers and patients will be further compromised and we will all become more vulnerable. Contrary to popular belief and practice, CULTURALCOMPETENCY is not a "condition" that is rapidly achieved. Rather, it is an ongoing process of growth and the development of knowledge that takes a considerable amount of time to ingest, digest, assimilate, circulate, and master. The content is readily available:

- Countless books and articles have been published in nursing, medicine, public health, and the popular media over the past 40 years that contain invaluable information relevant to CULTURALCOMPETENCY.
- Innumerable workshops and meetings have been available where the content is presented and discussed.
- "Self-study" programs on the Internet have been developed that provide continuing education credits to nurses, physicians, and other providers.

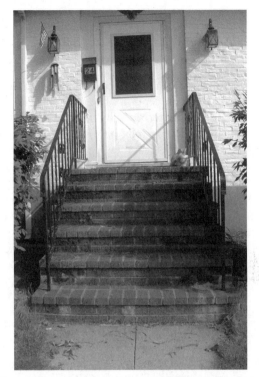

Figure P-4   The steps to CULTURALCOMPETENCY.

However, the process of becoming CULTURALLYCOMPETENT is not generally provided for. Issues persist, such as

- Demographic disparity exists in the profile of health care providers and in health status.
- Patient needs, such as modesty, space, and gender-specific care, are not universally met.
- Religious-specific needs are not met in terms of meal planning, procedural planning, conference planning, and so forth.
- Communication and language barriers exist.

As this knowledge is built, you are on the way to CULTURALCOMPETENCY. As it matures and grows, you become an advocate of CULTURALCARE, as it will be described in Chapter 1.

This book has been developed to provide an overview of the information necessary to climb these steps and examples of the process.

■ Overview

Unit I focuses on the background knowledge one must recognize as the foundation for developing CULTURALCOMPETENCY.

- Chapter 1 explores the concept of cultural heritage and history and the roles they play in one's perception of health and illness. This exploration is first outlined in general terms: What is culture? How is it transmitted? What is ethnicity? What is religion? How do they affect a person's health? What major sociocultural events occurred during the life trajectory of a person that may influence his or her personal health beliefs and practices?

- Chapter 2 presents a discussion of the diversity—demographic, immigration, and poverty—that impacts on the delivery of and access to health care. The backgrounds of each of the U.S. Census Bureau's categories of the population, an overview of immigration, and an overview of issues relevant to poverty are presented.

- Chapter 3 reviews the provider's knowledge of his or her own perceptions, needs, and understanding of health and illness.

Unit II explores the domains of HEALTH, blends them with one's personal heritage, and contrasts them with the Allopathic Philosophy.

- Chapter 4 introduces the concept of HEALTH and develops the concept in broad and general terms. The HEALTH Traditions Model is presented, as are natural methods of HEALTH maintenance and protection.

- Chapter 5 explores the concept of HEALTH restoration or HEALING and the role that faith plays in the context of HEALING, or magico-religious, traditions. This is an increasingly important issue, which is evolving to a point where the health care provider must have some understanding of this phenomenon.

- Chapter 6 discusses family heritage and explores personal and familial HEALTH traditions. It includes an array of familial health/HEALTH beliefs and practices shared by people from many different heritages.

- Chapter 7 focuses on the health care provider culture and the allopathic health care delivery system.

Once the study of each of these components has been completed, Unit III moves on to explore selected population groups in more detail, to portray a panorama of traditional HEALTH and ILLNESS beliefs and practices, and to present relevant health care issues.

Each chapter in the text opens with images—amulets, remedies, and/or shrines—relevant to the chapter's topic.

These pages cannot do full justice to the richness of any one culture or any one health belief system. By presenting some of the beliefs and practices and suggesting background reading, however, the book can begin to inform and sensitize the reader to the needs of a given group of people. It can also serve as a model as to how to develop cultural knowledge in populations that are not included.

The Epilogue is devoted to an overall analysis of the book's contents and how best to apply this knowledge in health care delivery, health planning, and health education, for both the patient and the health care professional.

There is so much to be learned. Countless books and articles have now appeared that address these problems and issues. It is not easy to alter attitudes and beliefs or stereotypes and prejudices—to change a person's philosophy. Some social psychologists state that it is almost impossible to lose all of one's prejudices, yet alterations can be made. I believe the health care provider *must* develop the ability to deliver CULTURALCARE and knowledge regarding personal fundamental values regarding health/HEALTH and illness/ILLNESS. With acceptance of one's own values come the framework and courage to accept the existence of differing values. This process of realization and acceptance can enable the health care provider to be instrumental in meeting the needs of the consumer in a collaborative, safe, and professional manner.

The shattering events of September 11, 2001, and the continuing wars in Afghanistan and Iraq, represent in many ways the clarion call for all of us to wake up and listen to the voices of all people. Indeed, the events are symptomatic of global polarization in such conflicts as

- Traditionalism vs. modernism
- Fundamentalism vs. universalism
- Heritage vs. secular
- Minimalism vs. excessism
- Self-denialism vs. materialism
- Fatalism vs. determinism
- Allopathy vs. homeopathy
- Curing vs. HEALING

Each of these terms is defined in the glossary—Appendix A.

Global polarization is culturally based and seems to be the engine driving recent events. CULTURALCARE is an attempt to look at the big picture that encompasses health care and attempts to find cultural meaning in daily life. In our world, that of health care delivery, it mandates that we must develop the knowledge and skills of CULTURALCARE.

This book is written primarily for the student in basic allied health professional programs, nursing, medical, social work, and other health care provider disciplines. I believe it will be helpful also for providers in all areas of practice, especially community health, long-term oncology, chronic care settings, and geriatric and hospice centers. I am attempting to write in a direct manner and to use language that is understandable by all. The material is sensitive, yet I believe that it is presented in a sensitive manner. At no point is my intent to create a vehicle for stereotyping. I know that one person will read this book and nod, "Yes, this is how I see it," and someone else of the same background will say, "No, this is not correct." This is the way it is meant to be. It is incomplete by intent. It is written in the spirit of open inquiry, so that an issue may be raised and so that clarification of any given point will be sought from the patient as health care is provided. The deeper I travel into this world of cultural diversity, the more I wonder at the variety. It is wonderfully exciting. By gaining insight into the traditional attitudes that people have toward health and health care, I find my own nursing practice is enhanced, and I am better able to understand the needs of patients and their families. It is thrilling to be able to meet, to know, and to provide care to people from all over the world. It is the excitement of nursing. As we now go forward in time, I hope that these words will help you, the reader, develop CULTURALCARE skills and help you provide the best care to all.

You don't need a masterpiece to get the idea.

—Pablo Picasso

■ Features

- **Research on Culture.** As evidence-based practice grows in importance, its application is expected in all aspects of health care. This special feature, new to this edition, spotlights how current research informs and impacts cultural awareness and competence.
- **Unit and Chapter Objectives.** Each unit and chapter opens with objectives to direct the reader when studying. The chapter objectives are new to this edition.
- **Unit Exercises and Activities.** The beginning of each unit provides exercises and activities related to the topic. Questions stimulate reflective consideration of the reader's own family and cultural history as well as to develop an awareness of one's own biases.
- **Figures, Tables, and Boxes.** Throughout the book are photographs, illustrations, tables, and boxes that exemplify and expand on information referenced in the chapter.
- **HEALTH Traditions Imagery.** These symbolic images are used to link the chapters. The images were selected to awaken you to the richness of a given heritage and the practices inherent within both modern and traditional cultures, as well as the beliefs surrounding health and HEALTH. (HEALTH, when written this way, is defined as the balance of the person, both within one's being—physical, mental, spiritual—and in the outside world—natural, familial and communal, metaphysical.)

Preface ■ xix

▦ Supplemental Resources

- **CulturalCare Guide.** Previously available as a separate booklet, the contents of this helpful guide are now available for downloading on the Companion Website. The guide includes the Heritage Assessment Tool, Cultural Phenomena Affecting Health Care, CulturalCare Etiquette, and other assessment tools and guides.

- **Companion Website.** www.prenhall.com/spector. The Companion Website includes a wealth of supplemental material to accompany each chapter. In addition to the complete contents of the **CulturalCare Guide**, the site presents chapter-related review questions, case studies, exercises, and MediaLinks to provide additional information. Panorama of Health and Illness videos accompany many chapters, and a glossary of terms appears for each chapter. Also included is a collection of the author's photographs and culturally significant images in the **CulturalCare Museum**.

- **Instructor's Resource Center.** Available to instructors adopting the book are PowerPoint Lecture Slides and a complete testbank available for downloading from the Instructor's Resource Center, which can be accessed through the online catalog.

- **Online Course Management.** Built to accompany *Cultural Diversity in Health and Illness* are online course management systems available for Blackboard, WebCT, Moodle, Angel, and other platforms. For more information, contact your Pearson Education sales representative.

About the Author

Dr. Rachel E. Spector has been a student of culturally diverse HEALTH and ILLNESS beliefs and practices for 35 years and has researched and taught courses on culture and HEALTH care for the same time span. Dr. Spector has had the opportunity to work in many different communities, including the American Indian and Hispanic communities in Boston, Massachusetts. Her studies have taken her to many places: most of the United States, Canada, and Mexico; several European countries, including Denmark, England, Finland, Iceland, Italy, France, Russia, Spain, and Switzerland; Israel and Pakistan; and Australia and New Zealand. She was fortunate enough to collect traditional amulets and remedies from many of these diverse communities and to meet practitioners of traditional HEALTH care in several places. She was instrumental in the creation and presentation of the exhibit "Immigrant HEALTH Traditions" at the Ellis Island Immigration Museum, May 1994 through January 1995. She has exhibited HEALTH-related objects in several other settings. Recently, she served as a *Colaboradora Honorífica* (Honorary Collaborator) in the University of Alicante in Alicante, Spain, and Tamaulipas, Mexico. In 2006, she was a Lady Davis Fellow in the Henrietta Zold-Hadassah Hebrew University School of Nursing in Jerusalem, Israel. This text was translated into Spanish by Maria Munoz and published in Madrid by Prentice Hall as *Las Culturas de la SALUD* in 2003. She is a Fellow in the American Academy of Nursing and a Scholar in Transcultural Nursing Society. The Massachusetts Association of Registered Nurses, the state organization of the American Nurses' Association, honored her as a "Living Legend" in 2007. In 2008 she received the Honorary Human Rights Award from the American Nurses Association. This award recognized her contributions and accomplishments that have been of national significance to human rights and have influenced health care and nursing practice.

Acknowledgments

I have had a 35-year adventure of studying the forces of culture, ethnicity, and religion and their profound influence on HEALTH, ILLNESS, and HEALING beliefs and practices. Many, many people have contributed generously to the knowledge I have acquired over this time as I have tried to serve as a voice for traditional people and the HEALTH, ILLNESS, and HEALING beliefs and practices derived from their given heritage. It has been a continuous struggle to insure that this information be included not only in nursing education but in the educational content of all helping professions—including medicine, the allied health professions, and social work.

I particularly wish to thank the following people for their guidance, professional support, and encouragement over the 32 years that this book, now in its seventh edition, has been an integral part of my life. They are people from many walks of life and have touched me in many ways. The people from Appleton-Century-Crofts, which became Appleton & Lang and then became Prentice Hall. They include Nancy Anselment, Sally Barhydt, Dave Caroll, Elisabeth Garafalo, Marion Kalstein-Welch, Pamela Lappies, Cathy O'Connell, Julie Stern, Patrick Walsh, and countless people involved in the production of the text. My first encounter with publishing was with Leslie Boyer, an acquisition editor from Appleton-Century-Crofts, who simply said "write a book" in 1976. For this edition I have worked closely with Michael Giacobbe, development editor, as not only an editor but a friend, a cheerleader, an encourager, and so forth. Without his patient help and guidance, this book would not be here today. Thanks to Teresa O'Neill of Our Lady of Holy Cross College for writing chapter review questions. The many people who helped with advice and guidance to resources over the years include Elsi Basque, Billye Brown, Louise Buchanan, Julian Castillo, Leonel J. Castillo, Jenny Chan, Dr. P. K. Chan, Joe Colorado, Miriam Cook, Elizabeth Cucchiaro, Mary A. Dineen, Norine Dresser, Celeste Dye, Laverne Gallman, Raymond and Madeline Goodman, Marjory Gordon, Orlando Isaza, Henry and Pandora Law, Hawk Littlejohn, Father Richard McCabe, S. Dale McLemore, Anita Noble, Carl Rutberg, Sister Mary Nicholas Vincelli, Nora Wang, David Warner, Ann Marie Yezzi-Shareef, and the late Irving K. Zola.

I wish to thank my friends and family, who have tolerated my absence at numerous social functions, and the many people who have provided the numerous support services necessary for the completion of an undertaking such as this.

A lot has happened in my life since the first edition of this book was published in 1979. My family has shrunk with the deaths of all four parents, and it has greatly expanded with a new daughter, Hilary, and a new son, Perry, and five granddaughters—Julia, Emma, Naomi, Rose, and Miriam. The generations have gone, and come.

■ Reviewers

Michelle Gagnon, BS, RUT, RDCS
Bunker Hill Community College
Boston, MA

Marie Gates, PhD
WMU Bronson School of Nursing
Kalamazoo, MI

Janette McCrory, MSN
Delta State University
Cleveland, MS

Anita Noble, DNSc
Hebrew University School of Nursing, Henrietta Zold-Hadassah School of Nursing
Jerusalem, Israel

A Word About HEALTH

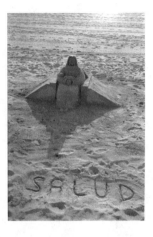

Sand Sculpture—Postiquet
Beach, Alicante, Spain

HEALTH connotes the balance of a person, both within one's being—physical, mental, and spiritual—and in the outside world—natural, familial and communal, and metaphysical. The model is a method for describing beliefs and practices used to **maintain** through daily HEALTH practices, such as diet, activities, and clothing; to **protect** through special HEALTH practices, such as food taboos, seasonal activities, and protective items worn, carried, or hung in the home or workplace; and/or to **restore** through special HEALTH practices, such as diet changes, rest, special clothing or objects, **physical, mental, and/or spiritual** HEALTH. The accompanying image, SALUD, is a metaphor for HEALTH in countless ways. Here, it is whole and emerging from the shadows of early morning. Just as the sand sculpture is fragile, disappearing overnight, so, too, is HEALTH. It brings to mind the reality that each of us has the internal responsibility to maintain, protect, and restore our HEALTH; the reciprocal holds true for the external familial, environmental, and societal forces—they, too, must look after and safeguard our HEALTH. This book, in part, is a mirror that reflects the countless ways by which people are able to maintain, protect, and/or restore their HEALTH. Just as there is an interplay between a sand sculpture and the natural forces that can create and harm and destroy it, so, too, it is with HEALTH and the forces of the outside world.

ILLNESS is the imbalance of the person, both within one's being—physical, mental, and spiritual—and in the outside world—natural, familial and communal, and metaphysical. HEALING is the restoration of this balance. The relationships of the person to the outside world are reciprocal.

When these terms, HEALTH, ILLNESS, AND HEALING are used in small capitals in this text, it is to connote that they are being used holistically. When they are written *health, illness,* and *healing,* they are to be understood in the common way.

The cover uses the sculpture as its focal point surrounded by selected segments of HEALTH related images. The segments are from the opening images of several chapters of this book and the explanations for each image can be found in the opening paragraphs of the chapters.

Cultural Diversity
in Health and Illness

Unit

I

Cultural Foundations

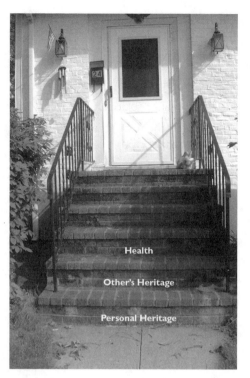

Health

Other's Heritage

Personal Heritage

Unit I creates the foundation for this book and enables you to become aware of the importance of cultural heritage and history—both your own and those of other people; the importance of understanding diversity—demographic, immigration, and economic—and importance of the standard concepts of health and illness.

The chapters in Unit I will present an overview of relevant historical and contemporary theoretical content that will help you climb the first three steps to CulturalCompetency. You will

1. Identify and discuss the factors that contribute to heritage consistency—culture, ethnicity, religion, acculturation, and socialization.

2. Identify and discuss sociocultural events that may influence the life trajectory of a given person.

3. Understand diversity in the population of the United States by observing
   - Demographic changes in the population of the United States
   - Immigration patterns
   - Economic issues relevant to poverty

4. Understand health and illness and the sociocultural and historical phenomena that affect them.

5. Reexamine and redefine the concepts of health and illness.

6. Understand the multiple relationships between health and illness.

7. Associate the concepts of good and evil and light and dark with health and illness.

Before you read Unit I, please answer the following questions:

1. What is your sociocultural heritage?
2. What major sociocultural events have occurred in your lifetime?
3. What is the demographic profile of the community you grew up in? How has it changed?
4. How would you acquire economic help if necessary?
5. How do you define *health*?
6. How do you define *illness*?
7. What do you do to maintain your health?
8. What do you do to protect your health?
9. What do you do when you experience a noticeable change in your health?
10. Do you diagnose your own health problems? If yes, how do you do so? If no, why not?
11. From whom do you seek health care?
12. What do you do to restore your health? Give examples.

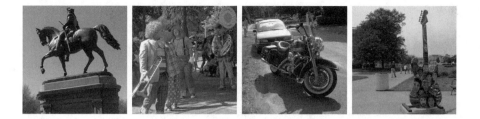

Chapter 1

Cultural Heritage and History

When there is a very dense cultural barrier, you do the best you can, and if something happens despite that, you have to be satisfied with little success instead of total successes. You have to give up total control. . . .

—Anne Fadiman (1997)

■ Objectives

1. Describe the National Standards for Culturally and Linguistically Appropriate Services in Health Care.
2. Articulate the attributes of CulturalCompetency and CULTURALCARE.
3. Explain the factors that contribute to heritage consistency—culture, ethnicity, religion, acculturation, and socialization.
4. Explain acculturation themes.
5. Determine and discuss sociocultural events that may influence the life trajectory of a given person.
6. Explain the factors involved in the cultural phenomena affecting health.

The images in the chapter opener are representative samples of the culture I acculturated into as a child and young adult in the process of being socialized into the American society of the 1950s. The first figure is a statue of George Washington, the first president, always a dominant figure in the public school classroom. The next is a segment of the July 4th parade, a national holiday heartily celebrated all my life. The Harley-Davidson motorcycle, created in 1903, is a metaphor for the 20th century. It embodies independence, rebellion, freedom, and even danger

(Carroll, 2003, p. 5). The guitar is in front of the Museum of Rock and Roll in Cleveland, Ohio—it celebrates the birth of rock—the 1950s. These are symbols and icons representative of my social heritage; what are the symbols and icons of your generation and heritage? If you had to choose four images to blend together to tell of your social heritage, what would you choose?

In May 1988, Anne Fadiman, editor of *The American Scholar*, met the Lee family of Merced, California. Her subsequent book, *The Spirit Catches You and You Fall Down*, published in 1997, tells the compelling story of the Lees and their daughter Lia and their tragic encounter with the American health care delivery system. This book has now become a classic and is used by many health care educators and providers in situations where there is an effort to demonstrate the need for developing cultural competence.

When Lia was 3 months old, she was taken to the emergency room of the county hospital with epileptic seizures. The family was unable to communicate in English; the hospital staff did not include competent Hmong interpreters. From the parents' point of view, Lia was experiencing "the fleeing of her soul from her body and the soul had become lost." They knew these symptoms to be *quag dab peg*—"the spirit catches you and you fall down." The Hmong regard this experience with ambivalence, yet they know that it is serious and potentially dangerous, as it is epilepsy. It is also an illness that evokes a sense of both concern and pride.

The parents and the health care providers both wanted the best for Lia, yet a complex and dense trajectory of misunderstanding and misinterpreting was set in motion. The tragic cultural conflict lasted for several years and caused considerable pain to each party (Fadiman, 1997). This moving incident exemplifies the extreme events that can occur when two antithetical cultural belief systems collide within the overall environment of the health care delivery system. Each party comes to a health care event with a set notion of what ought to happen—and, unless each is able to understand the view of the other, complex difficulties can arise.

The catastrophic events of September 11, 2001; the wars in Afghanistan and Iraq; and our preoccupation with terrorist threats have pierced the consciousness of all Americans in general and health care providers in particular. Now, more than ever, providers *must* become informed about and sensitive to the culturally diverse subjective meanings of **health/HEALTH, illness/ILLNESS**,[1] caring, and healing practices. Cultural diversity and pluralism are a core part of the social and economic engines that drive the country, and their impact at this time has significant implications for health care delivery and policymaking throughout the United States (Office of Minority Health, 2001, p. 25).

In all clinical practice areas—from institutional settings, such as acute and long-term care settings, to community-based settings, such as nurse prac-

---

[1]This style of combining terms, such as **health/HEALTH**, will be used throughout the text to convey that there is a blending of modern and traditional connotations for the terms. The terms are defined within the text and in the glossary.

titioner's and doctor's offices and clinics, schools and universities, public health, and occupational settings—one observes diversity every day. The compelling need for culturally and linguistically competent health care services for diverse populations has attracted increased attention from health care providers and those who judge their quality and efficiency for many years. The mainstream health care provider is treating a more diverse patient population as a result of demographic changes and participation in insurance programs, and the interest in designing culturally and linguistically appropriate services that lead to improved health care outcomes, efficiency, and patient satisfaction has increased.

One's personal cultural background, heritage, and language have a considerable impact on both how patients access and respond to health care services and how the providers practice within the system. **Cultural** and **linguistic comptence** suggests an ability by health care providers and health care organizations to understand and respond effectively to the cultural and linguistic needs brought to the health care experience. This is a phenomenon that recognizes the diversity that exists among the patients, physicians, nurses, and caregivers. This phenomenon is not limited to the changes in the patient population in that it also embraces the members of the workforce—including providers from other countries. Many of the people in the workforce are new immigrants and/or are from ethnocultural backgrounds that are different from that of the dominant culture.

In addition, health and illness can be interpreted and explained in terms of personal experience and expectations. We can define our own health or illness and determine what these states mean to us in our daily lives. We learn from our own cultural and ethnic backgrounds how to be healthy, how to recognize illness, and how to be ill. Furthermore, the meanings we attach to the notions of health and illness are related to the basic, culture-bound values by which we define a given experience and perception.

This first chapter presents an overview of the salient content and complex theoretical content related to one's heritage and their impact on health beliefs and practices. Two sets of theories are presented, the first of which analyzes the degree to which people have maintained their traditional heritage; the second, and opposite, set of theories relates to socialization and acculturation and the quasi creation of a melting pot or some other common threads that are part of an American whole. It then becomes possible to analyze health beliefs by determining a person's ties to his or her traditional heritage, rather than to signs of acculturation. The assumption is that there is a relationship between people with strong identities—either with their heritage or the level at which they are acculturated into the American culture—and their health beliefs and practices. Hand in hand with the concept of ethnocultural heritage is that of a person's ethnocultural history, the journey a person has experienced predicated on the historical sociocultural events that have touched his or her life directly or indirectly.

Box 1–1

National Standards for Culturally and Linguistically Appropriate Services in Health Care

1. Health care organizations should ensure that patients/consumers receive from all staff members effective, understandable, and respectful care that is provided in a manner compatible with their cultural health beliefs and practices and preferred language.
2. Health care organizations should implement strategies to recruit, retain, and promote at all levels of the organization a diverse staff and leadership that are representative of the demographic characteristics of the service area.
3. Health care organizations should ensure that staff at all levels and across all disciplines receive ongoing education and training in culturally and linguistically appropriate service delivery.
4. Health care organizations must offer and provide language assistance services, including bilingual staff and interpreter services, at no cost to each patient/consumer with limited English proficiency at all points of contact, in a timely manner during all hours of operation.
5. Health care organizations must provide to patients/consumers in their preferred language both verbal offers and written notices informing them of their right to receive language assistance services.
6. Health care organizations must assure the competence of language assistance provided to limited English-proficient patients/consumers by interpreters and bilingual staff. Family and friends should not be used to provide interpretation services (except on request by the patient/consumer).
7. Health care organizations must make available easily understood patient-related materials and post signage in the languages of the commonly encountered groups and/or groups represented in the service area.
8. Health care organizations should develop, implement, and promote a written strategic plan that outlines clear goals, policies, operational plans, and management accountability/oversight mechanisms to provide culturally and linguistically appropriate services.
9. Health care organizations should conduct initial and ongoing organizational self-assessments of CLAS-related activities and are encouraged to integrate cultural and linguistic competence–related measures into their internal audits, performance improvement programs, patient satisfaction assessments, and outcomes-based evaluations.
10. Health care organizations should ensure that data on the individual patient's/consumer's race, ethnicity, and spoken and written language are collected in health records, integrated into the organization's management information systems, and periodically updated.
11. Health care organizations should maintain a current demographic, cultural, and epidemiological profile of the community as well as a needs assessment

to accurately plan for and implement services that respond to the cultural and linguistic characteristics of the service area.

12. Health care organizations should develop participatory, collaborative partnerships with communities and utilize a variety of formal and informal mechanisms to facilitate community and patient/consumer involvement in designing and implementing CLAS-related activities.

13. Health care organizations should ensure that conflict and grievance resolution processes are culturally and linguistically sensitive and capable of identifying, preventing, and resolving cross-cultural conflicts or complaints by patients/consumers.

14. Health care organizations are encouraged to regularly make available to the public information about their progress and successful innovations in implementing the CLAS standards and to provide public notice in their communities about the availability of this information.

Source: National Standards for Culturally and Linguistically Appropriate Services in Health Care. Final Report. Washington, DC, March 2001. For full report and discussion, contact the Office of Minority Health: Guadalupe Pacheco, MSW, Special Assistant to the Director, Project Officer, Office of Minority Health, Office of Public Health and Science, U.S. Department of Health and Human Services, Rockwall II, Suite 1000, 5515 Security Lane, Rockville, MD 20852, phone: 301-443-5084, gpacheco@osophs.dhhs.gov.

■ National Standards for Culturally and Linguistically Appropriate Services in Health Care

In 1997, the Office of Minority Health undertook the development of national standards to provide a much needed alternative to the patchwork that has been undertaken in the field of Cultural Diversity. It developed the National Standards for Culturally and Linguistically Appropriate Services (CLAS) in Health Care. These 14 standards (Box 1–1) must be met by most health care–related agencies. The standards are based on an analytical review of key laws, regulations, contracts, and standards currently in use by federal and state agencies and other national organizations. They were developed with input from a national advisory committee of policymakers, health care providers, and researchers.

Accreditation and credentialing agencies can assess and compare providers who say they provide culturally competent services and assure quality care for diverse populations. This includes the Joint Commission on Accreditation of Healthcare Organizations (JCAHO); the National Committee on Quality Assurance; professional organizations, such as the American Medical and Nurses Associations; and quality review organizations, such as peer review organizations.

In order to ensure both equal access to quality health care by diverse populations and a secure work environment, all health care providers must "promote and support the attitudes, behaviors, knowledge, and skills necessary for staff to work respectfully and effectively with patients and each other in a culturally diverse work environment" (Office of Minority Health, 2001, p. 7). This is the first and fundamental standard of the 14 standards that have been recommended as national standards for culturally and linguistically appropriate services (CLAS) in health care.

■ Cultural Competence

Cultural competence implies that professional health care must be developed to be culturally sensitive, culturally appropriate, and culturally competent. Culturally Competent Care is critical to meet the complex culture-bound health care needs of a given person, family, and community. It is the provision of health care across cultural boundaries and takes into account the context in which the patient lives, as well as the situations in which the patient's health problems arise.

- **Culturally competent**—within the delivered care, the provider understands and attends to the total context of the patient's situation and this is a complex combination of knowledge, attitudes, and skills.
- **Culturally appropriate**—the provider applies the underlying background knowledge that must be possessed to provide a patient with the best possible health/HEALTH care.
- **Culturally sensitive**—the provider possesses some basic knowledge of and constructive attitudes toward the health/HEALTH traditions observed among the diverse cultural groups found in the setting in which he or she is practicing.

■ Linguistic Competence

Linguistic competence embraces the concept of linguistically appropriate services and espouses the implementation of competent interpreter services when the patient and family do not understand, speak, or read English. Under the provisions of Title VI of the Civil Rights Act of 1964, people with Limited English Proficiency (LEP) who are cared for in both institutional and community health facilities, such as

- Hospitals
- Day care centers
- Mental health centers
- Senior citizen centers
- Family health centers and clinics

and are eligible for Medicaid, other health care, or human services cannot be denied assistance because of their race, color, or national origin. There are many forms of illegal discrimination that frequently limit the opportunities of people to gain equal access to health care services. The language barriers experienced by Limited English Proficiency (LEP) persons can result in limiting access to critical public health, hospital, and other medical and social services.

■ CulturalCare

The term CULTURALCARE expresses all that is inherent in the development of health care delivery to meet the mandates of the CLAS standards, and CULTURALCARE is holistic. There are countless conflicts in the health care delivery arenas that are predicated on cultural misunderstandings. Although many of these misunderstandings are related to universal situations—such as verbal and nonverbal language misunderstandings, the conventions of courtesy, the sequencing of interactions, the phasing of interactions, and objectivity—many cultural misunderstandings are unique to the delivery of health care. The need to provide CULTURALCARE is essential, and providers must be able to assess and interpret a patient's health beliefs and practices and cultural needs. CULTURALCARE alters the perspective of health care delivery as it enables the provider to understand, from a cultural perspective, the manifestations of the patient's cultural heritage and life trajectory. The provider must serve as a bridge in the health care setting between the patient and people who are from different cultural backgrounds.

■ Heritage Consistency

Heritage consistency is a concept developed by Estes and Zitzow (1980, p. 1) to describe "the degree to which one's lifestyle reflects his or her respective tribal culture." The theory has been expanded in an attempt to study the degree to which a person's lifestyle reflects his or her traditional culture, such as European, Asian, African, or Hispanic. The values indicating heritage consistency exist on a continuum, and a person can possess value characteristics of both a consistent heritage (traditional) and an inconsistent heritage (acculturated). The concept of heritage consistency includes a determination of one's cultural, ethnic, and religious background (Figure 1–1).

Culture

The word *culture* shows 436 million hits on the Internet and hundreds of articles. An overview of the content on these sites, however, is certainly in harmony with the forthcoming discussion.

There is no single definition of *culture*, and all too often definitions omit salient aspects of culture or are too general to have any real meaning. Of the countless ideas of the meaning of this term, some are of particular note. The classical definition of Fejos (1959, p. 43) describes culture as "the sum total of socially inherited characteristics of a human group that comprises everything which one generation can tell, convey, or hand down to the next; in other words, the nonphysically inherited traits we possess." Another way of understanding the concept of culture is to picture it as the luggage that each of us carries around for our lifetime. It is the sum of beliefs, practices, habits, likes, dislikes, norms, customs, rituals, and so forth that we learned from our families during the years of socialization. In turn, we transmit cultural luggage to our

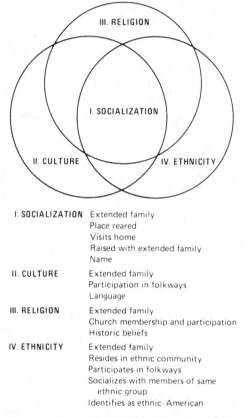

Figure 1-1 Model of heritage consistency.

children. A third way of defining *culture*, and one that is most relevant in areas of traditional health, is that culture is a "metacommunication system," wherein not only the spoken words have meaning but everything else does as well (Matsumoto, 1989, p. 14).

All facets of human behavior can be interpreted through the lens of culture, and everything can be related to and from this context. Culture includes all the following characteristics:

1. Culture is the medium of personhood and social relationships.
2. Only part of culture is conscious.
3. Culture can be likened to a prosthetic device because it is an extension of biological capabilities.
4. Culture is an interlinked web of symbols.
5. Culture is a device for creating and limiting human choices.
6. Culture can be in two places at once—it is found in a person's mind and exists in the environment in such form as the spoken word or an artifact. (Bohannan, 1992, p. 12)

Culture is a complex whole in which each part is related to every other part. It is learned, and the capacity to learn culture is genetic, but the subject matter is not genetic and must be learned by each person in a family and social community. Culture also depends on an underlying social matrix, and included in this social matrix are knowledge, belief, art, law, morals, and custom (Bohannan, 1992, p. 13).

Culture is learned in that people learn the ways to see their environment—that is, they learn from the environment how to see and interpret what they see. People learn to speak, and they learn to learn. Culture, as the medium of our individuality, is the way in which we express ourselves. It is the medium of human social relationships in that it must be shared and creates social relationships. The symbols of culture—sound and acts—form the basis of all languages. Symbols are everywhere—in religion, politics, and gender—these are cultural symbols, the meanings of which vary between and within cultural groups (Bohannan, 1992, pp. 11–14). The society in which we live and political, economic, and social forces tend to alter the way in which some aspects of a culture are transmitted and maintained. Many of the essential components of a culture, however, pass from one generation to the next unaltered. Consequently, much of what we believe, think, and do, both consciously and unconsciously, is determined by our cultural background. In this way, culture and ethnicity are handed down from one generation to another. These classic definitions of *culture* continue to serve as a basis for understanding the term in the present time. In fact, the definition developed by the Office of Minority Health in 1998 incorporates many of these central themes. It defines *culture* as "the thoughts, communications, actions, customs, beliefs, values, and institutions of racial, ethnic, religious, or social groups" (Office of Minority Health, 2001, p. 131).

Ethnicity

The word *ethnicity* shows 44 million hits and hundreds of articles on the Internet. A random exploration of selected sites did not provide information different from the classical information in the following discussion.

Cultural background is a fundamental component of one's ethnic background. Before we proceed with this discussion, though, we need to define some terms, so that we can proceed from the same point of reference. The classic reference defines *ethnic* as an adjective "of or pertaining to a social group within a cultural and social system that claims or is accorded special status on the basis of complex, often variable traits including religious, linguistic, ancestral, or physical characteristics (*American Heritage Dictionary*, 1976, p. 247). The contemporary definition applied by the Office of Minority Health is that of "a group of people that share a common and distinctive racial, national, religious, linguistic, or cultural heritage" (Office of Minority Health, 2001, p. 131). O'Neil (2008) described *ethnicity* as selected cultural and sometimes physical characteristics used to classify people into groups or categories considered to be significantly different from others.

The term *ethnic* has for some time aroused strongly negative feelings and often is rejected by the general population. One can speculate that the upsurge in the use of the term stems from the recent interest of people in discovering their personal backgrounds, a fact used by some politicians who overtly court "the ethnics." Paradoxically, in a nation as large as the United States and comprising as many different peoples as it does—with the American Indians being the only true native population—we find ourselves still reluctant to speak of ethnicity and ethnic differences. This stance stems from the fact that most foreign groups that come to this land often shed the ways of the "old country" and quickly attempt to assimilate themselves into the mainstream, or the so-called melting pot (Novak, 1973). Other terms related to ethnic include:

- Ethnicity: (1) the condition of belonging to a particular ethnic group; (2) ethnic pride (American Heritage Dictionary, 1976, p. 247)
- Ethnocentrism: (1) belief in the superiority of one's own ethnic group; (2) overriding concern with race
- Xenophobe: a person unduly fearful or contemptuous of strangers or foreigners, especially as reflected in his or her political or cultural views
- Xenophobia: a morbid fear of strangers

The behavioral manifestations of these phenomena occur in response to people's needs, especially when they are foreign born and must find a way to function (1) before they are assimilated into the mainstream and (2) in order to accept themselves. The people cluster together against the majority, who in turn may be discriminating against them.

Indeed, the phenomenon of ethnicity is "complex, ambivalent, paradoxical, and elusive" (Senior, 1965, p. 21). Ethnicity is indicative of the following characteristics a group may share in some combination:

1. Geographic origin
2. Migratory status
3. Race
4. Language and dialect
5. Religious faith or faiths
6. Ties that transcend kinship, neighborhood, and community boundaries
7. Traditions, values, and symbols
8. Literature, folklore, and music
9. Food preferences
10. Settlement and employment patterns
11. Special interest, with regard to politics, in the homeland and in the United States
12. Institutions that specifically serve and maintain the group
13. An internal sense of distinctiveness
14. An external perception of distinctiveness

There are at least 106 ethnic groups and more than 500 American Indian Nations in the United States that meet many of these criteria. People from every country in the world have immigrated to this country. Some nations, such as Germany, England, Wales, and Ireland, are heavily represented; others, such as Japan, the Philippines, and Greece, have smaller numbers of people living here (Thernstrom, 1980, p. vii). People continue to immigrate to the United States, with the present influx coming from Haiti, Mexico, South and Central America, India, and China.

Religion

The word *religion* shows well over 44 million hits and countless articles on the Internet. Again, a random review of the material yielded information that was similar to existing data.

The third major component of heritage consistency is religion. Religion, "the belief in a divine or superhuman power or powers to be obeyed and worshipped as the creator(s) and ruler(s) of the universe; and a system of beliefs, practices, and ethical values," is a major reason for the development of ethnicity (Abramson, 1980, pp. 869–875). The Office of Minority Health has adopted the definition of *religion* as "a set of beliefs, values, and practices based on the teachings of a spiritual leader" (Office of Minority Health, 2001, p. 132). The practice of religion is revealed in numerous cults, sects, denominations, and churches. Ethnicity and religion are clearly related, and one's religion quite often determines one's ethnic group. Religion gives a person a frame of reference and a perspective with which to organize information. Religious teachings in relation to health help present a meaningful philosophy and system of practices within a system of social controls having specific values, norms, and ethics. These are related to health in that adherence to a religious code is conducive to spiritual harmony and health. Illness is sometimes seen as a punishment for the violation of religious codes and morals.

Religion plays a fundamental role in the health beliefs and practices of many people. An additional way of understanding the relationship of religion to health is to conceptualize religion as

1. particular churches or organized religious institutions
2. scholarly field of study and
3. the domain of life that deals with things of the spirit and matters of "ultimate concern"

In addition, religious affiliation and membership benefit health by promoting healthy behavior and lifestyles in the following ways:

1. Regular religious fellowship benefits health by offering support that buffers and affects stress and isolation.
2. Participation in worship and prayer benefits health through the physiological effects of positive emotions.
3. Religious beliefs benefit health by their similarity to health promoting beliefs and personality styles.

4. Simple faith benefits health by leading to thoughts of hope, optimism, and positive expectation.

5. Mystical experiences benefit health by activating a healing bioenergy or life force or altered state of consciousness.

6. Absent prayer for others is capable of healing by paranormal means or by divine intervention. (Levin, 2001, p. 9)

Unlike some countries, the United States does not include a question about religion in its census and has not done so for over 50 years. Religious adherent statistics in the United States are obtained from surveys and organizational reporting. However, it is also noteworthy that "'we the people' of the United States now form the most profusely religious nation on earth" (Eck, 2001, p. 4). Each year the annual *Yearbook of American and Canadian Churches* publishes information on North America's largest religious bodies. The yearbook is a publication of the National Council of Churches (NCC). The membership counts published in this work are primarily based on organizational reporting. The yearbook's data are used in U.S. government publications and various almanacs. The following are the largest U.S. religious bodies (distinct churches) according to the *2005 Yearbook*. These figures are based primarily on 2003 denominational reporting data:

1. Roman Catholic Church: 67.2 million
2. Southern Baptist Convention: 16.4 million
3. United Methodist Church: 8.2 million
4. Church of Jesus Christ of Latter-day Saints: 5.5 million
5. Church of God in Christ: 5.4 million
6. National Baptist Convention USA: 5 million
7. Evangelical Lutheran Church in America: 4.9 million
8. National Baptist Convention of America: 3.5 million
9. Presbyterian Church (USA): 3.2 million
10. Assemblies of God: 2.7 million

Another source of religious affiliation is the Pew Research Council. In February and March 2002, the Pew Research Council conducted a survey of 2,002 adults. Questions about religious preference were included and the results are in Table 1–1.

Examples of Heritage Consistency

The factors that constitute heritage consistency are listed in Table 1–2. The following are examples of each factor:

1. The person's childhood development occurred in the person's country of origin or in an immigrant neighborhood in the United States of like ethnic group.

Table 1–1   U.S. Religious Affiliation, 2002 (%)

Religious Preference	June 1996	March 2001	March 2002
Christian	84	82	82
Jewish	1	1	1
Muslim	——	1	——
Other non-Christian	3	2	1
Atheist	——	1	1
Agnostic	——	2	2
Something else	——	1	2
No preference	11	8	10
Don't know/refused	1	2	1
Total	100	100	100

Source: Kohut, A., & Rogers, M. (2002). "Americans struggle with religion's role at home and abroad." Retrieved from http://www.adherents.com/rel_USA.html

The person was raised in a specific ethnic neighborhood, such as Italian, Black, Hispanic, or Jewish, in a given part of a city and was exposed to only the culture, language, foods, and customs of that group.

2. Extended family members encouraged participation in traditional religious and cultural activities.

   The parents sent the person to religious school, and most social activities were church-related.

3. The individual engages in frequent visits to the country of origin or returns to the "old neighborhood" in the United States.

Table 1–2   Factors Indicating Heritage Consistency

1. The person's childhood development occurred in the person's country of origin or in an immigrant neighborhood in the United States of like ethnic group.
2. Extended family members encouraged participation in traditional religious or cultural activities.
3. The individual engages in frequent visits to the country of origin or returns to the "old neighborhood" in the United States.
4. The individual's family home is within the ethnic community.
5. The individual participates in ethnic cultural events, such as religious festivals or national holidays, sometimes with singing, dancing, and special garments.
6. The individual was raised in an extended family setting.
7. The individual maintains regular contact with the extended family.
8. The individual's name has not been Americanized.
9. The individual was educated in a parochial (nonpublic) school with a religious or ethnic philosophy similar to the family's background.
10. The individual engages in social activities primarily with others of the same ethnic background.
11. The individual has knowledge of the culture and language of origin.
12. The individual possesses elements of personal pride about heritage.

The desire to return to the old country or to the old neighborhood is prevalent in many people; however, many people, for various reasons, cannot return. The people who came here to escape religious persecution or whose families were killed during world war or the Holocaust may not want to return to European homelands. Other reasons people may not return to their native country include political conditions in the homeland and lack of relatives or friends in that land.

4. The individual's family home is within the ethnic community of which he or she is a member.

   As an adult, the person has elected to live with family in an ethnic neighborhood.

5. The individual participates in ethnic cultural events, such as religious festivals or national holidays, sometimes with singing, dancing, and costumes.

   The person holds membership in ethno- or religious-specific organizations and primarily participates in activities with the groups.

6. The individual was raised in an extended family setting.

   When the person was growing up, there may have been grandparents living in the same household, or aunts and uncles living in the same house or close by. The person's social frame of reference was the family.

7. The individual maintains regular contact with the extended family.

   The person maintains close ties with members of the same generation, the surviving members of the older generation, and members of the younger generation who are family members.

8. The individual's name has not been Americanized.

   The person has restored the family name to its European original if it had been changed by immigration authorities at the time the family immigrated or if the family changed the name at a later time in an attempt to assimilate more fully.

9. The individual was educated in a parochial (nonpublic) school with a religious or ethnic philosophy similar to the family's background.

   The person's education plays an enormous role in socialization, and the major purpose of education is to socialize a person into the dominant culture. Children learn English and the customs and norms of American life in the schools. In the parochial schools, they not only learn English but also are socialized in the culture and norms of the religious or ethnic group that is sponsoring the school.

10. The individual engages in social activities primarily with others of the same religious or ethnic background.

    The major portion of the person's personal time is spent with primary structural groups.

11. The individual has knowledge of the culture and language of origin.

    The person has been socialized in the traditional ways of the family and expresses this as a central theme of life.

12. The individual expresses pride in his or her heritage.

    The person may identify him- or herself as ethnic American and be supportive of ethnic activities to a great extent.

It is not possible to isolate the aspects of culture, religion, and ethnicity that shape a person's worldview. Each is part of the others, and all three are united within the person. When one writes of religion, one cannot eliminate culture or ethnicity, but descriptions and comparisons can be made. Referring to Figure 1–1 and Figures 1–2A and 1–2B to assess heritage consistency can help determine ethnic group differences in health beliefs and practices. Understanding such differences can help enhance your understanding of the needs of patients and their families and the support systems that people may have or need.

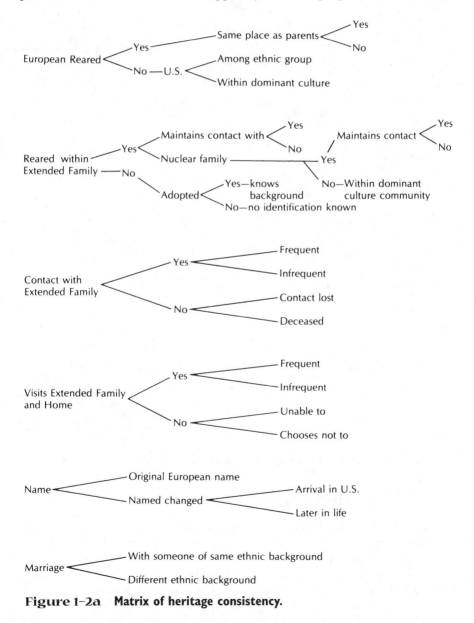

Figure 1-2a   Matrix of heritage consistency.

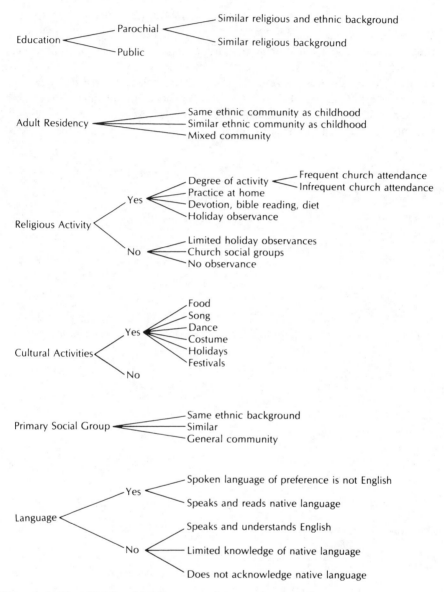

Figure 1-2b   Matrix of heritage consistency, continued.

■ Acculturation Themes

Several facets are relevant to the overall experience of acculturation. *Acculturation* is the broad term used to describe the process of adapting to and becoming absorbed into the dominant social culture. The overall process of acculturation into a new society is extremely difficult. Have you ever moved to a new community? Imagine moving to a new country and society. The three facets to the process of overall acculturation are socialization, acculturation, and assimilation.

Socialization

Socialization is the process of being raised within a culture and acquiring the characteristics of that group. Education—be it elementary school, high school, college, or a health care provider program—is a form of socialization. For many people who have been socialized within the boundaries of a "traditional culture" or a non-Western culture, modern American culture becomes a second cultural identity. Those who immigrate here, legally or illegally, from non-Western or nonmodern countries may find socialization into the American culture, whether in schools or in society, to be an extremely difficult and painful process. They may experience biculturalism, which is a dual pattern of identification and one often of divided loyalty (LaFrombose, Coleman, & Gerton, 1993).

Understanding culturally determined health and illness beliefs and practices from different heritages requires moving away from linear models of process to more complex patterns of cultural beliefs and interrelationships.

Acculturation

While becoming a competent participant in the dominant culture, a member of the nondominant culture is always identified as a member of the original culture. The process of acculturation is involuntary, and a member of the nondominant cultural group is forced to learn the new culture to survive. Individuals experience second-culture acquisition when they must live within or between cultures (LaFrombose et al., 1993). *Acculturation* also refers to cultural or behavioral assimilation and may be defined as the changes of one's cultural patterns to those of the host society. In the United States, people assume that the usual course of acculturation takes three generations; hence, the adult grandchild of an immigrant is considered fully Americanized.

Assimilation

Acculturation also may be referred to as assimilation, the process by which an individual develops a new cultural identity. Assimilation means becoming in all ways like the members of the dominant culture. The process of assimilation encompasses various aspects, such as cultural or behavioral, marital, identification, and civic. The underlying assumption is that the person from a given cultural group loses this cultural identity to acquire the new one. In fact, this is not always possible, and the process may cause stress and anxiety (LaFrombose et al., 1993). Assimilation can be described as a collection of subprocesses: a process of inclusion through which a person gradually ceases to conform to any standard of life that differs from the dominant group standards and, at the same time, a process through which the person learns to conform to all the dominant group standards. The process of assimilation is considered complete when the foreigner is fully merged into the dominant cultural group (McLemore, 1980, p. 4).

There are four forms of assimilation: cultural, marital, primary structural, and secondary structural. One example of cultural assimilation is the ability to speak excellent American English. It is interesting to note that, according to the 2000 census, in the United States 33.9 million people speak a language other than English as their primary language (U.S. Bureau of the Census, 2003). Marital assimilation occurs when members of one group intermarry with members of another group. The third and fourth forms of assimilation, those of structural assimilation, determine the extent to which social mingling and friendships occur between groups. In primary structural assimilation, the relationships between people are warm, personal interactions between group members in the home, the church, and social groups. In secondary structural assimilation, there is nondiscriminatory sharing—often of a cold, impersonal nature—between groups in settings such as schools and workplaces (McLemore, 1980, p. 39).

The concepts of socialization, assimilation, and acculturation are complex and sensitive. The dominant society expects that all immigrants are in the process of acculturation and assimilation and that the worldview we share as health care practitioners is shared by our patients. Because we live in a pluralistic society, however, many variations of health beliefs and practices exist.

The debate still rages between those who believe that America is a melting pot and that all groups of immigrants must be acculturated to an American norm and those who dispute theories of acculturation and believe that the various groups maintain their own identities within the American whole. The concept of heritage consistency is one way of exploring whether people are maintaining their traditional heritage and of determining the depth of a person's traditional cultural heritage.

■ Ethnocultural Life Trajectories

Generational differences have been described as deep and gut-level ways of experiencing and looking at the cultural events that surround us. "The differences between generations—and the determination of who we are—are more than distinct ways of looking at problems and developing solutions for problems" (Hicks & Hicks, 1999, p. 4). Changes in the past several decades have created cultural barriers that openly or more subtly create misunderstandings, tensions, and often conflicts between family members, co-workers, and other individuals—as well as between patients and caregivers, especially in the practice of gerontology. The cycle of our lives is an ethnocultural journey and many of the aspects of this journey are derived from the social, religious, and cultural context in which we grew up. Factors that imprint our lives are the characters and events that we interacted with at 10 years of age, more or less (Hicks & Hicks, 1999, p. 25).

One example of generational conflict between health care providers and patients is within institutional settings where the patients are cared for not only by people who are immigrants but also by those who are much younger and have limited knowledge as to what has been a patient's life trajectory. The patient may also be an immigrant who experienced a much different life trajectory than others of the same age and the caregivers. Imagine your life today and what it may have been like to live without a television, a computer, a cell phone, or an iPod. For too many people, these commonplace objects may be seen as "strangers" rather than "friends"; or "digital natives" rather than "digital immigrants."

Table 1–3 describes selected seminal events of the past 75 years that have had a profound impact on the lives of patients throughout the life span and

Table 1–3 Selected Seminal Sociocultural Events of the Past 75 Years, Workplace Ethos, Lifestyle, and Social Values

Generation	Seminal Events	Workplace Ethos	Lifestyle	Social Values
Pre-boomers b. 1934–1945 10*-1944–1955	WWII Hiroshima World's first electronic computer assembled	Traditional work ethic Employer loyalty Born to lead Conventional Believe in mission	Work first Expect to lead Care for religion Buy decent home	Community service Vote Family first
Boomers b. 1946–1959 10-1956–1969	Television— *I Love Lucy* TV dinners Elvis Presley Marilyn Monroe Rosa Parks Sputnik	Money/work Expect to lead What do others think? Lip service to mission	Work/play hard Religion acceptable Buy most house you can	Reluctant community service Vote only if convenient Family and friends
Cuspers b. 1960–1968 10-1970–1978	Kent State Watergate Nixon resigned	Money/ principle Lead and follow Independent and care what others think Care about mission	Work/play hard Religion a hobby Do I need a house?	I do not give Vote if you want to Family and friends
Busters b. 1969–1978 10-1979–1988	Vietnam Memorial Wall HIV/AIDS epidemic *Challenger* explosion	Principle/ satisfaction Lifestyle first Loyal to skills Must have mission Individual first	Work hard if it does not interfere What is religion? Gentrify inner city	May donate Vote privately Friends are family
Nesters b. 1979–1984+ 10-1989–1994+	Tiananmen Square Desert Storm President Clinton impeached World Trade Center Afghanistan Iraq	Principle/ satisfaction Lifestyle first Must have a mission Individual first	Make others pay Comparative religions Live with parents	Community service equals punishment Vote my issues Want extended families

*Decade when person turns ten. This is the decade that influences a person's culture identity.

Sources: Hicks, R., & Hicks, K. (1999). *Boomers, Xers, and other strangers.* Wheaton, IL: Tyndale House and Jennings, P. (1998). *The century.* Copyright 1998 by ABC Television.

examples of workplace ethos, lifestyle, and social values of different age cohorts, as a cumulative experience and then in more recent years have impacted their providers and caregivers. Depending on the heritage and history of the caregivers, too, the experiences differ. Many people describe the ages from 10 to 19 years as the time when one's sociocultural orientation is established. The first column, "Generation," places the person in the year he or she was born; in boldface are the years the person aged from 10 to 19.

■ Commingling Variables

Five commingling variables relate to this overall situation of social and generational divisions as they are potential sources of conflict:

1. **Decade of birth.** People's life experiences vary greatly, depending on the events of the decades in which they were born and the cultural values and norms of the times. People who tend to be heritage consistent—that is, have a high level of identification and association with a traditional heritage—tend to be less caught up in the secular fads of the time and popular sociocultural events.

2. **Generation in United States.** Worldviews differ greatly between the immigrant generation and subsequent generations and people who score high as heritage consistent and mainstream people who may score low on the heritage consistency assessment and have been born into families who have resided in the United States for multiple generations.

3. **Class.** Social class is an important factor. The analysis of one's education, economics, and background is an important observation of people. There are countless differences among people predicated on class. The United States Department of Labor produces employment and wage estimates for over 800 occupations (Table 1–4). These are esti-

Table 1–4   May 2007 National Occupational Employment and Wage Estimates for Selected Major Occupational Groups

Major Occupational Group	Employment Estimate	Mean Annual Wage
Management	6,003,930	$96,150
Legal	998,590	$88,450
Computer and mathematical	3,191,360	$72,190
Architecture and engineering	2,486,020	$68,880
Healthcare practitioners	6,877,680	$65,020
Registered Nurses	2,468,340	$62,480
Community and social services	1,793,040	$40,540
Production occupations	10,146,560	$29,890

Source: U.S. Department of Labor Statistics. Washington DC: United States Department of Labor. Retrieved from http://www.bls.gov/oes/current/oes_nat.htm#b00-0000, May 16, 2008.

mates of the number of people employed in certain occupations, and estimates of the wages paid to them. Self-employed persons are not included in the estimates.

The unemployment rate in January 2008 was 4.9%. The annual average rate for unemployment in 2007 was 4.6%.

These figures demonstrate the differences in economic class and play heavily in relation to issues of health care access and insurance coverage.

4. **Language.** There are countless conflicts when people who are hard of hearing attempt to understand people with limited English-speaking skills, and many cultural and social misunderstandings can develop. There are also frequent misunderstandings when people who do not understand English must help and care for or take direction from English speakers.

5. **Education.** Increasing percentages of students have completed high school (from 69% in 1980 to 84% in 2000). At the same time, among persons aged 25 or older, fewer Black and Hispanic students eventually complete high school (U.S. Department of Education, 2007).

In 2002, President Bush signed into law the No Child Left Behind Act. The early evaluations of this law seem to indicate that the educational gaps are narrowing. The No Child Left Behind Act is designed to provide additional tools to our schools and educators to close the achievement gap and help America's students read and do math at grade level by 2014. Among the changes are

■ The achievement gap between White and Hispanic fourth graders narrowed, reaching an all-time low in reading and matching its all-time low in math.

■ The achievement gaps in eighth-grade math between White and African American students, and between White and Hispanic students, narrowed to their lowest points since 1990.

■ The achievement gap between White and Hispanic students in eighth-grade reading narrowed to its lowest point since 1998.

It will be several more years before the true efficacy of this law can be evaluated. If successful, it will make a new cohort of students eligible for college admission (U.S. Department of Education, 2007).

■ Cultural Conflict

Hunter (1994) describes cultural conflicts as events that occur when there is polarization between two groups and the differences are intensified by the way they are perceived. The struggles are centered on the control of the symbols of culture. In the case of the conflict between the Lee family and the health care system, discussed earlier in this chapter, the scope of the conflict is readily apparent

Table 1-5   Common "Isms" Plus One Non-"Ism"

Belief	Definition
Racism	The belief that members of one race are superior to those of other races
Sexism	The belief that members of one gender are superior to the other gender
Heterosexism	The belief that everyone is or should be heterosexual and that heterosexuality is best, normal, and superior
Ageism	The belief that members of one age group are superior to those of other ages
Ethnocentrism	The belief that one's own cultural, ethnic, or professional group is superior to that of others; one judges others by one's "yardstick" and is unable or unwilling to see what the other group is really about—"My group is best!"
Xenophobia	The morbid fear of strangers

Source: American Nurses' Association. (1993). *Proceedings of the invitational meeting, multicultural issues in the nursing workforce and workplace.* Washington, DC: Author.

and lends itself to further analysis. Hunter describes the fields of conflict as found in family, education, media and the arts, law, and electoral politics. Health care is a sixth field, and the conflict is between those who actively participate in traditional health care practices—that is, the practices of their given ethnocultural heritage—and those who are progressive and see the answers to contemporary health problems in the science and technology of the present.

When cultures clash, many misanthropic feelings, or "isms," can enter into a person's consciousness (Table 1-5). Just as Hunter proclaimed that the "differences" must be confronted, so, too, must stereotypes, prejudice, and discrimination be confronted. It is impossible to describe traditional beliefs without a temptation to stereotype, but each person is an individual; therefore, levels of heritage consistency differ within and between ethnic groups, as do health beliefs.

Another issue that manifests itself in this arena is prejudice. Prejudice occurs either because the person making the judgment does not understand the given person or his or her heritage or because the person making the judgment generalizes an experience of one individual from a culture to all members of that group. Discrimination occurs when a person acts on prejudice and denies another person one or more of his or her fundamental rights.

■ Cultural Phenomena Affecting Health

Giger and Davidhizar (1995) have identified six cultural phenomena that vary among cultural groups and affect health care: environmental control, biological variations, social organization, communication, space, and time orientation.

Environmental Control

Environmental control is the ability of members of a particular cultural group to plan activities that control nature or direct environmental factors. Included in this concept are the complex systems of traditional health and illness beliefs, the practice of folk medicine, and the use of traditional healers. This cultural phenomenon plays an extremely important role in the way patients respond to health-related experiences, including the ways in which they define *health* and *illness* and seek and use health care resources and social supports.

Biological Variations

The several ways in which people from one cultural group differ biologically (i.e., physically and genetically) from members of other cultural groups constitute their biological variations. The following are significant examples:

- Body build and structure, including specific bone and structural differences between groups, such as the smaller stature of Asians
- Skin color, including variations in tone, texture, healing abilities, and hair follicles
- Enzymatic and genetic variations, including differences in response to drug and dietary therapies
- Susceptibility to disease, which can manifest as a higher morbidity rate of certain diseases within certain groups
- Nutritional variations, countless examples of which include the "hot and cold" preferences among Hispanic Americans, the yin and yang preferences among Asian Americans, and the rules of the kosher diet among Jewish and Islamic Americans; a relatively common nutritional disorder, lactose intolerance, is found among Mexican, African, Asian, and Eastern European Jewish Americans

Social Organization

The social environment in which people grow up and live plays an essential role in their cultural development and identification. Children learn their culture's responses to life events from the family and its ethnoreligious group. This socialization process is an inherent part of heritage—cultural, religious, and ethnic background. *Social organization* refers to the family unit (nuclear, single-parent, or extended family) and the *social group organizations* (religious or ethnic) with which patients and families may identify. Countless social barriers, such as unemployment, underemployment, homelessness, lack of health insurance, and poverty, can also prevent people from entering the health care system.

Communication

Communication differences present themselves in many ways, including language differences, verbal and nonverbal behaviors, and silence. Language differences are possibly the most important obstacle to providing multicultural health care because they affect all stages of the patient-caregiver relationship. Clear and effective communication is important when dealing with any patient, especially if language differences create a cultural barrier. When deprived of the most common medium of interaction with patients—the spoken word—health care providers often become frustrated and ineffective. Accurate diagnosis and treatment is impossible if the health care professional cannot understand the patient. When the provider is not understood, he or she often avoids verbal communication and does not realize the effect of nonverbal communication, which is all too often the painful isolation of patients who do not speak the dominant language and who are in an unfamiliar environment. Consequently, patients experience cultural shock and may react by withdrawing, becoming hostile or belligerent, or being uncooperative.

Language differences can be bridged, however, with the use of competent interpreters. If the patient does not speak the dominant language, a skilled interpreter is mandatory.

Space

Personal space refers to people's behaviors and attitudes toward the space around themselves. Territoriality is the behavior and attitude people exhibit about an area they have claimed and defend or react emotionally about when others encroach on it. Both personal space and territoriality are influenced by culture, and thus different ethnocultural groups have varying norms related to the use of space. Space and related behaviors have different meanings in the following zones:

- Intimate zone—extends up to 1½ feet. Because this distance allows adults to have the most bodily contact for perception of breath and odor, incursion into this zone is acceptable only in private places. Visual distortions also occur at this distance.
- Personal distance—extends from 1½ to 4 feet. This is an extension of the self that is like having a "bubble" of space surrounding the body. At this distance, the voice may be moderate, body odor may not be apparent, and visual distortion may have disappeared.
- Social distance—extends from 4 to 12 feet. This is reserved for impersonal business transactions. Perceptual information is much less detailed.
- Public distance—extends 12 feet or more. Individuals interact only impersonally. Communicators' voices must be projected, and subtle facial expressions may be lost.

It must be noted that these generalizations about the use of personal space are based on studies of the behavior of European North Americans. The use of personal space varies among individuals and ethnic groups. The extreme modesty practiced by members of some cultural groups may prevent members from seeking preventive health care.

Time Orientation

The viewing of time in the present, past, or future varies among cultural groups. Certain cultures in the United States and Canada tend to be future-oriented. People who are future-oriented are concerned with long-range goals and with health care measures in the present to prevent the occurrence of illness in the future. They prefer to plan by making schedules, setting appointments, and organizing activities. Others are oriented more to the present than the future and may be late for appointments because they are less concerned about planning to be on time. This difference in time orientation may become important in health care measures such as long-term planning and explanations of medication schedules.

Figure 1–3 illustrates how a person, with a unique ethnic, religious, and cultural background, is affected by cultural phenomena. The discussions in Chapters 8 through 12 highlight these phenomena, and examples are presented within the text and in tabular form. The examples used in the text to illustrate

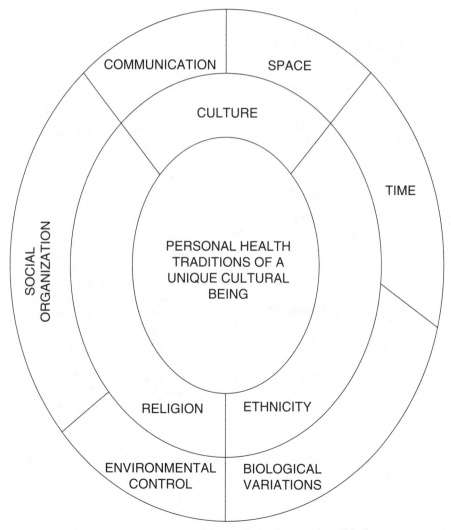

Figure 1–3 Personal health traditions of a unique cultural being.

Table 1-6   Examples of Etiquette as Related to Selected Cultural Phenomena

Time	Visiting Being on time	Inform person when you are coming Avoid surprises Explain your expectations about time
	Taboo times	Ask people from other regions and cultures what they expect Be familiar with the times and meanings of person's ethnic and religious holidays
Space	Body language and distances	Know cultural and/or religious customs regarding contact, such as eye and touch, from many perspectives
Communication	Greetings	Know the proper forms of address for people from a given culture and the ways by which people welcome one another Know when touch, such as an embrace or a handshake, is expected and when physical contact is prohibited
	Gestures	Gestures do not have universal meaning; what is acceptable to one cultural group is taboo with another
	Smiling	Smiles may be indicative of friendliness to some, taboo to others
	Eye contact	Avoiding eye contact may be a sign of respect
Social organization	Holidays	Know what dates are important and why, whether to give gifts, what to wear to special events, and what the customs and beliefs are
	Special events Births Weddings Funerals	Know how the event is celebrated, the meaning of colors used for gifts, and expected rituals at home or religious services
Biological variations	Food customs	Know what can be eaten for certain events, what foods may be eaten together or are forbidden, and what and how utensils are used
Environmental control	Health practices and remedies	Know what the general HEALTH traditions are for person and question observations for validity

Source: Adapted from Dresser, N. (1996). *Multicultural manners*. New York: Wiley. Copyright © 1996 John Wiley & Sons, Inc. Reprinted by permission of John Wiley & Sons. Inc.

health traditions in different cultures are not intended to be stereotypical. With careful listening, observing, and questioning, the provider should be able to sort out the traditions of a given person. Table 1–6 suggests examples of etiquette relevant to each of the cultural phenomena.

This chapter has served as the foundation that delineates the multiple, interrelating phenomena that underlie the cultural conflict that occurs between health care providers and patients, many of whom have difficulty interacting with the health care providers and system. It has presented both classical and contemporary definitions and explanations relevant to the foundation of this conflict and sets the stage for further discussion.

Explore 🌐 MediaLink

Go to the Companion Website at www.prenhall.com/spector for chapter-related review questions, case studies, and activities. Contents of the CulturalCare Guide and CulturalCare Museum can also be found on the Companion Website. Click on Chapter 1 to select the activities for this chapter.

■ Internet Sources

Kohut, A., and Rogers, M. (2002) Americans Struggle with Religion's Role at Home and Abroad. Washington, DC: Pew Research Center. Retrieved from http://www.adherents.com/rel_USA.html. July 22, 2007.

Kohut, A., and Rogers, M. (2002). Largest Religions in the United States. Washington, DC: The Pew Research Center. Retrieved from http://www.adherents.com/rel_USA.html#religions, July 24, 2007.

Linder, E. W. (Ed.) (2008). Yearbook of American and Canadian Churches. NY: National Council of Churches. Retrieved from http://www.electronicchurch.org. July 22, 2007.

O'Neil, D. (2008). Ethnicity and Race: An Introduction to the Nature of Social Group Differentiation and Inequality. San Marcos, CA: Palomar College. Retrieved from http://anthro.palomar.edu/ethnicity/Default.htm. February 18, 2008.

United States Census Bureau, Census 2000. Summary File 3, Tables P19, PCT13, and PCT14. Internet Release data: February 25, 2003. Retrieved from http://www.census.gov/population/cen2000/phc-t20/tab01.pdf, April 16, 2008.

United States Department of Education. (2007). No child left behind – High School Facts at a Glance. Retrieved from http://www.ed.gov/about/offices/list/ovae/pi/hs/hsfacts.html, October 18, 2007.

United States Department of Labor Statistics. (2008). Washington DC: United States Department of Labor. Retrieved from http://www.bls.gov/oes/current/oes_nat.htm#b00-0000, May 16, 2008.

United States Department of Health and Human Services. Fact Sheet – Your rights under Title VI of the Civil Rights Act. Retrieved from http://www.hhs.gov/ocr/generalinfo.html, July 15, 2007.

■ References

Abramson, H. J. (1980). Religion. In S. Thernstrom (Ed.), *Harvard encyclopedia of American ethnic groups*. Cambridge: Harvard University Press.

American Nurses' Association. (1993). *Proceedings of the invitational meeting, multicultural issues in the nursing workforce and workplace*. Washington, DC: Author.

Bohannan, P. (1992). *We, the alien—An introduction to cultural anthropology*. Prospect Heights, IL: Waveland Press.

Carroll, J. (2003). *Harley-Davidson: The living legend*. Edison, NJ: Edison Books.

Eck, D. L. (2001). *A new religious America: How a "Christian country" has become the world's most religious diverse nation*. San Francisco: Harper.

Estes, G., & Zitzow, D. (1980, November). *Heritage consistency as a consideration in counseling Native Americans*. Paper read at the National Indian Education Association Convention, Dallas, TX.

Fadiman A. (1997). *The spirit catches you and you fall down*. New York: Farrar, Straus, Giroux.

Fejos, P. (1959). Man, magic, and medicine. In L. Goldston (Ed.), *Medicine and anthropology*, New York: International University Press.

Giger, J. N., & Davidhizar, R. E. (1995). *Transcultural nursing assessment and intervention* (2nd ed.). St. Louis: Mosby-Year Book.

Hicks, R., & Hicks, K. (1999). *Boomers, Xers, and other strangers*. Wheaton, IL: Tyndale House.

Hunter, J. D. (1994). *Before the shooting begins—Searching for democracy in America's culture wars*. New York: Free Press.

LaFrombose, T., Coleman, L. K., & Gerton, J. (1993). Psychological impact of biculturalism: Evidence and theory. *Psychological Bulletin, 114*(3), 395.

Levin, J. (2001). *God, faith, and health*. New York: John Wiley & Sons.

Matsumoto, M. (1989). *The unspoken way*. Tokyo: Kodahsha International.

McLemore, S. D. (1980). *Racial and ethnic relations in America*. Boston: Allyn & Bacon.

Novak, M. (1973). How American are you if your grandparents came from Serbia in 1888? In S. Te Selle (Ed.), *The rediscovery of ethnicity: Its implications for culture and politics in America*. New York: Harper & Row.

Office of Minority Health. (2001). *National standards for culturally and linguistically appropriate services in health care*. Washington, DC: U.S. Department of Health and Human Services.

Senior, C. (1965). *The Puerto Ricans: Strangers then neighbors*. Chicago: Quadrangle Books.

Thernstrom, S. (Ed.). (1980). *Harvard encyclopedia of American ethnic groups*. Cambridge: Harvard University Press.

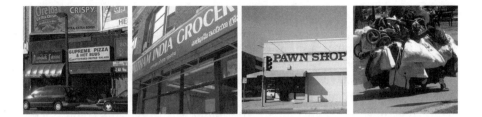

Chapter *2*

Diversity

Demography is destiny.

—*Hodgkinson (1986)*

■ Objectives

1. Describe the total population characteristics of the United States as presented in Census 2000.
2. Compare the population characteristics of the United States from 1970 to 2000.
3. Discuss the changes in points of origin of recent and past immigrants.
4. Discuss the meanings of terms related to immigration, such as *citizen* and *refugee*.
5. Discuss the facets of poverty.
6. Analyze the cycle of poverty.
7. Describe poverty guidelines.

The images in the chapter opener are representative of the demographic and socioeconomic diversity that exists in countless communities in this nation. The first image is that of a typical city block in Boston, Massachusetts, where you can see restaurant with Bangkok cuisine, an Italian pizza restaurant, and an Indian restaurant side by side. The next image depicts an Indian grocery store in Waltham, Massachusetts. The next images depict the poverty in this land of plenty—this pawn shop, where one can dispose of treasured items for desperately needed cash, is located in Bakersfield, California; the homeless woman, pushing her cart of possessions, can be found in countless cities across this land. An infinite number of images could be placed in these chapter opening images. What comes to your mind when you think about the demographic diversity in your home community? What are your images of poverty and homelessness?

This is now the 21st century and health care providers are entangled in the revolutionary consequences of enormous demographic, social, and cultural change. Many of these changes are playing a dramatic role both in the delivery of health care to patients, their families, and communities and in the workforce and environment in which the provider practices. The emerging majority—people of color—that constituted 19.7% of the population in 1990 in 2000 constituted 25% of the population; in 2005, the figure was 32% and is rapidly growing (U.S. Bureau of the Census, 1992, 2006). The comments and data presented in this chapter are designed to provide you with an image of the demographic features, derived from Census 2000, recent immigration, labor, and economic backgrounds of the American population.

In order to understand the profound changes that are taking place in the health care system, both in the delivery of services and in the profile of the people who are receiving and delivering services, we must look at the changes in the American population. The White majority is aging and shrinking; the Black, Hispanic, Asian, and American Indian populations are young and growing. It is imperative for those who deliver health care to be understanding of and sensitive to cultural differences and to the effect of the differences on a person's health and illness beliefs and practices and health care needs.

■ Census 2000

Every census adapts to the decade in which it is conducted. One of the most important changes for Census 2000 was the revision of the questions that were asked regarding race and Hispanic origin. The federal government considers race and Hispanic origin to be two separate concepts and the questions on race and Hispanic origin were asked of all people living in the United States. The changes were developed to reflect the country's growing diversity. The respondents were given the option of selecting one or more race categories to indicate their racial identities. Given these changes, the Census 2000 data on race are not directly comparable with data from the 1990 Census or earlier censuses. However, for the purpose of comparison in this text, the data from the tables that factor in Hispanic origin and use the categories White and Black, alone, *non-Hispanic* will be used. Another factor that presents confusion is that people were free to define themselves as belonging to many groups. However, the overwhelming majority of the population reported one race.

In 1997 the Office of Management and Budget established federal guidelines to collect and present data on race and Hispanic origin. Census 2000 adhered to the guidelines, and established minimal categories as follows:

1. **White**—A person having origins in any of the original peoples of Europe, the Middle East, or North Africa. It includes people who indicate their race as "White" or report on entries such as Irish, German, Italian, or Arab.

2. **Black or African American**—A person having origins in any of the original black racial groups of Africa. It includes, for example, people who indicate their race as Black, African American, or Negro.

3. **American Indian and Alaska Native**—A person having origins in any of the original people of North and South America (including Central America) and who maintain tribal affiliation or community attachment.

4. **Asian**—A person having origins in any of the original people of the Far East, Southeast Asia, or the Indian subcontinent, including, for example, China, India, and the Philippine Islands.

5. **Native Hawaiian and Other Pacific Islander**—People who have origins in any of the original peoples of Hawaii, Guam, Samoa, or other Pacific Islands or who provided a write-in response of a Pacific Islander group. This group has been clustered in the category of "other," as the percentages in the general population and age are small (Grieco & Cassidy, 2001, p. 2).

6. **Hispanic or Latino**—People who identify in categories such as Mexican, Puerto Rican, or Cuban, as well as those who indicate they are of other Spanish origin. Origin can be viewed as heritage, nationality group, lineage, or country of birth of the person or person's parents, or their ancestors before their arrival in the United States. People who identify their origin as Spanish can be of any race (Grieco & Cassidy, 2001, p. 2; Lew, 2000).

These terms of classification will be used throughout this chapter and the text. Since the census does not break down the population by gender, except male/female and by abled/disabled, this text will not include these variables in its discussions.

Total Population Characteristics

The 2000 census percentages are compared with the 1980 and 1990 census percentages in Table 2–1. The figures demonstrate both the growth of the American population in general and the growth of people of color specifically. The changes are as follows:

1. In 1990, despite an accepted head count shortfall of 4.7 million people, the population count of the United States represented an increase of 22,167,670 people over the 1980 census and 19.8% of

Table 2-1   **Resident Population by Race and Hispanic Origin: 1980, 1990, and 2000**

Year	Total Resident Population	White	Black or African American	Asian	American Indian and Alaska Native	Hispanic or Latino	White Alone
1980	226,546	83.20%	11.70%	1.50%	0.60%	6.40%[1]	
1990	248,791	80.20%	12.20%	2.90%	0.80%	9.00%[1]	
2000	282,193	75.10%	12.30%	3.60%	0.90%	12.50%	72.10%

[1] 1970 Hispanic included in overall data.

Sources: U.S. Bureau of the Census. (1981, February 23). 1980 census population. Press release CB81-32 and Supplementary report PC80-S1-1. Washington, DC: U.S. Government Printing Office; U.S. Bureau of the Census (1992, November). *1990 census of the population, general population characteristics United States* (p. 4). Washington, DC: U.S. Government Printing Office; Meyer, J. (2001). *Age: 2000 Census 2000 brief* (p. 3). Washington, DC: U.S. Department of Commerce, with permission, Retrieved from http://www.census.gov/popest/estimates.php., June 2006.

the population was comprised of people of color. Again, it may also be noted that 9.0% of the population claimed Hispanic or Spanish origin but could be of any race. Note that the European American majority had shrunk by about 3%, and there is an "emerging majority" of people of color.

2. In 2000, the population of the United States was counted as 281,421,906 (U.S. Bureau of the Census, 2006), which represented an increase of 32,712 (in thousands) from 1990, and 25% of the population was comprised of people of color. It may also be noted that 12.5% of the population claimed Hispanic or Latino origin but could be of any race.

3. During the fall of 2006, the population reached 300 million. In March 2008 the total population for the United States was 303,536,174. (U.S. Census Bureau, Retrieved March 1, 2008 from http://www.census.gov/index.html).

Age. The age classification is based on the age of the person in complete years as of April 1, 2000. The age was derived from the date of birth information requested on the census form. It is critical to note the following points regarding age in 2000:

- Twenty-six percent, or 72.3 million, of the U.S. population were under 18.
- Twenty-six percent, or 174.1 million, of the population were between 18 and 64.
- The percentage of the under-18-year-old populations was greater than the total population among Blacks, American Indians, and Hispanics.
- Twelve percent, or 35 million people, were age 65 or over.
- The percentage of the 65+ population was the greatest among White non-Hispanics (U.S. Bureau of the Census, 2001, p. 1 retrieved from http://www.census.gov).

Table 2–2   Mean and Median Ages of the Resident Population, 2000 and 2005

Population Group	Mean Age		Median Age	
	2000	**2005**	**2000**	**2005**
American Indian (alone)	29.4 years	31.6 years	27.7 years	29.5 years
Asian/Pacific Islander (alone)	33.3 years	34.9 years	32.5 years	34.5 years
Black (alone)	31.4 years	32.4 years	30.0 years	30.9 years
Hispanic	27.6 years	28.7 years	25.8 years	27.2 years
White (alone—not of Hispanic heritage)	38.4 years	39.3 years	38.6 years	40.3 years

Source: U.S. Census Bureau. (2006, May 10). Annual estimates of the population by sex, age and race for the United States: April 1, 2000 to July 1, 2005. Retrieved from http://www.census.gov/popest/national/asrh/NC-EST2005-asrh.html, July 3, 2007.

American Indian, Aleut, and Eskimo Populations (Alone).   The American Indian, Eskimo, and Aleut populations alone in the United States constituted 0.9% of the total population in 2000 and in 2005. The percentage of the population in 2000, as illustrated in Table 2–2, under 18 was 33.9%; 18–24, 11%; 25–44, 30.9%; 45–64, 18.0%; and 65 and over, 5.6%. The median age of the population was 27.7 years in 2000.

Asian/Pacific Islander Population (Alone).   Members of the Asian/Pacific Island communities made up 3.6% of the population in 2000 and 4.7% in 2005. The percentage of the population under 18 in 2000, as illustrated in Table 2–2, was 24.1%; 18–24, 11.1%; 25–44, 36.0%; 45–64, 21%; and 65 and over, 7.8%. The median age of the Asian/Pacific Island population was 32.5 years in 2000.

Black Population (Alone).   The Black population alone in the United States constituted 12.3% of the total population in 2000 and 12.8% in 2005. The percentage of the population under 18 in 2000, as illustrated in Table 2–2, was 31.4%; 18–24, 11.0%; 25–44, 30.9%; 45–64, 18.6%; and 65 and over, 8.1%. The median age of the Black population was 30.0 years in 2000.

Hispanic Population (of Any Race).   Hispanic Americans (of any race) made up 12.5% of the total population in 2000 and 14.4% in 2005. The percentage of the population under 18, as illustrated in Table 2–2, was 35%; 18–24, 13.4%; 25–44, 33.0%; 45–64, 13.7%; and 65 and over, 4.9%. The median age of the Hispanic population was 25.8 years in 2000.

White Population (Alone).   In 2000 the White population in the United States constituted 72.1% of the total population and 68% in 2005. The percentage of the population under 18 in 2000, as illustrated in Table 2–2, was 23.5%; 18–24, 8.9%; 25–44, 29.6%; 45–64, 23.7%; 65 and over, 14.4%. The median age of the population was 38.6 years in 2000.

The U.S. Census Bureau produces estimates of the resident population for the United States on an annual basis. It revises the estimates time series each year as final input data become available. These postcensal estimates from April 1, 2000, through July 1, 2006, supersede all previous estimates produced since Census 2000. On March 30, 2007, the U.S. Census Bureau submitted to Congress the subjects it plans to address in the 2010 Census, which include gender, age, race, ethnicity, relationship, and whether you own or rent your home. It is estimated that the questions will take less than 10 minutes to complete. This indicates that the 2010 Census will be one of the shortest and easiest to complete since the nation's first census in 1790. There will also be a yearly American Community Survey, which will eliminate the need for a long-form questionnaire and will provide key socioeconomic and housing data about the nation's rapidly changing population.

■ Immigration

Immigrants and their descendants constitute most of the population of the United States, and Americans who are not themselves immigrants have ancestors who came to the United States from elsewhere. The only people considered native to this land are the American Indians, the Aleuts, and the Inuit (or Eskimos), for they migrated here thousands of years before the Europeans (Thernstrom, 1980, p. vii).

Immigrants come to the United States seeking religious and political freedom and economic opportunities. The life of the immigrant is fraught with difficulties—going from an "old" to a "new" way of life, learning a new language, and adapting to a new climate, new foods, and a new culture. Socialization of immigrants occurs in American public schools, and Americanization, according to Greeley (1978), is for some a process of "vast psychic repression," wherein one's language and other familiar trappings are shed. In part, the concept of the melting pot has been created in schools, where children learn English, reject family traditions, and attempt to take on the values of the dominant culture and "pass" as Americans (Novak, 1973). This difficult experience, as noted and described by Greeley and Novak in the 1970s, continues today.

A **citizen** of the United States is a native-born, foreign-born child of citizens, or a naturalized person who owes allegiance to the United States and who is entitled to its protection. "All persons born or naturalized in the United States, are citizens of the United States and of the state wherein they reside." A **refugee** is any person who is outside his or her country of nationality who is unable or unwilling to return to that country because of persecution or a well-founded fear of persecution. Persecution or the fear thereof must be based on the alien's race, religion, nationality, membership in a particular social group, or political opinion. People with no nationality must generally be outside their country of last habitual residence to qualify as a refugee. Refugees are subject to ceilings by geographic area set annually by the president in consultation with Congress and are eligible to adjust to lawful permanent resident status after 1 year of continuous presence in the United States. A permanent resident alien is an alien admitted to the United States as a lawful permanent resident. A "green card" provides official immigra-

Box 2–1

Sample Questions and Answers for New Pilot Naturalization Test

1. What does "We the People" mean in the Constitution?
2. What do we call changes to the Constitution?
3. Name one right or freedom from the First Amendment.
4. How many amendments does the Constitution have?
5. What are the three branches or parts of the government?
6. How many United States Senators are there?
7. How many justices are on the Supreme Court?
8. Name one responsibility that is only for United States citizens.
9. Name two rights that are only for United States citizens.
10. When was the Declaration of Independence adopted?

Answers
1. The power of government comes from the people.
2. Amendments
3. Speech Religion Assembly Press Petition the government
4. Twenty-seven (27)
5. Executive, legislative, and judicial (Congress, the president, the courts)
6. 100
7. Nine (9)
8. Vote Serve on a jury
9. The right to apply for a federal job The right to vote The right to run for office The right to carry a U.S. passport
10. July 4, 1776

Source: Department of Homeland Security. Retrieved March 1, 2008 from http://www.dhs.gov/ximgtn/statistics/publications/index.shtm

tion status (lawful permanent residency) in the United States. Immigrants are now referred to as Legal Permanent Residents; however, the Immigration and Nationality Act (INA) broadly defines an immigrant as "any alien in the United States, except one legally admitted under specific nonimmigrant categories." An illegal alien, or undocumented person, who entered the United States without inspection, for example, would be strictly defined as an immigrant under the INA but is not a Legal Permanent Resident. Legal Permanent Residents are legally accorded the privilege of residing permanently in the United States. Box 2–1 contains an example of the questions a person is asked when taking the examination for naturalization. There are estimated (2007) to be 12 million undocumented people living in the United States.

In 2006, a total of 1,266,264 people became Legal Permanent Residents of the United States. The majority, 65%, already resided here. Among the LPRs

**Table 2-3   Five Leading Metropolitan Areas
of Residence**

1. New York, northern New Jersey–Long Island: 17.7%
2. Los Angeles–Long Beach–Santa Ana, California: 9.5%
3. Miami–Fort Lauderdale–Miami Beach, Florida: 7.8%
4. Washington, DC–Maryland–Virginia: 4.3%
5. Chicago–Joliet, Illinois, Indiana, Wisconsin: 3.9%

Source: Jefferys, K. (2007). U.S. Legal Permanent Residents, 2006. Washington, D.C.
Department of Homeland Security. Retrieved March 1, 2008 from http://www.dhs.
gov/ximgtn/statistics/publications/index.shtm

Mexico, 14%; China, 7%; and the Philippines, 6% were the leading countries of
birth (Jefferys, 2007, p. 1). In 1970, the highest percentage of people were from
Europe, whereas in 2000 people from Mexico, China, and the Philippines were
the highest in percentage.

Table 2–3 lists the primary metropolitan areas for Legal Permanent Residents in 2006, and Table 2–4 lists the top 10 states where Legal Permanent Residents are residing. Table 2–5 shows the leading 10 countries of origin for Legal
Permanent Residents Flow by Country of Birth in 2006. Table 2–6 compares
selected characteristics of the native and foreign-born populations in 2005. The
following are examples:

- Fewer foreign-born people are likely to have a vehicle than native born
  residents.
- More are likely to graduate from high school than natives.
- More are likely to speak English less than well.
- More are likely to be unemployed.
- More are likely to earn less than natives.
- More are likely to live in poverty than natives.

**Table 2-4   Permanent Resident Flow by State
of Residence: 2006**

1.	California	20.9%
2.	New York	14.2%
3.	Florida	12.3%
4.	Texas	7.0%
5.	New Jersey	5.2%
6.	Illinois	4.1%
7.	Virginia	3.0%
8.	Massachusetts	2.8%
9.	Georgia	2.5%
10.	Maryland	2.4%
	Other states	25.4%

Source: Jefferys, K. (2007). U.S. Legal Permanent Residents, 2006. Washington, DC:
Department of Homeland Security. Retrieved March 1, 2008 from http://www.dhs.
gov/ximgtn/statistics/publications/index.shtm

Table 2–5 Leading 10 Countries of Origin for Legal Permanent Resident Flow by Country of Birth: 2006

1.	Mexico	13.7%
2.	People's Republic of China	6.9%
3.	Philippines	5.9%
4.	India	4.8%
5.	Cuba	3.6%
6.	Colombia	3.4%
7.	Dominican Republic	3.0%
8.	El Salvador	2.5%
9.	Vietnam	2.4%
10.	Jamaica	2.0%

Source: Jefferys, K. (2007) U.S. Legal Permanent Residents, 2006. Washington, DC: Department of Homeland Security. Retrieved March 1, 2008 from http://www.dhs.gov/ximgtn/statistics/publications/index.shtm

In addition to the number of people entering the United States legally, there were 4.6 to 5.4 million undocumented immigrants residing here in 1996. It is extremely difficult to count the number of people who are hiding because they are not documented and estimated to be 12 million in 2007. It is widely recognized that the population is growing by about 275,000 people each year. California is the leading state of residence for undocumented people. Other states include Texas, New York, and Florida.

Table 2–6 Selected Characteristics of the Native and Foreign-Born Populations

Characteristic	Native Population	Naturalized Citizens	Not a U.S. Citizen
Population	252.7 million	15 million	20.7 million
Median age	35.7 years	47.9 years	33.9 years
Asian	1.6%	31.1%	18%
Hispanic	9.9%	31.4%	58.2%
Population 25 years and older, less than high school	15.8%	23.3%	40.3%
Speak language other than English	9.5%	78.1%	88.4%
Speak English less than well	8.6%	38.7%	61.9%
Family poverty rates	9.3%	9.3%	22.2%
Poverty status below 100% of poverty level	12.8%	10.4%	21.6%
Renting household unit	31%	31.5%	62.6%
Vehicle unavailable	8.1%	11.9%	15.8%
No telephone service	5.1%	3%	8.5%

Source: American fact finder selected characteristics of the native and foreign-born population, American community survey. (2005). Retrieved from http://factfinder.census.gov/servlet/STTable?_bm=y&-geo_id=01000US&-qr_name=ACS_2005_EST_G00_S0602&-ds_name=ACS_2005_EST_G00

There has been an effort by the government to tighten both immigration and travel access to the United States since the terrorist attacks in September 2001. On July 22, 2002, the Justice Department announced that it will use criminal penalties against immigrants and foreign visitors who fail to notify the government of change of address within 10 days. This requirement is not a new one, but it has not been strictly enforced. This will have an impact on at least 11 million people and visitors who stay in the United States more than 30 days (Davis & Furtado, 2002, p. A2). In addition, this will have an impact on the health care system and on providers of health care both directly and indirectly. For example, it will be more difficult for people to work here and to visit family members who are ill. In addition, the passage of Proposition 187 in California in November 1994, and earlier laws relating to bilingual education in Texas, demonstrates that many citizens are no longer willing to provide basic human services, such as health care and education, to the new residents. Thus far, the implementation of these laws has been held up in the courts. Despite such efforts, however, it is evident that immigration to this country will continue. It is predicted that by the year 2020 immigration will be a major source of new people for the United States and will be responsible for whatever growth occurs in the United States after 2030. The United States will continue to attract about two thirds of the world's immigrants, and 85% will be from Central and South America. Other immigration events are noted in Box 2–2.

On May 17, 2007, the U.S. president and a bipartisan group of senators reached bipartisan agreement on comprehensive immigration reform. The proposal included the following points:

1. Putting border security and enforcement first
2. Providing tools for employers to verify the eligibility of the workers they hire
3. Creating a temporary worker program
4. No amnesty for illegal immigrants
5. Strengthening the assimilation of new immigrants: the proposal declares that English is the language of the United States
6. Establishing a merit system for future immigration
7. Ending chain migration
8. Clearing the family backlog in 8 years (Homeland Security, May 17, 2007)

This legislation did not pass, however, and will not be addressed until after the next presidential election. In addition, there are an estimated 11.6 million unauthorized immigrants living in the United States as of January, 2006. (Hoefer, M., Rytina, N., and Campbell, C., 2007, p. 1)

Table 2–6 lists and compares several selected characteristics of the Native population, naturalized citizens, and not a U.S. citizen.

The need for strict enforcement of Title VI and the CLAS standards becomes self evident when you realize the high numbers of people who do not understand and speak English.

Box 2–2

Highlights of Immigration History: 1798–2007

Year	Event
1798	Alien and Sedition Acts passed
1808	African slave trade prohibited
1819	First immigrant data collected
1824	Naturalization set at 2 years
1844	Nativist riots in Philadelphia
1846	Potato famine in Ireland, resulting in massive Irish influx
1849	California gold rush; imported Chinese labor
1862	Homestead Act opens land to immigrants
1870	Naturalization extended to Africans
1882–1943	Chinese Exclusion Act
1886	Statue of Liberty opens
1892	Ellis Island Immigration Station opens
1898	Immigrants classified by "race"
1903	Political radicals banned from entering the United States
1907	1,004,756 people—a record—pass through Ellis Island
1908	"Gentleman's Agreement" restricts Japanese immigration
1910	Entrance barred to criminals, paupers, and diseased
1917	Literacy required for immigrants over 16
1924	Annual racial quotas established; Border Patrol established
1942–1964	Bracero Program allows temporary workers
1975	Vietnam War ends; Indochinese refugee program
1980	Mariel boatlift from Cuba—125,000 people
1986	Amnesty for illegal aliens
1990	Ellis Island immigration museum opens
1996	Illegal Immigration Reform and Immigrant Responsibility Act of 1996
1996	Personal Responsibility and Work Opportunity Reconciliation Act of 1996
1996	Antiterrorism and Effective Death Penalty Act of 1996
1999	Nursing Relief for Disadvantaged Areas Act of 1999
2001	USA Patriot Act of 2001
2002	Family Sponsor Immigration Act of 2002
2002	Enhanced Security and Visa Entry Reform Act of 2002
2003	Extension of the Special Immigrant Religious Worker Program
2003	Department of Homeland Security Begins
2005	Disadvantaged Areas Reauthorization Act
2006	Secure Fence Act
2006	National Defense Authorization Act for Fiscal Year 2006
2007	Failure of immigration reform

Sources: Lefcowitz, E. (1990). *The United States immigration history timeline.* New York: Terra Firma Press. Reprinted with permission; Retrieved from http://www.uscis.gov/propub/ProPubVAP.jsp?dockey=2b289cf41dd6b70a61a078a9fbfbc379 and Homeland Security (2003). Retrieved from http://www.dhsgov/index.shtm

■ Poverty

There are countless ways to answer the question "What is poverty?" Poverty may be viewed through many lenses and from anthropological, cultural, demographic, economical, educational, environmental, historical, medical, philosophical, policy, political, racial, sexual, sociological, and theological points of view. The consequences of poverty are ubiquitous. They include, but are not limited to, battering, bullying, child abuse, gaming, obesity, spousal abuse, substance abuse, and violence. Poverty may also be viewed in a "holistic" way. Here, the physical, mental, and spiritual aspects of poverty are self-evident. Examples include, but are not limited to,

- Physical—substandard housing, no telephone or vehicle, limited access to health care
- Mental—inadequate education, poor opportunity
- Spiritual—despair, the experience of being disparaged

In 2005, 37 million people, approximately 13% of the population, lived below the poverty level (DeNavas-Walt, Proctor, & Lee, 2006, p. 8). Poverty rates dif-

Table 2-7 Selected Federal Poverty Programs

Purpose	Program	Federal Cash Outlay	Description
Cash aid	Temporary Assistance for Needy Families (TANF)	$10.4 billion	Basic cash aid through state Requires work
Food and nutrition	Food Stamps	$27.2 billion	Provides, depending on need, funding for food
	Special Supplemental Nutrition Program for Women, Infants, and Children (WIC)	$4.5 million	Provides benefits for low-income mothers, infants, and children considered to be "at risk"
Medical	Medicaid	$176 billion	Provides payments to health care providers in full or in a co-pay for eligible low-income families and individuals and for long-term care to those eligible who are aged or disabled
Housing	Section 8 Low-Income Housing Assistance	$22.4 billion	Provides rental assistance through vouchers or rental subsidies to eligible low-income families

Source: Nilsen, S. (2007). Poverty in America. Retrieved from www.gao.gov/cgi_bin/qetrpt

fer by age, gender, race, and ethnicity. For example, the rates of poverty in 2005 were

- 24.9% for Blacks
- 21.8% for Hispanics
- 8.3% for non-Hispanic Whites
- 17.6% for children
- 10.1% for adults over 65

The federal government has an extensive history of efforts to improve the conditions of people living with limited incomes and material resources. Since the 1850s, there have been countless initiatives enacted to help citizens who were "poor." The programs described in Table 2–7 are examples of federal cash assistance programs available to low-income families.

Another way of answering this question ("what is poverty?") is with the description used by the U.S. Bureau of Labor Statistics, which counts the poor and describes them by age, education, location, race, family composition, and employment status. A third answer is the federal government's definition of the poverty threshold. This poverty threshold, developed in 1965, is based on pre-tax income only, excluding capital gains, and does not include the value of non-cash benefits, such as employer-provided health insurance, food stamps, or Medicaid. The poverty-level figures are used by programs such as Head Start, Low-Income Home Energy, and National School Lunch, to determine eligibility. The poverty level for an average family of four was $19,971 in 2005.

Table 2–8 lists the poverty guidelines for persons and families for selected years.

Table 2-8 Poverty Guidelines for the Years 1986–2005 for the Contiguous States and the District of Columbia

Year	First Person	Additional Person	Four-Person
1986	$5,360	$1,880	$11,000
1988	5,770	1,960	11,650
1990	6,280	2,140	12,700
1992	6,810	2,380	13,950
1994	7,360	2,480	14,800
1996	7,740	2,620	15,600
1998	8,050	2,800	16,450
2002	8,860	3,080	18,100
2005	9,973	2,782	19,971

Sources: *Federal Register 63*, no. 36. (1998, February 24). 9235–9238, and (2002, February 14), 6931–6933; U.S. Census Bureau. (2006, August 29). Current population survey, 2006 annual social and economic supplement. Retrieved from http://pubdb3.census.gov/macro/032006/pov/new35_000.htm

The association between socioeconomic status and health status of a person or family may be explained in part by the reduced access to health care among those with lower socioeconomic status. Income may be related to health because it

- Increases access to health care
- Enables the person or family to live in a better neighborhood
- Enables the person or family to afford better housing
- Enables the person or family to reside in locations not abutting known environmentally degraded locations (heavy industrial pollution or known hazardous waste sites)
- Increases the opportunity to engage in health promoting behaviors

Health also may affect income by restricting the type and amount of employment a person may seek or by preventing a person from working.

There has been an increase in earning inequality over the last 25 years. The income for all races rose, then dipped, in this time period. For Blacks and Hispanics, it was much lower than for Whites and Asians and for people from the Pacific Islands. Much of this change and inequality was due to technological changes that increased income to highly skilled labor. At the same time, less skilled workers saw their wages decrease or stagnate. The other factors responsible for this phenomenon include

- Globalization of the economy
- Decline in the real minimum wage
- Decline in unionization
- Increase in immigration
- Increase in families headed by women (from 10% in 1970 to 18% in 1996 and 24.7% in 2000) (households headed by women generally have lower incomes) (Dalaku, 2001, p. 2)

The following are examples of the poverty in the United States:

- The official poverty rate in 2005 was 12.6%.
- In 2005, 37 million people were in poverty.
- The poverty rate has increased in recent years among people under 65 years.
- In 2005, 17.6% of the children under 18 lived in poverty.
- In 2005, 43.9% of the people living in poverty were non-Hispanic White families; non-Hispanic White families constitute 66.7% of the total population.
- Children in households headed by females had the highest rates of poverty, and these rates were higher among Black and Hispanic children.

The poverty rate in 2005 for

- Blacks was 24.9%
- Non-Hispanic Whites was 8.3%
- Female-householder families with no husband present was 52.9%
- People 65 years old and over was 10.2%

- Asians and Pacific Islanders was 11.1%
- Hispanics was 21.2%
- Non-Hispanic Whites was 7.5% (DeNavas-Walt et al., 2006, p. 13)

Cycle of Poverty

Poverty is more than the absence of money. One way of analyzing the phenomenon is by observing the effects of the "cycle of poverty," as illustrated in Figure 2–1. In this cycle, the poor person lives in a situation that may create poor intellectual and physical development and poor economic production, and in which the birth rate is high; this living situation in turn causes poor production, which creates insufficient salaries and a subsistence economy that often forces the person to reside in densely populated areas or remotely located rural areas where adequate shelter and potable water are scarce, and the person suffers from chronically poor nutrition. These conditions all too often lead to high morbidity and accident rates, precipitating high health care costs, which, in turn, prevent the person

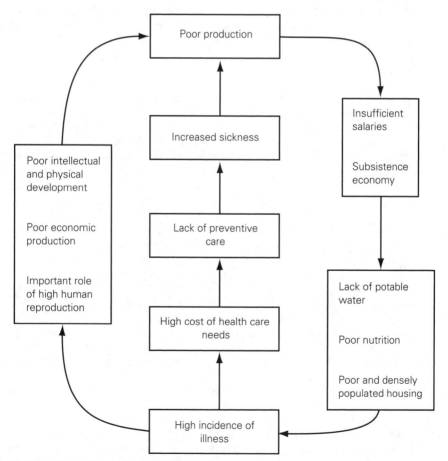

Figure 2–1 The cycle of poverty.

from seeking health care services. Thus, there is an increase in sickness and poor production, in a cycle that has yet to be broken. Other barriers that are interrelated to this cycle are the lack of access to health care services, language issues, and transportation issues (Spector, 1979, pp. 148–152).

The issues of overcrowded housing, poor sanitation, homelessness, and so forth that are part of the cycle of poverty have a profound and prolonged impact on the health status of people.

This chapter has presented an overview of the major phenomena contributing to the profound diversity existing within the United States—demographic; population and immigration; and poverty. Additional issues will be explored in more depth in the chapters relating to each of the major population groups described in Census 2000.

Explore 🌐 MediaLink

Go to the Companion Website at www.prenhall.com/spector for chapter-related review questions, case studies, and activities. Contents of the CulturalCare Guide and CulturalCare Museum can also be found on the Companion Website. Click on Chapter 2 to select the activities for this chapter.

■ Internet Sources

American Fact Finder Selected Characteristics of the Native and Foreign-Born Population, American Community Survey, 2005. (http://factfinder.census.gov/servlet/STTable?_bm=y&-geo_id=01000US&-) http://www.uscis.gov/propub/ProPubVAP.jsp?dockey=2b289cf41dd6b70a61a078a9fbfbc379

Bernstein, R., Census Bureau, August 9, 2007, http://www.census.gov/Press-Release/www/releases/, August 9, 2007.

Grieco, E. and Cassidy, R. C. (2001). Overview of Race and Hispanic Origin. Census Brief. Washington, DC: Census Bureau. Retrieved from http://www.census.gov/prod/2001pubs/c2kbr01-1.pdf, July 25, 2007.

Hoefer, M., Rytina, N., and Campbell, C. (2007). Estimates of the Unauthorized Immigrant Population in the United States: January, 2006. Washington, DC: Department of Homeland Security. Retrieved March 1, 2008 from http://www.dhs.gov/ximgtn/statistics/publications/index.shtm

Jefferys, K. (2007). U.S. Legal Permanent Residents, 2006. Washington, DC: Department of Homeland Security. Retrieved March 1, 2008 from http://www.dhs.gov/ximgtn/statistics/publications/index.shtm

Lew, J. J. (2000). Guidance on Aggregation and Allocation of Data on Race for use in Civil Rights Monitoring and Enforcement. Washington, DC, Office of Management and Budget. Retrieved March 1, 2008 from http://www.whitehouse.gov/omb/bulletins/b00-02.html

Nilsen, S. (2007). Poverty in America – Report to Congrssional Requesters. Washington, DC: United States Government Accountability Office. Retrieved July 21, 2007 from www.gao.gov/cgi-bin/getrpt

U.S. Census Bureau, "Annual Estimates of the Population by Sex, Age and Race for the United States: April 1, 2000 to July 1, 2005(NC-EST2005-04)"; published 10 May 2006; http://www.census.gov/popest/national/asrh/NCEST2005-asrh.

html, http://www.uscis.gov/portal/site/uscis/menuitem.5af9bb95919 f35e66 f614176543f6dla/?vgnextoid=dcf5eldf53b2f010VgnVCM1000000ecd190a RCRD &vgnextchannel=d1fc9f9934741110VgnVCM1000000ecd190aRCRD

U.S. Census Bureau, Current Population Survey, 2006 Annual Social and Economic Supplement. *Last revised: August 29, 2006* http://pubdb3.census.gov/macro/032006/pov/new35_000.htm

United States Department of Homeland Security. (2007). United States History and Government Questions. Washington, DC: United States Citizenship and Immigration Services. Retrieved March 1, 2008 from http://www.dhs.gov/index.shtm

United States Department of Homeland Security. (2007). Press Release. Administration and Bipartisan Group of Senators Reach Bipartisan Agreement on Comprehensive Immigration Reform. Washington, DC: Department of Homeland Security. P. 1. Retrieved on March 1, 2008 from http://www.dhs.gov/xnews/releases/pr_1179511978687.shtm

United States Department of Homeland Security. (2007). United States History and Government Questions. Washington, DC: United States Citizenship and Immigration Services. Retrieved March 1, 2008 from http://www.uscis.gov/portal/site/uscis/menuitem.5af9bb95919f35e66f614176543f6d1a/?vgnextoid=12e596981298d010VgnVCM10000048f3d6a1RCRD&vgnextchannel=96719c7755cb9010VgnVCM10000045f3d6a1RCRD

■ References

Dalaku, J. (2001). *Poverty in the United States: 2000.* U.S. Census Current Population Reports Series P60–214. Wahington, DC: U.S. Government Printing Office.

Davis, F., & Furtado, C. (2002, July 22). INS to enforce change-of-address rule. *Boston Globe,* p. A2.

DeNavas-Walt, C., Proctor, B., & Lee, C. (2006). *Income, poverty, and health insurance coverage in the United States: 2005.* Washington, DC: U.S. Government Printing Office.

Greeley, A. (1978). *Why can't they be like us? America's white ethnic groups.* New York: E. P. Dutton.

Grieco, E. M., & Cassidy, R. C. (2001). *Overview of race and Hispanic origin.* Washington, DC: U.S. Census Bureau.

Hodgkinson, H. L. (1986, December). Reform? Higher education? Don't be absurd! *Higher Education,* 273.

Novak, M. (1973). How American are you if your grandparents came from Serbia in 1888? In S. Te Selle (Ed.), *The rediscovery of ethnicity: Its implications for culture and politics in America.* New York: Harper & Row.

Spector, M. (1979). Poverty: The barrier to health care. In R. E. Spector (Ed.), *Cultural diversity in health and illness* (pp. 141–162). New York: Appleton, Century & Crofts.

Thernstrom, S. (Ed.). (1980). *Harvard encyclopedia of American ethnic groups.* Cambridge: Harvard University Press.

U.S. Bureau of the Census. (1981, February 23). *1980 census population.* Press release CB81-32 and Supplementary report PC80-S1-1. Washington, DC: U.S. Government Printing Office.

U.S. Bureau of the Census. (1992, November). *1990 census of the population, general population characteristics United States.* Washington, DC: U.S. Government Printing Office.

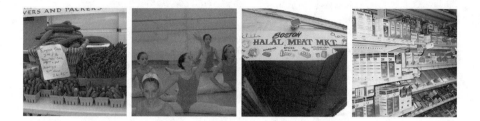

Chapter 3

Health and Illness

All things are connected. Whatever befalls the earth befalls the children of the earth.

—Chief Seattle Suqwamish and Duwamish

 **Objectives**

1. Understand health and illness and the sociocultural and historical phenomena that affect them.
2. Reexamine and redefine the concepts of health and illness.
3. Understand the multiple relationships between health and illness.
4. Associate the concepts of good and evil and light and dark with health and illness.
5. Analyze the Health Belief Model from both the provider and patient points of view.
6. Analyze the sick roles as described by Parsons, Alksen, and Suchman.
7. Generate experiential examples of the illness trajectory.

The images in the chapter opener represent facets of health and illness in various stages along the health/illness continuum. This first image is suggestive of maintaining health and the fresh, well-balanced food that must be included in a healthy diet. One of the greatest signs of the healthy person is that of being able to accomplish demanding physical challenges; in the second image, the youngsters are practicing ballet, an art that not only demands good health but also requires discipline and agility. The third image represents a resource from within a religious community for purchasing the proper food. The Islamic Halal market sells meats such as beef and lamb, no pig products, from animals that are ritually slaughtered. Over-the-counter remedies in the fourth image are representing remedies that may be used to restore health when everyday ailments occur.

There are countless images we can imagine to ponder comprehensive notions of health and illness. What do you do daily to maintain your health? What do you do when you experience a self-limiting ailment? How are ideas of health and illness reflected throughout the contemporary dominant culture in your home community? The community you work in? If you could pick four images relating to health and illness from your heritage, what would they be?

■ Health

The answers to the question "What is health?" are not as readily articulated as you might assume. One response may be a flawless recitation of the World Health Organization (WHO) definition of *health* as a "state of complete physical, mental, and social well being and not merely the absence of disease." This answer may be recited with great assurance—a challenge is neither expected nor welcomed but may evoke an intense dispute in which the assumed right answer is completely torn apart. Answers such as "homeostasis," "kinetic energy in balance," "optimal functioning," and "freedom from pain" are open to discussion. Experienced health care providers may be unable to give a comprehensive, acceptable answer to such a seemingly simple question. It is difficult to give a definition that makes sense without the use of some form of medical jargon. It is also challenging to define *health* in terms that a layperson can understand. (We lack skill in understanding "health" from the layperson's perspective.)

When you "Google" *health*, the response on the World Wide Web is well over 1.15 billion hits. One basic dictionary definition for the term is 1 : the condition of an organism or one of its parts in which it performs its vital functions normally or properly : the state of being sound in body or mind <dental *health*> <mental *health*>; *especially* : freedom from physical disease and pain <nursed him back to *health*> 2 : the condition of an organism with respect to the performance of its vital functions especially as evaluated subjectively or nonprofessionally <how is your *health* today>. Another one of the many classical definitions of *health* is in the *American Heritage Dictionary* (1976, p. 328):

> n. 1. The state of an organism with respect to functioning, disease, and abnormality at any given time. 2. The state of an organism functioning normally without disease or abnormality. 3. Optimal functioning with freedom from disease and abnormality. 4. Broadly, any state of optimal functioning, well being, or progress. 5. A wish for someone's good health, expressed as a toast.

As long ago as 1860, Florence Nightingale described health as "being well and using one's powers to the fullest extent." Murray and Zentner (1975) have classically defined *health* as "a purposeful, adaptive response, physically, mentally, emotionally, and socially, to internal and external stimuli in order to maintain stability and comfort." Rogers (1989) described health as "symbolic of wellness, a value term defined by culture or individual."

These definitions—varying in scope and context—are essentially those that the student practitioner, and educator within the health professions agree convey the meaning of *health*. The most widely used and recognized definition is that of WHO. Within the socialization process of the health care deliverer, the denotation of the word is that contained in the WHO definition. For other students, the meaning of the word *health* becomes clear through the educational experience.

In analyzing these definitions, we are able to discern subtle variations in denotation. In fact, the connotation does not essentially change over time. If this occurs in the denotation of the word, what of the connotation? That is, are health care providers as familiar with implicit meanings as with more explicit ones? Historically, Irwin M. Rosenstock (1966) commented that the health professions are becoming increasingly aware of the lack of clarity in the definition of *health*. Surely this is a contemporary and an accurate thought on the educational process, which is indeed deficient. He concluded, "Whereas health itself is in reality an elusive concept, in much of research, the stages involved in seeking medical care are conceived as completely distinct" (p. 49).

The framework of both education and research in the health professions continues to rely on the more abstract definitions of the word *health*. When taken in a broader context, health can be regarded not only as the absence of disease but also as a reward for "good behavior." In fact, a state of health is regarded by many people as the reward one receives for "good" behavior and illness as punishment for "bad" behavior. You may have heard something like "She is so good; no wonder she is so healthy" or a mother admonishing her child, "If you don't do such and such, you'll get sick." Situations and experiences may be avoided for the purpose of protecting and maintaining one's health. Conversely, some people seek out challenging, albeit dangerous, situations with the hope that they will experience the thrill of a challenge and still emerge in an intact state of health. One example of such behavior is driving at high speeds.

Health can also be viewed as the freedom from and the absence of evil. In this context, health is analogous to day, which equals good light. Conversely, illness is analogous to night, evil, and dark. Illness, to some, is seen as a punishment for being bad or doing evil deeds; it is the work of vindictive evil spirits. In the modern education of health care providers, these concepts of health and illness are rarely if ever discussed, yet, if these concepts of health and illness are believed by some consumers of health care services, understanding these varying ideas is important for the provider. Each of us enters the health care community with our own culturally based concept of health. During the educational and socialization process in a health care provider profession—nursing, medicine, or social work—we are expected to shed these beliefs and adopt the standard definitions. In addition to shedding these old beliefs, we learn, if only by unspoken example, to view as deviant those who do not accept the prevailing, institutional connotation of the word *health*.

The material that follows illustrates the complex process necessary to enable providers to return to and appreciate our former interpretations of health, to understand the vast number of meanings of the word *health*, and to be aware of the difficulties that exist with definitions such as that of WHO.

How Do YOU Define Health?

You have been requested to describe the term *health* in your own words. You may initially respond by reciting the WHO definition. What does this definition really mean? The following is a representative sample of actual responses:

1. Being able to do what I want to do
2. Physical and psychological well-being: *physical* meaning that there are no abnormal functions with the body—all systems are without those abnormal functions that would cause a problem physically—and *psychological* meaning that one's mind is capable of a clear and logical thinking process and association
3. Being able to use all of your body parts in the way that you want to— to have energy and enthusiasm
4. Being able to perform your normal activities, such as working, without discomfort and at an optimal level
5. The state of wellness with no physical or mental illness
6. I would define health as an undefined term: it depends on the situations, individuals, and other things.

In the initial step of the unlocking process, it begins to become clear that no single definition fully conveys what health really is.[1] We can all agree on the WHO definition, but when asked "What does that mean?" we are unable to clarify or to simplify that definition. As we begin to perceive a change in the connotation of the word, we may experience dismay, as that emotional response accompanies the breaking down of ideas. When this occurs, we begin to realize that as we were socialized into the provider culture by the educational process our understanding of health changed, and we moved a great distance from our older cultural understanding of the term. The following list includes the definitions of *health* given by students at various levels of education and experience. The students ranged in age from 19-year-old college juniors to graduate students in both nursing and social work.

---

[1]The unlocking process includes those steps taken to help break down and understand the definitions of both terms—*health* and *illness*—in a living context. It consists of persistent questioning: What is health? No matter what the response, the question "What does that mean?" is asked. Initially, this causes much confusion, but in classroom practice—as each term is written on the chalkboard and analyzed—the air clears and the process begins to make sense.

Junior Students

■ A system involving all subsystems of one's body that constantly work on keeping one in good physical and mental condition

Senior Students

■ Ability to function in activities of daily living to optimal capacity without requiring medical attention
■ Mental and physical wellness
■ The state of physical, mental, and emotional well-being

Graduate Students

■ Ability to cope with stressors; absence of pain—mental and physical
■ State of optimal well-being, both physical and emotional
■ State of well-being that is free from physical and mental distress; I can also include in this social well-being, even though this may be idealistic
■ Not only the absence of disease but a state of balance or equilibrium of physical, emotional, and spiritual states of well-being

It appears that the definition becomes more abstract and technical as the student advances in the educational program. The terms explaining health take on a more abstract and scientific character with each year of removal from the lay mode of thinking. Can these layers of jargon be removed, and can we help ourselves once again to view heath in a more tangible manner?

In further probing this question, let us think back to the way we perceived health before our entrance into the educational program. I believe that the farther back we can go in our memory of earlier concepts of health, the better. Again, the question "What is health?" is asked over and over. Initially, the responses continue to include such terms and phrases as "homeostasis," "freedom from disease," or "frame of mind." Slowly, and with considerable prodding, we are able to recall earlier perceptions of health. Once again, health becomes a personal, experiential concept, and the relation of health to being returns. The fragility and instability of this concept also are recognized as health gradually acquires meaning in relation to the term *being*.

This process of unlocking a perception of a concept takes a considerable amount of time and patience. It also engenders dismay that briefly turns to anger and resentment. You may question why the definitions acquired and mastered in the learning process are now being challenged and torn apart. The feeling may be that of taking a giant step backward in a quest for new terminology and new knowledge.

With this unlocking process, however, we are able to perceive the concept of health in the way that a vast number of health care consumers may perceive it. The following illustrates the transition that the concept passed through in an unlocking process from the WHO definition to the realm of the health care consumer.

Initial Responses

- Feeling of well-being, no illness
- Homeostasis
- Complete physical, mental, and social well-being

Secondary Responses

- Frame of mind
- Subjective state of psychosocial well-being
- Activities of daily living can be performed.

Experiential Responses

Health becomes tangible; the description is illustrated by using qualities that can be seen, felt, or touched.

- Shiny hair
- Warm, smooth, glossy skin
- Clear eyes
- Shiny teeth
- Being alert
- Being happy
- Freedom from pain
- Harmony between body and mind

Even this itemized description does not completely answer the question "What is health?" The words are once again subjected to the question "What does that mean?" and once again the terms are stripped down, and a paradox begins to emerge. For example, *shiny hair* may, in fact, be present in an ill person or in a person whose hair has not been washed for a long time, and a healthy person may not always have clean, well-groomed, lustrous hair. It becomes clear that, no matter how much we go around in a circle in an attempt to define *health*, the terms and meanings attributed to the state can be challenged. As a result of this prolonged discussion, we never really come to an acceptable definition of *health*, yet, by going through the intense unlocking process, we are able finally to understand the ambiguity that surrounds the word. We are, accordingly, less likely to view as deviant those people whose beliefs and practices concerning their own health and health care differ from ours.

Health Maintenance and Protection

Health can be seen from many other viewpoints, and many areas of disagreement arise with respect to how *health* can be defined. The preparation of health care workers tends to organize their education from a perspective of illness.

Rarely (or superficially) does it include a study of the concept of health. The emphasis in health care delivery has shifted from acute care to preventive care. The need for the provider of health services to comprehend this concept is therefore crucial. As this movement for preventive health care continues to take hold, to become firmly entrenched, and to thrive, multiple issues must be constantly addressed in answering the question "What is health?" Unless the provider is able to understand health from the viewpoint of the patient, a barrier of misunderstanding is perpetuated. It is difficult to reexamine complex definitions dutifully memorized at an earlier time, yet an understanding of health from a patient's viewpoint is essential to the establishment of comprehensive primary health care services inclusive of health maintenance and protection services because the perception of health is a complex psychological process. There tends to be no established pattern in what individuals and families see as their health needs and how they go about practicing their own health care.

Health maintenance and protection or the prevention of illness are by no means new concepts. As long as human beings have existed, they have used a multitude of methods—ranging from magic and witchcraft to present-day immunization and lifestyle changes—in an ongoing effort to maintain good health and prevent debilitating illness. Logic suggests that in order to maintain health we must prevent disease, and that is best accomplished by complying with immunization schedules, enforced by school policies; eating balanced meals, including avoiding salt and cholesterol; exercising regularly; and seeing a nurse practitioner or physician once a year for a checkup. The annual ritual of visiting a nurse practitioner or physician has been extensively promoted by the nursing and medical establishments and is viewed as effective by numerous laypeople, primarily those who have access to these services. A provider's statement often is required by a person seeking employment or life insurance. Furthermore, the annual physical examination has been advertised as the key to good health. A "clean bill of health" is considered essential for social, emotional, and even economic success. This clean bill of health is bestowed only by members of the health care profession. The general public has been conditioned to believe that health is guaranteed if a disease that may be developing is discovered early and treated with the ever-increasing varieties of modern medical technology. Although many people believe in and practice the annual physical and screening for early detection of a disease, there are some—both within and outside the health care professions—who do not subscribe to it. Preventive medicine grew out of clinical practice associated either with welfare medicine or with industrial or occupational medical practice. The approach of preventive medicine and health maintenance is the focus of health care practice in the United States among many segments of the population at large. However, countless disparities in overall health, and in access and utilization of the health care delivery system, exist and these will become increasingly evident as we progress through this text.

Health Status and Determinants

The 10 leading health indicators are used to measure the health of the nation. Each of the following indicators reflects a major health concern in the United States:

1. Physical activity
2. Overweight and obesity
3. Tobacco use
4. Substance abuse
5. Responsible sexual behavior
6. Mental health
7. Injury and violence
8. Environmental quality
9. Immunization
10. Access to health care

These indicators were selected by developers of *Healthy People 2010* on the basis of their ability to motivate action, the availability of data to measure progress, and their importance as public health issues. Box 3–1 further explains the *Healthy People 2010* program and a brief report on the midyear evaluation of this effort follows.

Healthy People 2010 developed a simple but powerful idea: "provide health objectives in a format that enables diverse groups to combine their efforts and work as a team." It is a "road map to better health" for all and can be used by many different people, states, communities, professional organizations, and groups to improve health. It is a plan for improving the health of all people in the United States during the first decade of the 21st century. The midcourse review provides an opportunity to examine the progress that has been made during the first half of the decade. The plan was predicated on two overarching goals and 955 objectives and subobjectives. A total of 67 objectives and subobjectives were dropped at the midpoint, and 381 objectives and subobjectives lacked tracking data. Monitoring the health of the nation is an extremely complex endeavor, as the timely availability of data is an issue. There are data and progress that can be assessed for the 281 objectives:

- Twenty-nine objectives (10%) met the target.
- One hundred thirty-eight objectives (49%) moved toward the target.
- Forty objectives (14%) demonstrated mixed progress.
- Seventeen objectives (6%) were unchanged from the baseline.
- Fifty-seven objectives (20%) moved away from the target.

The status of the two overarching goals is as follows.

Goal 1 is to increase quality and years of healthy life. *Healthy People 2010: Understanding and Improving Health* highlighted the importance of increasing and

Box 3–1

Healthy People 2010

Just as *Healthy People 2000: National Health Promotion and Disease Prevention and Objectives* was a statement of national opportunities, *Healthy People 2010* was adjusted to continue in this trajectory. These prevention initiatives present a national strategy for significantly improving the health of the American people in the decade preceding the year 2000 and in the decades to follow. These documents recognize that lifestyle and environmental factors are major determinants in disease prevention and health promotion. They provide strategies for significantly reducing preventable death and disability, for enhancing quality of life, and for reducing disparities in health status among various population groups within our society.

　　Both *Healthy People 2000* and *Healthy People 2010* define two broad goals:

1. *Increase the span of healthy life for all Americans.* The first goal of *Healthy People 2000,* and now of 2010, was to increase the quality as well as the years of healthy life. Here the emphasis is on the health status and nature of life, not just longevity. The life expectancy of Americans has steadily increased. In 1979, when the first *Healthy People: The Surgeon General's Report on Health Promotion and Disease Prevention* was published, the average life expectancy was 73.7 years. Based on current mortality experience, babies born in 1995 are expected to live 75.8 years. There is now increasing interest in other health goals, such as preventing disability, improving functioning, and relieving pain and the distress caused by physical and emotional symptoms.

2. *Eliminate health disparities.* This is a critical objective, as disparities are prominent between Whites and the emerging majority. During the 1997 *Healthy People* progress reviews for Hispanics and Asian Americans and Pacific Islanders, a consensus emerged to do away with differential targets for racial and ethnic minority groups in *Healthy People 2010.* Subsequently, this recommendation was extended to people with low income, people with disabilities, women, and people in different age groups. The elimination of disparities is a bold step forward from the goal of *Healthy People 2010,* which was to reduce disparities in health status, health risks, and use of preventive interventions among population groups. *Healthy People 2010* special population targets were established for racial and ethnic minority groups, women, people with low incomes, people with disabilities, and specific age groups (i.e., children, adolescents, and the elderly). Targets were set, calling for greater improvements for each of these groups than for the total population. However, with the exception of service interventions, these targets rarely aimed at achieving equity by 2000. *Healthy People 2010,* in contrast, has set the goal of eliminating these disparities by 2010.

　　The elimination of disparities by the year 2010 requires new knowledge about the determinants of disease and effective interventions for prevention and treatment. It also requires improved access for all to the resources that influence health. Research and a knowledge base dedicated to a better understanding of the relationships among health status and income, education, race and ethnicity, cultural influences, environment, and access to quality medical services is now imperative. It is well known that the improvement of access to quality health care and the delivery of preventive care and treatment requires that health care professionals work closely with communities, they must identify culturally sensitive implementation strategies.

CULTURALCOMPETENCE, which is defined as a set of knowledge, skills, and attitudes that allows individuals, organizations, and systems to work effectively with diverse racial, ethnic, religious, and social groups, is an inherent component of this mandate. It follows that CULTURALCARE is the mode of care that will develop within the scope of CULTURALCOMPETENCE.

maximizing both years and quality of healthy life. The progress toward meeting this goal is currently assessed by measuring life expectancy and healthy life expectancies. These assessments result in the following conclusions:

- Life expectancy continues to improve for the populations that could be assessed.
- Women continue to have a longer life expectancy than men.
- The White population has a longer life expectancy than the Black population.

There are three different measures of healthy life expectancy:

1. expected years in good or better health,
2. expected years free of activity limitations, and
3. expected years free of selected chronic diseases demonstrate gender and racial differences.

Goal 2 is to eliminate health disparities. The second goal of *Healthy People 2010* stems from the observation that there are substantial disparities among populations in specific measures of health, life expectancy, and quality of life. The second goal is to eliminate health disparities that occur by race and ethnicity, gender, education, income, geographic location, disability status, or sexual orientation. There has been widespread improvement in objectives for nearly all of the populations associated with these characteristics. However, progress toward the target for individual populations and progress toward the goal to eliminate disparities are independent of each other. Improvements for individual populations—even improvements for all of the populations for a characteristic—do not necessarily ensure the elimination of disparities. Disparities between populations and the persistence of disparities over time have been well documented.

For specific population characteristics, it has been reported that

- Among 195 objectives and subobjectives with trend data for racial and ethnic groups, disparities decreased for 24 and increased for 14.
- Among 238 objectives and subobjectives with trend data for males and females, disparities decreased for 25 and increased for 15. Females more

often had the best group rate, and reductions in disparity were more frequent among males.

■ Among education groups, disparities decreased for 3 objectives and subobjectives and increased for 14.

■ Among income groups, between geographic groups, and between persons with disabilities and persons without disabilities, there were few changes in disparities.

The ambitious goals and objectives formulated in *Healthy People 2010* have a long way to go. Indeed, there has been some progress made in improvement in the overall health of our nation. Further information regarding *Healthy People 2010* can be found at http://www.healthypeople.gov/data/midcourse/pdf/ExecutiveSummary.pdf and http://www.healthypeople.gov/Implementation. Box 3–1 presents further information about *Healthy People 2010*.

Health, United States, 2007, is the 31st report on the health status of the nation submitted by the secretary of health and human services to the president and Congress of the United States. It presents national trends in public health statistics. The following examples are relevant to this overall text:

1. Infant mortality rates were higher in 2004 for infants of non-Hispanic Black mothers (13.6 deaths per 1,000 live births), American Indian mothers (8.4 per 1,000), and Puerto Rican mothers (7.8 per 1,000) than for infants of other groups.

2. In 2004 life expectancy at birth for the total population was 77.8 years.

3. In 2004 age-adjusted death rates were one-third higher for Black Americans than for White Americans—46% higher for stroke, 32% higher for heart disease, 23% higher for cancer, and more than 787% higher for HIV.

4. In 2005 almost one third of adults 18 years and older engaged in regular physical activity.

5. Between 1976 and 1980 and 2003 and 2004, the prevalence of overweight among children 6–11 years of age increased from 11% to 19% and the prevalence of overweight among adolescents 12–19 years of age increased from 11% to 17%.

The Health Belief Model

The Health Belief Model (Figures 3–1A and 3–1B) is useful for transitioning from a discussion of health to that of illness. It illustrates the patient's perceptions of health and illness and can be modified to reflect the viewpoint of health care providers. When implemented from the provider's viewpoint, the material provides a means of reinspecting the differences between professional and lay beliefs and expectations. Forging a link between the two helps one better understand how people perceive themselves in relation to illness and what motivates them seek medical help and then follow that advice.

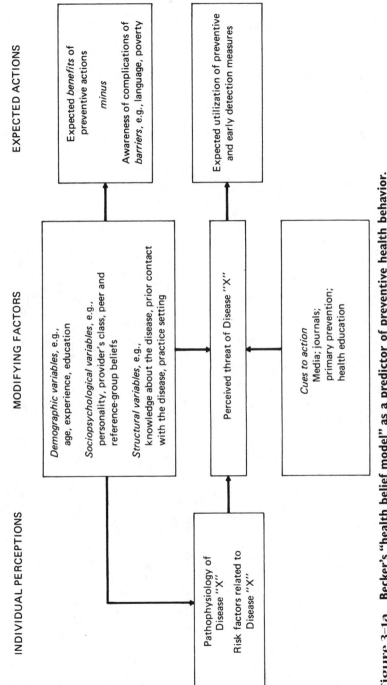

INDIVIDUAL PERCEPTIONS   MODIFYING FACTORS   EXPECTED ACTIONS

Demographic variables, e.g., age, experience, education

Sociopsychological variables, e.g., personality, provider's class, peer and reference-group beliefs

Structural variables, e.g., knowledge about the disease, prior contact with the disease, practice setting

Expected *benefits* of preventive actions

minus

Awareness of complications of *barriers*, e.g., language, poverty

Expected utilization of preventive and early detection measures

Perceived threat of Disease "X"

Cues to action
Media; journals; primary prevention; health education

Pathophysiology of Disease "X"
Risk factors related to Disease "X"

Figure 3–1a   Becker's "health belief model" as a predictor of preventive health behavior.

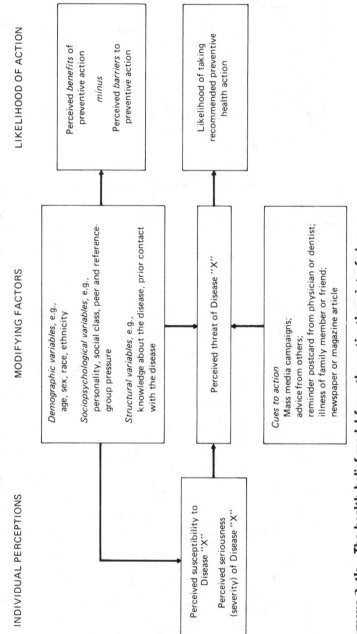

INDIVIDUAL PERCEPTIONS   MODIFYING FACTORS   LIKELIHOOD OF ACTION

Demographic variables, e.g.,
age, sex, race, ethnicity

Sociopsychological variables, e.g.,
personality, social class, peer and reference-
group pressure

Structural variables, e.g.,
knowledge about the disease, prior contact
with the disease

Perceived susceptibility to
Disease "X"

Perceived seriousness
(severity) of Disease "X"

Perceived threat of Disease "X"

Cues to action
Mass media campaigns;
advice from others;
reminder postcard from physician or dentist;
illness of family member or friend;
newspaper or magazine article

Perceived *benefits* of
preventive action

minus

Perceived *barriers* to
preventive action

Likelihood of taking
recommended preventive
health action

Figure 3–1b   The health belief model from the patient's point of view.

Perceived Susceptibility

How susceptible to a certain condition do people consider themselves to be? For example, a woman whose family does not have a history of breast cancer is unlikely to consider herself susceptible to that disease. A woman whose mother and maternal aunt both died of breast cancer may well consider herself highly susceptible, however. In this case, the provider may concur with this perception of susceptibility on the basis of known risk factors.

Perceived Seriousness. The perception of the degree of a problem's seriousness varies from one person to another. It is in some measure related to the amount of difficulty the patient believes the condition will cause. From a background in pathophysiology, the provider knows—within a certain range—how serious a problem is and may withhold information from the patient. The provider may resort to euphemisms in explaining a problem. The patient may experience fear and dread by just hearing the name of a problem, such as cancer.

Perceived Benefits: Taking Action. What kinds of actions do people take when they feel susceptible, and what are the barriers that prevent them from taking action? If the condition is seen as serious, they may seek help from a doctor or some other significant person, or they may vacillate and delay seeking and using help. Many factors enter into the decision-making process. Several factors that may act as barriers to care are cost, availability, and the time that will be missed from work.

From the provider's viewpoint, there is a protocol governing who should be consulted when a problem occurs, when during that problem's course help should be sought, and what therapy should be prescribed.

Modifying Factors. The modifying factors shown in Figures 3–1A and 3–1B indicate the areas of conflict between patient and provider.

The variables of race and ethnicity are cited most often as complex problem areas when the provider is White and middle-class (or from one sociocultural economic class and the patient is from another) and the patient is a member of the emerging majority. The issues are complex and include overtones of personal and institutional racism. Such perceptions vary not only among groups but also among individuals.

Social class, peer group, and reference group pressures also vary between the provider and patient and among different ethnic groups. For example, if the patient's belief about the causes of illness is "traditional" and the provider's is "modern," an inevitable conflict arises between the two viewpoints. This conflict is even more evident when the provider either is unaware of the patient's traditional beliefs or is aware of the manifestation of traditional beliefs and practices and devalues them. Quite often, class differences exist between the patient and provider. The reference group of the provider may well be that of the "technological health system," whereas the reference group of the patient may well be that of the "traditional system" of health care and health care deliverers.

Structural variables also differ when the provider and the patient see the problem from different angles. Often, each is seeing the same thing but is using different terms (or jargon) to explain it. Consequently, neither understands the other. Reference group problems also are manifested in this area, and the news and broadcast media are an important structural variable.

In summary, this section has attempted to deal solely with the concept of health. The multiple denotations and connotations of the word have been explored. A method for helping you tune in to your health has been presented, a transitional discussion illustrating the plethora of issues to be raised later in the text has been included, and an overview of *Healthy People 2010* has set the tone for the remainder of the text.

■ Illness

It is a paradox that the world of illness is the one that is most familiar to the providers of health care. It is in this world that the provider feels most comfortable and useful. Many questions about illness need to be answered:

- What determines illness?
- How do you know when you are ill?
- What provokes you to seek help from the health care system?
- At what point does self-treatment seem no longer possible?
- Where do you go for help? And to whom?

We tend to regard illness as the absence of health, yet we demonstrated in the preceding discussion that *health* is at best an elusive term that defies a specific definition. Let us look at the present issue more closely. Is illness the opposite of health? Is it a permanent condition or a transient condition? How do you know if you are ill?

When you "Google" *illness,* the response on the World Wide Web is well over 95.7 million hits. One basic dictionary definition for this term is an unhealthy condition of body or mind: SICKNESS (© 2005 by Merriam-Webster Incorporated). Another definition is found in the *American Heritage Dictionary* defines *illness* as "Sickness of body or mind. b. sickness. 2. obsolete. Evil; wickedness" (Davies, 1976, p. 351). A more contemporary definition of *illness* is "a highly personal state in which the person feels unhealthy or ill, may or may not be related to disease" (Kozier, Erb, Berman, & Burke 2000, p. 176). As with the word *health,* the word *illness* can be subjected to extensive analysis. What is illness? A generalized response, such as "abnormal functioning of a body's system or systems," evolves into more specific assessments of what we observe and believe to be wrong. Illness is a "sore throat," a "headache," or a "fever"—the last one determined not necessarily by the measurement on a thermometer but by a flushed face; a warm-to-hot feeling of the forehead, back, and abdomen; and overall malaise. The diagnosis of "intestinal obstruction" is described as pain in the stomach (abdomen), a greater pain than that caused by "gas," accompanied by severely upset stomach, nausea, vomiting, and marked constipation.

Essentially, we are being pulled back in the popular direction and encouraged to use lay terms. We initially resist this because we want to employ professional jargon. (Why use lay terms when our knowledge is so much greater?) It is crucial that we be called to task for using jargon. We must learn to be constantly conscious of the way in which the laity perceive illness and health care.

Another factor emerges as the word *illness* is stripped down to its barest essentials. Many of the characteristics attributed to health occur in illness, too. You may receive a rude awakening when you realize that a person perceived as healthy by clinical assessment may then—by a given set of symptoms—define him- or herself as ill (or vice versa). For example, in summertime, one may see a person with a red face and assume that she has a sunburn. The person may, in fact, have a fever. A person recently discharged from the hospital, pale and barely able to walk, may be judged ill. That individual may consider himself well, however, because he is much better than when he entered the hospital—now he is able to walk! Thus, perceptions are relative and, in this instance, the eyes of the beholder have been clouded by inadequate information. Unfortunately, at the provider's level of practice, we do not always ask the patient, "How do you view your state of health?" Rather, we determine the patient's state of health by objective and observational data.

As is the case with the concept of health, we learn in nursing or medical school how to determine what illness is and how people are expected to behave when they are ill. Once these terms are separated and examined, the models that health care providers have created tend to carry little weight. There is little agreement as to what, specifically, illness is, but we nonetheless have a high level of expectation as to what behavior should be demonstrated by both the patient and the provider when illness occurs. We discover that we have a vast amount of knowledge with respect to the acute illnesses and the services that ideally must be provided for the acutely ill person. When contradictions surface, however, it becomes apparent that our knowledge of the vast gray area is minimal—for example, whether someone is ill or becoming ill with what may later be an acute episode. Because of the ease with which we often identify cardinal symptoms, we find we are able to react to acute illness and may have negative attitudes toward those who do not seek help when the first symptom of an acute illness appears. The questions that then arise are "What is an acute illness, and how do we differentiate between it and some everyday indisposition that most people treat by themselves?" and "When do we draw the line and admit that the disorder is out of the realm of adequate self-treatment?"

These are certainly difficult questions to answer, especially when careful analysis shows that even the symptoms of an acute illness tend to vary from one person to another. In many acute illnesses, the symptoms are so severe that the person experiencing them has little choice but to seek immediate medical care. Such is the case with a severe myocardial infarction, but what about the person who experiences mild discomfort in the epigastric region? Such a symptom could lead the person to conclude he or she has "indigestion" and to self-medicate with baking soda, an antacid, milk, or Alka-Seltzer. A person who experiences mild pain in the left arm may delay seeking care, believing the pain will disappear. Obviously, this person may be as ill as the person who seeks help during the onset of symptoms but will, like most people, minimize these small aches because of not wanting to assume the sick role.

The Sick Role

The seminal work of Talcott Parsons (1966) helps explain the phenomenon of "the sick role." In our society, a person is expected to have the symptoms viewed as illness confirmed by a member of the health care profession. In other words, the sick role must first be legitimately conferred on this person by the keepers of this privilege. You cannot legitimize your own illness and have your own diagnosis accepted by society at large. There is a legitimate procedure for the definition and sanctioning of the adoption of the sick role and it is fundamental for both the social system and the sick individual. Thus, illness is not only a "condition" but also a social role. Parsons describes four main components of the sick role:

1. "The sick person is exempted from the performance of certain of his/her normal social obligations." An example is a student or worker who has a severe sore throat and decides that he or she does not want to go to classes or work. For this person to be exempted from the day's activities, he or she must have this symptom validated by someone in the health care system, a provider who is either a physician or a nurse practitioner. The claim of illness must be legitimized or socially defined and validated by a sanctioned provider of health care services.

2. "The sick person is also exempted from a certain type of responsibility for his/her own state." For example, an ill person cannot be expected to control the situation or be spontaneously cured. The student or worker with the sore throat is expected to seek help and then to follow the advice of the attending physician or nurse in promoting recovery. The student or worker is not responsible for recovery except in a peripheral sense.

3. "The legitimization of the sick role is, however, only partial." When you are sick, you are in an undesirable state and should recover and leave this state as rapidly as possible. The student's or worker's sore throat is acceptable only for a while. Beyond a reasonable amount of time—as determined by the physician or nurse, peers, and the faculty or supervisors—legitimate absence from the classroom or work setting can no longer be claimed.

4. "Being sick, except in the mildest of cases, is being in need of help." Bona fide help, as defined by the majority of American society and other Western countries, is the exclusive realm of the physician or nurse practitioner. A person seeking the help of the provider now not only bears the sick role but in addition takes on the role of patient. Pa-

tienthood carries with it a certain, prescribed set of responsibilities, some of which include compliance with a medical regimen, cooperation with the health care provider, and the following of orders without asking too many questions, all of which leads to the illness experience.

The Illness Experience

The experience of an illness is determined by what illness means to the sick person. Furthermore, *illness* refers to a specific status and role within a given society. Not only must illness be sanctioned by a physician for the sick person to assume the sick role, but it also must be sanctioned by the community or society structure of which the person is a member. Alksen and colleagues (n.d.) divide this experience into four stages, which are sufficiently general to apply to any society or culture.

The first stage, onset, is the time when the person experiences the first symptoms of a problem. This event can be slow and insidious or rapid and acute. When the onset is insidious, the patient may not be conscious of symptoms or may think that the discomfort will eventually go away. If, however, the onset is acute, the person is positive that illness has occurred and that immediate help must be sought. This stage is seen as the prelude to legitimization of illness. It is the time when the person with a sore throat in the preceding discussion may have experienced some fatigue, a raspy voice, or other vague symptoms.

In the second stage of the illness experience, diagnosis, the disease is identified or an effort is made to identify it. The person's role is now sanctioned, and the illness is socially recognized and identified. At this point, the health care providers make decisions pertaining to appropriate therapy. During the period of diagnosis, the person experiences another phenomenon: dealing with the unknown, which includes fearing what the diagnosis will be.

For many people, going through a medical workup is an unfamiliar experience. It is made doubly difficult because they are asked and expected to relate to strange people who are doing unfamiliar and often painful things to their bodies and minds. To the layperson, the environment of the hospital or the provider's office is both strange and unfamiliar, and it is natural to fear these qualities. Quite often, the ailing individual is faced with an unfamiliar diagnosis. Nonetheless, the person is expected to follow closely a prescribed treatment plan that usually is detailed by the health care providers but that, in all likelihood, may not accommodate a particular lifestyle. The situation is that of a horizontal-vertical relationship, the patient being figuratively and literally in the former position, the professional in the latter.

During the third stage, patient status, the person adjusts to the social aspects of being ill and gives in to the demands of his or her physical condition. The sick role becomes that of patienthood, and the person is expected to shift into this role as society determines it should be enacted. The person must make any necessary lifestyle alterations, become dependent on others in some circumstances for the basic needs of daily life, and adapt to the demands of the physical condition as well as to treatment limitations and expectations. The environment of the patient is highly structured. The boundaries of the patient's world are determined by the providers of the health care services, not by the patient. Herein lies the conflict.

Much has been written describing the environment of the hospital and the roles that people in such an institution play. As previously stated, the hospital is typically unfamiliar to the patient, who, nevertheless, is expected to conform to a predetermined set of rules and behaviors, many of which are unwritten and undefined for the patient—let alone by the patient.

The fourth stage—recovery—is generally characterized by the relinquishing of patient status and the assumption of prepatient roles and activities. There is often a change in the roles a person is able to play and the activities able to be performed once recovery takes place. Often, recovery is not complete. The person may be left with an undesirable or unexpected change in body image or in the ability to perform expected or routine activities. One example is a woman who enters the hospital with a small lump in her breast and who, after a surgery, returns home with only one breast. Another example is that of a man who is a laborer and enters the hospital with a backache and returns home after a laminectomy. When he returns to work, he cannot resume his job as a loader. Obviously, an entire lifestyle must be altered to accommodate such newly imposed changes.

From the viewpoint of the provider, this person has recovered. His or her body no longer has the symptoms of the acute illness that made surgical treatment necessary. In the eyes of the former patient, illness persists because of the inability to perform as in the past. So many changes have been wrought that it should come as no surprise if the person seems perplexed and uncooperative. Here, too, there is certainly conflict between society's expectations and the person's expectation. Society releases the person from the sick role at a time when, subjectively, the person may not be ready to relinquish it.

Table 3–1 is a tool designed for the assessment of the patient during the four stages of illness. Originally designed as a sociological measuring tool, the material has been altered here to meet the needs of the health care provider in achieving a better understanding of patient behavior and expectations. If the provider is able to obtain answers from the patient to all the questions raised in Table 3–1, understanding the patient's behavior and perspective and subsequent attempts to provide safe, effective care become easier.

Another method of dividing the illness experience into stages was developed by Edward A. Suchman (1965). He described the following five components:

1. **The symptom experience stage.** The person is physically and cognitively aware that something is wrong and responds emotionally.
2. **The assumption of the sick role stage.** The person seeks help and shares the problem with family and friends. After moving through the lay referral system, seeking advice, reassurance, and validation, the person is temporarily excused from such responsibilities as work, school, and other activities of daily living as the condition dictates.

Table 3-1 A Tool for the Assessment of the Patient during the Four Stages of Illness

Onset	Diagnosis	Patient Status	Recovery
A. The Meaning of the Illness			
1. What symptoms does this patient complain of?	1. Does he or she understand the diagnosis?	1. Has his or her perception of the illness changed?	1. What are signs of recovery?
2. How does he or she judge the extent and kind of disease?	2. How does he or she interpret the illness?	2. What are the changes in his or her life as a consequence of it?	2. Can he or she resume prepatient role and functions?
3. How does this illness fit with his or her image of health? Him- or herself?	3. How can he or she adapt to the illness?	3. What is his or her goal in recovery—the same level of health as before the illness, attainment of a maximal level of wellness, or perfect health?	3. Has his or her self-image been changed?
4. How does the disease threaten him or her?	4. How does he or she think others feel about it?	4. How does he or she relate to medical professionals?	4. How does he or she see present state of health—as more vulnerable or resistant?
5. Why does he or she seek medical help?		5. What are his or her social pressures leading to recovery?	
		6. What is motivating him or her to recover?	
B. Behavior in Response to Illness			
1. How does he or she control anxiety?	1. What treatment agents were used?	1. How does he or she handle the patient role?	1. Are there any permanent aftereffects from this illness?
2. How are affective responses to concerns expressed?		2. How does he or she relate to the medical personnel?	2. How does he or she resume old roles?
3. Did he or she seek some form of health care before seeking medical care?			

Source: Alksen, L., Wellin, E., Suchman, E., et al. (n.d.). *A conceptual framework for the analysis of cultural variations in the behavior of the ill.* Unpublished report. New York City Department of Health. Reprinted with permission.

3. **The medical care contact stage.** The person then seeks out the "scientific" rather than the "lay" diagnosis, wanting to know the following: Am I really sick? What is wrong with me? What does it mean? At this point, the sick person needs some knowledge of the health care system, what the system offers, and how it functions. This knowledge helps the person select resources and interpret the information received.

4. **The dependent-patient role stage.** The patient is now under the control of the physician and is expected to accept and comply with the prescribed treatments. The person may be quite ambivalent about this role, and certain factors (physical, administrative, social, or psychological) may create barriers that eventually will interfere with treatment and the willingness to comply.

5. **The recovery or rehabilitation stage.** The role of the patient is given up at the recovery stage, and the person resumes—as much as possible—his or her former roles.

The Illness Trajectory

Yet another way of explaining illness is to follow the trajectory of a given illness that a given person may experience. The term *trajectory* is applied to the following phases as they summarize the social science approaches that have been discussed to answer our second fundamental question—"What is illness?"—and begin to shift our focus to the responses and experiences people have to and with illness. The focus now begins to move to the active role the patient plays in shaping and experiencing the course of a given illness. For example, the person with an illness may experience the following trajectory: acute illness; comeback, or recovery; stable status; unstable or chronic status; deterioration; and death. The acute phase most often is treated in the acute care hospital, and the early phases of comeback and rehabilitation occur in this setting. The management of the chronic phase, except for acute episodes, is performed at home or in an institution that is either a rehabilitation facility or a long-term care institution (Figure 3–2). The illness profoundly affects the lives of the ill and their families in the scope of day-to-day living and hopes for the future. Further consideration of this phenomenon is found in later chapters.

As you can see, there have been countless explanatory words and models developed over time to define *health* and *illness*. Each of these is valid; each of these is time-tested; each of these is relevant as we go forward into the new century and into the millennium.

In summary, this chapter has introduced the dominant culture's perception of health and illness through countless lenses. The writings of a number of theorists and sociologists have been examined in terms of applicability to health care delivery.

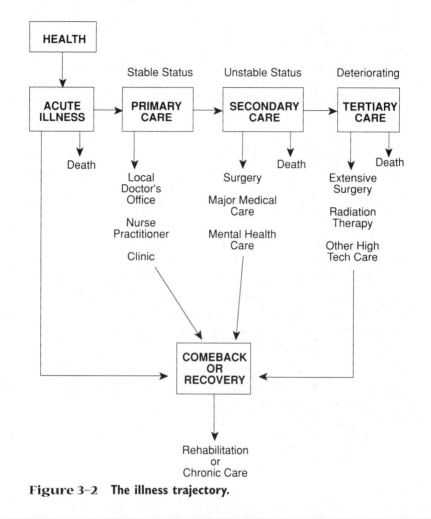

Figure 3-2 The illness trajectory.

Explore MediaLink

Go to the Companion Website at www.prenhall.com/spector for chapter-related review questions, case studies, and activities. Contents of the CulturalCare Guide and CulturalCare Museum can also be found on the Companion Website. Click on Chapter 3 to select the activities for this chapter.

■ Internet Sources

Office of Disease Prevention and Health Promotion. (2005). Healthy People 2010 Rockville, MD: U.S. Department of Health and Human Service. Retrieved from http://www.healthypeople.gov/, June 22, 2007.

■ References

Alksen, L., Wellin, E., Suchman, E., et al. (n.d.). *A conceptual framework for the analysis of cultural variations in the behavior of the ill.* Unpublished report (p. 2). New York: New York City Department of Health.

Davies, P. (Ed.). (1976). *The American heritage dictionary of the English language.* New York: Dell.

Kozier, B., Erb, G., Berman, A. J., & Burke, K. (2000). *Fundamentals of nursing concepts, process, and practice.* Upper Saddle River, NJ: Prentice Hall Health.

Mechanic, D. (1968). *Medical sociology* (p. 80). New York: Free Press of Glencoe.

Murray, R., & Zentner, J. (1975). *Nursing concepts for health promotion.* Englewood Cliffs, NJ: Prentice Hall.

National Center for Health Statistics [NCHS]. (2007). *Health United States 2007.* Hyattsville, MD: Author.

Nightingale, F. (1860, 1946). (A fascimile of the first edition published by D. Appleton and Co.). *Notes on nursing—What it is, what it is not.* New York: Appleton-Century.

Parsons, T. (1966). Illness and the role of the physician: A sociological perspective. In W. R. Scott & E. H. Volkart (Eds.), *Medical care: Readings in the sociology of medical institutions* (p. 275). New York: John Wiley & Sons.

Rogers, M. (1989). Nursing: A science of unitary human beings. In Riehl-Sisca, J. (Ed.), *Conceptual models for nursing practice* (3rd ed., pp. 181–188). Norwalk, CT: Appleton & Lange.

Rosenstock, I. M. (1966, July). Why people use health services. *Millbank Memorial Fund Quarterly, 44*(3), 94–127.

Suchman, E. A. (1965, fall). Stages of illness and medical care. *Journal of Health and Human Behavior, 6*(3), 114.

Unit

II

HEALTH
Domains

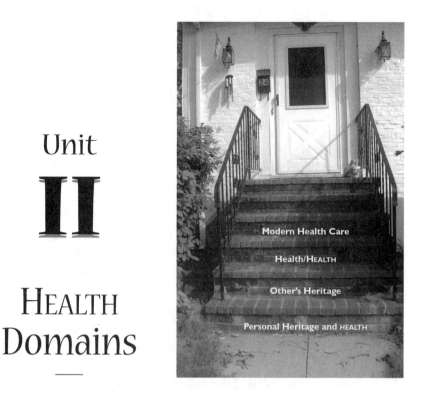

Modern Health Care

Health/HEALTH

Other's Heritage

Personal Heritage and HEALTH

Unit II develops the "plot" of this book by providing background material for the central themes discussed in this text. Imagine climbing the stairs in the opening figure and this unit will bring you to the fifth step. Chapters 4 and 5 will explore the concepts of HEALTH and will describe **traditional** ways of maintaining, protecting, and restoring HEALTH and magico-religious traditions related to HEALING and HEALING practices. Chapter 6 will explore your heritage and historical health/HEALTH and curing/HEALING beliefs and practices in particular.

Chapter 7 will present an overview of the issues related to the modern, scientific, high-technological health care delivery system in general and will discuss why an analytical understanding of the modern allopathic philosophy relevant in this arena is so vital in regard to the development of a holistic philosophy of HEALING and CULTURALCARE.

The chapters in Unit II will present an overview of relevant historical and contemporary theoretical content that will help you to

1. Describe traditional aspects of HEALTH care.[1]

2. Describe traditional HEALTH care philosophies and systems.

3. Discuss various forms of HEALING practices.

[1]Small capital letters are used to differentiate traditional definitions of HEALTH, ILLNESS, and HEALING from contemporary definitions.

4. Trace your family's beliefs and practices in
   a. Health/HEALTH maintenance
   b. Health/HEALTH protection
   c. Health/HEALTH restoration
   d. Curing/HEALING

5. Discuss the interrelationships of sociocultural, public health, and medical events that have produced the crises in today's modern health care system.

6. Trace the complex web of factors that
   a. Contribute to the high cost of health care
   b. Discuss ways of paying for health care services
   c. Impede a person's passage through the health care system
   d. Describe common barriers to utilization of the health care system

7. Compare and contrast the modern and traditional systems of health/ HEALTH care.

As you proceed through this unit, you will encounter several activities that link Unit I to Unit II and will help the content resonate and come alive. These are activities in which several people may participate and share their experiences.

1. Re-answer questions 5–12 from Unit I, thinking of HEALTH rather than health. (Remember, when HEALTH is in small capital letters, it is to designate it as a holistic phenomenon, rather than dualistic, as is the common way it is defined.) They are the following questions:
   How do you define *HEALTH*?
   How do you define *ILLNESS*?
   What do you do to maintain your HEALTH?
   What do you do to protect your HEALTH?
   What do you do when you experience a noticeable change in your HEALTH?
   Do you diagnose your own HEALTH problems? If yes, how do you do so? If no, why not?
   From whom do you seek HEALTH care?
   What do you do to restore your HEALTH? Give examples.

2. To whom do you turn first when you are ILL? Where do you go next?

3. You have just moved to a new location. You do not know a single person in this community. How do you find health/HEALTH care resources?

4. Visit an emergency room in a large city hospital. Visit an emergency room in a small community hospital. Spend some time quietly observing what occurs in each setting.
   a. How long do patients wait to be seen?
   b. Are patients called by name—first name, surname—or number?
   c. Are relatives or friends allowed into the treatment room with the patient?

5. Determine the cost of a day of hospitalization in an acute care hospital in your community.
   a. How much does a room cost? How much is a day in the intensive care unit or coronary care unit? How much is time in the emergency room? How is a surgical procedure charged?
   b. How much is charged for diagnostic procedures, such as a computed tomography (CT) scan or an ultrasound? How much is charged for such equipment as a simple intravenous (IV) setup?
   c. What are the pharmacy charges?
   d. How many days, or hours, are women kept in the hospital after delivery of a child? Is the newborn baby sent home at the same time? If not, why not? What is the cost of a normal vaginal delivery or cesarean section and normal newborn care?

6. Visit a homeopathic pharmacy or a natural food store and examine the shelves that contain herbal remedies and information about alternative or complementary HEALTH care.
   a. What is the cost of a variety of herbal remedies used to maintain HEALTH or to prevent common ailments?
   b. What is the cost of a variety of herbal remedies used to treat common ailments?
   c. What is the range of costs for the books and other reading and instructional materials sold in the store?

7. Attend a service in a house of worship with which you are not familiar. Inquire of the clergyperson what is taught or done within the faith tradition to maintain, protect, and restore HEALTH.

8. Visit a community HEALER other than a physician.

9. Attend a HEALING service.

10. Explore other methods of HEALING, such as massage, herbal therapy, or prayer.

11. Explore birth and birthing practices in traditions other than those derived from your own sociocultural heritage.

12. Explore end-of-life beliefs and practices and mourning in traditions other than those derived from your own sociocultural heritage.

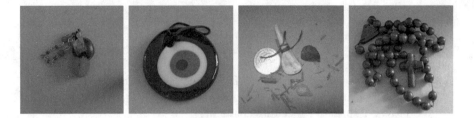

Chapter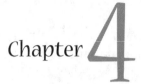

HEALTH Traditions

You can do nothing to bring the dead to life; but you can do much to save the living from death.

—B. Frank School (1924)

■ Objectives

1. Describe traditional aspects of HEALTH care.
2. Describe the interrelated components of the HEALTH Traditions Model.
   a. Give examples of the traditional ways people maintain their physical, mental, and spiritual HEALTH.
   b. Give examples of the traditional ways people protect their physical, mental, and spiritual HEALTH.
   c. Give examples of the traditional ways people restore their physical, mental, and spiritual HEALTH.
3. Describe the factors that constitute traditional epidemiology.
4. Give examples of the choices that people have in health care.
5. Give examples of the traditional HEALTH care philosophies and systems.
6. Discover information available from the National Center for Complementary and Alternative Medicine.

The images in the chapter opener reflect HEALTH-related objects that may be used to protect, maintain, and/or restore physical, mental, or spiritual HEALTH by people of many different heritages. These images contain items that are symbolic of the HEALTH traditions model and its themes, which will be discussed later in the chapter. The small beaded bracelet from Mexico, with a deer's eye with an image of the Virgin of Guadalupe and a red pom-pom, is placed on an infant to protect his or her HEALTH. The second image, a glass eye from Turkey, may be pinned on clothing, pinned on a crib or bed, or hung in the home to protect the HEALTH of the person or family. The third image represents items that may be carried in a person's pocket. These items are contained in a small pouch that could be carried by a *coyote,* a person who leads people across the United States/Mexico border. It contains a coyote tooth, a chachayotel (large seed), red string, and a crystal—all items believed to protect the person and bring good luck. The fourth image, rosary beads from Italy, symbolizes prayer and meditation methods used in both the spiritual maintenance and the restoration of HEALTH.

What are the sacred objects that you and your family may have hung in your home, placed on your bed, or worn? If you could pick four images from your heritage that are used to protect your HEALTH, what would they be? Do you know where the objects can be purchased? Do you continue to use sacred objects to protect your HEALTH?

Health care providers have the opportunity to observe the most incredible phenomenon of life: health/HEALTH and the recovery, in most cases, from illness/ILLNESS. In today's society, the healer is primarily thought by many to be the physician, and the other members of the health team all play a significant role in the maintenance and protection of HEALTH and the detection, and treatment of ILLNESS. However, human beings have existed, some sources suggest, for 2 million years. How, then, did the species *Homo sapiens* survive before the advent of the scientific methods and modern technology? What did the people of other times do to maintain, protect, and restore their health/HEALTH? It is quite evident that numerous forms of health/HEALTH care and healing/HEALING existed long before the technological methodologies that we apply today.

In the natural course of any life, a person can expect to experience the following set of events: He or she becomes ill/ILL; the illness/ILLNESS may be acute, with concomitant symptoms or signs, such as pain, fever, nausea, bleeding, depression, anxiety, or despair. On the other hand, the illness/ILLNESS may be insidious, with a gradual progression and worsening of symptoms, which might encompass slow deterioration of movement or a profound intensification of pain or desperation. Or the person may not experience symptoms, seek care for a routine ailment, and discover he or she has a near-fatal illness/ILLNESS.

If the illness/ILLNESS is mild, the person relies on self-treatment or, as is often the case, does nothing and gradually the symptoms disappear. If the illness/ILLNESS is more severe or is of longer duration, the person may consult expert help from a healer—usually, in contemporary times a physician or nurse practitioner.

The person recovers or expects to recover. As far back as historians and interested social scientists can trace in the history of humankind, this phenomenon of recovery has occurred. In fact, it made very little difference what mode of treatment was used; recovery was expected and usual. It is this occurrence of natural recovery that has given rise to all forms of therapies and healing/HEALING beliefs and practices that attempt to explain a phenomenon that is natural. That is, one may choose to rationalize the success of a healing/HEALING method by pointing to the patient's recovery. Over the generations, natural healing/HEALING has been attributed to all sorts of rituals, including trephining (puncturing the skull), cupping, magic, leeching, and bleeding. From medicine man to sorcerer, the arts of maintaining, protecting, restoring health/HEALTH, and healing/HEALING have passed through succeeding generations. People knew the ailments of their time and devised treatments for them. In spite of ravaging plagues, disasters (both natural and those caused by humans), and pandemic and epidemic diseases, human beings as a species have survived!

This chapter explores the concepts of HEALTH and ILLNESS and the HEALTH Traditions Model; the choices people have in terms of folk medicine, natural or magico-religious medicine; complementary and alternative methods of health/HEALTH maintenance, protection, and/or restoration; and other schools of health/HEALTH care in contemporary American society. Just as the understanding of health and illness are fundamental in the socialization process into the health care professions, the understanding of HEALTH and ILLNESS within the traditional context is fundamental to the development of CULTURAL COMPETENCY and the skills necessary to deliver CULTURALCARE.

■ HEALTH and ILLNESS

In this section, the "steps and bricks" of HEALTH and ILLNESS are going to be explored in greater depth. Once again, HEALTH is defined as "the balance of the person, both within one's beings—physical, mental, and spiritual—and in the outside world—natural, communal, and metaphysical, is a complex, interrelated phenomenon." On the other hand, ILLNESS is "the imbalance of one's being—physical, mental, and spiritual—and in the outside world—natural, communal, and meta-physical." When the terms *HEALTH* and *ILLNESS* are used in the remainder of this text, they denote the preceding definitions; small capitals are used to differentiate them from the terms *health* and *illness*, as defined in Chapter 3. *Health/HEALTH* and *illness/ILLNESS* are used in the text when there is an overlap between the terms.

The physical aspect of the person includes: anatomical organs, such as the skin, skeleton, and muscles. It is our genetic inheritance, body chemistry, gender, age, and nutrition. The mind, mental, includes cognitive process, such as thoughts, memories, and knowledge. This includes emotional processes as feelings, defenses, and self-esteem. The spiritual facet includes both positive and negative learned spiritual practices and teachings, dreams, symbols, and stories;

gifts and intuition; grace and protecting forces; and positive and negative metaphysical or innate forces. These facets are in constant flux and change over time, yet each is completely related to the others and related to the context of the person. The context includes the person's family, culture, work, community, history, and environment. There is also an overlap of the mental and spiritual facets of the person.

The person must be in a state of balance with the family, community, and the forces of the natural world around him or her. This *balance* is what is perceived as HEALTH in a traditional sense and the way in which it is determined within most traditional cultures, as you will note in Chapters 8 through 12. ILLNESS, as stated, is the *imbalance* of one or all parts of the person (body, mind, and spirit); this person may be in a state of *imbalance* with the family, the community, or the forces of the natural world. The ways in which this *balance*, or harmony, is achieved, maintained, protected, or restored often differ from the prevailing scientific health philosophy of our modern societies. However, many of the traditional HEALTH- ILLNESS- and HEALING-related beliefs and practices exist today among people who know and live by the traditions of their own ethnocultural and/or religious heritage.

■ HEALTH Traditions Model

The HEALTH Traditions Model uses the concept of holistic HEALTH and explores what people do from a traditional perspective to maintain HEALTH, protect HEALTH or prevent ILLNESS, and restore HEALTH. HEALTH, in this traditional context, has nine interrelated facets, represented by

1. Traditional methods of maintaining HEALTH—physical, mental, and spiritual
2. Traditional methods of protecting HEALTH—physical, mental, and spiritual
3. Traditional methods of restoring HEALTH—physical, mental, and spiritual

The traditional methods of HEALTH maintenance, protection, and restoration require the knowledge and understanding of HEALTH-related resources from within a person's ethnoreligious cultural heritage. These methods may be used instead of or along with modern methods of health care. They are not alternative methods of health care because they are methods that are an integral part of a person's ethnocultural and religious heritage. Alternative, or complementary, medicine is a system of health care that persons may elect to use that is generic and not a part of their personal heritage. The burgeoning system of alternative medicine must not be confused with traditional HEALTH and ILLNESS beliefs and practices. In subsequent chapters of this book, traditional HEALTH and ILLNESS beliefs and practices are discussed, following (in part) the models

	PHYSICAL	MENTAL	SPIRITUAL
MAINTAIN HEALTH	Proper clothing Proper diet Exercise/Rest	Concentration Social and Family support systems Hobbies	Religious worship Prayer Meditation
PROTECT HEALTH	Special foods and food combination Symbolic clothing	Avoid certain people who can cause illness Family activities	Religious customs Superstitions Wearing amulets and other symbolic objects to prevent the "Evil Eye" or defray other sources of harm
RESTORE HEALTH	Homeopathic remedies liniments Herbal teas Special foods Massage Acupuncture/ moxibustion	Relaxation Exorcism Curanderos and other traditional healers Nerve teas	Religious Rituals—special prayers Meditation Traditional healings Exorcism

Figure 4-1 The nine interrelated facets of HEALTH (physical, mental, and spiritual) and personal methods of maintaining HEALTH, protecting HEALTH, and restoring HEALTH.

(Figures 4–1 and 4–2). This model is two-dimensional in that it examines HEALTH as the internal perceptions of a person and addresses the ways by which a person can externally obtain the objects and/or substances necessary for his or her HEALTH. Tradition is the essential element in this model, and the model recognizes the fact that the role of tradition is fundamental. "When tradition is no longer adequate, human life faces the gravest crises" (Smith, 1991, p. 163). Given that the United States has been a melting pot, it has frequently weakened the traditions of immigrants during the processes of acculturation, especially where HEALTH beliefs and practices are concerned. For many people, modern medicine has not provided a compelling replacement. Examples of the barriers to modern health care are further explored in Chapter 7.

Traditional HEALTH Maintenance

The traditional ways of maintaining HEALTH are the active, everyday ways people go about living and attempting to stay well or HEALTHY—that is, ordinary

	PHYSICAL	MENTAL	SPIRITUAL
MAINTAIN HEALTH	Availability of Proper shelter, clothing, and food Safe air, water, soil	Availability of traditional sources of entertainment, concentration, and "rules" of the culture	Availability and promulgation of rules of ritual and religious worship Meditation
PROTECT HEALTH	Provision of the knowledge of necessary special foods and food combinations, the wearing of symbolic clothing, and avoidance of excessive heat or cold	Provision of the knowledge of what people and situations to avoid, family activities; Family activities	The teaching of: Religious customs Superstitions Wearing amulets and other symbolic objects to prevent the "Evil Eye" or how to defray other sources of harm
RESTORE HEALTH	Resources that provide Homeopathic remedies, liniments, Herbal teas, Special foods, Massage, and other ways to restore the body's balance of hot and cold	Traditional healers with the knowledge to use such modalities as: relaxation exorcism, storytelling, and/or Nerve teas	The availability of healers who use magical and supernatural ways to restore health: including religious rituals, special prayers, meditation, traditional healings, and/or Exorcism

Figure 4-2 **The nine interrelated facets of HEALTH (physical, mental, and spiritual) and personal methods of maintaining HEALTH, protecting HEALTH, and restoring HEALTH.**

functioning within their family, community, and society. These include such actions as wearing proper clothing—boots when it snows and sweaters when it is cold, long sleeves in the sun, and scarves to protect from drafts and dust. Many traditional ethnic or religious groups may also prescribe garments, such as special clothing or head coverings. Many "special objects," such as hats to protect the eyes and face, long skirts to keep the body clean, down comforters to keep warm, special shoes for work and comfort, glasses to improve vision, and canes to facilitate walking, are used to maintain HEALTH, and they can be found in many traditional homes.

The food that is eaten and the methods for preparing it contribute to people's HEALTH. Here, too, one's ethnoreligious heritage plays a strong role in the determination of how foods are cooked, what combinations they may be eaten in, and what foods may be eaten. Foods are prepared in the home and follow the recipes from the family's tradition. Traditional cooking methods do not use preservatives. Most foods are fresh and well prepared. Traditional diets are followed, and food taboos and restrictions are obeyed. Cleanliness of the self and the environment is vital. Hand washing and praying before and after meals are examples of necessary rituals.

Mental HEALTH in the traditional sense is maintained by concentrating and using the mind—reading and crafts are examples. There are countless games, books, music, art, and other expressions of identity that help in the maintenance of mental well-being. Hobbies also contribute to mental well-being.

The keys to maintaining HEALTH are, however, the family and social support systems. Spiritual HEALTH is maintained in the home with family closeness—prayer and celebrations. Rights of passage and kindred occasions are also family and community events. The strong identity with and connections to the "home" community are a great part of traditional life and the life cycle, as well as factors that contribute to HEALTH and well-being.

■ HEALTH Protection

The protection of HEALTH rests in the ability to understand the cause of a given ILLNESS or set of symptoms. Most of the traditional HEALTH and ILLNESS beliefs regarding the causation of ILLNESS differ from those of the modern epidemiological model. In modern epidemiology, we speak of viruses, germs, and other pathogens as the causative agents. In "traditional" epidemiology, factors such as the "evil eye," envy, hate, and jealousy may be the agents of ILLNESS.

Traditional Epidemiology

ILLNESS is most often attributed to the "evil eye." The evil eye is primarily a belief that someone can project harm by gazing or staring at another's property or person (Maloney, 1976, p. 14). The belief in the evil eye is probably the oldest and most widespread of all superstitions, and it is found to exist in many parts of the world, such as southern Europe, the Middle East, and North Africa (Maloney, 1976, p. vi).

The evil eye is thought by some to be merely a superstition, but what is seen by one person as superstition may well be seen by another as religion. Various evil-eye beliefs were carried to this country by immigrant populations. These beliefs have persisted and may be quite strong among newer immigrants and heritage-consistent peoples (Maloney, 1976, p. vii).

The common beliefs in the evil eye assert that

1. The power emanates from the eye (or mouth) and strikes the victim.
2. The injury, be it illness or other misfortune, is sudden.

3. The person who casts the evil eye may not be aware of having this power.
4. The afflicted person may or may not know the source of the evil eye.
5. The injury caused by the evil eye may be prevented or cured with rituals or symbols.
6. This belief helps explain sickness and misfortune. (Maloney, 1976, p. vii)

The nature of the evil eye is defined differently by different populations. The variables include how it is cast, who can cast it, who receives it, and the degree of power it has. In the Philippines, the evil is cast through the eye or mouth; in the Mediterranean, it is the avenging power of God; in Italy, it is a malevolent force, like a plague, and is warded off by wearing amulets.

In different parts of the world, various people cast it: in Mexico—strangers; in Iran—kinfolk; and in Greece—witches. Its power varies, and in some places, such as the Mediterranean, it is seen as the "devil." In the Near East, it is seen as a deity and, among Slovak Americans, as a chronic but low-grade phenomenon (Maloney, 1976, p. xv).

Among Germans, the evil eye is known as *aberglobin* or *aberglaubisch* and it causes preventable problems, such as evil, harm, and illness/ILLNESS. Among the Polish, the evil eye is known as *szatan*, literally, "Satan." Some "evil spirits" are equated with the devil and can be warded off by praying to a patron saint or guardian angel. *Szatan* also is averted by prayer and repentance and the wearing of medals and scapulars. These serve as reminders of the "Blessed Mother and the Patrons in Heaven" and protect the wearer from harm. The evil eye is known in Yiddish as *kayn aynhoreh*. The expression *kineahora* is recited by Jews after a compliment or when a statement of luck is made to prevent the casting of an evil spell on another's health/HEALTH. Often, the speaker spits three times after uttering the word (Spector, 1983, pp. 126–127).

Agents of disease may also be "soul loss," "spirit possession," "spells," and "hexes." Here, prevention becomes a ritual of protecting oneself and one's children from these agents. Treatment requires the removal of these agents from the afflicted person (Zola, 1972, pp. 673–679).

ILLNESS also can be attributed to people who have the ability to make others ILL—for example, witches and practitioners of voodoo. The ailing person attempts to avoid these people to prevent ILLNESS and to identify them as part of the treatment. Other "agents" to be avoided are "envy," "hate," and "jealousy." A person may practice prevention by avoiding situations that could provoke the envy, hate, or jealousy of a friend, an acquaintance, or a neighbor. The evil-eye belief contributes to this avoidance.

Another source of evil can be of human origin and occurs when a person is temporarily controlled by a soul not his or her own. In the Jewish culture, this controlling spirit is known as *dybbuk*. The word comes from the Hebrew word meaning "cleaving" or "holding fast." A *dybbuk* is portrayed as a "wandering, disembodied soul which enters another person's body and holds fast" (Winkler, 1981, pp. 8–9).

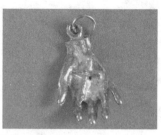

Figure 4–3 Mano milagroso.

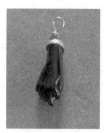

Figure 4–4 Mano negro.

Traditional practices used in the protection of HEALTH include, but are not limited to,

1. The use of protective objects—worn, carried, or hung in the home
2. The use of substances that are ingested in certain ways and amounts or eliminated from the diet, and substances worn or hung in the home
3. The practices of religion, such as the burning of candles, the rituals of redemption, and prayer

Objects That Protect HEALTH

Amulets are sacred objects, such as charms, worn on a string or chain around the neck, wrist, or waist to protect the wearer from the evil eye or the evil spir-

Figure 4–5 The Jerusalem amulet. This amulet serves as protection from pestilence, fire, bad wounds and infection, the evil eye, bad decrees and decisions, curses, witchcraft, and from everything bad; to heal nervous illness, weakness of body organs, children's diseases, and all kinds of suffering from pain; as a talisman for livelihood for success, fertility, honesty, and honor; and for charity, love, mercy, goodness, and grace. It also has the following admonition: "Know before whom you stand—the King of Kings, The Holy One, Blessed be He."
(Translated by B. Koff, Jerusalem, Israel, 26 December, 1988. From the author's personal collection. Photographed by Stephen Vedder.)

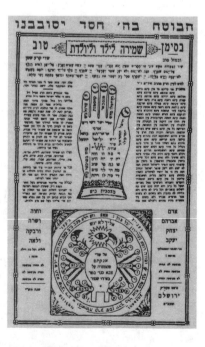

its that could be transmitted from one person to another or have supernatural origins. For example, the *mano milagroso* (miraculous hand) (Figure 4–3) is worn by many people of Mexican origin for luck and the prevention of evil. A *mano negro* (black hand) (Figure 4–4) is placed on babies of Puerto Rican descent to ward off the evil eye. The *mano negro* is placed on the baby's wrist on a chain or pinned to the diaper or shirt and is worn throughout the early years of life.

Amulets may also be written documents on parchment scrolls, and these are hung in the home. Figure 4–5 is an example of a written amulet acquired in Jerusalem. It is hung in the home or workplace to protect the person or family from the evil eye, famine, storms, diseases, and countless other dangers. Table 4–1 describes several practices found among selected ethnic groups to protect themselves from or to ward off the evil eye.

Table 4–1 Practices to Ward Off the Evil Eye

Origin	Practices
Eastern European Jews	Red ribbon woven into clothes or attached to crib
Greece	Blue "eye" bead, crucifix, charms Phylact—a baptismal charm placed on a baby Cloves of garlic pinned to shirt
Guatemala	Small red bag containing herbs placed on baby or crib
India	Wearing a red string on the wrist
India/Pakistan Hindus or Muslims	Copper plates with magic drawings rolled in them Slips of paper with verses from the Koran Black or red string around a baby's wrist
Iran	Child covered with amulets—agate, blue beads Children left filthy and never washed to protect them from the evil eye
Italians	Wearing a red ribbon or the corno (horn)
Mexico	Amulet or seed wrapped with red yarn
Philippines	Charms, amulets, medals
Puerto Rico	*Mano negro*
Scotland	Red thread knotted into clothing Fragment of Bible worn on body
Sephardic Jews	Blue ribbon or blue bead worn
South Asia	Knotted hair or fragment of Koran worn on body
Tunisia	Amulets pinned on clothing consisting of tiny figures or writings from the Koran Charms of the fish symbol—widely used to ward off evil

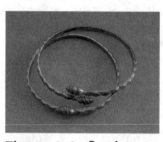

Figure 4-6 Bangles.

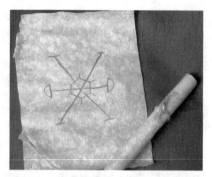

Figure 4-7 Talisman.
(From the author's personal collection.
Photographed by R. Schadt)

Bangles (Figure 4–6) are worn by people originating from the West Indies. The silver bracelets are open to "let out evil" yet closed to prevent evil from entering the body. They are worn from infancy, and as the person grows they are replaced with larger bracelets. The bracelets tend to tarnish and leave a black ring on the skin when a person is becoming ILL. When this occurs, the person knows it is important to rest, to improve the diet, and to take other needed precautions. Many people believe they are extremely vulnerable to evil, even to death, when the bracelets are removed. Some people wear numerous bangles. When they move an arm, the bracelets tinkle. It is believed that this sound frightens away the evil spirit. Health care providers should realize that, when the bracelets are removed, the person experiences a great deal of anxiety.

In addition to amulets, there are talismans (Figure 4–7). A talisman is believed to possess extraordinary powers and may be worn on a rope around the waist or carried in a pocket or purse. The talisman illustrated in Figure 4–7 is a marionette, and it protects the wearer from evil. It is recommended that people who wear amulets or carry a talisman be allowed to do so in health care institutions. The person who uses an amulet determines and interprets the meaning of the object.

Substances That Protect HEALTH

The second practice uses diet to protect HEALTH and consists of many different observances. People from many ethnic backgrounds eat raw garlic or onions (Figure 4–8) in an effort to prevent ILLNESS. Garlic or onions also may be worn on the body or hung in the Italian, Greek, or Native American home. Chachayotel (Figure 4–9), a seed, may be tied around the waist by a Mexican person to prevent arthritic pain. Among traditional Chinese people, thousand-year-old eggs are eaten with rice to keep the body HEALTHY and to prevent ILLNESS. The ginseng root is the most famous of Chinese medicines. It has universal medicinal applications and is used preventively to "build the blood," especially after childbirth. Tradition states that, the more the root looks like a man, the more

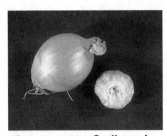

Figure 4–8 Garlic and onion.
(From the author's personal collection. Photographed by Stephen Nedder)

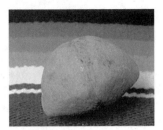

Figure 4–9 Chachayotel.
(From the author's personal collection. Photographed by Stephen Nedder)

effective it is. Ginseng is also native to the United States and is used in this country as a restorative tonic (Figure 4–10).

Diet regimens also are used to protect HEALTH. It is believed that the body is kept in balance, or harmony, by the type of food one eats.

Traditionalists have strong beliefs about diet and foods and their relationship to the protection of HEALTH. The rules of the kosher diet practiced among Jewish people mandate the elimination of pig products and shellfish. Only fish with scales and fins are allowed, and only certain cuts of meat from animals with a cleft hoof and that chew cud can be consumed. Examples of this kind of animal are cattle and sheep. Many of the dietary practices, such as the avoidance of pig products, are also adhered to by Muslims and the meats are "Halal." Jews also believe that milk and meat must never be mixed and eaten at the same meal.

In traditional Chinese homes, a balance must be maintained between foods that are *yin* or *yang*. These are eaten in specified proportions. In Hispanic homes, foods must be balanced as to "hot" and "cold." These foods, too, must be eaten in the proper amounts, at certain times, and in certain combinations. There are also foods that are consumed at certain times of the week or year and not during other times.

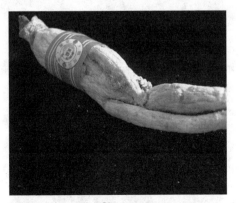

Figure 4–10   Ginseng root.
(From the author's personal collection. Photographed by Stephen Nedder)

Spiritual Practices That Protect HEALTH

A third traditional approach toward HEALTH protection centers in part on religion. The words *spirituality* and *religion* are frequently used synonymously, but they are not the same. *Spirituality* connotes the way we orient ourselves toward the Divine, the way we make meaning out of our lives, the recognition of the presence of Spirit (breath) within us, a cultivation of a lifestyle consistent with this presence, and a perspective to foster purpose, meaning, and direction to life. It may find expression through religion, or religion may be a tool for finding one's spirit (Hopkins et al., 1995, p. 11).

Religion strongly affects the way people choose to protect HEALTH, and it plays a strong role in the rituals associated with HEALTH protection. It dictates social, moral, and dietary practices that are designed to keep a person in balance. Many people believe that ILLNESS and evil are prevented by strict adherence to religious codes, morals, and practices. They view ILLNESS as a punishment for breaking a religious code. For example, I once interviewed a woman who believed she had cancer because God was punishing her for stealing money when she was a child. An example of a protective religious figure is the Virgin of Guadalupe (Figure 4–11), the patron saint of Mexico, who is pictured on medals that people wear or in pictures or icons hung in the home. She is believed to protect the person and home from evil and harm, and she serves as a figure of hope.

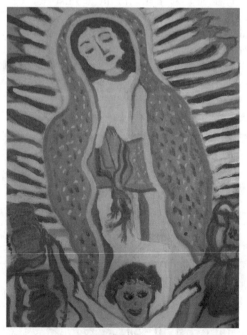

Figure 4–11   The Virgin of Guadalupe.

Religion can, therefore, help provide the believer with an ability to understand and interpret the events of the environment and life. This discussion continues in Chapter 5.

HEALTH Restoration

HEALTH restoration in the physical sense can be accomplished by the use of countless traditional remedies, such as herbal teas, liniments, special foods and food combinations, massage, and other activities.

The restoration of HEALTH in the mental domain may be accomplished by the use of various techniques, such as performing exorcism, calling on traditional healers, using teas or massage, and seeking family and community support.

The restoration of HEALTH in the spiritual sense can be accomplished by healing rituals; religious healing rituals; or the use of symbols and prayer, meditation, special prayers, and exorcism. This will be further discussed in Chapter 5.

■ Health/HEALTH Care Choices

There are countless ways to describe and label health/HEALTH care beliefs, practices, and systems. "Health care" may be labeled as "modern," "conventional," "traditional," "alternative," "complementary," "allopathic," "homeopathic," "folk," and so forth. The use of the word *traditional* to describe "modern health care" is, by definition, a misnomer. *Traditional* connotes a tradition—"the delivery of opinions, doctrines, practices, rites, and customs from generation to generation by oral communication" or "a long-established custom or practice that has the effect of an unwritten law handed down through the generations and generally observed that is old and has been passed down for generations" (*American Heritage Dictionary*, 1976, p. 732). The use of *traditional* to connote modern health care is a misnomer, as modern, allopathic, health care is a new science and has been passed down in writing for a relatively short amount of time, rather than orally over many generations.

There are also many reasons people may choose to use HEALTH care systems other than modern medical care. These include, but are not limited to, access issues, such as poverty, language, availability, and lack of insurance, and preference for familiar and personal care. *Traditional* here connotes HEALTH care beliefs and practices observed among peoples who have steadfastly maintained their heritage and observe HEALTH care practices derived from their ethnocultural or religious heritage.

As stated earlier, in nearly every situation when a person becomes ill there is an expectation for the restoration of health/HEALTH, and the person usually recovers. As far back as historians and interested social scientists can trace in the extended history of humankind, the phenomenon of recovery has occurred. It made little difference what mode of treatment was used; health/HEALTH restoration was usual and expected. Established cultural norms have been attributed to the recovery from illness, and over time the successful methods for treating various maladies were preserved and passed down to each new generation within a traditional ethnocultural community. It is the occurrence of natural recovery that has given rise to all forms of therapeutic treatments and the attempts to explain a phenomenon that is natural. Over the generations, natural recovery has been attributed to all sorts of rituals, including cupping, magic, leeching, and bleeding. Today, the people who are members of many different native, immigrant, and traditional cultural communities in the United States—American Indian, Black, Asian, European, and Hispanic—may continue to utilize the practices found within their tradition.

■ Folk Medicine

Folk medicine today is related to other types of medicine that are practiced in our society. It has coexisted, with increasing tensions, alongside modern medicine and was derived from academic medicine of earlier generations. There is ample evidence that the folk practices of ancient times have been abandoned only in part by modern health care belief systems, for many of these beliefs and practices continue to be observed today. Many may be practiced in secret, under ground. Today's popular medicine is, in a sense, commercial folk medicine. Yoder (1972) describes two varieties of folk medicine:

1. Natural folk medicine—or rational folk medicine—is one of humans' earliest uses of the natural environment and utilizes herbs, plants, minerals, and animal substances to prevent and treat illnesses.
2. Magico-religious folk medicine—or occult folk medicine—is the use of charms, holy words, and holy actions to prevent and cure illnesses/ ILLNESSES.

Natural Folk Medicine

Natural folk medicine has been widely practiced in the United States and throughout the world. In general, this form of prevention and treatment is found in old-fashioned remedies and household medicines. These remedies have been passed down for generations, and many are in common use today. Much folk medicine is herbal, and the customs and rituals related to the use of the herbs vary among ethnic groups. Specific knowledge and usages are addressed throughout this text. Commonly, across cultures, the herbs are found in nature and are used by humans as a source of therapy, although how these medicines are gathered and specific modes of use vary from group to group and place to place. In general, folk medical traditions prescribed the time of year in which the herb was to be picked; how it was to be dried; how it was to be prepared; the method, amount, and frequency of taking; and so forth.

In addition, an infinite number of maladies have, over the generations, cultivated an assortment of folk methods for thwarting or curing them. Boxes 4–1 and 4–2 describe these phenomena as related to cholera and choking. All too frequently, the practices consist of both natural and magico-religious forms.

Box 4–1

Choking

Choking, an often fatal mishap, occurs when air is prevented access to the lungs by compression or obstruction of the windpipe.

Folk Beliefs
It is widely believed that, throughout life, a person is at risk of all sorts of encounters with spirits and witches that may cause choking. The alp (incubus, nightmare) strangles people to death; the glacial demon springs on a boy's shoulders and strangles him to death; the poltergeist strangles a victim until it is half dead; witches pinch and attempt to strangle a person in bed; and Naamah, who is described in the Kabbala as a semi-human, deathless being, seduces men and strangles children in their sleep. If children are left outside on purpose, fairies strangle them, and mothers are warned to beware of the striglas, a wild and bad woman, that can catch hold of a baby and strangle it. It is widely believed that many activities, when undertaken by pregnant women, can cause the umbilical cord to be twisted around the unborn baby's neck, choking and strangling it to death.

Prevention
An expectant mother must avoid cords, such as by not wearing necklaces, or "wind string, yarn, or other material"; for that matter, she should "avoid seeing other women who do this" or stretching, and she is instructed never to "raise her hands above her head," "hang up curtains," "sit with crossed legs," "scrub floors," or "walk through a hole in a fence."

    The Catholic ritual of The Blessing of the Throats on Saint Blaise (third century) Day (February 3) is related to the prevention of choking. Two burning candles are crossed over the throat and the following prayer is recited: "May the Lord deliver you from the evils of the throat, and from every other evil." Other methods of prevention include the belief that

1. It is wise never to drink milk after eating choke-cherries.
2. One should not be eating while going over the threshold of a door.
3. If a person chokes without eating, it means that he or she told a lie, someone has told lies about the person, he or she is begrudging someone food, or the person's demise might entail choking on the gallows.

Treatment
Examples of advice regarding the treatment of choking include

1. If you swallow a fish bone, drink lemon juice or eat a biscuit; if you had choked in the early 1900s, you would have probably had to swallow a string with cotton on the end, which was pulled back up.

2. Swallow rice water or a raw egg.

(continued)

3. Have someone pat or slap you hard between the shoulders.

4. Rub your nose.

5. Go on all fours and cough.

Choking is often a sign that foreshadows death, since it interrupts breathing and breath is the sign of life.

Sources: Thurston, H. (1955). Ghosts & poltergeists. *Journal of American Folklore Society, 68,* 97; Thompson, K. (1964). Body, boots, britches. *Journal of American Folklore Society, 77,* 305; Lee, K. (1951). Greek supernatural. *Journal of American Folklore Society, 64,* 309; Rivas, A. (1990). *Devotions to the saints* (p. 22). Los Angeles: International Imports; and UCLA Department of Folklore Archives.

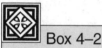

Box 4–2

Cholera

Cholera is an acute diarrheal, infectious disease, caused by a bacterium. It is fatal 10 to 50% of the time.

Folk Beliefs
Cholera generates senses of mystery, fear, and dread; around the world, it was imagined in the form of a personified spirit and attributed to spiritual or human causes. The Eastern Europeans believed that a cat bringing home a baby stork after it fell out of the nest signaled the arrival of cholera, and Slavs saw cholera as a small woman with only one eye, one ear, and two long teeth.

In India, cholera had many identities: the red flower mother and Marhai Devi, the goddess of cholera and the sister of the goddess Devi. In Italy it was caused by the evil eye and/or an evil spirit, and in Sicily it was spread by rulers to get rid of people. In the American folk tradition, a change of the moon or a rainbow appearing in the west in the sign of the Twins signaled the arrival of cholera, and it was said that someone staring at a baby caused it. Others rationalized cholera outbreaks by regarding dead oak trees in the yard or foods—such as dried beans, green apples, green fruit, and food combinations such as cucumbers and ice cream—as the probable cause.

Prevention
Cholera was thought to be prevented by wearing wooden shoes to stop the seeping through of telluric poisons. A minister actually requested President Jackson to declare a day of fasting and prayer to halt a cholera epidemic. Fire and heat were popular methods, and when an epidemic hit Fort Riley, Kansas, in 1855 a physician burned barrels of pure tar beneath open hospital windows. Onions were a charm against cholera, and a bunch of onions could be hung in front of the threshold of the house. Tobacco smoke was found to slow the growth of many kinds of microbes, particularly those of Asiatic cholera.

Treatment

The range of homemade therapeutic remedies consisted of the use of a single agent, simple combinations, and some rather complex concoctions.

1. Simple substances—such as castor oil; nutmeg; camedative balsam, a patent medicine; wormwood tea; muskrat root; lettuce milk; dewberry or low blackberry—were praised by a 19th-century physician. Pyroligneous acid, used to cure hams, was also thought to cure cholera.

2. When the simple substances failed to halt the excessive diarrhea, herbal remedies were combined and/or used with popular patent medicines, such as calomel followed by castor oil; a teaspoon of wood ash was added to a cup of warm water; and nutmeg was added to milk. Powerful pills were rolled with red pepper and asafetida, or a large spoonful of pepper was added to a cup of boiled milk.

3. More elaborate concoctions contained such ingredients as turpentine, camphor, capsicum, cajeput, and tincture of flies or a combination of opium, charcoal, quinine, tobacco juice, and burning moxa.

4. A very exotic ritual consisted of chopping off the head of a black hen, ripping the gizzard from its body, and putting it into boiling water for a few minutes. The gizzard was discarded and the patient had to drink the boiling liquid.

Sources: Gifford, E. S. (1957, August). Evil eye in medicine. *Amer. J. Opth.,* 44(2), 238; Lorenz, A. J. (1957). Scurvy in the gold rush. *Journal History of Medicine, 12,* p. 503; Koschi, B. *UCLA archive of California and western folklore,* unpublished, Cannon, UT, no. 3173; Erickson (1941). Tarboro Free Press, *SFQ, 5,* 123; Karolevitz, R. F. (1967). *Doctors of the Old West* (p. 71). Seattle: Superior; Van-Ravenswaay (1955) Pioneer medicine. In Missouri, *South Medical Journal, 48,* 36; Kell (1965). Tobacco cures. *Journal of American Folklore Society, 78,* 106; VanWart (1948). Native cures. *Canadian Medical Association Journal, 59*(342), 575; N.N., Collection, Hyatt, H. M. (1935). *Folk-lore from Adams County Illinois* (p. 433). New York, other materials in the archives of UCLA Folklore Department; (2002).

Natural Remedies

The use of natural products, such as wild herbs and berries, accessible to healers developed into today's science of pharmacology. Early humankind had a wealth of knowledge about the medicinal properties of the plants, trees, and fungi in their environment. They knew how to prepare concoctions from the bark and roots of trees and from berries and wildflowers. As an example, purple foxglove, which contains the cardiotonic digitalis, was used for centuries to slow the heart rate. There are a number of medicinal teas and herbs. A listing of commonly used herbs is presented in Table 4–2. Almost 100 herbal teas are listed in a small paperback entitled *Herbal Tea Book* (Adrian & Dennis, 1976). The herbs are listed alphabetically, and the source and use of each are given.

Table 4-2 Commonly Used Herbal Remedies

Herb	Action	Use	Administration
Alfalfa (or lucerne)	Stimulant; nutritive	Arthritis; weight gain; strength-giving	1 oz herb to 1 pint water; drink one cupful as tea
Anise (seed used)	Stimulant; aromatic; relaxant	Flatulence; dry coughs	2 tsp seed to 1/2 pint water; dose: 1–3 tsp often
Bayberry (bark used)	Astringent; stimulant; emetic	Sore-throat gargle; cleanses stomach; douche; rinse for bleeding gums	1 oz powdered bark to 1 pint water; drink as tea
Blessed thistle	Diaphoretic; stimulant; emetic	Reduces fevers; breaks up colds; alleviates digestive problems	1 oz herb to 1 pint water; small doses as desired
Bugleweed	Romatic; sedative; tranquilizer; astringent	Suppresses coughs; relieves pulmonary bleeding; increases appetite	1 oz herb to 1 pint water; drink by glassful often
Catnip (leaves)	Diaphoretic; tonic; antispasmodic	Helpful in convulsions; produces perspiration	1 oz leaves to 1 pint water (measured by teaspoonful)
Cayenne pepper (fruit and seed)	Stimulant	Purest and most positive stimulant in herbal medicine; heals burns and other wounds; relieves toothaches	Powder in small doses; by mouth or topical
Chestnut, horse (bark and fruit)	Astringent; narcotic; tonic	Bark used for fevers; fruit used to treat rheumatism	Bark: 1 oz to 1 pint water, tsp 4 times per day; fruit: tincture 10 drops twice per day
Chicory (root)	Diuretic; laxative	Liver enlargement; gout; rheumatic complaints	1 oz root to 1 pint water; take freely
Corn silk	Diuretic; mild stimulant	Irritated bladder; urinary stones; trouble with prostate gland	2 oz in 1 pint water; take freely

Dandelion (root)	Diuretic; tonic	Used in many patent medicines; general body stimulant; used chiefly with kidney and liver disorders	Roasted roots are ground and used like coffee; small cup once or twice per day
Ergot (fungus)	Uterine stimulant; sedative hemostatic	Menstrual disorders; stops hemorrhage	Liquid extract 10–20 minims by mouth
Eucalyptus	Antiseptic; antispasmodic, stimulant	Inhale for sore throat; apply to ulcers and other wounds	Local application or fluid extract in small doses by mouth
Fennel (seeds)	Aromatic; carminative (expels air from bowels)	Gas; gout; colic in infants; increases milk in nursing mothers	Pour water (1/2 pint) or 1 tsp of seeds; take freely
Garlic (juice)	Diaphoretic; diuretic; stimulant; expectorant	Treats colds; diuretic; antiseptic	Juice, 10–30 drops
Goldenrod (leaves)	Aromatic; stimulant	Sore throat; general pain; colds; rheumatism	1 oz leaves to 1 pint water; small dose often
Hollyhock (flowers)	Diuretic	Chest complaints	1 oz flowers to 1 pint water; drink as much as needed
Ivy (leaves)	Cathartic; diaphoretic	Poultices on ulcers and abscesses	As a poultice
Ivy, poison (leaves)	Irritant; stimulant; narcotic	Rheumatism; sedative for the nervous system	Liquid extract 5–30 drops
Juniper berries	Diuretic; stimulant	Bladder and kidney problems; gargles; digestive aid	Oil of berries 1–5 drops
Licorice (root)	Demulcent	Coughs; prevents thirst	Powdered root
Lily of the valley (flower)	Cardiac stimulant; diuretic; stimulant	Headaches	1/2 oz flowers to 1 pint water; tablespoon doses

(continued)

Table 4-2 Commonly Used Herbal Remedies (continued)

Herb	Action	Use	Administration
Marigold (flowers and leaves)	Diaphoretic; stimulant	Flowers and leaves made into a salve for skin eruptions; relieves sore muscles, amenorrhea	1 oz herbs and petals to 1 pint water; 1 tbsp on mouth or topical application
Mistletoe (leaves)	Nervine; antispasmodic; tonic; narcotic	Epilepsy and hysteria; painful menstruation; induces sleep	2 oz to 1/2 pint water; tsp often
Mustard (leaves)	Cooling; sedative	Hoarseness (excellent aid in recovering the voice)	Liquid extract; small doses
Nightshade, deadly (poison) (leaves and root)	Narcotic; diuretic; sedative; antispasmodic	Eye diseases; increases urine; stimulates circulation	Powdered leaves and root; small amounts
Papaya leaves	Digestive	Digestive disorders; fresh leaves; dry wounds	Papain; small doses
Rosemary (leaves) (herb)	Astringent; diaphoretic; tonic; stimulant	Prevents baldness; cold; colic; nerves; strengthens eyes	1 oz herb to 1 pint water; small doses
Saffron (flower pistils)	Carminative; diaphoretic	Amenorrhea; dysmenorrhea; hysteria	1 dram flower pistils in 1 pint water; teacup doses
Thyme (dried herb)	Antiseptic; antispasmodic; tonic	Perspiration; colds; coughs; cramps	1 oz herb to 1 pint water; 1 tsp doses often

Source: Leek S. (1975). *Herbs and mysticism* (pp. 73–235). Chicago: Henry Regnery. Reprinted with permission.

Magico-religious Folk Medicine

The magico-religious form of folk medicine has existed for as long as humans have sought to maintain, protect, and/or restore their HEALTH. It has now, in this modern age of science and technology, come to be labeled by some as "superstition," "old-fashioned nonsense," or "foolishness," yet for believers it may go so far on the continuum as to take the form of religious practices related to HEALTH maintenance, protection, restoration, and healing. Chapter 5 addresses these belief systems in more detail.

■ Health/HEALTH Care Philosophies

Two distinctly different health/HEALTH care philosophies determine the scope of health/HEALTH beliefs and practices: dualistic and holistic. Each of these philosophies espouses effective methods of maintaining, protecting, and restoring health/HEALTH, and the "battles for dominance" between the allopathic and hemopathic philosophies have been hard fought in this country (Starr, 1982) over the past century. One manifestation of these struggles is an emerging preference for homeopathic or holistic, complementary or alternative medicine among people from all walks of life.

The Allopathic (Dualistic) Philosophy, the dominant health care system in the United States is predicated on the allopathic philosophy. The word *allopathy* has two roots. One comes from the Greek meaning "other than disease" because drugs are prescribed on a basis that has no consistent or logical relationship to the symptoms. The second root of *allopathy* is derived from the German meaning "all therapies." Allopathy is a "system of medicine that embraces all methods of **proven,** that is, empirical science and scientific methodology is used to prove the value in the treatment of diseases" (Weil, 1983, p. 17). After 1855, the American Medical Association (AMA) adopted the "all therapies" definition of *allopathy* and has exclusively determined who can practice medicine in the United States. For example, in the 1860s the AMA refused to admit women doctors to medical societies, practiced segregation, and demanded the purging of homeopaths. Today, allopaths may show little or limited tolerance or respect for other providers of health care, such as homeopaths, osteopaths, and chiropractors, and for such traditional healers as lay midwives, herbalists, and American Indian medicine men and women (Weil, pp. 22–25). The allopathic health care system is further discussed in Chapter 7.

The Homeopathic (Holistic) Philosophy is the other health care philosophy in the United States. Homeopathic medicine was developed between 1790 and 1810 by Samuel C. Hahnemann in Germany and is extremely popular in much of Europe and other parts of the world. It is becoming, once again, more popular in the United States.

Homeopathy, or homoeopathy, comes from the Greek words *homoios* ("similar") and *pathos* ("suffering"). In the practice of homeopathy, the person, not the disease, is treated (Starr, 1982). This system has not been "tolerated" by

Table 4–3 Selected Examples of Health/HEALTH Care Choices.

Health Care Allopathic Conventional	HEALTH Care Homeopathic Complementary	
	Alternative (Integrative)	Traditional (Ethnocultural)
	Aromatherapy	Ayurveda
Acute care	Biofeedback	Curanderismo
Chronic care	Hypnotherapy	Qi gong
Rehabilitation	Macrobiotics	Reiki
Psychiatric/mental health	Massage therapy	Santeria
Community/public health	Reflexology	Voodoo

the allopaths, yet it continues to thrive and is used by countless people. It espouses a holistic philosophy—that is, it sees health as a balance of the physical, mental, and spiritual whole. Homeopathic care encompasses a wide range of health care practices and is often referred to as "complementary medicine" or "alternative medicine." Complementary, alternative, unconventional, or unorthodox therapies are medical practices that do not conform to the scientific standards set by the allopathic medical community; they are not taught widely in the medical and nursing communities and are not generally available in the allopathic health care system, including the hospital settings. These include such therapies as acupuncture, massage therapy, and chiropractic medicine. Presently, this situation is changing, and the use of services such as acupuncture is more wide spread in modern health care settings.

Table 4–3 demonstrates the health/HEALTH care choices, or pathways a person may follow when an illness occurs. The allopathic system comprises the conventional or familiar services within the dominant health care culture—acute care, chronic care, rehabilitation, psychiatric/mental health, public/community health care, and so forth.

There are two types of care in the holistic system that are classified as complementary. These break down again into two categories, either alternative, or integrative, and traditional, or ethnocultural. Alternative therapies are those that are not a part of one's ethnocultural or religious heritage, interventions neither taught widely in medical schools nor generally available in U.S. hospitals and other health care settings; traditional therapies are those that are part of one's traditional ethnocultural or religious heritage. In other words, a European American electing to use acupuncture as a method of treatment is seeking alternative treatment; a Chinese American using this treatment modality is using traditional medicine.

Homeopathic Schools

The period 1870 through 1930 was when the allopathic health care model as we know it today was established. During the time that the roots of this system of health care were becoming firmly established, the ideas of the eclectic and other schools of medical thought were also prevalent.

Homeopathic Medicine. As stated earlier in this chapter, homeopathic medicine was developed between 1790 and 1810 by Samuel C. Hahnemann in Germany. In the practice of homeopathy, the person, not the disease, is treated. The practitioner treats a person by using minute doses of plant, mineral, or animal substances. The medicines are selected using the principle of the "law of similars." A substance that is used to treat a specific set of symptoms is the same substance that, if given to a healthy person, would cause the symptoms. The medicines are administered in extremely small doses. These medicines are said to provide a gentle but powerful stimulus to the person's own defense system, helping the person recover.

Homeopathy was popular in 19th-century America and Europe because it was successful in treating the raging epidemics of those times. In 1900, 20 to 25% of physicians were homeopaths. Due to allopathic efforts to wipe out the homeopaths beginning in 1906, the movement has dissipated. A small group of homeopaths still exists in the United States, however, and there are larger practices in India, Great Britain, France, Greece, Germany, Brazil, Argentina, and Mexico (Homeopathic Educational Services).

Osteopathic Medicine. Osteopathy, developed in 1874 by Dr. A. T. Still in Kirksville, Missouri, is the art of curing without the use of surgery or drugs. Osteopathy attempts to discover and correct all mechanical disorders in the human machine and to direct the recuperative power of nature that is within the body to cure the disease. It claims that, if there is an unobstructed blood and nerve supply to all parts of the body, the effects of a disease will disappear.

Doctors of osteopathy (D.O.s) are fully qualified physicians who can practice in all areas of medicine and surgery. They, like medical doctors, have completed 4 years of medical school, 1 year of internship, and generally a further residency in a specialty area. They take the same course work as do medical doctors, often use the same textbooks, and often take the same licensing examinations. There are 23 osteopathic medical schools in the United States. The lines of distinction between the medical doctor and the osteopath arise because the osteopath, in addition to using modern scientific forms of medical diagnosis and treatment, uses manipulation of the bones, muscles, and joints as therapy. Osteopaths also employ structural diagnosis and take into account the relationship between body structure and organic functioning when they determine a diagnosis. The osteopathic doctor has the same legal power to treat patients as a medical doctor (Dolgan, 2006).

Chiropractic. Chiropractic is a controversial form of healing that has been in existence for well over a century. It, too, adheres to a disease theory and a method of therapy that differ from allopathy. It was developed as a form of healing in 1895 in Davenport, Iowa, by a storekeeper named Daniel David Palmer, also known as a "magnetic healer." Palmer's theory underlying the practice of chiropractic was that an interference with the normal transmission of "mental impulses" between the brain and body organs produced diseases. The interference is caused by misalignment, or subluxation, of the vertebrae of the spine, which decreases the flow of "vital energy" from the brain through the nerves and spinal cord to all parts of the body. The treatment consists of manipulation to eradicate the subluxation.

Chiropractic is practiced in two ways. One form is that of the "mixers," who use heat therapy, enemas ("colonic irrigation"), exercise programs, and other therapeutic practices. The other group, the "straight" chiropractors, who use only manipulation, disapprove of the practices of the "mixers." They believe that the other techniques are a form of allopathic medicine (Cobb, 1977).

Eclectic Medicine. The word *eclectic* means "choosing," and it refers to choosing the means for treating disease. Methods and remedies are selected from all other systems. This school of medicine believes that nature has curative powers, and practitioners seek to remove the causes of disease through the natural outlets of the body. They treat the cause of disease, rather than the symptoms, and do not use bleeding, antimony, or poisons to treat diseases (School, 1924, pp. 1545–1546).

Hydrotherapy. The use of water for the maintenance of health or the treatment of disease is one of the oldest known therapies. It is an ancient method of treatment that has been used to treat disease and injury by many different peoples. A German farmer, Vincent Priessnitz, reintroduced hydrotherapy in 1840. It includes the application of water, internally and externally, in any form at any temperature, with the belief that the water can have a very profound effect on the body (School, 1924, p. 1527). A popular form of hydrotherapy can be found in today's popular SPAs—*SPA* is an acronym for the Latin *salus per aquam*—"health by water."

There were also many popular theories of healing during this era that focused only on the mind. Some examples follow.

Mesmerism. In the late 18th century, mesmerism was a popular form of healing by touch and was named for its founder, Friedrich Anton Mesmer. Mesmer believed that illness was a condition in which the body and mind of a person were influenced by a mysterious force emanating from another person. He further believed that the stars exerted an influence on people and that this force was the same as electricity and magnetism. Initially, he believed that stroking the body with magnets would bring about a cure for illness. He later modified this to the belief that touch alone could heal (School, 1924, p. 1592).

Hypnotism. Hypnotism artificially creates a condition in which the person appears to be asleep and acts in obedience to the will of the operator as regards both motion and sensation. It was developed in 1841 by James Braid, an English surgeon (School, 1924, p. 1595).

Mind Cure. Mind cure is the cure of disease by means of the mind alone, in which faith influences the cure of disease. Two prerequisites in faith healing are the desire to get well and faith in the treatment (School, 1924, p. 1598).

Christian Science. The religious philosophy of scientism lies outside allopathic and most homeopathic philosophies and delivery systems. Christian Science, as a system of spiritual healing, was first explained in 1875 in Mary Baker Eddy's book *Science and Health with Key to the Scriptures.* Eddy introduced the term *Christian Science* to designate the scientific system of divine healing. Eddy's revelation consists of two parts:

1. "The discovery of this divine Science of Mind-healing, through a spiritual sense of the Scriptures, and
2. The proof, by present demonstration, that the so-called miracles of Jesus did not specially belong to a dispensation now ended, but that they illustrated an ever-operative divine Principle (Eddy, 1875, p. 123:16–27).

Eddy's own early research and experiments in homeopathy, allopathy, and diet preceded her discoveries about spiritual healing. Ultimately, she found that "a mental method produces permanent health" (Eddy, 1875, p. 79:8–9).

Christian Scientists are free to choose the method of health care they feel is most effective. Their choice is not compelled by a church. Individuals and families make their own decisions. Christian Scientists, like others, grapple with the moral, social, and cultural implications of modern medical approaches and technological developments—including gene therapy, cloning, and artificial life support systems. They are free to make their own choices on important social health matters, such as abortion, birth control, blood transfusions and organ donations. Those who consider themselves Christian Scientists may have studied and practiced Christian Science for up to five generations. Or they may be reading *Science and Health* for the first time, for a better understanding of how spirituality is linked to health and well-being. Christian Scientists turn to the Bible and the pages of *Science and Health* for answers to humanity's deepest questions (Graunke, 2003).

National Center for Complementary and Alternative Medicine

The National Center for Complementary and Alternative Medicine (NCCAM) at the National Institutes of Health was founded in 1998 and is the federal government's lead agency for scientific research on complementary and alternative medicine, or CAM. The agency describes the different approaches to health care that are outside the realm of conventional medicine as either complementary or alternative. Conventional medicine is health care that is practiced by M.D.s or D.O.s and allied health professionals, such as registered nurses, physical therapists, and psychologists. The NCCAM differentiates between complementary and alternative medicine in that complementary medicine is used together with conventional medicine. An example of a complementary therapy is using aromatherapy to help lessen a patient's discomfort following surgery or while undergoing cancer therapies. Alternative medicine is used in place of conventional medicine. An example of an alternative therapy is using a special diet or medication to treat cancer instead of undergoing the surgery, radiation, or chemotherapy that has been recommended by a conventional doctor. The list of what is considered to be CAM changes continually, as the therapies that are proven to be safe and effective become adopted into conventional health care and as new approaches to health care emerge. The agency conducts ongoing research in many areas of complementary and alternative medicine.

Complementary and alternative medicines are classified into five categories. The following are the categories with an example of each intervention:

1. **Alternative medical systems**—homeopathic medicine
2. **Mind-Body interventions**—patient support groups
3. **Biologically based therapies**—herbal products
4. **Manipulative and body-based methods**—massage
5. **Energy therapies**—reiki (http://nccam.nih.gov)

The following are selected examples of alternative care:

1. **Aromatherapy**—an ancient science, presently popular, that uses essential plant oils to produce strong physical and emotional effects in the body
2. **Biofeedback**—the use of an electronic machine to measure skin temperatures; the patient controls bodily responses that are usually involuntary
3. **Hypnotherapy**—the use of hypnosis to stimulate emotions and involuntary responses, such as blood pressure
4. **Macrobiotics**—a diet and lifestyle from the Far East and adapted for the United States by Michio Kushi; the principles of this vegetarian diet consist of balancing the yin and yang energies of food
5. **Massage therapy**—the use of manipulative techniques to relieve pain and return energy to the body, now popular among many groups, both modern and traditional
6. **Reflexology**—the natural science dealing with the reflex points in the hands and feet that correspond to every organ in the body; the goal is to clear the energy pathways and the flow of energy through the body

The objectives of the NCCAM have been to

1. Explore complementary and alternative healing practices in the context of rigorous science
2. Train complementary and alternative medicine researchers
3. Disseminate authoritative information to the public and professionals

Tables 4–4 and 4–5 summarize selected findings of currently funded research projects.

Table 4-4   Selected Health Problems Studied by the National Center for Complementary and Alternative Medicine When CAM Is Utilized

Health Problem	Therapy
Arthritis, rheumatoid	Preparations made from botanicals (plants and their products, including herbs) • Vitamins and minerals in unconventional amounts • Other products taken by mouth, such as fish oil • Dietary approaches • Preparations applied to the skin, such as balms and liniments • Hydrotherapy • Items that are worn (for example, magnetic clothing or copper bracelets) • Mind-body therapies, such as relaxation techniques, meditation, prayer for health purposes, and tai chi • Whole medical systems, such as Ayurveda (a traditional medicine of India), traditional Chinese medicine, homeopathy, and chiropractic
Cancer	• Acupuncture to relieve neck and shoulder pain following surgery for head or neck cancer • Ginger as a treatment for nausea and vomiting caused by chemotherapy • Massage for the treatment of cancer pain • Mistletoe extract combined with chemotherapy for the treatment of solid tumors
Depression Menopausal symptoms	St. John's wort for treating mild to moderate depression • Six botanicals—black cohosh, red clover, dong quai root, ginseng, kava, and soy • Dehydroepiandrosterone (DHEA), a dietary supplement • Exercise • Paced respiration • Health education • Dietary Supplements

Sources: http://nccam.nih.gov/health/RA/; http://nccam.nih.gov/health/camcancer/;
http://nccam.nih.gov/health/stjohnswort/sjwataglance.htm; http://nccam.nih.gov/health/menopauseandcam/

Table 4-5 **Selected Remedies Studied by the National Center for Complementary and Alternative Medicine**

Remedy	Use
Black cohosh	• Rheumatism (arthritis and muscle pain) • Hot flashes • Night sweats • Vaginal dryness • Other symptoms that can occur during menopause • Menstrual irregularities and premenstrual syndrome
Echinacea	• Treat or prevent colds, flu, and other infections • Stimulate the immune system to help fight infections • Wounds and skin problems, such as acne or boils
Ginkgo	• Asthma • Bronchitis • Fatigue • Tinnitus • Improve memory • Prevent Alzheimer's disease and other types of dementia • Decrease intermittent claudication • Sexual dysfunction
St. John's wort	• Mental disorders and nerve pain • Balm for wounds, burns, and insect bites • Depression • Anxiety • Sleep disorders

Sources: http://nccam.nih.gov/health/blackcohosh/; http://nccam.nih.gov/health/echinacea/; http://nccam.nih.gov/health/ginkgo/; http://nccam.nih.gov/health/stjohnswort/

Traditional, or Ethnocultural, Care

The following list describes selected traditional HEALTH care systems:

1. **Ayurvedic.** This 4,000-year-old method of healing originated in India and is the most ancient existing medical system that uses diet, natural therapies, and herbs. Its chief aim is longevity and quality of life. It formed the foundation of Chinese medicine.

2. **Curanderismo.** This traditional Hispanic (Mexican) system of HEALTH care originated in Spain and is derived, in part, from traditional practices of indigenous Indian and Spanish HEALTH practices.

3. **Qi gong.** This form of Chinese traditional medicine combines movement, meditation, and regulation of breathing to enhance the flow of qi (the vital energy), improve circulation, and enhance the immune system.

4. **Reiki.** This Japanese form of therapy is based on the belief that, when spiritual energy is channeled through a practitioner, the patient's spirit is healed, in turn healing the physical body.

5. **Santeria.** This form of traditional HEALTH care is observed among the practitioners of a syncretic religion that comprises both African and Catholic beliefs, also called Santeria. This religion is practiced among Puerto Ricans and Dominicans.

6. **Voodoo.** This form of traditional HEALTH care is observed among the practitioners of a religion that is a combination of Christian and African Yoruba religious beliefs, called Voodoo.

The use of alternative therapies is growing rapidly. Astin (1998) reported that three theories have been offered to explain why people seek alternative care:

1. **Dissatisfaction.** Patients are not satisfied with allopathic care because it is seen as ineffective, it produces adverse effects, or it is impersonal, too costly, or too technological.

2. **Need for personal control.** The providers of alternative therapies are less authoritarian and more empowering, as they offer the patient the opportunity to have autonomy and control in their health care decisions.

3. **Philosophical congruence.** The alternative methods of therapy are compatible with the patients' values, worldview, spiritual philosophy, or beliefs regarding the nature and meaning of *health*/HEALTH and *illness*/ILLNESS. These therapies are now frequently used by patients with cancer, arthritis, chronic back or other pain, stress-related problems, AIDS, gastrointestinal problems, and anxiety.

Since 1990, Eisenberg and colleagues have studied the trends in the use of alternative medicine in the United States. They reported the results of a national survey of 1,539 subjects in 1993 and reported the findings of a 1997 survey in 1998. They found in 1991 that about a third of all American adults use some form of unconventional medical treatment; this number rose to 42.1% in 1997. A more recent study, in May 2004, CAM Use in America: Up Close, found that, in the United States, 40% of adults are using some form of CAM. The most frequent users in both the early studies were educated upper-income White Americans in the 25–49 age group who were most likely to live on the West Coast. CAM use presently spans people of all backgrounds. However, according to the 2004 survey, some people are more likely than others to use CAM. Overall, CAM use is greater by

■ Women than men

■ People with higher educational levels

■ People who have been hospitalized in the past year

■ Former smokers, compared with current smokers or those who have never smoked

The recent CAM Use in America survey was the first to yield substantial information on CAM use by minorities, and the major findings so far show that, when vitamins and prayer were presented as one of the options for use, 61% of the Hispanic respondents and 71% of the Black respondents used CAM. The analyses of the data are ongoing and further research needs to be done in the area.

The total projected out-of-pocket expenditure for unconventional therapy was $10.3 billion in 1990 and was conservatively estimated to be $27 billion. Between $36 to $47 billion was spent on CAM therapies in 1997. Of this amount, between $12 billion and $20 billion was paid out of pocket for the services of professional CAM health care providers. It is interesting to note that the amount of money paid out of pocket for CAM is greater than the fees paid for hospitalization out of pocket in 1997. Five billion dollars out of pocket was spent on herbal remedies. The various types of alternative therapies included relaxation techniques, chiropractic, imagery, commercial weight-loss programs, lifestyle diets (such as macrobiotics), megavitamin therapy, self-help groups, biofeedback, and hypnosis. Neither recent study examined the use of traditional healers and therapies by members of the immigrant and traditional communities (Barnes & Powell-Griner, 2004, p. 4; Eisenberg et al., 1998, p. 1574).

It is difficult to sort out which aspects of complementary and traditional medicine have merit and which are a hoax. From the viewpoint of the patient if he or she has faith in the efficacy of an herb, a diet, a pill, or a healer, it is not a hoax. From the viewpoint of the medical establishment, jealous of its territorial claim, the same herb, diet, pill, or healer is indeed a hoax if it is "scientifically" ineffective and prevents the person from using the method of treatment the physician-healer or other health care provider believes is effective.

The tensions between allopathic and homeopathic philosophies have been going on since the late 19th century. In this chapter, we have explored traditional ways of maintaining, protecting, and restoring HEALTH the choices available to patients, and health/HEALTH care philosophies.

Explore 🌐 MediaLink

Go to the Companion Website at www.prenhall.com/spector for chapter-related review questions, case studies, and activities. Contents of the CulturalCare Guide and CulturalCare Museum can also be found on the Companion Website. Click on Chapter 4 to select the activities for this chapter.

▓ Internet Sources

Broe, R., and Broe, K. (n.d.). Hydrotherapy. Retrieved from http://tuberose.com/Hydrotherapy.html, June 22, 2007.

Christian Science Publishing Society. (2008). Writings of Mary Baker Eddy. Boston, MA: Author. P. 1. Retrieved from http://www.spirituality.com, February 29, 2008.

Dolgan, E. (2006). Addressing Osteopathy: The Osteopathic Home Page. Santa Monica, CA: Osteopathic Physicians. P. 1. Retrieved from http://www.osteo-home.com/, June 22, 2006.

National Center for Complimentary and Alternative Medicine (NCCAM). (2008). Health Information. Washington, DC: National Institutes of Health. Retrieved from http://nccam.nih.gov/health/, February 29, 2008.

National Center for Complimentary and Alternative Medicine (NCCAM). (2007). Questions and Answers About Homeopathy. Washington, DC: National Institutes of Health. Retrieved from http://nccam.nih.gov/health/homeopathy/, June 22, 2007.

National Center for Complimentary and Alternative Medicine (NCCAM). (2007). CAM at the NIH Newsletter. Washington, DC: National Institutes of Health. V. XIV, No. 3, Summer, 2007. P. 1. Retrieved from http://nccam.nih.gov/news/newsletter/2007_summer/stakeholders.htm, June, 2007.

National Center for Complimentary and Alternative Medicine (NCCAM). (2004). Herbs at a Glance; Blackcohosh. Washington, DC: National Institutes of Health. Retrieved from http://nccam.nih.gov/health/blackcohosh/, July, 2007.

National Center for Complimentary and Alternative Medicine (NCCAM). (2005). Herbs at a Glance, Echinacea. Washington, DC: National Institutes of Health. p. 1. Retrieved from http://nccam.nih.gov/health/echinacea/, July, 2007.

National Center for Complimentary and Alternative Medicine (NCCAM). (2005). Herbs at a Glance: Ginkgo. Washington, DC: National Institutes of Health. p. 1. Retrieved from http://nccam.nih.gov/health/ginkgo/, July, 2007.

National Center for Complimentary and Alternative Medicine (NCCAM). (2005). Herbs at a Glance: St. John's Wort. Washington, DC: National Institutes of Health. p. 1. Retrieved from http://nccam.nih.gov/health/St. John's Wort/, July, 2007.

National Center for Complimentary and Alternative Medicine (NCCAM). (2005). Rheumatoid Arthritis and Complementary Medicine. Washington, DC: National Institutes of Health. p. 1. Retrieved from http://nccam.nih.gov/health/RA/, July, 2007.

National Center for Complimentary and Alternative Medicine (NCCAM). (2007). Cancer and CAM. Washington, DC: National Institutes of Health. p. 1. Retrieved from http://nccam.nih.gov/health/camcancer/, July, 2007.

National Center for Complimentary and Alternative Medicine (NCCAM). (2008). Menopausal Symptoms and CAM. Washington, DC: National Institutes of Health. p. 1. Retrieved from http://nccam.nih.gov/health/menopauseandcam/, February 29, 2008.

World Chiropractic Alliance (n.d.). Chiropractic – What is it *really* about? Retrieved from http://www.worldchiropracticalliance.org, June 23, 2007.

▮ References

Adrian, A. & Dennis, J. (1976). *Herbal Tea Book.* San Francisco: Health.

Astin, J. A. (1998, May 20). Why patients use alternative medicine: Results of a national study. *Journal of the American Medical Association, 279*(19), 1548–1553.

Barnes, P. M., & Powell-Griner, E. (2004). *Complimentary and alternative medicine use among adults: United States, 2002.* Washington, DC: National Center for Health Statistics.

Cobb, A. K. (1977). Pluralistic legitimation of an alternative therapy system: The case of chiropractic. *Medical Anthropology, 6*(4), 1–23.

Eddy, M. B. (1875). *Science and health with key to the scriptures.* Boston: Christian Science Publishing.

Eisenberg, D. M., Davis, R. B., Ettner, S. L., et al. (1998). Trends in alternative medicine use in the United States, 1990–1997. *Journal of the American Medical Association, 280*(18), 1569–1575.

Graunke, K. Personal Interview. Boston, Massachusetts, January 8, 2003.

Hopkins, E., Woods, L., Kelley, R., Bentley, K., and Murphy, J. (1995). *Working with groups on spiritual themes.* Duluth, MN: Whole Person Associates.

Maloney, C. (Ed.). (1976). *The evil eye.* New York: Columbia University Press.

School, B. F. (Ed.). (1924). *Library of health complete guide to prevention and cure of disease.* Philadelphia: Historical.

Smith, H. (1991, original 1958). *The world's religions.* San Francisco: Harper.

Spector, R. E. (1983). *A description of the impact of medicare on health–illness beliefs and practices of white ethnic senior citizens in central Texas* (pp. 126–127). Ph.D. dissertation. University of Texas at Austin School of Nursing. Ann Arbor, MI: University Microfilms International.

Starr, P. (1982). *The social transformation of American medicine* (pp. 79, 145). New York: Basic Books.

Weil, A. (1983). *Health and healing.* Boston: Houghton Mifflin.

Winkler, G. (1981). *Dybbuk.* New York: Judaica Press.

Yoder, D. (1972). Folk medicine. In R. H. Dorson (Ed.), *Folklore and folklife* (pp. 191–193). Chicago: University of Chicago Press.

Zola, I. K. (1972). The concept of trouble and sources of medical assistance to whom one can turn with what. *Social Science and Medicine, 6,* 673–679.

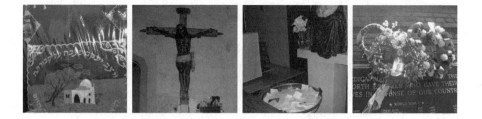

Chapter 5

Healing Traditions

■ Objectives

1. Discover practices that were part of ancient forms of HEALING.
2. Distinguish ways that one's religion influences HEALING.
3. Identify saints related to HEALTH problems.
4. Discuss the various destinations and purposes of spiritual journeys.
5. Discuss the relationship of HEALING to today's health beliefs and practices.
6. Describe various forms of HEALING.
7. Differentiate rituals of birth and death among people of different religions.

The images in the chapter opener are representative of sacred places, shrines, from selected destinations of pilgrimages or spiritual tourism. These are places where people may travel to seek HEALTH or HEALING from deep within their traditional spiritual heritage or from a secular source of memory, solace, or HEALING. The images here are locations that I have personally visited, both in the United States and abroad. The first image is from the Tomb of Rachel in Bethlehem, Israel, and is a place where Jewish pilgrims may go seeking HEALTH protection, HEALING, and help, especially for fertility. The journey to Rachel's Tomb is currently a difficult experience, as you must travel there on a bulletproof bus and pass through layers of barbed wire fences, tunnels, and security due to the current hostilities between the Israelis and Palestinians. People visit the Black Jesus in the San Fernando Cathedral in San Antonio, Texas, to petition for favors and HEALING and attest to countless miraculous HEALINGS. Petitions are placed at the Saint Ann's Shrine in Cleveland, Ohio. The last image represents the small secular shrines that may be set up at the scene of a fatal accident or at a memorial in a public setting, such as this one that is a veterans' memorial.

Are you having difficulties in your life that you would like to change? Are you seeking answers to questions that you cannot easily answer? Do you know about the HEALING traditions within your ethnoreligious heritage or the places you may visit to find the help you need? What are the HEALING practices within your family and ethnocultural heritage? What are the shrines, or sacred places, that are a part of your tradition or that you have visited? In the minds of countless people, shrines such as the ones in the chapter opener are an invaluable resource. If you could pick four images from your heritage that are related to HEALING, what would they be?

What is *HEALING*? What is the connotation of this word from a magico-religious or traditional perspective? What compels people to travel to shrines in the United States or in other parts of the world? Could it be that people who experience the need to seek consolation and solutions for overpowering events for which they cannot find rational answers turn to sources such as these Holy Shrines? The phenomenon of seeking HEALING is observed worldwide, and every religion and ethnic group offers substantive beliefs and practices in this genre. Are these examples of magic or of faith in a form of HEALTH care that is obtained from sources other than those that are conventional medicine? This chapter explores these questions by introducing a wide range of magico-religious and religious beliefs and practices regarding HEALING. It also discusses the traditions cross-culturally related to life cycle crises—birth, dying, and death—as these phenomena are closely linked to the beliefs and practices inherent in HEALING.

■ HEALING

The professional history of nursing was born with Florence Nightingale's knowledge (1860) that "nature heals." In more recent times, Blattner (1981) has written a text designed to help nurses assist patients in upgrading their lives in a holistic sense and in healing the person—body, mind, and spirit. Krieger (1979), in *The Therapeutic Touch*, has developed a method for teaching nurses how to use their hands to heal. Wallace (1979) has described methods of helping nurses diagnose and deliver spiritual care. She points out that the word *spiritual* is often used synonymously with *religion* but that the terms are not the same. If they are used synonymously as a basis for the health care and nursing assessment of needs, some of the patient's deepest needs may be glossed over. *Spiritual care* implies a much broader grasp of the search for meanings that goes on within every human life. In addition to answers to these questions from nursing raised in the introduction to this chapter, one is able to explore the concept from the classical and historical viewpoints of anthropology, sociology, psychology, and religion.

From the fields of anthropology and sociology come texts that describe rituals, customs, beliefs, and practices that surround healing. Shaw (1975, p. 121) contends that, "for as long as man has practiced the art of magic, he has sought to find personal immortality through healing practices." Buxton (1973) describes traditional beliefs and indigenous HEALING rituals in Mandari and relates the source of these rituals with how humans view themselves in relation to God and Earth. In this culture, the healer experiences a religious calling to become a healer. HEALING is linked to beliefs in evil and the removal of evil from the sick person. Naegele (1970, p. 18) describes healing in our society as a form of "professional practice." He asserts, however, that "healing is not wholly a professional monopoly and that there are several forms of nonprofessional healing such as the 'specialized alternatives.'" These include Christian Science and the marginally professional activities of varying legitimacy, such as chiropractic, folk medicine, and quackery. He states: "To understand modern society is to understand the tension between traditional patterns and self-conscious rational calculations devoted to the mastery of everyday life."

Literature from the field of psychology abounds with references to HEALING. Shames and Sterin (1978) describe the use of self-hypnosis to HEAL, and Progoff (1959), a depth psychologist, describes depth as the "dimension of wholeness in man." He has written extensively on how one's discovery of the inner self can be used for both HEALING and CREATION.

Krippner and Villaldo (1976, p. viii) contend that there is a "basic conflict between healing and technology" and that "the reality of miracles, of healing, of any significant entity that could be called God is not thought to be compatible with the reality of science." They further contend that healings are psychosomatic in origin and useful only in the sense of the placebo effect.

The literature linking religion to HEALING is bountiful. The primary source is the Bible (both the Old and New Testament) and prayers. Bishop (1967, p. 45) discusses miracles and their relationship to healing. He states that the "miracles must be considered in relation to the time and place in which they occur." He further describes faith and its relationship to healing and states that "something goes on in the process of faith healing." He also points out that healing "is the exception rather than the rule." HEALING through faith generally is not accepted as a matter of plain fact, but it is an event to rejoice over.

Ford (1971, p. 6) describes healing of the spirit and methods of spiritual healing for spiritual illness. He describes suffering in three dimensions: body, mind, and spirit. He fully describes telotherapy—spiritual healing—which is both a means and an invitation. His argument is that full healing takes place only when there is agape love—divine love—and no estrangement from God. Russell (1937, p. 221) and Cramer (1923, p. 11) assert that healing is the work of God alone. Russell asserts that "God's will normally expresses itself in health," and Cramer focuses on the unity of human beings with God and claims that permanent health is truth, that healing is the gift of Jesus, and that it is a spiritual gift.

■ Ancient Forms of HEALING

Illness was considered to be a crisis and the people of ancient times developed elaborate systems of HEALING. The cause of an ILLNESS was attributed to the forces of evil, which originated either within or outside the body. Early forms of HEALING dealt with the removal of evil. Once a method of treatment was found effective, it was passed down through the generations in slightly altered forms.

If the source of sickness-causing evil was within the body, treatment involved drawing the evil out of the body. This may have been accomplished through the use of purgatives, which caused either vomiting or diarrhea, or by blood-letting: "bleeding" the patient or "sucking out" blood. (The barbers of medieval Europe did not originate this practice; bleeding was done in ancient times.) Leeching was another method used to remove corrupt humors from the body.

If the source of the evil was outside the body, there were a number of ways to deal with it. One source of external evil was witchcraft. In a community, there were often many people or a single person who was "different" from the other people. Quite often, when an unexplainable or untreatable illness occurred, it was these people who were seen as the causative agents. In such a belief system, successful treatment depended on the identification and punishment of the person believed responsible for the disease. (Certainly, the practice of scapegoating is in part derived from this belief.) By removing or punishing the guilty person from the community, the disease would be cured. In some communities, the HEALERS themselves were seen as witches and the possessors of evil skills. How easy it was for ancient humankind to turn things around and blame the person with the skills to treat the disease for causing the disease!

Various rituals were involved in the treatment of ILL people. Often, the sick person was isolated from the rest of the family and community. In addition, it was customary to chant special prayers and incantations on the invalid's behalf. Sacrifices and dances often were performed in an effort to cure the ILLS. Often, the rituals of the healer involved reciting incantations in a language foreign to the ears of the general population ("speaking in tongues") and using practices that were strange to the observers. Small wonder, then, as superstition abounded, that at times the healers themselves were ostracized by the population.

Given that another cause of ILLNESS was believed to be the envy of people within the community, the best method, consequently, of preventing such an ILLNESS was to avoid provoking the envy of one's friends and neighbors. The treatment was to do away with whatever was provoking the envy—even though the act might have prevented a person from accomplishing a "mission in life," and the fear of being "responsible" might have been psychologically damaging.

Today, we tend to view the HEALING beliefs and methods of ancient people as primitive, yet to fully appreciate their efficacy we need only make the simple observation that these methods in many forms exist today and have aided the survival of humankind.

▧ Religion and HEALING

Religion plays a vital role in one's perception of HEALTH and ILLNESS. Just as culture and ethnicity are strong determinants in an individual's interpretation of the environment and the events within the environment, so, too, is religion. In fact, it is often difficult to distinguish between those aspects of a person's belief system arising from a religious background and those that stem from an ethnic and cultural heritage. Some people may share an ethnicity yet be of different religions; a group of people can share a religion yet have a variety of ethnic and cultural backgrounds. It is never safe to assume that all individuals of a given ethnic group practice or believe in the same religion. The point was embarrassingly driven home when I once asked a Chicano woman if she would like me to call the priest for her while her young son was awaiting a critical operation. The woman became angry with me. I could not understand why until I learned that she was a Methodist and not a Catholic. I had made an assumption, and I was wrong. She later told me that not all Chicanos are Catholic. After many years of hearing people make this assumption, she had learned to react with anger.

Religion strongly affects the way people interpret and respond to the signs and symptoms of ILLNESS. So pervasive is religion that the diets of many people are determined by their religious beliefs. Religion and the piety of a person determine not only the role that faith plays in the process of recovery but also in many instances the response to a given treatment and to the HEALING process. Each of these threads—religion, ethnicity, and culture—is woven into the fabric of each person's response to treatment and HEALING.

There are far too many religious beliefs and practices related to HEALING to include in this chapter. An introductory discussion of religious HEALING beliefs from the Judeo-Christian background, however, is possible.

The Old Testament does not focus on HEALING to the extent the New Testament does. God is seen to have total power over life and death and is the HEALER of all human woes. God is the giver of all good things and of all misfortune, including sickness. Sickness represented a break between God and humans. In Exodus 15:26, God is proclaimed the supreme HEALER ("I will put none of the diseases upon you which I put upon the Egyptians; for I am the Lord, your healer.") In a passage from Deuteronomy 32:39, it is stated "I kill, and I make alive. I have wounded and I heal." The traditionalist Jew believes that the "HEALING of illness comes from God through the mediation of His 'messenger,' the doctor." The Jew who is ill combines hope for a cure with faith in God and faith in the doctor (Ausubel, 1964, pp. 192–195). A prayer is recited for HEALING each Sabbath and other times throughout the week, and people are invited to submit or speak the names of people for whom they are petitioning for a restoration of their HEALTH.

The HEALING practices of the Roman Catholic tradition include a variety of beliefs and numerous practices of both a preventive and a HEALING nature. For example, St. Blaise, an Armenian bishop who died in A.D. 316 as a martyr, is revered as the preventer of sore throats. The blessing of the throats on his feast day (February 3) derives from the tradition that he miraculously saved the life of a boy by removing a fishbone he had swallowed (*Monthly Missalette*, 1980, p. 38).

The saints concerned with other aspects of ILLNESS include the following (Foy, 1980, pp. 305–313; Hallam, 1994):

Saint	Problem
St. Anthony of Padua	Barrenness
St. Odilia	Blindness
Our Lady of Lourdes	Bodily ills
St. Peregrine	Cancer
St. Francis de Sales	Deafness
St. Joseph	Dying
St. Vitus	Epilepsy
St. Raymond Nonnatus	Pregnancy
St. Lucy	Eye disease
St. Teresa of Avila	Headache
St. John of God	Heart disease
St. Roch	Being bedridden
St. Dymphna	Mental illness
St. Bruno	Possession

Many more saints could be included. I refer you to other sources for information, and I also recommend that you ask patients for information. I was caring for a young woman with terminal colon cancer. We began a conversation about St. Peregrine. She shared with me her belief in this saint, showed me a medal that she had carried with her, and expressed that she was comforted by sharing this information.

Spiritual Journeys

There are countless places in this world where people make spiritual journeys, or pilgrimages, for the purpose of giving thanks or petitioning for favors. The shrines are related to magico-religious folk medicine and the use of charms, holy words, and holy actions. For example, at many shrines petitioners leave amulets or written petitions or light candles. Shrines range from small memorials—such as shrines that are created at the sites where accidents have occurred and people were killed to large, famous shrines where people who are part of a given religious tradition or a follower of a given healer may go to pray or petition at the site. In the United States, and throughout the world, people make pilgrimages to a number of shrines in search of special favors and HEALING. Shrines are not limited to any one-faith tradition and they can be secular as well as religious. Over the years, I have visited many shrines and have learned that they are indeed extraordinary places. The essentials that each of the shrines have in common are a feeling of peacefulness and serenity to the visitor; a calm, soothing atmosphere; and a place where petitions and/or objects are left for HEALING. Most, but not all, have a source of water as part of the milieu, and it is a part of the tradition to take home water from the shrine.

The following are examples of shrines located in the United States.

The Tomb of Menachem Mendel Schneerson in Queens, New York, is a holy shrine where Jewish people from around the world gather to leave petitions and seek HEALING. People have reported healings when they visit his tomb (Figure 5–1).

The oldest shrine in the United States is the Shrine of Our Lady of La Leche, located in St. Augustine, Florida (Figure 5–2). The shrine was founded

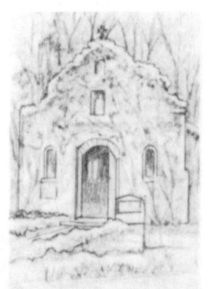

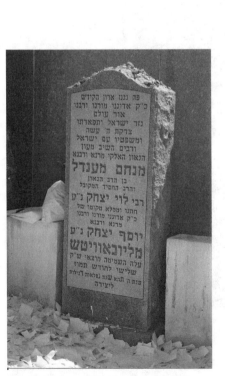

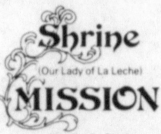

Figure 5-1 The Tomb of Rabbi Menachem Mendel Schneerson in Queens, New York.

Figure 5-2 Our Lady of La Leche Shrine and Mission.

in 1620 by Spanish settlers as a sign of their love for the Mother of Christ. The shrine is visited by thousands of mothers to ask for the blessings of motherhood, a safe and happy delivery, a healthy baby, and holy children. Countless letters can be read at the shrine attesting to the powers of Our Lady of La Leche (Informational brochure, 1953).

The Shrine of Our Lady of San Juan (Figure 5–3) is located in San Juan, Texas. This shrine houses a statue of the Virgin that was taken to Mexico by Spanish missionaries in 1623. The statue was responsible for causing a miracle,

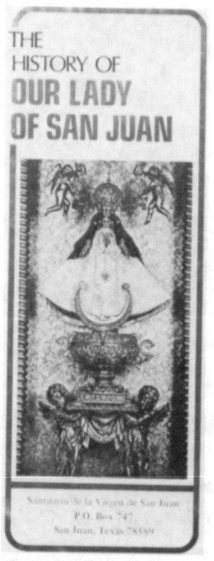

Figure 5-3 Our Lady of San Juan Shrine.

and devotion to *La Virgin de San Juan* spread. The statue was taken to Texas in the 1940s after a woman claimed to have seen an image of the Virgin in the countryside around San Juan. The statue is presently housed in a beautiful new church, and pilgrims arrive daily to ask for HEALING and other favors. Countless letters are displayed attesting to the HEALING powers of this statue and crutches and other artifacts are left at the church, to attest to the miracles that happened there (Informational brochure, 1999).

The Shrine of St. Peregrine for Cancer Sufferers (Figure 5–4) is located in the Old Mission San Juan Capistrano in California. This statue is housed in a small grotto in the shrine. St. Peregrine was born in Italy in 1265 and died in 1345. He was believed to have miraculous powers against sickness and could cure cancer. This won for him the title "official patron for cancer victims." Once a woman was afflicted with cancer and a lady gave her a prayer to St. Peregrine. The woman prayed for 6 months, and her cancer was arrested. In gratitude for this, the woman had a statue of the saint placed in the mission. Today, the belief in this saint has spread, and countless documents attesting to his healing powers are on display in the mission.

Chimayo, New Mexico, is the home of the Shrine of our Lord of Esquipulas. The shrine was built between 1814 and 1816 and is visited by thousands of people each year. The shrine has been called the "Lourdes of America"

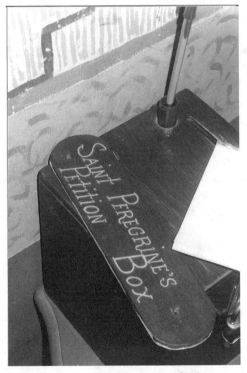

Figure 5–4   Saint Peregrine Shrine.

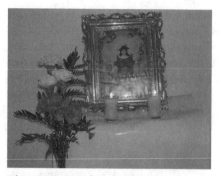

Figure 5-5 An altar in the shrine in Chimayo, New Mexico, known as "Lourdes of America."

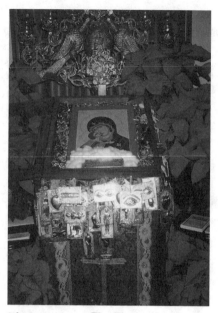

Figure 5-6 The Virgin at the Shrine of the Blessed Virgin Mary in Blanco, Texas.

and countless healings have been reported in this location (Figure 5–5). There is a hole in the shrine and it is believed that eating the mud from this hole will cure many illnesses. The mud may also be mixed with water and rubbed on the body (Informational brochure, 1994).

It has been reported that the Virgin at the Shrine of the Blessed Virgin Mary in Blanco, Texas, cries tears of myrrh (Figure 5–6). Pilgrims report that they have had mystical and HEALING experiences here (Informational brochure, 2000).

The National Shrine of Our Lady of the Snows (Figure 5–7) is located in Belleville, Illinois. It is a site that provides an atmosphere where people of all faiths have the opportunity to pray for HEALING and hope. There are numerous locations where petitions may be placed.

Other Shrines

The following are examples of shrines located in Israel and Europe.

The Tomb of King David is in Jerusalem, Israel, and is located in the same building as the room of the Last Supper. It is a frequented place of HEALING. The Tomb of the Nebbe Sabalam (Figure 5–8) is the historic father of the Druze Faith. People visit this shrine in the northern part of Israel to petition and give

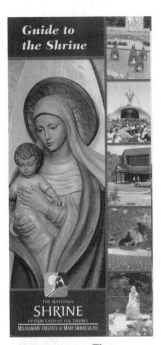

Figure 5-7 **The National Shrine of Our Lady of the Snows.**

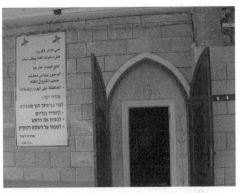

Figure 5-8 **The Tomb of the Nebbe Sabalam.**

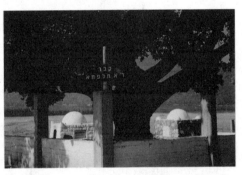

Figure 5-9 **Tombs in northern Israel.**

thanks for HEALTH. In addition, there are several tombs (Figure 5–9) scattered throughout northern Israel where people of all faiths visit to seek HEALING.

Three of the most revered and known shrines worldwide are located in France, Spain, and Portugal. Lourdes, in France, is believed to be a site where the Virgin Mary visited Bernadette Soubirous. In 1858, she observed a vision of St. Mary in a grotto. The Virgin was reported to have visited her several times. There have been 67 accepted miracle cures at this site and countless pilgrims continue to go there.

"*Enagradecimiento por devolver la vida a neustro sobrino, I. G. R. 14-9-01*": this translates to "Praise [or exaltation] for returning the life of our nephew." This brief note was found at the shrine in Montserrat, near Barcelona, Spain. The immediate image was that of a couple making the difficult pilgrimage to Montserrat and placing this petition there. Note that the date is September 14, 2001—3 days after the attacks on the United States. Could it be that this person, the nephew, survived the attack on either the Pentagon or the World

Trade Center? Could it be that the family sought and found a way to express their gratitude? The journey to Montserrat is difficult; the image this note evoked was one of sacrifice and homage.

Fatima is located in a small village in central Portugal, a short distance from Lisbon. It is a site of a shrine dedicated to the Virgin Mary. In 1917, three peasant children reported a vision of a woman who identified herself as the "Lady of the Rosary." The first national pilgrimage to the site occurred in 1927. Many miraculous cures have been reported at this site.

One need only visit these remarkable places and bear witness to the display of faith that can be observed to begin to understand their important contributions in the complex areas of HEALING and faith.

Many people will not be fortunate enough to actually participate in a pilgrimage. However, there are countless Web sites that bring information and images to you. One such site, *El Nino Fidencio*, The *Curanderismo* Research Project from the University of Texas at Brownsville and Texas Southmost College, contains pertinent information about *El Nino Fidencio*. Fidencio Constantine, a folk curer, practiced in Nuevo Leon, Mexico from the early 1920s until his death in 1938, and is presently the central figure in a widespread curing cult. Twice each year, on the anniversaries of his birth and death, Espinazo (a town of about 300 population) is inundated by 10,000 to 15,000 people from Mexico and the United States who make pilgrimages in hopes of a cure and/or help from the *Niño* (The University of Texas at Brownsville and Texas Southmost University [2006]).

Believers combine elements of traditional Catholicism, Indian dances, herbology, and laying on of hands in effecting cures. It is believed that certain individuals receive the *Niño's* power to heal. They are called "*Cajitas*" or "*Materias*" (women) (Figure 5–10) and "*Cajones*" (men)—"receptacles" of the *Niño's* power—and they cure in the name of *Niño Fidencio* and God. During the celebrations, they roam Espinazo curing all who wish a cure-blessing. There are several "holy places" in Espinazo where curing is conducted: Fidencio's tomb, "temple," and deathbed; two trees; a cemetery hill; the hill of the bell; and the "charco" or mudpond, where Fidencio conducted baptisms to cure his patients. The pilgrimage to Espinazo has increased in popularity over recent years and extensive studies have been conducted in Espinazo (Gardner, 1992).

Table 5–1 summarizes the beliefs of people from several religious backgrounds with respect to health/HEALTH, healing/HEALING, and several events related to health care delivery. Remember, this is a summary, and you are urged not to generalize from this guide when relating to an individual patient and family. It is important to show respect, sensitivity, and an awareness and understanding of the different perspectives that may exist and to be able to convey to the patient and family your desire to understand their viewpoint on health care.

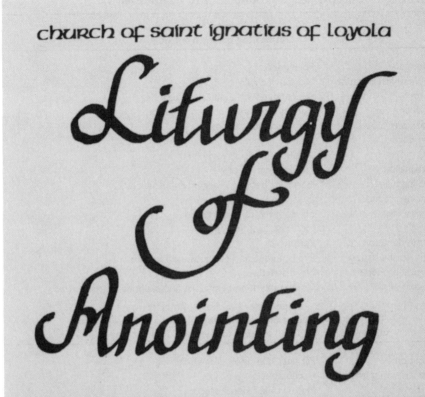

church of saint ignatius of loyola

Liturgy of Anointing

THE CHURCH OF ST. IGNATIUS WILL PRAY FOR THE SICK AND ELDERLY IN THE PARISH ON THE FEAST OF CHRIST THE KING, NOVEMBER 20th AT THE LITURGY FOR ANOINTING AT 9:30 A.M.. AREA RESIDENTS, ESPECIALLY THOSE WHO ARE SICK, DISABLED OR ELDERLY, ARE WELCOME TO TAKE PART. EACH PERSON WHO DESIRES IT WILL BE BLESSED OR ANOINTED WITH HOLY OIL.

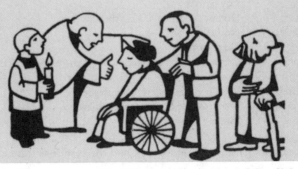

Figure 5-10   Announcement for Liturgy of Anointing of the Sick.

Table 5–1   Selected Religions' Responses to Health Events

	Baha'i "All healing comes from God."
Abortion	Forbidden
Artificial insemination	No specific rule
Autopsy	Acceptable with medical or legal need
Birth control	Can choose family planning method
Blood and blood products	No restrictions for use
Diet	Alcohol and drugs forbidden
Euthanasia	No destruction of life
Healing beliefs	Harmony between religion and science
Healing practices	Pray
Medications	Narcotics with prescription No restriction for vaccines
Organ donations	Permitted
Right-to-die issues	Life is unique and precious—do not destroy
Surgical procedures	No restrictions
Visitors	Community members assist and support

	Buddhist Churches of America "To keep the body in good health is a duty— otherwise we shall not be able to keep our mind strong and clear."
Abortion	Patient's condition determines
Artificial insemination	Acceptable
Autopsy	Matter of individual practice
Birth control	Acceptable
Blood and blood products	No restrictions
Diet	Restricted food combinations Extremes must be avoided
Euthanasia	May permit
Healing beliefs	Do not believe in healing through faith
Healing practices	No restrictions
Medications	No restrictions
Organ donations	Considered act of mercy; if hope for recovery, all means may be taken
Right-to-die issues	With hope, all means encouraged
Surgical procedures	Permitted, with extremes avoided
Visitors	Family, community

	Roman Catholicism "The prayer of faith shall heal the sick, and the Lord shall raise him up."
Abortion	Prohibited
Artificial insemination	Illicit, even between husband and wife
Autopsy	Permissible
Birth control	Natural means only
Blood and blood products	Permissible

Table 5–1 *Continued*

Diet	Use foods in moderation
Euthanasia	Direct life-ending procedures forbidden
Healing beliefs	Many within religious belief system
Healing practices	Sacrament of sick, candles, laying on of hands
Medications	May be taken if benefits outweigh risks
Organ donations	Justifiable
Right-to-die issues	Obligated to take ordinary, not extraordinary, means to prolong life
Surgical procedures	Most are permissible except abortion and sterilization
Visitors	Family, friends, priest
	Many outreach programs through church to reach sick

Christian Science

Abortion	Incompatible with faith
Artificial insemination	Unusual
Autopsy	Not usual; individual or family decide
Birth control	Individual judgment
Blood and blood products	Ordinarily not used by members
Diet	No solid food restrictions
	Abstain from alcohol and tobacco, some from tea and coffee (caffeine)
Euthanasia	Contrary to teachings
Healing beliefs	Accepts physical and moral healing
Healing practices	Full-time healing ministers
	Spiritual healing practiced
Medications	None
	Immunizations/vaccines to comply with law
Organ donations	Individual decides
Right-to-die issues	Unlikely to seek medical help to prolong life
Surgical procedures	No medical ones practiced
Visitors	Family, friends, and members of the Christian Science community and Healers, Christian Science nurses

Church of Jesus Christ of Latter-day Saints

Abortion	Forbidden
Artificial insemination	Acceptable between husband and wife
Autopsy	Permitted with consent of next of kin
Birth control	Contrary to Mormon belief
Blood and blood products	No restrictions
Diet	Alcohol, tea (except herbal teas), coffee, and tobacco are forbidden
	Fasting (24 hours without food and drink) is required once a month
Euthanasia	Humans must not interfere in God's plan
Healing beliefs	Power of God can bring healing
Healing practices	Anointing with oil, sealing, prayer, laying on of hands

(continued)

Table 5–1 *Continued*

Medications	No restrictions; may use herbal folk remedies
Organ donations	Permitted
Right-to-die issues	If death inevitable, promote a peaceful and dignified death
Surgical procedures	Matter of individual choice
Visitors	Church members (Elder and Sister), family, and friends
	The Relief Society helps members

Hinduism
"Enricher, Healer of disease, be a good friend to us."

Abortion	No policy exists
Artificial insemination	No restrictions exist but not often practiced
Autopsy	Acceptable
Birth control	All types acceptable
Blood and blood products	Acceptable
Diet	Eating of meat is forbidden
Euthanasia	Not practiced
Healing beliefs	Some believe in faith healing
Healing practices	Traditional faith healing system
Medications	Acceptable
Organ donations	Acceptable
Right-to-die issues	No restrictions
	Death seen as "one more step to nirvana"
Surgical procedures	With an amputation, the loss of limb is seen as due to "sins in a previous life"
Visitors	Members of family, community, and priest support

Islam
"The Lord of the world created me—and when I am sick, He healeth me."

Abortion	Not accepted
Artificial insemination	Permitted between husband and wife
Autopsy	Permitted for medical and legal purposes
Birth control	Acceptable
Blood and blood products	No restrictions
Diet	Pork and alcohol prohibited
Euthanasia	Not acceptable
Healing beliefs	Faith healing generally not acceptable
Healing practices	Some use of herbal remedies and faith healing
Medications	No restrictions
Organ donations	Controversial; must be discussed with family
Right-to-die issues	Attempts to shorten life prohibited
Surgical procedures	Most permitted
Visitors	Family and friends provide support

Table 5-1 *Continued*

Jehovah's Witnesses	
Abortion	Forbidden
Artificial insemination	Forbidden
Autopsy	Acceptable if required by law
Birth control	Sterilization forbidden
	Other methods individual choice
Blood and blood products	Forbidden
Diet	Abstain from tobacco, moderate use of alcohol
Euthanasia	Forbidden
Healing beliefs	Faith healing forbidden
Healing practices	Reading Scriptures can comfort the individual and lead to mental and spiritual healing
Medications	Accepted except if derived from blood products
Organ donations	Forbidden
Right-to-die issues	Use of extraordinary means an individual's choice
Surgical procedures	Not opposed, but administration of blood during surgery is strictly prohibited
Visitors	Members of congregation and elders pray for the sick person

Judaism "O Lord, my God, I cried to Thee for help and Thou has healed me."	
Abortion	Therapeutic permitted; some groups accept abortion on demand; seek rabbinical consultation
Artificial insemination	Permitted
Autopsy	Permitted under certain circumstances
	All body parts must be buried together—seek rabbinical consultation
Birth control	Permissible, except with orthodox Jews—seek rabbinical consultation
Blood and blood products	Acceptable
Diet	Strict dietary laws followed by many Jews—milk and meat not mixed; predatory fowl, shellfish, and pork products forbidden; kosher products only may be requested
Euthanasia	Active Euthanasia Prohibited—passive euthanasia—not prolonging life may be acceptable—nutrition a basic need—not withheld— seek rabbinic consultation
Healing beliefs	Medical care expected
Healing practices	Prayers for the sick
Medications	No restrictions
Organ donations	Complex issue; some practiced—seek rabbinic consultation
Right-to-die issues	Right to die with dignity
	If death is inevitable, no new procedures need to be undertaken, but those ongoing must continue
Surgical procedures	Most allowed
Visitors	Family, friends, rabbi, many community services

(continued)

Table 5-1 *Continued*

Mennonite	
Abortion	Therapeutic acceptable
Artificial insemination	Individual conscience; husband to wife
Autopsy	Acceptable
Birth control	Acceptable
Blood and blood products	Acceptable
Diet	No specific restrictions
Euthanasia	Not condoned
Healing beliefs	Part of God's work
Healing practices	Prayer and anointing with oil
Medications	No restrictions
Organ donations	Acceptable
Right-to-die issues	Do not believe life must be continued at all cost
Surgical procedures	No restrictions
Visitors	Family, community

Seventh-day Adventists	
Abortion	Therapeutic acceptable
Artificial insemination	Acceptable between husband and wife
Autopsy	Acceptable
Birth control	Individual choice
Blood and blood products	No restrictions
Diet	Encourage vegetarian diet
Euthanasia	Not practiced
Healing beliefs	Divine healing
Healing practices	Anointing with oil and prayer
Medications	No restrictions
	Vaccines acceptable
Organ donations	Acceptable
Right-to-die issues	Follow the ethic of prolonging life
Surgical procedures	No restrictions
	Oppose use of hypnotism
Visitors	Pastor and elders pray and anoint sick person
	Worldwide health system includes hospitals and clinics

Unitarian/Universalist Church	
Abortion	Acceptable, therapeutic and on demand
Artificial insemination	Acceptable
Autopsy	Recommended
Birth control	All types acceptable
Blood and blood products	No restrictions
Diet	No restrictions
Euthanasia	Favor nonaction
	May withdraw therapies if death imminent

Table 5-1 *Continued*

Healing beliefs	Faith healing: seen as "superstitious"
Healing practices	Use of science to facilitate healing
Medications	No restrictions
Organ donations	Acceptable
Right-to-die issues	Favor the right to die with dignity
Surgical procedures	No restrictions
Visitors	Family, friends, church members

Source: Adapted with permission from Andrews, M. M., & Hanson, P. A. (1995). Religion, culture, and nursing, In J. S. Boyle & M. M. Andrews (Eds.), *Transcultural concepts in nursing care* (2nd ed.) (pp. 371–406). Philadelphia: J. B. Lippincott. Used with permission.

■ HEALING and Today's Beliefs

It is not an accident or a coincidence that today, more so than in recent years, we are not only curious but vitally concerned about the ways of HEALING that our ancestors employed. Some critics of today's health care system choose to condemn it, with more vociferous critics, such as Illich (1975), citing its failure to create a utopia for humankind. It is obvious to those who embrace a more moderate viewpoint that diseases continue to occur and that they outflank our ability to cure or prevent them. Once again, many people are seeking the services of people who are knowledgeable in the arts of HEALING and folk medicine. Many patients may elect, at some point in their lives, more specifically during an ILLNESS, to use modalities outside the medical establishment. It is important to understand the HEALERS.

Types of HEALING

A review of HEALING and spiritual literature reveals that there are four types of HEALING:

1. **Spiritual HEALING.** When a person is experiencing an illness of the spirit, spiritual HEALING applies. The cause of suffering is personal sin. The treatment method is repentance, which is followed by a natural healing process.
2. **Inner HEALING.** When a person is suffering from an emotional (mental) illness, inner HEALING is used. The root of the problem may lie in the person's conscious or unconscious mind. The treatment method is to heal the person's memory. The HEALING process is delicate and sensitive and takes considerable time and effort.
3. **Physical HEALING.** When a person is suffering from a disease or has been involved in an accident that resulted in some form of bodily damage, physical HEALING is appropriate. Laying on hands and speaking in tongues usually accompany physical HEALING. The person is prayed over by both the leader and members of a prayer group (Figure 5–10).
4. **Deliverance, or exorcism.** When the body and mind are victims of evil from the outside, exorcism is used. In order to effect treatment,

the person must be delivered, or exorcised, from the evil. The ongoing popularity of films such as *The Exorcist* gives testimony to the return of these beliefs. Incidentally, the priest who has lectured in my classes stated that he does not, as yet, lend credence to exorcisms; however, he was guarded enough not to discount it, either.

The people who HEAL, both in the past and in the present, often have been those who received the gift of HEALING from a "divine" source. Many receive this gift in a vision and have been unable to explain to others how they know what to do. Other HEALERS learned their skills from their parents. Most of the HEALERS with acquired skills are women, who subsequently pass their knowledge on to their daughters. People who use herbs and other preparations to remove the evil from the sick person's body are known as herbalists. Other HEALERS include bone setters and midwives, and although early humankind did not separate ILLS of the body from those of the mind, some HEALERS were more adept at solving problems by using early forms of "psychotherapy."

There are numerous HEALERS in the general population, some of whom are legitimate and some of whom are not. They range from housewives and priests to gypsies and "witches." Many people seek their services. There are numerous stylistic differences between the scope of practice of a modern health care practitioner and that of a traditional HEALER (Table 5–2). I have visited with several

Table 5–2 Comparisons: Traditional Homeopathic HEALER Versus Modern Allopathic Physician

HEALER	Physician
1. Maintains informal, friendly, affective relationship with the entire family	1. Businesslike, formal relationship; deals only with the patient
2. Comes to the house day or night	2. Patient must go to the physician's office or clinic, and only during the day; may have to wait for hours to be seen; home visits are rarely, if ever, made
3. For diagnosis, consults with head of house, creates a mood of awe, talks to all family members, is not authoritarian, has social rapport, builds expectation of cure	3. Rest of family usually is ignored; deals solely with the ill person and may deal only with the sick part of the person; authoritarian manner creates fear
4. Generally less expensive than the physician	4. More expensive than the healer physician
5. Has ties to the "world of the sacred"; has rapport with the symbolic, spiritual, creative, or holy force	5. Secular; pays little attention to the religious beliefs or meaning of an illness
6. Shares the worldview of the patient— that is, speaks the same language, lives in the same neighborhood, or lives in some similar socioeconomic conditions; may know the same people; understands the lifestyle of the patient	6. Generally does not share the worldview of the patient—that is, may not speak the same language, live in the same neighborhood, or understand the socioeconomic conditions; may not understand the lifestyle of the patient

traditional healers. One man I visited was a *Santero*, a traditional HEALER from Puerto Rico. He enjoyed a reputation as a person who can "bring comfort to those most in need." I had an appointment for an interview but, when I arrived, he informed me that if I wanted to learn about his practice I had to "sit." I did. He examined me by asking questions, (history); examining my head and hands (palpation and observation); and casting cowarie shells (in-depth examination). He then told me a story, asked me to interpret it, and then, based on my interpretation, told me how to treat my "problem."

■ Ancient Rituals Related to the Life Cycle

Today, just as it did in antiquity, religion also plays a role in the rites surrounding both birth and death. Many of the rituals that we observe at the time of birth and death have their origins in the practices of ancient human beings. Close your eyes for a few moments and picture yourself living thousands and thousands of years ago. There is no electricity, no running water, no bathroom, no plumbing. The nights are dark and cold. The only signs of the passage of time are the changing seasons and the apparent movement of the various planets and stars through the heavens. You are prey to all the elements, as well as to animals and the unknown. How do you survive? What sort of rituals and practices assist you in maintaining your equilibrium within this often hostile environment? It is from this milieu that many of today's practices sprang.

Generally speaking, three critical moments occur in the life of almost every human being: birth, marriage, and death (Morgenstern, 1966, p. 3). One needs to examine the events and rites that were attendant on birth and death in the past and to demonstrate how many of them not only are relevant to our lives today but also are still practiced. Rites related to marriage are not included in this text but certainly are related, in the long term, to a person's HEALTH.

Birth Rituals

In the minds of early human beings, the number of evil spirits far exceeded the number of good spirits, and a great deal of energy and time was devoted to thwarting these spirits. They could be defeated by the use of gifts or rituals or, when the evil spirits had to be removed from a person's body, with redemptive sacrifices. Once these evil spirits were expelled, they were prevented from returning by various magical ceremonies and rites. When a ceremony and an incantation were found to be effective, they were passed on through the generations. It has been suggested and supported by scholars that, from this primitive beginning, organized religion came into being. Today, many of the early rites have survived in altered forms, and we continue to practice them.

The power of the evil spirits was believed to endure for a certain length of time. The 3rd, 7th, and 40th days were the crucial days in the early life of a child and the new mother. Hence, it was on these days, or on the 8th day, that most of the rituals were observed. It was believed that, during this period, the newborn and the mother were at the greatest risk from the power of supernatural beings and thus in a taboo state. "The concept underlying taboo is that all things created by or emanating from a supernatural being are his, or are at least in his power" (Morgenstern, 1966, p. 31). The person was freed from this taboo by certain rituals, depending on the practices of a given community. When the various rites were completed and the 40 days were over, both the mother and child were believed to be redeemed from evil. The ceremonies that freed the person had a double character: They were partly magic and partly religious.

I have deliberately chosen to present the early practices of Semitic peoples because their beliefs and practices evolved into the Judaic, Christian, and Islamic religions of today. Because the newborn baby and mother were considered vulnerable to the threats of evil spirits, many rituals were developed to protect them. For example, in some communities, the mother and child were separated from the rest of the community for a certain length of time, usually 40 days. Various people performed precautionary measures, such as rubbing the baby with different oils or garlic, swaddling the baby, and lighting candles. In other communities, the baby and mother were watched closely for a certain length of time, usually 7 days. (During this time span, they were believed to be intensely susceptible to the effects of evil—hence, close guarding was in order.) Orthodox Jews still refer to the seventh night of life as the "watch night" (Morgenstern, 1966, pp. 22–30).

The birth of a male child was considered more significant than that of a female, and many rites were practiced in observance of this event. One ritual sacrifice was cutting off a lock of the child's hair and then sprinkling his forehead with sheep's blood. This ritual was performed on the eighth day of life and may be practiced today among Muslims. In other Semitic countries, when a child was named, a sheep was sacrificed and asked to give protection to the infant. Depending on regional or tribal differences, the mother might be given parts of the sheep. It was believed that, if this sacrificial ritual was not performed on the 7th or 8th day of life, the child would die (Morgenstern, 1966, p. 87). The sheep's skin was saved, dried, and placed in the child's bed for 3 or 4 years as protection from evil spirits.

Both the practice of cutting a lock of a child's hair and the sacrifice of an animal served as a ceremony of redemption. The child could also be redeemed from the taboo state by giving silver—the weight of which equaled the weight of the hair—to the poor. Although not universally practiced, these rites are still observed in some form in some communities of the Arab world.

Circumcision is closely related to the ceremony of cutting the child's hair and offering it as a sacrifice. Some authorities hold that the practice originated as a rite of puberty: a body mutilation performed to attract the opposite sex. (Circumcision was practiced by many peoples throughout the ancient world. Alex Haley's *Roots* describes it as a part of initiating boys into manhood in Africa.) Other sources attribute circumcision to the concept of the sanctity of the male organ and claim that it was derived from the practice of ancestor worship. The Jews of ancient Israel, as today, practiced circumcision on the 8th day of life. The Muslims circumcise their sons on the 7th day in the tradition that Mohammed established. In other Muslim countries, the ritual is performed anywhere from the 10th day to the 7th year of life. Again, this sacrifice redeemed the child from being taboo in his early stages of life. Once the sacrifice was made, the child entered the period of worldly existence. The rite of circumcision was accompanied by festivals of varying durations. Some cultures and kinship groups feasted for as long as a week.

The ceremony of baptism is also rooted in the past. It, too, symbolically expels the evil spirits, removes the taboo, and is redemptive. It is practiced mainly among members of the Christian faith, but the Yezidis and other non-Christian sects also perform the rite. Water was thought to possess magical powers and was used to cleanse the body from both physical and spiritual maladies, which included evil possession and other impurities. Usually, the child was baptized on the 40th day of life. In some communities, however, the child was baptized on the 8th day. The 40th (or 8th) day was chosen because the ancients believed that, given performance of the particular ritual, this day marked the end of the evil spirits' influence (Morgenstern, 1966).

Some rituals also involved the new mother. For example, not only was she (along with her infant) removed from her household and community for 40 days, but in many communities she had to practice ritual bathing before she could return to her husband, family, and community. Again, these practices were not universal, and they varied in scope and intensity from people to people. Table 5–3 illustrates examples of birth-related religious rituals.

Table 5–3   Birth-Related Religious Rituals

Religion	Practice	Time	Method
Baptist (27 bodies)	Baptism	Older child	Immersion
Church of Christ	Baptism	8 years	Immersion
Church of Jesus Christ of Latter-day Saints (Mormons)	Baptism	8 years or older	Immersion
Eastern Orthodox	Baptism	Infants	Total immersion
Episcopalian	Baptism	Infant	
Friends (Quaker)	No baptism	Named	
Greek Orthodox	Baptism	40 days	Sprinkle or immersion
Islam	Circumcision	7th day	
Jewish	Circumcision	8th day	
Lutheran	Baptism	6–8 weeks	Pouring, sprinkling, immersion
Methodist	Baptism	Childhood	
Pentecostal	Baptism	Age of accountability	
Roman Catholic	Baptism	Infant	Pour water
Russian Orthodox	Baptism	Infant	Immerse three times
Unitarian	Baptism	Infant	

Extensions of Birth Rituals to Today's Practices

Early human beings, in their quest for survival, strove to appease and prevent the evil spirits from interfering with their lives. Their beliefs seem simple and naive, yet the rituals that began in those years have evolved into those that exist today. Attacks of the evil spirits were warded off with the use of amulets, charms, and the like. People recited prayers and incantations. Because survival was predicated on people's ability to appease evil spirits, the prescribed rituals were performed with great care and respect. Undoubtedly, this accounts in part for the longevity of many of these practices through the ages. For example, circumcision and baptism still exist, even when the belief that they are being performed to release the child from a state of being taboo may not continue to be held. It is interesting also that adherence to a certain timetable is maintained. For example, as stated, the Jewish religion mandates that the ritual of circumcision be performed on the 8th day of life as commanded by Jewish law in the Bible.

The practice of closely guarding the new mother and baby through the initial hours after birth is certainly not foreign to us. The mother is closely watched for hemorrhage and signs of infection; the infant initially is watched for signs of choking or respiratory distress. This form of observation is very intense. Could factors such as these have been what our ancestors watched for? If early human beings believed that evil spirits caused the frequent complications that surrounded the birth of a baby, it stands to reason that they would seek to control or prevent these complications by adhering to astute observation, isolation, and rituals of redemption.

Table 5–4 lists birth rites from selected nations.

Death Rituals

It was believed that the work of evil spirits and the duration of their evil—whether it was 7 or 40 days—surrounded the person, family, and community at the time of and after death. Rites evolved to protect both dying and dead persons and the remaining family from these evil spirits. The dying person was cared for in specific ways (ritual washing), and the grave was prepared in set ways (storing food and water for the journey after death). Further rituals were performed to protect the deceased's survivors from the harm believed to be rendered by the deceased's ghost. It was believed that this ghost could return from the grave and, if not carefully appeased, harm surviving relatives (Morgenstern, 1966, pp. 117–160).

Countless ethnocultural and religious differences can be found in the ways we observe dying, death, and mourning. Table 5–5 displays a sampling of the ways death is talked about at various locations in the United States. The expressions for death have been collected over several years of randomly reading the

Table 5–4   Cross-Cultural Guide to Birth Rites from Selected Nations

National Origin of Your Client/Family	Rites You May Observe Before, When, and/or After Birth
Afghanistan (population 89% Muslim)	Use of traditional birth attendant (dais) Breast-feeding nearly universal BCG[a] at birth
Albania (population 70% Muslim, 20% Orthodox, 10% Catholic)	BCG at birth
Algeria (population 99% Muslim)	Father not present at delivery Baby wrapped in swaddling clothes Breast-feeding common, BCG at birth
Australia (population 76% Christian)	Physician delivers, father usually present Breast-feeding BCG at birth
Bahrain (population 100% Muslim)	BCG at birth
Bangladesh (population 83% Muslim, 16% Hindu, 1% other)	Mother prays postpartum, remains indoors up to 40 days Only husband visits Objects placed over door to prevent evil spirits Breast-feeding BCG at birth
Belize (population 90% Christian)	Fifty percent of children born out of wedlock Christened before visitors allowed, to prevent evil eye Bottle-feeding preferred
Brazil (population 70% Catholic, 30% other)	Fathers not present during labor and delivery Forty-day rest period for mother Short-term breast-feeding BCG at birth
Cambodia	Seek prenatal care at 5 to 6 months of pregnancy
Kampuchea (population 95% Buddhist)	Do not compliment newborn to prevent evil spirits Breast-feeding BCG at birth
Chad (population 44% Muslim)	Female circumcision BCG at birth
China (population 97% atheist and eclectic)	Fathers do not come into labor and delivery Newborn considered 1 year at birth Breast-feeding

(continued)

Table 5–4 *Continued*

Cuba (population 85% Catholic)	Avoid loud noises and looking at deformed people when pregnant Stay home for 41 days Breast-feeding BCG at birth
Egypt (population 94% Muslim)	Sugar water and foods offered after 40 days Newborn swaddled Celebration held on 7th day of life
Ethiopia (population 45% Muslim, 35% Ethiopian Orthodox, 20% animist and other)	Pregnancy is a dangerous time because of evil eye Unfulfilled cravings may cause miscarriage Mother confined 14–40 days postpartum Father may not attend labor and delivery
France (population 90% Catholic)	BCG at birth
Germany (population predominantly Christian)	Breast-feeding BCG at birth
Greece (population 98% Greek Orthodox)	Amulets may be placed on baby or crib BCG at 5–6 years
Haiti (population 80% Catholic, 10% Protestant, 10% Voodoo)	Avoid exposure to cold air during pregnancy May bury placenta beneath the doorway to the home or burn it Infants named after a 1-month confinement Nutmeg, castor oil, or spider webs may be placed on umbilical stump; bellybands may be used
India (population 83% Hindu, 11% Muslim, 6% other)	Cravings during pregnancy are satisfied Birth of son may be festively celebrated BCG at birth
Indonesia (population 88% Muslim)	Many children valued Breast-feeding BCG at birth
Iran (population 98% Muslim)	May place amulets on baby or in room BCG at birth
Iraq (population 97% Muslim)	Fertility of five children rewarded May place amulets on baby or in room BCG at birth
Ireland (population 94% Catholic)	BCG at birth Baptism at 40 days
Israel (population 80% Jewish)	Orthodox Jews do not allow men into labor and delivery Newborn vulnerable to evil 1st week of life—amulets used Male circumcision on 8th day of life

Table 5-4 *Continued*

Italy (population 99% Catholic)	Grandmother may want to give grandson his birth bath Amulets and/or medals may be placed on the baby or in room
Japan (population 84% Buddhist)	Midwives may be used Mother may stay confined up to 100 days Mother may not shower or wash hair for a week
Jordan (population 95% Muslim)	Mother has a 40-day confinement postpartum Males are circumcised on the 7th day Infant rubbed with salt and oil after birth and swaddled
Korea (South) (population 72% Buddhist and Confucianist, 28% Christian)	Father not present at birth Mother avoids exposure to cold and does not drink cold liquids Breast-feeding
Kuwait (population 85% Muslim)	Breast-feeding Amulets used to prevent evil eye BCG at 3½–4 years
Laos (population 85% Buddhist)	Newborns not complimented to avoid evil spirits Colostrum believed to cause diarrhea BCG at birth
Malaysia (population 58% Muslim, 30% Buddhist, 8% Hindu)	Many birth taboos Amulets used Breast-feeding BCG at birth
Mali	BCG at birth
Mexico (population 97% Catholic)	Avoid cold air Be active to have a small, easy-to-deliver baby Coin may be strapped to navel to keep it attractive
Morocco (population 99% Muslim)	BCG at birth
Netherlands	Home births common
Nigeria (population 50% Muslim)	Traditional birth attendants are frequently used BCG at birth
Norway (population 94% Lutheran)	Kangaroo care (baby is carried in a "pocket" that the mother wears) Father may attend delivery Breast-feeding

(continued)

Table 5-4 *Continued*

Pakistan (population 97% Muslim)	Traditional birth attendants BCG at birth
Philippines (population 83% Catholic, 9% Protestant, 5% Muslim)	Symbolic unlocking ritual performed during labor Showers and bathing prohibited for 10 days postpartum New mother dresses in warm clothing BCG at birth
Portugal (population 97% Catholic)	Midwives Mother may consume chicken soup or melted butter after delivery to help uterus return to normal
Russia	Breast-feeding May use amulets
Sweden (population 94% Lutheran)	Low infant mortality rate Breast-feeding
Thailand (population 95% Buddhist)	Mother keeps warm to increase milk supply BCG at birth
Tunisia (population 98% Muslim)	Use of henna to decorate body before going into labor BCG at birth
Vietnam (population 60% Buddhist, 13% Confucianist, 12% Taoist, 3% Catholic, 12% other)	Some type of blossom may be used during labor to symbolically open the cervix Mother drinks only warm liquids during labor Child 1 year old at birth BCG at birth

ªBacillus Calmette-Guérin (BCG) vaccine is used routinely to prevent tuberculosis. The vaccine is not used in the United States, but it is administered in countless other countries.

Source: Adapted from Geissler, E. M. (1998). *Pocket guide: Cultural assessment* (2nd ed.). St. Louis, MO: Mosby. Used with permission.

local newspapers' death notices. It is interesting to observe the regional differences in expressions and that in some locations deaths are merely listed by the person's name and in other locations the event of death evokes comments such as "sunrise. . . sunset" and "departed this life." Table 5–6 is a guide to death rites from selected nations. Table 5–7 lists beliefs that people from different religious backgrounds may have regarding death. Finally, Table 5–8 lists selected cultural traditions in after-death rituals and mourning.

Table 5–5 **Ways of Expressing Death, from Bangor, Maine; Boston, Massachusetts; Dallas, Houston, and San Antonio, Texas; Des Moines, Iowa; Elk Horn, Iowa; Los Angeles, California; and New York City**

Expression	Location	Religion[a]
"Nothing" (only the name of the person, family, and funeral details)	New York, Dallas, Boston, Los Angeles	Catholic, Episcopalian
Passed away	New York, Dallas, Boston, Houston, Elk Horn, Los Angeles	Catholic, Jewish, Baptist, Church of Christ
Died	New York, Dallas, Boston, San Antonio, Bangor, Houston, Des Moines	Baptist, Catholic, Congregational, Christian
Died peacefully	Houston, Bangor, Los Angeles	Catholic, Episcopalian, Jewish
Suddenly	New York	
Passed away peacefully	Houston, Los Angeles	
Entered into the arms of his Lord	San Antonio	Catholic
Departed this life	Dallas	
Went to be with her heavenly father	Houston	
Went to be with her (his, our) Lord	San Antonio	Catholic
Went home to be with God	Houston	
Sunrise ... sunset ...	Houston	Methodist
Departed this life	Houston	Baptist
Passed from this life	Houston	
Deceased	Dallas	Baptist
Expired	Houston	
Unexpectedly	Boston, Bangor	
With his Lord	Houston	
Entered into rest	Boston, San Antonio	Jewish, Catholic

[a]Most death notices do not list the religion of the deceased, and it is difficult to tell unless the funeral is held in a church or synagogue.

Table 5–6   Cross-Cultural Guide to Death Rites from Selected Nations

National Origin of Your Client/Family	Rites When Death Occurs
Afghanistan (population 89% Muslim)	Muslim rites: body generally remains at home—cared for, washed, wrapped in white cloth Mullah often in attendance Friends and family visit Buried in 24 hours Ceremony held 2 days after burial and is followed by a meal
Albania (population 70% Muslim, 20% Orthodox, 10% Catholic)	Muslim rites
Algeria (population 99% Muslim)	Muslim rites
Australia (population 76% Christian)	Cremation and burial both practiced Grieving may be reserved—crying with no wailing
Bahrain (population 100% Muslim)	Muslim rites
Bangladesh (population 83% Muslim, 16% Hindu, 1% other)	Muslim rites
Belize (population 90% Christian)	Demonstrative in grief May have spectacular funerals
Burma (population 85% Buddhist)	May prefer quality rather than quantity of life Dying person may be helped to recall past good deeds Cremation may be preferred
Cambodia Kampuchea (population 95% Buddhist)	Buddhist beliefs as above White clothing worn during 3-month mourning period Some mourners shave their heads
Chad (population 44% Muslim)	Muslim rites
China (population 97% atheist and eclectic)	Initial burial in a coffin; after 7 years, body is exhumed and cremated, and the urn is reburied in a tomb
Cuba (population 85% Catholic)	Family and friends stay with body through night Burial in 24 hours May have holy hour each night for 9 consecutive days
Egypt (population 94% Muslim)	Muslim rites
Ethiopia (population 45% Muslim, 35% Ethiopian Orthodox, 20% Animist and other)	Muslim rites Loud wailing may be a normal grief reaction

Table 5–6 *Continued*

National Origin of Your Client/Family	Rites When Death Occurs
France (population 90% Catholic)	Chrysanthemums used exclusively for funerals
Germany (population predominantly Christian)	Crying in private is expected Cremation may be selected
Greece (population 98% Greek Orthodox)	May isolate dying person and withhold truth Death at home important Person buried; exhumed in 5 years and bones reburied in urn or vault Widow wears dark mourning clothes for rest of life
Haiti (population 80% Catholic, 10% Protestant, 10% Voodoo)	Burial in 24 hours White clothing represents death
India (population 83% Hindu, 11% Muslim, 6% other)	Non-Hindus ought not touch body; wash body themselves Cremation is preferred Reincarnation is a Hindu belief
Indonesia (population 88% Muslim)	Muslim rites
Iran (population 98% Muslim)	Muslim rites Mourning may be loud, obvious, and expressive
Iraq (population 97% Muslim)	Muslim rites
Ireland (population 94% Catholic)	Practice of watching or "waking" the dead originates from keeping vigil to keep evil spirits away from the deceased—now a religious ritual
Israel (population 83% Jewish)	Relatives remain with dying person Eyes must be closed at death Body is never left alone Buried in ground in 24 hours except if Sabbath (Saturday)
Italy (population 99% Catholic)	Before death, fatal diagnosis is not discussed with patient and family
Japan (population 84% Buddhist)	Control public expressions of grief
Jordan (population 95% Muslim)	Muslim rites
Korea (North) (population 95% atheist)	Confucian funeral—elaborate Chief mourner and relatives weep
Korea (South) (population 72% Buddhist and Confucianist, 28% Christian)	Buddhists accept death as birth into another life Family members observe last breath; may respond with loud wailing and display intense emotion *(continued)*

Table 5–6 *Continued*

National Origin of Your Client/Family	Rites When Death Occurs
Kuwait (population 85% Muslim)	Muslim rites
Laos (population 85% Buddhist)	Beliefs in reincarnation White flowers or candles may be placed in the deceased's hands Cremation and burial are practiced
Lebanon (population 75% Muslim)	Muslim rites
Libya	Muslim rites
Malaysia (population 58% Muslim, 30% Buddhist, 8% Hindu)	Muslim rites
Mali	Muslim rites
Mexico (population 97% Catholic)	Family members stay with dying person around the clock Grief may be expressive "Day of the Dead" celebrated in November
Morocco (population 99% Muslim)	Muslim rites
Netherlands	Active euthanasia permitted under certain circumstances
Nigeria (population 50% Muslim)	Muslim rites
Norway (population 94% Lutheran)	Close family members stay with person; no one should die alone Cremation and/or burial
Oman	Muslim rites
Pakistan (population 97% Muslim)	Muslim rites
Philippines (population 83% Catholic, 9% Protestant, 5% Muslim)	Muslim rites Protect person from knowing prognosis Emotional grief may occur after death
Portugal (population 97% Catholic)	Widow wears black and never remarries Visit grave frequently
Russia	Family is told of serious illness and decides if patient should know
Sweden (population 94% Lutheran)	Quiet and open grief acceptable Dying person not left alone Body usually not viewed after death
Thailand (population 95% Buddhist)	Beliefs in reincarnation
Tunisia (population 98% Muslim)	Muslim rites

Table 5-6 *Continued*

National Origin of Your Client/Family	Rites When Death Occurs
Vietnam (population 60% Buddhist, 13% Confucianist, 12% Taoist, 3% Catholic, 12% other)	Death at home preferred Body washed and wrapped in white sheets Burial in ground

Source: Adapted from Geissler, E. M. (1994). *Pocket guide: Cultural assessment.* St. Louis, MO: Mosby; Lipson, J. G., Dibble, S. L., & Minarik, P. A. (1996). *Cultural and nursing care: A pocket guide.* San Francisco: UCSF Nursing Press. Used with permission.

Table 5-7 Religious Groups and Death Beliefs

Religious Group	Is There a Heaven?	What Is Heaven Like?	Belief in Resurrection?	Recognition of Friends and Relatives	Is Cremation Allowed?
Assemblies of God	Heaven is a real place	A pleasant place	Of the body	Yes	Not encouraged
Baha'is	Heaven designates spiritual proximity to God	An eternal spiritual evolution of the soul	Spiritual	Yes	No
Baptists	A place where the redeemed go	Filled with mansions and golden streets	Physical	Yes	Allowed but not encouraged
Buddhists	Numerous heavens	It has no independent existence	No future time is foreseen	See living friends and relatives but are not seen	Preferred
Churches of Christ	Dwelling place of God and future residence of the righteous	A realm of peace and love	Consciousness leaves body at death and takes rebirth until enlightened	Yes	Permitted
Hindus	A relative-plane of existence to which souls go to after death	Dwellers in heaven enjoy long life and are free from thirst, hunger, and old age	Liberation of the soul	Visions	Most common method for disposing of body

(continued)

Table 5-7 *Continued*

Religious Group	Is There a Heaven?	What Is Heaven Like?	Belief in Resurrection?	Recognition of Friends and Relatives	Is Cremation Allowed?
Jews	Place where anxiety and travail are ended	Quiet, peaceful intellectual activity takes place	Yes, some only in soul	Yes	Not practiced
Lutherans	Believe in heaven	Nature unknown	Physical	Yes	Yes
Mormons	There are three "degrees of glory"	Places of continuing growth and progress	Yes	Yes	Yes, but not encouraged
Muslims	Several layers, usually seven	A garden	Describe afterlife as physical pains and pleasures	Some believe families are reunited	Not practiced
Roman Catholics	A condition: eternal fullness of life	Supreme happiness flowing from intimacy with God	Physical	Entire community together	Disposal of body does not affect afterlife
Seventh-day Adventists	A being in the presence of God	Will be located in the renewed earth	Glorified body will be resurrected for life to come	Yes	No objection
United Methodists	Heaven exists	Being in the presence of God	Body and spirit	Yes	Yes

Source: Adapted from Johnson, C. J., & McGee, M. G. (Eds.). (1991). *How different religions view death and afterlife.* Philadelphia: The Charles Press.

Table 5-8 Cultural Traditions in Mourning and After-Death Rituals

Religion of Your Patient/Family	Rituals You May Observe When Death Occurs
American Indian religions	Beliefs and practices vary widely Seeing an owl is omen of death
Buddhism	Believe in impermanence Last-rite chanting at bedside Cremation common Pregnant women should avoid funerals to prevent bad luck for baby
Catholicism	Obligated to take ordinary, not extraordinary, means to prolong life Sacrament of the sick Autopsy, organ donation acceptable Burial usual
Christian Science	Euthanasia contrary to teachings Do not seek medical help to prolong life Do not donate body parts Disposal of body and parts decided by family
Hinduism	Seen as opposite of birth—a passage—expect rebirth Autopsy, organ donation—acceptable Religious prayers chanted before and after death Men and women display outward grief Cremation common; ashes disposed of in holy rivers Thread is tied around wrist to signify a blessing—do not remove
Islam	Euthanasia prohibited Organ donation acceptable Autopsy only for medical or legal reasons Body washed only by Muslim of same gender
Jehovah's Witnesses	Euthanasia forbidden Autopsy acceptable if legally necessary Donations of body parts forbidden Burial determined by family preference
Judaism	Autopsy, organ donation not acceptable Euthanasia prohibited Life support not mandated Body ritually washed Burial as soon as possible Seven-day mourning period
Mormonism	Euthanasia not practiced Promote peaceful and dignified death Organ donation individual choice Burial in "temple clothes"

(continued)

Table 5-8 *Continued*

Religion of Your Patient/Family	Rituals You May Observe When Death Occurs
Protestantism	Organ donation, autopsy, and burial or cremation usually individual decisions Prolonging life may have restrictions Euthanasia—varies
Seventh-day Adventism	Prefer prolonging life Euthanasia—no Autopsy, organ donation acceptable Disposal of body and burial—individual decisions

Source: Adapted from Lipson, J. G., Dibble, S. L., & Minarik, P. A. (1996). *Cultural and nursing care: A pocket guide.* San Francisco: UCSF Nursing Press. Used with permission.

Expressions of death and death rituals are also found in objects. Figure 5–11 depicts several objects that may be used.

■ Masks represent methods people use to hide from the "Angel of Death." Masks may also be placed on the face of the deceased. The mask is from Africa.

■ A bride and groom skeleton convey the message that marriage is forever, even unto death. The souls of the bride and groom are united for eternity. Statues such as the one in Figure 5–11 are frequently displayed during the celebration of *Dia de las Muertos,* the Mexican Day of the Dead, on November 2.

■ Candles are used by many people after a death as a way of lighting the way for the soul of the deceased.

■ Jade stone, from China, is placed in orifices of the body to block the entrance of evil spirits after death.

■ Ghost money, from China, is burned to send payments to a deceased person and to ensure his or her well-being in the afterlife.

Intersections of HEALTH, HEALING, and RELIGION

There are several areas in which there is an intersection of HEALTH, HEALING, and RELIGION. The following are examples of additional spiritual/religious factors that link with the myriad of facets that have been described earlier in

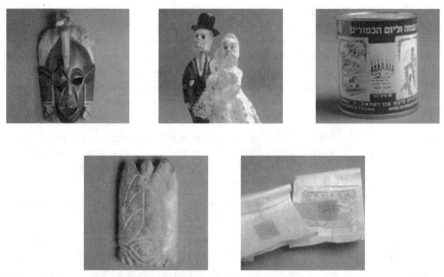

Figure 5-11 Death mask, Africa; couple—Day of the Dead, Mexico; candle, Israel; jade stone, China; and ghost money.

this chapter and in Chapter 4. One's religious affiliation may be seen as providing many links in a complex chain of life events. Religious affiliation frequently provides a background for a person regarding HEALTHY behavior and contributes to HEALTH. Participation in religious practices provides social support and this in turn brings HEALTH. In addition, religious worship may create positive emotions; this, too, contributes to HEALTH. Table 5–9 illustrates several of these intersections, which must be known by health care providers.

This chapter has been no more than an overview of the topics introduced. The amount of relevant knowledge could fill many books. The issues raised here are those that have special meaning to the practice of nursing, medicine, and health care delivery. We must be aware (1) of what people are thinking that may differ from our own thoughts and (2) that sources of help exist outside the modern medical community. As the beliefs of ethnic communities are explored in later chapters, the text discussions will attempt to delineate who are specifically recognized and used as HEALERS by the members of the communities, and will describe some of the forms of treatment used by each community.

Table 5-9 **Areas of Intersection Between the Provision of Health Care and HEALTH, HEALING, and RELIGION**

Communication	Spirituality and religion begin in silence; however, the need for adequate interpreters has been addressed, but it is also imperative to have available to people the members and leaders of their faith community who can reach out and interpret what is happening in regard to a health crisis at a deeper and spiritual level for the patient and family
Gender	Understand the "rules" for gender care; in many faith traditions—for example, among Orthodox Jews and Muslims—care must be gender-specific and people of opposite genders may be forbidden to be touched by someone of the opposite gender
Modesty	Religious and elderly people may be extremely modest and modesty *must* be safe-guarded at all times
Diet	There are many food taboos predicated by one's religion and consideration must be given to see that improper foods are not served to patients
Objects	Sacred objects, such as amulets and statues, must be allowed in the patient's space and all precautions must be observed to safeguard them
Social organization	Spirituality or a religious background contributes many positive factors to the health care situation; collaboration with the leaders of a faith community can result in strongly positive outcomes for a patient and family
Space	Space must be defined and allocated for the patient's and family's private use
Time	Health care providers must be knowledgeable about sacred time—for example, what day the patient and family observe as a day of rest—Friday for Muslims, Friday sunset until Saturday sunset for Jews and Seventh-day Adventists, and Sunday for Christians; calendars must be posted that note holidays for all the faith traditions of people served within a given institution; meetings should not be held on these dates; Appendix B contains a list of religious holidays that do not occur on the same date each year; clergy within the faith tradition must be contacted to provide the dates for the holidays on a yearly basis

Explore ⊕ MediaLink

Go to the Companion Website at www.prenhall.com/spector for chapter-related review questions, case studies, and activities. Contents of the CulturalCare Guide and CulturalCare Museum can also be found on the Companion Website. Click on Chapter 5 to select the activities for this chapter.

Internet Sources

Fatima, A grace for Mankind. (2006). http://www.ewtn.com/fatima

Lourdes-France.org. (2008). Numerous links to information and history of the site. Lourdes, France: Author. Retrieved March 2, 2008 from http://www.lourdesfrance.org/index.php?goto_centre=ru&contexte=en&id=405

The University of Texas at Brownsville and Texas Southmost University. (2006). *El Nino Fidencio, Curanderismo* Research Project. Brownsville, Texas: Author. Retrieved March 1, 2008 from http://vpea.utb.edu/elnino/fidencio.html

References

Ausubel, N. (1964). *The book of Jewish knowledge.* New York: Crown.

Bishop, G. (1967). *Faith healing: God or fraud?* Los Angeles: Sherbourne.

Blattner, B. (1981). *Holistic nursing.* Englewood Cliffs, NJ: Prentice Hall.

Buxton, J. (1973). *Religion and healing in Mandari.* Oxford: Clarendon.

Cramer, E. (1923). *Divine science and healing.* Denver: The Colorado College of Divine Science.

Ford, P. S. (1971). *The healing trinity: Prescriptions for body, mind, and spirit.* New York: Harper & Row.

Foy, F. A. (Ed.). (1980). *Catholic almanac.* Huntington, IN: Our Sunday Visitor.

Gardner, D. (1992). *Niño Fidencio: A heart thrown open.* Santa Fe: Museum of New Mexico Press.

Geissler, E. M. (1994). *Pocket guide: Cultural assessment.* St. Louis: Mosby.

Geissler, E. M. (1998). *Pocket guide: Cultural assessment* (2nd ed.). St. Louis: Mosby.

Hallam, E. (1994). *Saints.* New York: Simon & Schuster.

Illich, I. (1975). *Medical nemesis: The expropriation of health.* London: Marion Bogars.

Informational brochure. (1953). *Shrine of Our Lady of La Leche.* St. Augustine, FL, (personal visit, 1999).

Informational brochure. (1999). *Shrine of the Blessed Virgin Mary.* Christ of the Hills Monastery, Blanco, TX, (personal visit, 1997).

Informational brochure. (n.d.). *Chimayo, New Mexico, the Shrine of our Lord of Esquipulas.*

Johnson, C. J., & McGee, M. G. (Eds.). (1991). *How different religions view death and afterlife.* Philadelphia: Charles Press.

Kelsey, M. T. (1973). *Healing and Christianity.* New York: Harper & Row.

Krieger, D. (1979). *The therapeutic touch.* Englewood Cliffs, NJ: Prentice Hall.

Krippner, S., & Villaldo, A. (1976). *The realms of healing.* Millbrae, CA: Celestial Arts.

Lipson, J. G., Dibble, S. L., & Minarik, P. A. (1996). *Cultural and nursing care: A pocket guide.* San Francisco: UCSF Nursing Press.

Monthly Missalette, 15(13) (1980, February), 38.

Morgenstern, J. (1966). *Rites of birth, marriage, death and kindred occasions among the Semites.* Chicago: Quadrangle Books.

Naegele, K. (1970). *Health and healing.* San Francisco: Jossey-Bass.

Nightingale, F. (1860, 1946). (A facsimile of the first edition published by D. Appleton and Co.). *Notes on nursing—What it is, what it is not.* New York: Appleton-Century.

Progoff, I. (1959). *Depth psychology and modern man.* New York: McGraw-Hill.

Russell, A. J. (1937). *Healing in his wings.* London: Methuen.

Shames, R., & Sterin, C. (1978). *Healing with mind power.* Emmaus, PA: Rodale Press.

Shaw, W. (1975). *Aspects of Malaysian magic.* Kuala Lumpur, Malaysia: Nazibum Negara.

Wallace, G. (1979, November). Spiritual care—A reality in nursing education and practice. *The Nurses Lamp, 5*(2), 1–4.

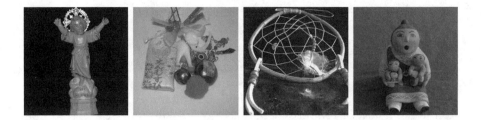

Chapter 6

Familial HEALTH Traditions

As modern medicine becomes more impersonal, people are recalling with some wistfulness old country cures administered by parents and grandparents over the generations.

—*F. Kennet (1976)*

■ Objectives

1. Trace your family's heritage.
2. Describe your family's beliefs and practices in
   a. Health/HEALTH maintenance
   b. Health/HEALTH protection
   c. Health/HEALTH restoration
   d. Curing/HEALING
3. Compare and contrast the difference and similarities between you and your peers in respect to beliefs and practices in
   a. Health/HEALTH maintenance
   b. Health/HEALTH protection
   c. Health/HEALTH restoration
   d. Curing/HEALING

A baby is born—a new life begins. The child may go home with birth parents, foster parents, or adoptive parents and to a nuclear, an extended, or a single-parent family with parents who have lived in this country for many generations or are immigrants, who are heritage consistent or heritage inconsistent. The images in the chapter opener portray several examples of objects used to protect family members' HEALTH and to transmit the family's traditional heritage. Many folk, or traditional, methods may be used to "create" a baby and safeguard it once born. The first image is that of the Infant of Prague and was purchased from a *Santera* in a *botanica* in the metropolitan Boston area. She recommended that this statue be placed in the room of a couple desiring to conceive and told of several women who had successfully used it for this purpose. The next image contains three items, from Japan, Armenia, and Mexico, that may be placed on a baby's crib for HEALTH protection. The dream catcher, in the third image, is from the American Indian Ojibway Nation. It is believed that dreams have magical qualities. The dream catcher is placed on an infant's cradleboard or hung in its room. When hung, the dream catcher captures dreams as they go by—good dreams drift gently through it, with the help of the feathers, to the sleeping baby; bad dreams are captured in the web and discarded. The crystal is hung in the center to enhance the dreams. The last image represents the need to pass heritage from one generation to the next—here an American Indian grandmother is telling the family's stories to the children.

What are your family's traditional HEALTH beliefs and practices? What family stories have been passed to you from your parents and grandparents? If you could choose four ways to present the HEALTH traditions from your family's heritage, what would they be?

Given the now apparent difficulty of defining *health*/HEALTH and *illness*/ILLNESS, it can be assumed that you may have little or no working knowledge of personally practiced "folk medicine," or traditional medicine, within your own family, or you may come from a family where traditional HEALTH and ILLNESS beliefs and practices constitute a significant part of your daily life.

In addition to exploring the already described questions regarding the definitions of *health* and *illness*, it is beneficial to your understanding to describe how you maintain, protect, and/or restore your *health*/HEALTH. Common forms of self-medication and treatment are the use of aspirin for headaches and colds and occasional vitamin supplements. Initially, one may admit to using tea, honey, and lemon and hot or cold compresses for headaches and minor aches and pains. For the most part, however, we tend to look to the health care system for the prevention and treatment of illness.

There is an extremely rich tradition in the United States related to self-care. This includes the early use of patent medicines. Throughout most of their history, patent medicines enjoyed a free existence and were very popular with the people of the times. Some of the most popular medicines of the early 20th century contained alcohol; others contained opium and cocaine. This increased their popularity, and the practice continued until passage of the Food, Drug, and Cosmetic Act of 1938 (Armstrong & Armstrong, 1991). Today, as our lives become more complex and the health care system becomes more complicated, costly, and difficult to access, we see a return to self-care and an increasing use of traditional and homeopathic health care systems (see Chapters 4 and 5).

■ Familial Health/HEALTH Traditions

We are now ready for a transition and it is time to begin climbing the steps to CULTURALCOMPETENCY. The foundation—a discussion of heritage, an overview of demographic issues, an exploration of terms such as *health* and *illness*, and a discussion of HEALTH and ILLNESS as they relate to religion and spirituality—has been created and what remains is the ascent! Before you read on, ask yourself the following questions regarding your health/HEALTH beliefs and practices:

- What remedies and/or methods do you use to maintain, protect, and restore your health/HEALTH?
- Do you know the health/HEALTH and illness/ILLNESS beliefs and practices that were or are a part of your heritage?
- Were you ever thought to be mortally ill/ILL?
- What did your familial caregiver do to take care of you?
- Did he or she consult someone in your own ethnic or religious community to find out what was wrong?

It has been mentioned earlier in this text that the first step for developing CULTURALCOMPETENCY is to know yourself, your heritage, and the health/HEALTH and illness/ILLNESS beliefs and practices derived from your heritage—ethnic, religious, or both. It was pointed out in Chapters 4 and 5 that many daily HEALTH practices have their origins in one's heritage yet may not be thought of in this context.

The following interview procedure is useful for making you aware of the overall history and health/HEALTH belief and practice–related folklore and ethnocultural knowledge of your family. Because the ethnocultural history of each family is unique, you may want to discover more than health/HEALTH beliefs and practices with this interview. Ask your parents or grandparents questions about your family surname, traditional first names, family stories, the history of family "characters" or notorious family members, how historical events affected your family in past generations, and so forth. Then, in interviewing your grandmothers, great-aunts, and mother, obtain answers to the following questions:

1. What is their family's heritage—their country of origin? Ethnic background? Religion?
2. What did they do to maintain health/HEALTH? What did their mothers do?
3. What did they do to protect health/HEALTH? What did their mothers do?
4. Do they wear, carry, or hang in their home objects that protect their HEALTH and home?
5. Do they follow a particular dietary regimen or refrain from eating restricted foods?

Physical, mental, and spiritual aspects are implicit in each of the next three questions:

6. What home remedies do they use to restore health/HEALTH? What did their mothers use?

7. What are their traditional beliefs regarding pregnancy and childbirth?
8. What are their traditional beliefs regarding dying and death?

There are two reasons for exploring your familial heritage. First, it draws your attention to your ethnocultural and religious heritage and HEALTH-related belief system. Many of your daily habits relate to early socialization practices that are passed on by parents or additional significant others. Many behaviors are both subconscious and habitual, and much of what you believe and practice is passed on in this manner. By digging into the past, remote and recent, you can recall some of the rituals you observed either your parents or your grandparents perform. You are then better able to realize their origin and significance. There are many beliefs and practices that are ethnically similar, and socialization patterns may tend to be similar among ethnic groups as well. Religion also plays a role in the perception of, interpretation of, and behavior in health/HEALTH and illness/ILLNESS.

The maternal side is ideal for your interview because, in today's society of interethnic and interreligious marriages and complex family structures, it is assumed that the ethnic beliefs and practices related to health/HEALTH and illness/ILLNESS of the family may be more in tune with the mother's family than with the father's. By and large, family nurturance and health/HEALTH maintenance, protection, and/or restoration have been the domain of women in most cultures and societies. The mother tends to be the person within a family who cares for family members when illness/ILLNESS occurs. She also tends to be the prime mover in protecting health/HEALTH and seeking health/HEALTH care. It is the mother who tells the child what and how much to eat and drink, when to go to bed, and how to dress in inclement weather. She shares her knowledge and experience with her offspring, but usually the daughter is singled out for such experiential sharing. However, this is not a "universal" circumstance and in many heritages it is the father who is the family caregiver. If that is true for your family, it is your paternal family whom you must interview. Given the complex familial changes and social changes related to family life, it behooves you to question both your maternal and your paternal relatives.

The second reason for this examination of familial health/HEALTH practices is to sensitize you to the role your ethnocultural and religious heritage has played. You must reanalyze the concepts of health/HEALTH and illness/ILLNESS and view your own definitions from another perspective. If your familial background is presented in a class or another group setting, the peer group is able to see the people in a different light. A group observes similarities and differences among its members. You discover peer beliefs and practices that you originally had no idea existed. You may then be able to identify the "why" behind many daily health/HEALTH habits, practices, and beliefs in your family.

You may be amazed to discover the origins of the health/HEALTH practices. The "mysterious" behavior of a roommate or friend may be explained by reflecting on its origin. It is interesting to discover cross-ethnic practices within one's own group, as some people believe that a given practice is an "original," done only by their family. Many religious customs, such as the blessing of the throat, are now conceptualized in terms of health/HEALTH behavior. Table 6–1

Table 6-1 **Family Health Histories Obtained from Students of Various Ethnic Backgrounds and Religions**

Austrian (United States), Jewish

HEALTH Maintenance

Bake own bread
Eat wholesome foods, homegrown fruits and vegetables

HEALTH Protection

Camphor around the neck (in the winter) in a small cloth bag to prevent measles and scarlet fever

HEALTH Restoration

Boils: fry chopped onions, make a compress, and apply to the infections
Sore throat: go to the village store, find a salted herring, wrap it in a towel, put it around the neck, and let it stay there overnight; gargle with salt water

Black and Native American, Baptist

HEALTH Maintenance

Dress right for the weather
Eat balanced meals three times a day

HEALTH Protection

Blackstrap molasses
Keep everything clean and sterile
Regular checkups
Stay away from people who are sick

HEALTH Restoration

Bloody nose: place keys on a chain around neck to stop
Sore throat: suck yolks out of eggshell; honey and lemon; baking soda, salt, warm water; onions around the neck; salt water to gargle

Black African (Ethiopia), Orthodox Christian

HEALTH Maintenance

Keep the area clean
Pray every morning when getting up from bed

HEALTH Protection

Eat hot food, such as pepper, fresh garlic, lemon

HEALTH Restoration

Eat hot and sour foods, such as lemons, fresh garlic, hot mustard, red pepper
Make a kind of medicine from leaves and roots of plants mixed together
Colds: hot boiled milk with honey
Evil eye: they put some kind of plant root on fire and make the man who has the evil eye smile and the man talks about his illness

(continued)

Table 6-1 *Continued*

Canadian, Catholic

HEALTH Maintenance

Cleanliness
Food: people should eat well (fat people used to be considered healthy)
Prayer: HEALTH was always mentioned in prayer

HEALTH Protection

Elixirs containing herbs and brewed, given as a vitamin tonic
Lots of good food
Sleep
Wear camphor around the neck to ward off any evil spirit; use Father John's medicine
  November to May

HEALTH Restoration

Aches and pains: hot Epsom salt baths
Colds: hot lemons
Cough: shot of whiskey
Eye infections: potatoes are rubbed on them or a gold wedding ring is placed on them and
  the sign of the cross is made three times
Fever: lots of blankets and heat make you sweat out a fever
Headache: lie down and rest in complete darkness
Infected wounds: raw onions placed on wounds
Kidney problems: herbal teas
Sinuses: camphor placed in a pouch and pinned to the shirt

Eastern Europe (United States), Jewish

HEALTH Maintenance

Doctor only when pregnant (grandmother)
Go to doctor when sick (mother)
Health care for others, not self (mother)
Health for self not a priority (grandmother)
Physician twice a year (mother)
Reluctantly sought medical help (grandmother)

HEALTH Protection

Not much to prevent illness—very ill today with chronic diseases (grandmother)
Observe precautions, such as dressing warmly, not going out with wet hair, getting enough
  rest, staying in bed if not feeling well (mother)
Vitamins and water pills

HEALTH Restoration

Colds: fluids, aspirin, rest
Insomnia: glass of wine
Muscle aches: massage with alcohol
Sore throat: gargle with salt water, tea with lemon and honey
Stomach upset: eat light and bland foods
Chicken soup used by mother and grandmother

Table 6–1 *Continued*

English, Baptist

HEALTH Maintenance

Daily walks
Eat well
Keep warm
Read

HEALTH Restoration

Cold: heat glass and put on back
Earache: honey and tea; warm cod-liver oil in ear; stay in bed

English, Catholic

HEALTH Maintenance

Bedroom window open at night
Good housekeeping
Immediate cleanup after meals; wash pan before meals
Lots of exercise, proper sleep; lots of walking; no drinking or smoking; hard work
Never wear dirty clothing
Rest
Take baths

HEALTH Protection

Keep kitchen at 90°F in winter and house will be warm
Maintain a good diet: fresh vegetables, vitamins, little meat, lots of fish, no fried foods; lots of
  sleep
Strict enforcement of lifestyle

HEALTH Restoration

Colds: chicken soup; herb tea made from roots; alcohol concoctions; Vicks and hot towels on
  chest; lots of fluids, rest; Vicks, sulfur and molasses
Cuts: wet tobacco
Rashes: burned linen and cornstarch
Sore throat: four onions and sugar steeped to heal and soothe the throat

English, Episcopal

HEALTH Maintenance

Cod-liver oil
Enough sleep
Thorough diet, vitamins

HEALTH Restoration

Colds and sore throats: camphor on chest and red scarves around chest

(continued)

Table 6-1 *Continued*

French (France), Catholic

HEALTH Maintenance

Proper food; rest; proper clothing; cod-liver oil daily

HEALTH Protection

Every spring give sulfur and molasses for 3 days as a laxative to get rid of worms

HEALTH Restoration

Colds: rub chest with Vicks; honey

French Canadian, Catholic

HEALTH Maintenance

Wear rubbers in the rain and dress warmly; take part in sports; active body; lots of sleep

HEALTH Protection

Cod-liver oil in orange juice
No "junk foods"; play outside; walk; daily use of Geritol; camphor on clothes; balanced meals
Sulfur and molasses in spring to clear the system

HEALTH Restoration

Back pain: mustard packs
Colds: brandy with warm milk; honey and lemon juice; hot poultice on the chest; tea,
    whiskey, and lemon
Rashes: oatmeal baths
Sore throat: wrap raw potatoes in sack and tie around neck; soap and water enemas
Warts: rub potato on wart, run outside and throw it over left shoulder

German (United States), Catholic

HEALTH Maintenance

Good diet
Take aspirin
Take shots
Wash before meals; change clothes often
Wear rubbers; never go barefoot; long underwear and stockings

HEALTH Protection

Cod-liver oil
Drink glass of water at meals
Exercise
No sweets at meals
Plenty of milk
Spring tonic; sulfured molasses

Table 6–1 *Continued*

HEALTH Restoration

Coughs: honey and lemon; hot water and Vicks; boiled onion water, honey and vinegar
Constipation: Ivory soap suppositories
Cramps: ginger tea
Earache: few drops of warm milk in the ear; laxatives when needed
Fever: mix whiskey, water, and lemon juice and drink before bed—causes person to perspire and break fever
Headache: boil a beef bone and break up toast in the broth and drink
Recovery diet: boil milk and shredded wheat and add a dropped egg—first thing eaten after an illness
Sore back: hot mustard plaster
Sore throat: saltwater gargle
Stye: cold tea-leaf compress
Swollen glands or mumps: put pepper on salt pork and tie around the neck

Iran (United States), Islam

HEALTH Maintenance

Cleanliness
Diet

HEALTH Protection

Dress properly for the season and weather; keep feet from getting wet in the rain
Inoculations

HEALTH Restoration

Cough: honey and lemon
Indigestion: baking soda and water
Rashes: apply cornstarch
Sore throat: gargle with vinegar and water
Sore muscles: alcohol and water

Irish (Catholic)

HEALTH Maintenance

Attitudes important: "good living habits and good thinking"; "eat breakfast—if late for school, eat a good breakfast and be a little late"; "don't be afraid to spend on groceries— you won't spend on the doctor later"
Avoid "fast foods"
Be clean, wear clean clothes
Blessing of the throat
Brush teeth; if out of toothpaste use table salt, or Ivory soap, or Dr. Lyon's Tooth Powder
Dress warmly
Early to bed ("rest is the best medicine")
Good food, balanced diet
Keep clean
Keep feet warm and dry

(continued)

Table 6-1 *Continued*

Health Maintenance *(continued)*

Outdoor exercise, enjoy fresh air and sunshine
Plenty of rest
Vitamins
Wear holy medals, green scapular

HEALTH Protection

Avoid sick people
Be goal-oriented
Clean out bowels with senna for 8 days
Drink senna tea at every vacation—cleans out the system
During flu season, tie a bag of camphor around the neck
Eat lots of oily foods
Every spring, drink a mixture of sulfur and molasses to clean blood
Maintain a strong family with lots of love
Never go to bed with wet hair
Nurture a strong religious faith
Onions under the bed to keep nasal passages clear
Prevent evil spirits: don't look in mirror at night and close closet doors
Take Father John's medicine every so often

HEALTH Restoration

Chicken soup for everything from colds to having a baby
See doctor only in emergency
Acne: apply baby's urine
Backache: apply hot oatmeal in a sock; place a silver dollar on the sore area, light a match to
  it; while the match is burning, put a glass over the silver dollar and then slightly lift the
  glass, and this causes a suction, which is said to lift the pain out
Boils: cooked oatmeal wrapped in a cloth (steaming hot) applied to drain pus; oatmeal
  poultice
Colds: tea and toast; chest rub; vaporizer; hot lemonade and a tablespoon of whiskey;
  mustard plasters; Vicks on chest; whiskey; Vicks in nostrils; hot milk with butter, soups,
  honey, hot toddies, lemon juice and egg whites; ipecac ("cruel but good medicine");
  whiskey with hot water and sugar; soak feet in hot water and sip hot lemonade; Boiled
  wines; coffee with anisette
Colic: warm oil on stomach
Coughs: cough syrup (available on stove all winter) made from honey and whiskey; Vicks on
  chest; mustard plaster on chest; onion-syrup cough medicine; steam treatment; swallow
  Vicks; linseed poultice on chest; flaxseed poultice on back, red flannel cloth soaked in hot
  water and placed on chest all night
Cramps: creme de menthe
Cuts: boric acid
Earache: heat salt, put in stocking behind the ear
Fever: spirits of niter on a dry sugar cube or mix with water: cold baths; alcohol rubdowns;
  cover with blankets to sweat it out

Table 6–1 *Continued*

Headache: fill a soup bowl with cold water and put some olive oil in a large spoon; hold the spoon over the bowl in front of the person with the headache; while doing this, recite words in Italian and place index finger in the oil in the spoon: drop three drops of oil from the finger into the bowl; by the diameter of the circle the oil makes when it spreads in the water, the severity of the headache can be determined (larger = more severe); after this is done three times, the headache is gone; or place a hot poultice on forehead; hot facecloth; cold, damp cloth to forehead; in general, stay in bed, get plenty of rest and sleep, a glass of juice about once an hour, aspirin, and lots of food to get back strength; kerchief with ice in it is wrapped around the head; mint tea

High blood pressure: in Italy for high blood pressure, colonies of blood suckers were kept in clay, where they were born; the person with high blood pressure would have a blood sucker put on his fanny, where it would suck blood; it was thought that this would lower his blood pressure; the blood suckers would then be thrown in ashes and would then throw up the blood they had sucked from the person. If the blood sucker died, it altered the person to see a doctor because it sometimes meant that there was something wrong with the person's blood

Insect bites: vaseline or boric acid

Menstrual cramps: hot milk sprinkled with ginger; shot of whiskey, glass of warm wine; warm teas; hot-water bottle on stomach

Muscle pain: heat up carbon leaves (herb) and bundle in a hot cloth to make a pack (soothes any discomfort)

Nausea and other stomach ailments: hot teas; castor oil; hot ginger ale; bay leaf; cup of hot boiled water; potato for upset stomach; baking soda; gruel

Pimples: to draw contents, apply hot flaxseed

Poison ivy: yellow soap suds

Sore throat: honey; apply Vicks on throat at bedtime and wrap up the throat; paint throat with iodine, honey and lemon, Karo syrup; paint with kerosene oil internally with a rag and then tie a sock around the neck; paint with iodine or Mercurochrome and gargle with salt and water, honey, melted Vicks

Splinters: flaxseed poultice

Sprains: beat egg whites, apply to part, wrap part

Stomachache: camilla and maloa (herbs) added to boiled water

Stye: hot tea bag to area

Sucking thumb: apply hot pepper to thumb

Sunburn: apply vinegar; put milk on cloth and apply to burn; a cold, wet tea bag on small areas such as eyelids

To build up blood: eggnog with brandy; marsala wine and milk

Toothache: whiskey applied topically

Upset stomach: herb tea made with herbs sent from Italy

Italian (United States), Catholic

HEALTH Maintenance

Eat (solved emotional and physical problems); fruit at end of meal cleans teeth; early to bed and early to rise

Hearty and varied nutritional intake; lots of fruit, pasta, wine (even for childern), cheese, home grown vegetables, and salads; exercise in form of physical labor; molasses on a piece of bread, or oil and sugar on bread; hard bread (good for the teeth)

(continued)

Table 6–1 *Continued*

HEALTH Maintenance *(continued)*

Pregnancy:
Two weeks early: girl
Two weeks late: boy
Heartburn: baby with lots of hair

Health Protection

Eat properly
Garlic cloves strung on a piece of string around the neck of infants and children to prevent colds and "evil" stares from other people, which they believed could cause headaches and a pain or stiffness in the back or neck (a piece of red ribbon or cloth on an infant served the same purpose)
If infants got their nights and days mixed up, they were tied upside down and turned all the way around
Keep feet warm
Keep warm in cold weather
Never wash hair before going outdoors or at night
Never wash hair or bathe during period
Stay out of drafts
To prevent bowlegs and keep ankles straight, up to the age of 6 to 8 months a bandage was wrapped around the baby from the waist to the feet
To prevent "evil" in the newborn, a scissor was kept open under the mattress of the crib

Norwegian (Norway), Lutheran

HEALTH Maintenance

Cleanliness
Cod-liver oil
Rest

Health Protection

Immunizations

Health Restoration

Colds and sore throat: hot peppermint drink and Vicks

Nova Scotian, Catholic

HEALTH Maintenance

Sleep; proper foods

HEALTH Protection

Cut up some onions and put them on back of stove to cook; feed them to all

Table 6-1 *Continued*

HEALTH Restoration

Cold: boil carrots until jellied, add honey; as expectorant boil onions, add honey

Cold in the back: alcohol was put in a small metal container, a piece of cotton on a stick was placed in the alcohol, ignited, and put in a *banky* (a type of glass resembling a whiskey glass); this was put on the back where the cold was and left for half an hour and a hickeylike rash would develop; it was believed that the rash would drain the cold

Earache: put few drops of heated camphorated oil in ear; melt chicken fat and sugar, put in ear

Earache with infection: to drain the infection, cut a piece of salt pork about 2 inches long and 3/4 inch thick and insert it into the infected ear and leave for a few days

Psoriasis: hang a piece of lead around the neck

Skin ulcer and infection: a sharp blade was sterilized and used to make a small incision in the skin, and live blood suckers were placed in the opening, they would drain the infection out; when the blood sucker was full, it would fall to a piece of paper, be bled, placed in alcohol, and reused

Sore throat: coat a tablespoon of molasses with black pepper

Polish (United States), Catholic

HEALTH Maintenance

Cod-liver oil
Eating good, nutritious foods
Plenty of rest
Use of physician

HEALTH Protection

Eat fresh, homegrown foods
Exercise
Good diet
Good personal hygiene
Work

HEALTH Restoration

Colds: drink hot liquids, chicken soup, honey
Headache: take aspirin, hot liquids
Sore muscles: heating pads and hot compresses

Swedish (United States), Protestant

HEALTH Maintenance

A lot of walking
Cod-liver oil
Eat well-balanced meals
Routine medical examinations

HEALTH Protection

Blessing of the throat on St. Blaise Day
Dress appropriately for weather
Eat an apple a day
Eat sorghum molasses for general, all around good health
"I don't do a blooming thing"; eat well

(continued)

Table 6-1 *Continued*

HEALTH Restoration

Anemia: cod-liver oil
Bee stings: poultice
Black eye: leeches
Congestion: steamy bathroom
Cough: warm milk and butter
Earache: warm oil
Fever: blankets to sweat it out
Lumbago: drink a yeast mixture
Rundown and tired: eat a whole head of lettuce
Sick: lots of juices and decarbonated ginger ale; lots of rest
Sore throat: gargle with salt and take honey in milk; herringbone wrapped in flannel around the neck
Upset stomach: baking soda

lists a sample of responses to the questions that students obtained from members of the maternal side of their families regarding the maintenance, protection, and restoration of health/HEALTH. Table 6–2 describes selected answers to questions regarding birth and death beliefs and practices. These methods, beliefs, and practices are examples to trigger your questions and help you to probe the memories of the person you are questioning.

■ Consciousness Raising

The experience of sharing one's familial HEALTH practices raises one's consciousness in several ways, and helps participants see themselves and others in a different context, and facilitates the understanding of patients' practices.

Recognizing Similarities

In my experience, as discussion continues, people realize that many personal beliefs and practices do, in fact, differ from what they are being taught in nursing or medical education to accept as the right way of doing things. Participants begin to admit that they do not seek medical care when the first symptoms of illness appear. On the contrary, they usually delay seeking care and often elect to self-treat at home. They also recognize that there are many preventive and health maintenance acts learned in school with which they choose not to comply. Sometimes they discover that they are following self-imposed regimen for health-related problems and are not seeking any outside intervention.

Another facet of a group discussion is the participants' exposure to the similarities that exist among them in terms of HEALTH maintenance and protection. To their surprise and delight, they find that many of their daily acts—routines they take for granted—directly relate to methods of maintaining and protecting HEALTH.

Table 6-2 **Examples of Selected Familial Ethnocultural and Religious Beliefs and Practices Related to Birth and Death**

Nation of Origin and Religion	Birth Beliefs	Death Beliefs
Cape Verde—Catholic	Baptism	Death is a part of life
England—Christian	Baptism Natural event	Body dying Everlasting life with Christ Funeral and prayer Person goes to heaven
Germany—Lutheran	Birth is sacred Do not take baby out until it is baptized Mother does not go to the baptism	Body dies when we die—souls go to heaven and enjoy everlasting life Celebrate person's life and the promise of eternal life God's will
Greece—Orthodox	After 40 days mother and newborn go to church—baby is blessed and prayers are said to keep away the evil spirits Baptized at 2 Gifts given to the baby to protect it from the evil eye—charms of white and blue beads are worn on the wrist If the baby cries excessively, exorcism may be performed Wrap the baby in blankets and pin to sheets to relax	After a death light a candle that burns all night Bones are unburied after 3 years, are put into a holy box, and are placed in the church or are reburied in the family grave In mourning, women wear black for the rest of their lives and men grow facial hair Hold a special service on the 40th day Some older people believe in ghosts The good go to paradise; the bad go to hell Visit grave daily
Ireland—Catholic	Baby shower before birth but never set up the crib until after birth Men not present at birth Tell of pregnancy after 3 months	After death, the body is washed and prepared for the wake at home by a neighbor and then the wake and mass Blessing with oils and receive the Eucharist for the last time Dying person wears a Rosary around the neck to keep evil spirits away and God closer

(continued)

Table 6-2 *Continued*

		Dying: pray the Rosary aloud as it is a stepping stone to the Virgin Mary, asking her to watch over this person and guide him or her to everlasting peace Final separation of the soul from the body—soul lives on and is transported to God Mourning: keening—a ritual of professional criers coming to the home and crying for hours over the death of a family member Wake—"a party with one less person"
Italy—Catholic	Life begins at conception	Closed casket Cremation
Japan—Shinto	Umbilical cord saved—a lasting bond between mother and child 100-day-old child taken to the Shrine	Cremation
Lithuania—Catholic	Baptism	Pray for the dead Visit graves
Portugal—Catholic	Throw a party for the birth of a boy (relates to the time when males were needed to work on the farms) Women during pregnancy get less pretty with a girl because the baby is taking her mother's looks	A party comforts the loved ones but if one dies in a painful way there is no celebration Celebrate a painless death—means the person has been good and is now with Jesus Widow must forever wear black—this serves as a warning to other men that she has suffered a loss and is not attractive to prevent shame from being brought to her
Sicily—Catholic	Baptism Gift from God	Close all shades and never go out during daylight The day you were born, it was known the day you were to die Women mourn for years, wearing only black and seldom going outside

As is common in most large groups, students seem to be shy at the beginning of this exploration. As more and more members of the group are willing to share their experiences, however, other students feel more comfortable and share more readily. A classroom tactic I have used to break the ice is to reveal an experience I had on the birth of my first child. My mother-in-law, an immigrant from Eastern Europe, drew a circle around the child's crib with her fingers and spat on the baby three times to prevent the evil spirits from harming him. Once such an anecdote is shared, other participants have less difficulty in remembering similar events that took place in their own homes.

Students have a variety of feelings about the self-care practices of their families. One feeling discussed by many students is shame. A number of students express conflict in their attitudes: They cannot decide whether to believe these old ways or to drop them and adopt the more modern ones they are learning in school. (This is an example of cognitive dissonance.) Many admit that this is the first time they have disclosed these HEALTH beliefs and practices in public, and they are relieved and amazed to discover similarities with other students. Frequently, there is a logical explanation as to why a given practice is successful. The acts may have different names or be performed in a slightly different manner, but the uniting thread among them is to prevent ILLNESS and to maintain HEALTH.

Transference to Patients and Others

The effects of such a verbal catharsis are long remembered and often quoted or referred to throughout the remainder of a course. The awareness we gain helps us understand the behavior and beliefs of patients and, for that matter, other people better. Given this understanding, we are comfortable enough to ask patients how they interpret a symptom and how they think it ought to be treated. We begin to be more sensitive to people who delay in seeking health care or fail to comply with preventive measures and treatment regimens. We come to recognize that we do the same thing. The increased familiarity with home health/HEALTH practices and remedies helps us project this awareness and understanding to the patients who are served.

Analyzed from a "scientific" perspective, the majority of these practices have a sound basis. In the area of health/HEALTH maintenance (see Table 6–1), one notes an almost universal adherence to activities that include rest, balanced diet, and exercise.

In the area of health/HEALTH protection, various differences arise, ranging from visiting a physician to wearing a clove of garlic around the neck. Although the purpose of wearing garlic around the neck is "to keep the evil spirit away," the act also forces people to stay away: what better way to cut down exposure to wintertime colds than to avoid close contact with people?

One person remembered that during her childhood her mother forced her to wear garlic around her neck. Like most children, she did not like to be different from the rest of her schoolmates. As time went on, she began to have frequent colds, and her mother could not understand why this was happening. The mother followed her child to school some weeks later and discovered that she removed the garlic on her way to school, hiding it under a rock and then replacing it on the way home. There was quite a battle between the mother and daughter! The youngster did not like this method of protection because her peers mocked her.

A discussion of home remedies is of further interest when each of the methods presented is analyzed for its possible "medical" analogy and for its prevalence among various religious and ethnic groups. Many of the practices and remedies, to the surprise and relief of students, tend to run throughout groups but have different names or contain different ingredients.

In this day of computers and sophisticated medicine, including transplants, cloning, and intricate surgery, the most prevalent need expressed by people who practice traditional medicine is to protect people and prevent "evil" from harming them or to remove the "evil" that may be the cause of their HEALTH problem. As students, we analyze and discuss a problem and its traditional treatments and we begin to see how evil continues to be considered the cause of ILLNESS and how often the treatment is then designed to remove it.

Each person testifies to the efficacy of a given remedy. Many state that, when their grandmothers and mothers shared these remedies with them, they experienced great feelings of nostalgia for the good old days, when things seemed so simple. Some people may express a desire to return to these practices of yesteryear, whereas others openly confess that they continue to use such measures—sometimes in addition to what a health care provider tells them to use or often without even bothering to consult a provider.

The goal of this kind of consciousness-raising session is to reawaken the participant to the types of health/HEALTH practices within her or his own family. The other purpose of the sharing is to make known the similarities and differences that exist as part of a cross-ethnocultural and religious phenomenon. We are intrigued to discover the wide range of beliefs that exists among our peers' families. We had assumed that people thought and believed as we did. For the first time, we individually and collectively realize that we all practice a certain amount of traditional medicine, that we all have ethnocultural-specific ways of treating ILLNESS, and that we, too, often delay in seeking professional health care. We learn that most people prefer to treat themselves at home and that they have their own ways of treating a particular set of symptoms—with or without a prescribed medical regimen. The previously held notion that "everybody does it this way" is shattered. The greatest challenge in this activity is to encourage students and others to think of HEALTH, rather than simply health. This exercise brings you to the window on the glass door pictured in the introduction.

Explore 🌐 MediaLink

Go to the Companion Website at www.prenhall.com/spector for chapter-related review questions, case studies, and activities. Contents of the CulturalCare Guide and CulturalCare Museum can also be found on the Companion Website. Click on Chapter 6 to select the activities for this chapter.

Folklife Centers

The following is a listing of selected folklife centers in the United States. From these centers, and others readily discovered on the World Wide Web, one may obtain films and literature related to folklife and medicine.

Alabama

The Alabama Folklife Program and The Alabama Folklife Association
410 N. Hull Street
Montgomery, AL 36104
334-242-3601
334-269-9098 Fax
http://www.arts.state.al.us/folklife/folklife.htm

Arizona

Southern Arizona Folklife Center
University of Arizona
Tucson, AZ 85721
520-621-2211
http://www.library.arizona.edu/images/folkarts/folkhome.html

California

Center for Study of Comparative Folklore and Mythology
University of California, Los Angeles
Los Angeles, CA 90024
http://www.folkmed.ucla.edu

Kentucky

Appalshop
P.O. Box 743A
Whitesburg, KY 41858
http://www.appalshop.org

Missouri

Missouri Folk Arts Program
157 McReynolds Hall
University of Missouri–Columbia
Columbia, MO 65211
573-882-6296
573-882-0360 Fax
http://museum.research.missouri.edu/mfap/

New England

Folk Arts Center of New England
42 West Foster Street
Melrose, MA 02176
http://www.facone

Utah

The Utah Arts Council
617 East South Temple
Salt Lake City, UT 84102-1177
801-236-7555 Voice
800-346-4128 TDD
801-236-7556 Fax
http://www.arts.utah.gov/folkarts/

Washington, DC

Within the federal government, resources for folklore and folklife endeavors in Washington, DC, are concentrated in four agencies:

1. The Library of Congress: http://www.loc.gov
2. The Smithsonian Institution: http://www.si.edu
3. National Endowment for the Arts: http://arts.endow.gov/
4. National Endowment of the Humanities: http://www.neh.gov/

American Folklife Center
The Library of Congress
Washington, DC 20540
202-287-6590
Folkline 202-287-2000: a telephone information service, http://www.loc.gov
Folklife Sourcebook: a resource guide to relevant organizations
This center was created by Congress in 1976 to "preserve and present" American folklife. It is an educational and research program.

Archive of Folk Culture
The Library of Congress
Washington, DC 20540
202-287-5510
http://www/loc.gov
This is the public reference and archival arm of the American Folklife Center.

The American Folklore Society
1703 New Hampshire Avenue, NW
Washington, DC 20009
Membership in this society, founded in 1888, is open to all persons interested in folklore. It serves as a forum for the preservation of folklore.

■ References

Armstrong, D., & Armstrong, E. M. (1991). *The great American medicine show.* New York: Prentice Hall.

Kennet, F. (1976). *Folk medicine—Fact and fiction: Age-old cures, alternative medicine, natural remedies.* New York: Crescent Books.

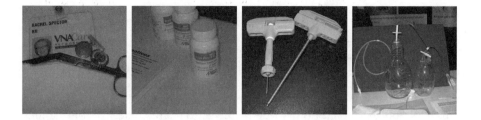

Chapter 7

Health Care Delivery and Issues

◼ Objectives

1. Discuss the professional socialization of nurses, physicians, and other members of the health care delivery system.
2. Describe the "culture" of the health care providers.
3. Compare the growth of the gross domestic product and national health care expenditures over time.
4. Compare the expenditures for health care in the United States with those of other nations.
5. Discuss the costs of health care both as a national issue and as an issue in the area you reside.
6. Itemize how the "dollar" spent for health care is allocated.
7. Recognize the interrelationships and trends of sociocultural, public health, and medical events that have produced the crises in today's modern health care system.
8. Break down the complex web of factors that impede a person's passage through the health care system.
9. Chart the "Amazing Maze of Health Care" and give examples of your personal and professional experience.
10. Describe barriers to health care.
11. Identify the factors that determine medicine to be an Institution of Social Control.
12. Compare and contrast Modern Medical Care and CULTURALCARE.

The chapter-opening images depict symbols related to the modern health care delivery culture and objects used to maintain or restore overall health. The first image portrays selected cultural objects—a nametag, bandage scissors, my school of nursing pin, and a volunteer pin from the American Red Cross. The second image symbolizes medications—whether given to maintain health (for example, vitamins or calcium) or to treat ailments from cardiovascular diseases to mental illnesses, one thing is certain—the costs are usually exorbitant. The third and fourth images depict thoracotomy instruments—the trochanters and underwater chest tube drainage bottles represent the tremendous amount of medical equipment now available that is disposable and the constantly rising costs of all aspects of health care. In fact, as will be discussed in this chapter, it has been frequently demonstrated that the high cost of health care is not proof of high quality (Abelson, 2007, p. A-1) What are the unique symbols of your profession within the overall culture of modern health care? What objects would you choose to represent your experiences of modern health care delivery?

The health care system of this nation has been in crisis, and the visionary words and observations of Dr. John Knowles in 1970 ring true today:

> American medicine, the pride of the nation for many years, stands on the brink of chaos. Our medical practitioners have their great moments of drama and triumph. But, much of U.S. medical care, particularly the everyday business of preventing and treating illness, is inferior in quality, wastefully dispensed, and inequitably financed.

What is it about our health care system and the people who practice within it that generated and continue to generate these comments? This chapter presents an overview of the issues inherent in the acculturation of health care providers and the health care delivery system in the United States. It begins by discussing the norms of the health care provider "cultures" and then examines many of the salient issues regarding the health care system in general.

■ The Health Care Provider's Culture

The providers of health care—nurses; physicians; social workers; dietitians; physical, occupational, respiratory, and speech therapists; laboratory and departmental professionals—are socialized into the culture of their profession. Professional socialization teaches the student a set of beliefs, practices, habits, likes, dislikes, norms, and rituals. Each of the professional disciplines has its own language and objects, rituals, garments, and myths, which become an inherent part of the scope of students' education, socialization, and practice. The providers view time in their own ways and they believe that their view of a health and illness situation and subsequent interventions are the only possible answers to the complex questions surrounding a health-related event. This newly learned information regarding health and illness differs in varying degrees from that of the individual's heritage. As students become more and more immersed and knowledgeable in the scientific and technological domains, they usually move further and further from their past belief systems and, indeed, futher from the population at large in terms of its understanding and beliefs regarding health/HEALTH and illness/ILLNESS. Just as it is not unusual to hear providers say, "Etoh, bid, tid, im, iv," and so forth, it is not uncommon to hear patients say things such as "I have no idea what the nurses and doctors are saying!" "They speak a foreign language!" "What they are doing is so strange to me." In addition, there exists an underlying cultural norm among health care providers that "all must be done to save a patient, regardless of the patient's and family's wishes" and regardless of the financial consequences to the patient and family, to the health care system, or to society in general. A consequence of this philosophy has been the rise of iatrogenic health problems and the escalation of out-of-control health care costs.

As a result, health care providers can be viewed as an alien or foreign culture or ethnic group. They have a social and cultural system; they experience "ethnicity" in the way they perceive themselves in relation to the health care consumer and often each other. Even if they deny the reality of the situation, health care providers must understand that they are ethnocentric. Not only are they ethnocentric, but also many of them are xenophobic. To appreciate this critical issue, consider the following. A principal reason for the difficulty experienced between the health care provider and the consumer is that health care providers, in general, adhere rigidly to the modern allopathic, or Western, system of health care delivery. (These terms may be used interchangeably to describe health care.) With few exceptions, they do not publicly sanction any methods of protection or healing other than scientifically proved ones. They ordinarily fail to recognize or use any sources of medication other than those that have been deemed effective by scientific means. The only types of healers that are sanctioned are those that have been educated, licensed, and certified according to the requirements of this culture.

What happens, then, when people of one belief system encounter people who have other beliefs regarding health and illness (either in protection or in treatment)? Is the provider able to meet the needs as perceived and defined by the patient? More often than not, a wall of misunderstanding arises between the two. At this point, a breakdown in communications occurs, and the consumer ends up at a disadvantage.

Providers think that they comprehend all facets of health and illness and may frequently take a xenophobic view to HEALTH and ILLNESS and traditional HEALERS. Although in training and education health care providers have a significant advantage over the consumer-patient, it is entirely appropriate for them to explore other ideas regarding health/HEALTH and illness/ILLNESS and to adjust their approach to coincide with the needs of the specific patient. Health care providers have tried to force Western medicine on one and all, regardless of results.

The following list outlines the more obvious aspects of the health care provider's culture. In connection with later chapters, it can be referred to as a framework for comparing various other ethnic and cultural beliefs and practices.

1. Beliefs
   a. Standardized definitions of *health* and *illness*
   b. The omnipotence of technology

2. Practices
   a. The maintenance of health and the protection of health or preven-tion of disease through such mechanisms as the avoidance of stress and the use of immunizations
   b. Annual physical examinations and diagnostic procedures, such as Pap smears, mammographies, and colonoscopies.
3. Habits
   a. Charting
   b. The constant use of jargon
   c. The use of a systematic approach and problem-solving methodology
4. Likes
   a. Promptness
   b. Neatness and organization
   c. Compliance
5. Dislikes
   a. Tardiness
   b. Disorderliness and disorganization
6. Customs
   a. Professional deference and adherence to the pecking order found in autocratic and bureaucratic systems
   b. Hand washing
   c. The use of certain procedures attending birth and death
7. The expectation of recovery no matter the cost or consequences of therapy

As noted, inherent in the socialization into the health care professions, nursing, medicine, social work, and the various therapies, there are countless cultural traits that are passed on both verbally and nonverbally. The doors in Figure 7–1 illustrate the closed aspects of the entire health care system.

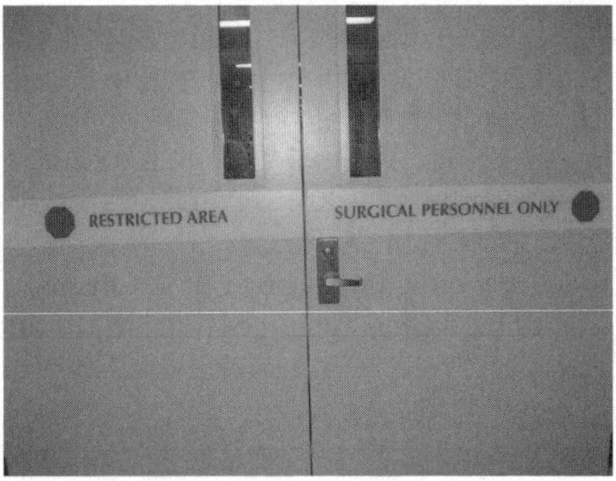

Figure 7–1 The doors to a surgical suite. In contrast to the transparent door found in the Preface, this door is symbolic of the closed culture of modern health care delivery. Few people outside of this system understand the intricacies of the cultures of the health care providers and the system within which they practice.

RESTRICTED AREA   SURGICAL PERSONNEL ONLY

Table 7-1 Gross Domestic Product and National Health Expenditures, Selected Years: 1960–2005

	Gross Domestic Product (GDP) in Billions of Dollars	National Health Expenditures in Billions of Dollars	Percentage of GDP in Health Expenditures
1960	527	26.7	5.1
1970	1,040	73.1	7.0
1980	2,796	245.8	8.8
1985	4,213	426.5	10.1
1990	5,803	695.6	12.0
1995	7,400	987.0	13.3
2000	9,817	1,358.5	13.8
2005	12,456	1,988	16.0

Source: National Center for Health Statistics. (2007). *Health, United States, 2007 with chartbook on trends in the health of Americans.* Hyattsville, MD: Author, p. 375.

We are now living in the 21st century, the third millennium; the problems of health care delivery have grown exponentially, and solutions are more elusive than ever. Doctors in the United States administer the world's most expensive medical (illness) care system. The costs of U.S. health care soared from $4 billion in 1940 to the 2000 figure of 1.4 trillion and to 1.9 trillion in 2005 (NCHS, 2007, p. 374). Health care is an enterprise that exceeds all the goods and services produced by half the states in the country. Health has become this country's biggest business, and it accounts for 16.0% of our gross domestic product, as shown in Table 7–1 and in Figure 7–2. In fact, $6,697 was spent in 2005 per capita on health care for every man, woman, child, and fetus (NCHS, 2007, pp. 374, 375). Table 7–2 displays the per capita health expenditures

Table 7-2 Per Capita Health Expenditures, Selected Years: 1960–2005

	National Health Expenditures	Private Health Expenditures	Public Health Expenditures
1960	$ 148	$ 111	$ 36
1970	356	222	134
1980	1,102	640	462
1990	2,813	1,684	1,130
1995	3,783	2,053	1,730
2000	4,790	2,680	2,110
2005	6,697	3,656	3,041

Source: National Center for Health Statistics. (2007). *Health, United States, 2007 with chartbook on trends in the health of Americans.* Hyattsville, MD: Author, p. 375.

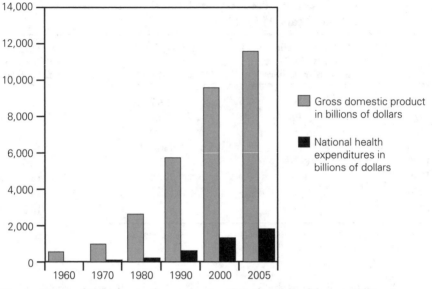

Figure 7-2 **Gross domestic product and national health expenditures: 1960–2005.**

Source: National Center for Health Statistics. (2007). *Health, United States, 2007, with chartbook on trends in the health of Americans* (p. 375). Hyattsville, MD: Author.

and breaks down the figures as to the amount of money coming from private and public funds. The increment of funds from 1960 to 2005 is distinct. Table 7–3 compares, over time, the amount of money paid per capita in the United States and several other nations for health care. In 2003, the amount of money paid per capita in the United States was double the amount spent in Denmark.

Table 7-3 **Per Capita Health Expenditures Adjusted to U.S. Dollars in Selected Countries and Selected Years: 1960–2004**

	1960	1970	1980	1990	2000	2004
United States	$144	$347	$1,055	$2,738	$4,539	$6,102
Switzerland	166	352	1,033	2,033	3,182	4,077
Norway	49	142	667	1,396	2,784	3,966
Germany	—	270	965	1,748	2,671	3,043
Canada	123	289	783	1,737	2,503	3,165
Luxembourg	—	163	643	1,547	2,722	5,089
Denmark	—	—	955	1,567	2,382	2,881
Iceland	57	165	708	1,614	2,625	2,596
Spain	16	96	365	875	1,525	2,094
Portugal	—	51	295	670	1,594	1,824

Source: National Center for Health Statistics. (2007). *Health, United States, 2007 with chartbook on trends in the health of Americans*. Hyattsville, MD: Author, p. 374.

A recently published study by the Kaiser Family Foundation points out that:

■ Health care costs have grown on average 2.5 percentage points faster than U.S. gross domestic product since 1970.

■ Almost half of health care spending is used to treat just 5 percent of the population.

■ Prescription drug spending is 10 percent of total health spending, but contributes to 14 percent of the growth in spending (Henry J. Kaiser Family Foundation, 2007, p.1).

■ Health Care Costs

The health care system is both a source of national pride—if one has an expensive and adequate health insurance package or the money, it certainly is possible to get the finest medical/technological care in the world—and a source of deep embarrassment—those who are poor or uninsured may be wanting for care. In fact, an estimated 16.4% of Americans under 65 years of age do not have health insurance (NCHS, 2006, p. 400). Other notable trends include

■ The number and percentage of people covered by employment-based health insurance declined in 2004, from 66.7% in 2000 to 63.5% in 2004 (NCHS, 2006, p. 396).

■ The percentage of uninsured children under 18 years dropped from 12.6% in 2000 to 9.2% in 2004 (NCHS, 2006, p. 400); however, children in low-income families remained more likely than children in higher-income families to lack coverage (NCHS, 2006, p. 12).

■ In 2004, 30% of young adults 18–24 years of age were uninsured at a point in time (NCHS, 2006, p. 12).

■ Of the people under 65 years old who were without health insurance in 2004,
  • 17.9% were male
  • 23.5% were between the ages of 18 and 44
  • 34.4% were Hispanic (NCHS, 2006, p. 400)

In addition

■ Many people under 65 years of age, particularly those with a low family income, do not have consistent health insurance.

■ The average percentage of the population with no health insurance coverage ranged from less than 10% in Minnesota, Hawaii, and Iowa to 25% in Texas.

■ About one-half of the uninsured population were non-Hispanic white persons with the other half being people of other races and ethnicities (NCHS, 2007, p. 14).

Almost 50% of the American public say they are very worried about having to pay more for their health care or health insurance, while 42% report they are very worried about not being able to afford health care services. Three questions then present themselves:

1. Is health care in America better than in any other place on Earth?
2. What really are the costs of health care?
3. Why is health care so expensive?

Despite the high expenditures for health care, we were not healthier in 2004 than people from other nations. Infant mortality rate is the figure used as a standard for measuring the overall health of a nation. Infant mortality rates in the United States have been steadily declining since 1960 and the national average stands at 6.8 deaths per 1,000 births, yet, some southern states are experiencing a rise in their infant mortality rates. For example, Mississippi has had the biggest increase in the number of babies dying in their first year of life, and between 2004 and 2005 the rate was 11.4 deaths per 1,000 births. In fact, 26 other nations had lower infant mortality rates than the United States. Table 7–4 illustrates infant mortality rates and international rankings from selected countries, 1960 and 2004. The United States ranked 12th in infant mortality rates in 1960 and 29th in 2004; Spain ranked 28th in 1960 and in 2004 ranked 7th; Portugal ranked 35th in 1960 and 10th in 2004. In 2004 the United States had 6.8 infant deaths per 1,000 live births; Spain had 3.5 and Portugal 4.0 (NCHS, 2007, p. 172). The greatest amount of money spent on health care *per capita* is in the United States, where we spent $6,697; Spain spent $2,094 and Portugal $1,824 in 2004. Many nations including Cuba have rates lower than the United States (Table 7–4).

Table 7–4 Infant Mortality Rates and International Rankings for Selected Countries: 2004 and 1960

Nation	Number of Infant Deaths/1,000 Live Births: 2004	Number of Infant Deaths/1,000 Live Births: 1960	Rank: 2004	Rank: 1960
	2004	1960	2004	1960
Singapore	2.0	34.8	1	21
Hong Kong	2.5	41.35	2	26
Japan	2.8	30.7	3	19
Sweden	3.1	16.6	4	1
Norway	3.2	18.9	5	3
Finland	3.3	21.0	6	6
France	3.9	27.5	9	16
Czech Republic	3.7	20.0	8	4
Portugal	4.0	77.5	10	35
Spain	3.5	43.7	7	28
Cuba	5.8	37.3	27	23
United States	6.8	26.0	29	12

Source: National Center for Health Statistics. (2007). *Health, United States, 2007 with chartbook on trends in the health of Americans.* Hyattsville, MD: Author, p. 172.

When I was studying nursing in 1960,

- National health expenditures were $27.6 billion; in 2005 they were $1,987.7 trillion.
- Hospital care expenditures were $9.2 billion; in 2005 they were $611.6 billion.
- Physician and clinical services expenditures were $5.4 billion; in 2005 they were $621.7 billion.
- Nursing home expenditures were $0.8 billion; in 2005 they were $169.3 billion.
- Research funding was $0.7 billion; in 2005 it was $40.0 billion (NCHS, 2007, p. 378).

Table 7–5 depicts the ways the health care dollar was spent from 1960 to 2005.

The sources for paying for care in 1960 were primarily personal, out of pocket or private insurance; Medicare and Medicaid did not yet exist—they were "born" in 1965. It is obvious that they now make over 50% of health care expenditures possible—coverage shifted from the private sector to the public sector and is presently shifting back to the private sector. Technology has exploded, the costs of health care have soared, and many of the health care–related programs are seen as "entitlements." The costs of services are blindly covered and quite often it is impossible for a patient to get an itemized bill, yet, when people get them, they are astonished at the costs but state, "My insurance covers it and it costs me nothing." However, for more and more people the costs of heath care have become so high that their health insurance companies either disallow desired procedures or stop payments after a certain amount is reached. Families are left bankrupt in many instances or finding it necessary to choose between care or financial insolvency.

The following examples illustrate the situation. As you read these examples, think about the events that may have occurred in the settings in which you deliver or receive care:

- Medication problems. In addition to the chronic, ongoing situation of medication errors, countless health care providers are "on the take and complicit with big business," gravely endangering our health and adding to the high costs of pharmaceuticals and other medical supplies (Kassirer, 2005, pp. 42–50).
- Quality of care errors. For example, one in three hospitals nationwide fail to ask patients on admission to list the medications they are taking (Kowalczyk, 2007b, p. A-1).
- Emergency room (department) errors. Patients may not be tended to in an appropriate manner. In fact, the wait in the emergency room can be as long as 8 hours and many patients may be left to wait in hallways (Kowalczyk, 2007a, p. A-1). In addition, the deeply embedded attitudes about race may influence the care doctors administer to African American patients in the emergency room (Smith, 2007, p. A-1).

Table 7-5 **National Health Expenditures: United States, Selected Years: 1960–2005**

	(Amount in Billions)					
	1960	1970	1980	1990	2000	2005
National health expenditures	$27.6	$75.1	$254.9	$717.3	$1,358.5	1,987.7
Health services and supplies	24.9	67.1	234.0	666.7	1,264.5	1,860.9
Personal health care	23.3	62.9	215.3	607.5	1,139.9	1,661.4
Hospital care	9.2	27.6	101.0	251.6	417.0	611.6
Professional services	8.3	20.6	67.3	216.8	426.7	621.7
Physicians and clinical services	5.4	14.0	47.1	157.5	288.6	421.2
Other professional services	0.04	0.7	3.6	18.2	45.7	56.7
Dental services	2.0	4.7	13.5	31.5	62.0	86.6
Other personal health care services	0.6	1.2	3.3	9.6	37.1	57.2
Nursing home and home health	0.9	4.3	21.4	65.2	125.8	169.3
Home health care	0.1	0.2	2.4	12.6	30.6	47.5
Nursing home care	0.8	4.0	19.0	52.6	95.3	121.9
Retail outlet sales of medical products	4.9	10.5	25.7	74.0	17.3	258.8
Prescription drugs	2.7	5.5	12.0	40.3	120.8	200.7
Other medical products	2.3	5.0	13.6	33.7	49.5	58.1
Government administration and net cost of private health insurance	1.2	2.8	12.2	39.2	81.2	143.0
Government public health activities	0.4	1.4	6.4	20.0	43.4	56.6
Investment	2.6	8.0	20.9	50.7	94.0	126.8
Research	0.7	2.0	5.4	12.7	25.6	40.0
Structures and Equipment	1.9	6.1	15.5	38.0	68.4	86.8

Source: National Center for Health Statistics. (2007). *Health, United States, 2007 with chartbook on trends in the health of Americans.* Hyattsville, MD: Author, p. 378.

■ Dumping. Recently, patients have been dumped by physicians, insurance plans, and/or exisiting health maintenance organizations. It is extremely difficult and frustrating to find new providers that are covered by an insurance company's network. This phenomena is particularly difficult for people over 65 and on Medicare.

■ Discredited medications, such as Avandia, used to treat diabetes. Patients given Avandia were found to have a 43% greater chance of developing a heart attack (Saul, 2007, p. A6).

- Diagnoses of bipolar disease in children. There has been a backlash on the frequent diagnosis of this disease (Allen, 2007, p. A-1), and the psychiatrists who have been ordering drugs, such as Risperdal, for children are being scrutinized (Harris, Carey, & Roberts, 2007, p. A1).
- False claims for OxyContin. The maker of OxyContin has been found guilty of making false claims of effects and misleading doctors about the chances of abuse of this drug and must pay a $600 million fine (Meier, 2007, p. A1).

At this writing, efforts are underway to pass legislation to protect patients from paying the costs of treatment for iatrogenic problems (Kowalczyk, 2007c, p. A-1).

The answer to the second question—"What really are the costs of health care?"—was not easy to discover. The most frequent answer was "insurance covers," and no further information was available. However, it is now possible to get some figures and to have a concrete idea as to what direct health care costs are. It is important to note that many costs are not included in the aggregate figures, such as doctors' fees, medications, visitors' needs (such as food), parking, travel, and amenities.

One example of a pragmatic way of measuring dollar costs for medical conditions, such as various cancers, and procedures, such as lung transplants and angioplasty, is to access the State of Florida's Web page, Florida Compare Care: http://www.floridahealthstat.com/index.shtml. The Agency for Health Care Administration's (AHCA's) Web site provides understandable information on quality, pricing, and performance. The total costs of an illness event are not calculated, but the costs of an incident are. The following are selected examples of costs in Florida's health care institutions delivered to all adults ages 18+ from January to December 2005, when there were

- 452 bone marrow transplant hospitalizations; the risk[1] average charge[2] was $155,425 and the risk average length of stay[3] was 23.7 days
- 5,245 liver/pancreatic cancer hospitalizations; the risk average charge was $30,823, and the average length of stay was 6.3 days
- 203 heart and/or lung transplant hospitalizations; the risk average charge was $387,432, and the risk average length of stay was 32.8 days
- 512 liver transplant hospitalizations; the risk average charge was $308,055, and the risk average length of stay was 21.1 days
- 65,472 angioplasty hospitalizations; the risk average charge was $56,118, and the average length of stay was 2.8 days

How did we get to this costly and critical situation? What factors converged to bring us to this dramatic breaking point? Because of the unprecedented growth of

---

[1]Risk adjustment is a method in which a complex set of data is put into terms by which one can compare apples to apples.

[2]The average charge is the average amount that the hospital billed for patients discharged from the hospital who had a particular condition or procedure. The hospital charge does not include physician fees, nor does it reflect the actual cost or the amount paid for the care. The amount that a patient pays depends on the type of insurance coverage.

[3]The average length of stay is the typical number of days a patient stayed in the hospital for a particular condition or procedure.

biomedical technology, we have witnessed the tremendous advancement in medical science and in the ability to perform an astounding variety of lifesaving procedures; now, not only can we no longer afford to finance these long-dreamed-of miracles, but the dream has become a nightmare. Figures 7–3A–F illustrate the changing distribution of dollars spent for health care from 1960 to 2004, as seen

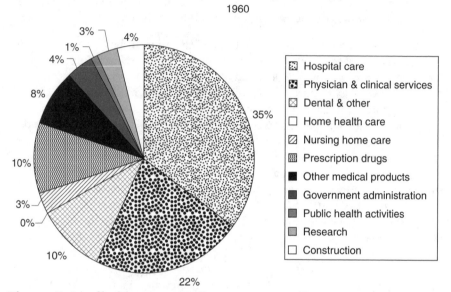

Figure 7–3a   Health care expenditure percentage distribution: United States, 1960, 1970, 1980, 1990, 1999

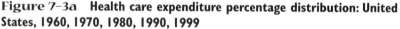

Source: National Center for Health Statistics (2007). Health, United States, 2007 with chartbook on trends in the health of Americans. Hyattsville, MD: Author, p. 378

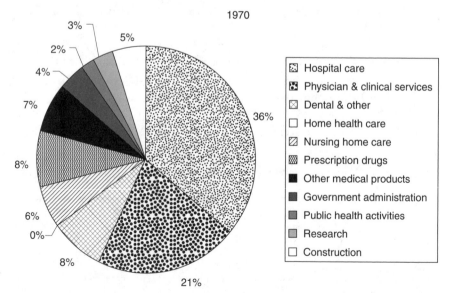

Figure 7–3b

1980

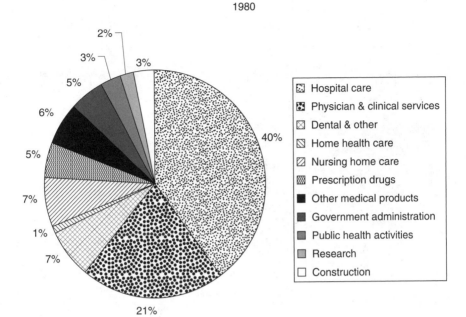

Figure 7–3c

1990

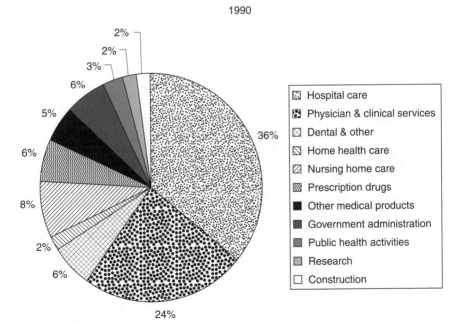

Figure 7–3d

2000

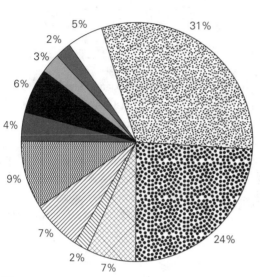
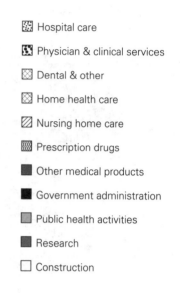

Figure 7–3e

2005

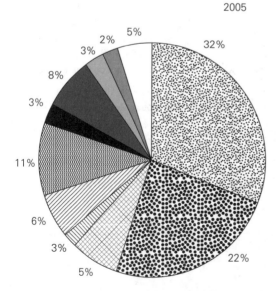
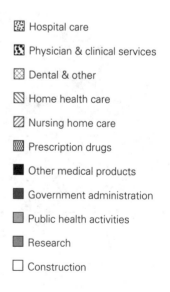

Figure 7–3f

in Table 7–5. The third question—"Why is it that health care is so expensive?"—may be answered by exploring the trends in the development of the health care system, but factored into this analysis is also the increase in the population; the desire by health care providers, researchers, and vendors to cure all diseases; and the public's expectation that all illnesses can be cured.

■ Trends in Development of the Health Care System

During the days of the early colonists, our health care system was a system of superstition and faith. It has evolved into a system predicated on a strong belief in science; the epidemiological model of disease; highly developed technology; and strong values of individuality, competition, and free enterprise. Two major forces—free enterprise and sciences—have largely shaped the problems we now face. Health problems have evolved from the epidemics of 1850 to the chronic diseases of today, notwithstanding the resurgence of tuberculosis and the AIDS epidemic. In 1850, health care technology was virtually nonexistent; today, it dominates the delivery of health care. We now take for granted such dramatic procedures as kidney, heart, and liver transplants. New technologies and biomedical milestones are materializing daily (Torrens, 1988, pp. 3–31). However, the consequences of these events are also rising daily in terms of extraordinary costs and countless practice issues and errors, discussed earlier.

Social organizations and peer review bodies to control the use of technology did not exist in 1850; today they proliferate, and the federal government is expected to play a dominant role. The belief that health care is a right for all Americans is still a prominent philosophy, yet the fulfillment of that right is still in question. The trends, begun in the 1980s and early 1990s, such as the cutbacks in federal funding for health services and the attempt to turn the clock back on social programs have led to a diminished and denigrated role for the government in people's health. On the other hand, the events of September 11, 2001, have pointed out the consequences of these cuts and the enormous and compelling need to boost public health and national security efforts.

There is growing and grave concern about the realization of this basic human right of health and health care. Mounting social problems, such as toxic waste, homelessness, and millions of people without health insurance, confound the situation. These factors all affect the delivery of health care. The problems of acquiring and using the health care system are legendary and ongoing.

The year 1960 is the benchmark being used to compare health care costs and significant events. A brief overview of these landmark events follows. These events have contributed to what we see today as the health care "nightmare." We are in a situation where health care delivery has become less and less personal and more and more technological in many health care settings. The barriers to health care are increasing and, as evidenced earlier, more and more people are unable to obtain health care, in spite of having health insurance. The events depicted that have occurred in the health care system, whether within the public health or medical sector, have happened within the context of the longer societal frame-work. The public sector events include those related to the collective responsi-bility for the health of large populations in many dimensions—prevention, surveillance, disease control, and so forth—and those events, positive and neg-ative, that affect large population cohorts. The medical events are those that in-clude the development of diagnostic and/or therapeutic methods that are problem-specific and affect limited numbers of people. The public health events include government laws and policies that were designed initially to increase the scope of the health care system and later to control medical costs.

This information is further embedded in the key health system issues of the century and the start of this decade, the key health problems, and selected key health strategies of the time. The key issues are professionalization, infrastruc-ture building, improved access, cost control, market forces, and the reinvention of government. The key health problems are reemerging infectious disease, chronic diseases, and the modern care changes. Key health strategies include ma-ternal and infant health, antibiotics, screen and treat, and managed care.

At the turn of the 20th century, 1900–1930, efforts were underway to identify medicine as a profession and to eradicate all philosophies of care that were not under the umbrella of the Flexner definition of a profession. Agents such as quinine for malaria and the diphtheria antitoxin for immunization were discovered, and the use of radium to treat cancer began.

Infectious diseases, including pneumonia and influenza, were pandemic. The main health strategy was maternal and child health, given the large numbers of new immigrants. In 1929, third-party payment for health care began with the creation of Blue Cross and Blue Shield.

Between 1930 and 1960, the health care system issue was infrastructure building. The passage of the Hill-Burton Act in 1946 provided funding for the building of hospitals and other health care resources. The system was on a roll—the development of today's extraordinarily costly tests and treatments began, and the settings for their use were built. The development of vaccines and an-tibiotics paved the way to a decrease in the occurrence of communicable disease, and a false sense of freedom from illness began to develop. At the same time, it began to become obvious that, for many, access to health care was becoming more and more difficult.

In 1965, President Lyndon B. Johnson's War on Poverty became the focal point of social and health policy and, among other laws, Medicare and Medicaid came into being. The Health Professionals Education Assistance Act was passed, which led to the proliferation of medical nursing and other allied health pro-grams. In 1967, the first heart transplant was performed by Dr. Christiaan Barnard in South Africa, and a whole new focus on science and technology was born. Today, transplants have become nearly ordinary events, and an entitlement philosophy is applied to receiving them.

The 1960s were an explosive time—there were too many assassinations, too many riots—yet strides were made in the struggle for civil rights. The war in Vietnam was a nightly television event until the truce in 1975. The 1970s, 1980s, and 1990s all had their share of strife and progress. Progress in health care was accompanied by the escalation of costs and the limiting of comprehensive care. The cases of HIV/AIDS continue to increase, and the threat of anthrax and other forms of bioterrorism are present in the minds of most people. In addition, the 1960s were a decade of profound change in the delivery of health care, public health, and available methods of treating health problems and funding new resources. Selected highlights include the

- Development of the vaccines for polio and rubella (1961 and 1963)
- Development of the methods for external cardiac pacing (1961)
- Development of liver transplant method (1963) and first human heart transplanted (1967)
- Surgeon General's Report on Smoking (1964)
- War on Poverty Medicare/Medicaid passed (1965)

The 1970s brought even greater strides in medical technology and public health:

- Professional Standards Review Organization established, Clean Water Act passed, and the Tuskegee experiment[4] ended (1972)
- Comprehensive Health Planning; "Certificate of Need" (1974)
- HBV—the hepatitis vaccine was developed (1978)
- First test tube baby born (1978)
- Biotechnical Explosion (1979)
- Cyclosporine developed (1979)

At the end of the 1970s, efforts were developed to "control" the costs of health care, yet the seductiveness of the "advances" in technology actually began the out-of-control escalation of the rise of health care costs. The following are examples of events in the 1980s that further fed the rising costs of health care and the emerging expectation of people to be entitled to better and better levels of technological diagnosis and illness care that would provide longer life expectancies:

- Nuclear magnetic resonance introduced (1980)
- The beginning of the HIV/AIDS epidemic and the HIV virus isolated at the Institute Pasteur, Paris (1981)
- Monoclonal antibodies (1984)
- Retroviral oncogenes (1985)

The 1990s to the present time have presented even greater challenges to the availability and affordability of health care. In 1993 and 1994, President and Mrs. Clinton made an extraordinary effort to study our complex health care system and sought ways to reform it. That effort did not materialize, and the present political energy has shifted from health care reform to welfare reform and the

---

[4]The Tuskegee syphilis experiment began in 1932.

saving of Social Security and Medicare. The nation's 76 million baby boomers will soon be able to retire, which will necessitate large payouts from Social Security and Medicare, but it is unknown how many workers there will be to contribute to the system. The size of the shortfall depends on the changes in longevity, the birth rate, and immigration rates (Zitner, 1999). Efforts such as managed care (Saltus, 1999) and the discounting of payments for medications for the elderly were short-term and controversial approaches to managing funds. These efforts, too, have not succeeded.

Meanwhile, the costs of health care continue to soar, causing some hospitals to downsize their nursing staff in an effort to reduce costs. Ultimately, it was believed that the Clinton plan would create a few giant insurers, and health maintenance organizations (HMOs) would dominate the market; most people would be forced into low-cost plans, doctors would be employed by the insurers or HMOs, hospitals would be controlled by insurers and HMOs, care would be multitiered, the bureaucracy would increase, costs would not be contained, and financing would be regressive. The overall goal of health care reform was to make health care accessible, comprehensive, and affordable—a right and not a privilege of all residents of the United States. However, technology is advancing and our use of it is increasing, and we continue to spend vast sums on the care of patients in the last year of life while delivering less and less preventive care. In addition, the costs of for-profit care continue to explode, and the dominant force in managed care is the for-profit HMO.

The following are examples of health care events in the 1990s and early 2000:

- Human Genome Project (1992)
- Assisted suicide; Dr. J. Kevorkian (1996)
- Hantavirus pulmonary syndrome (1993)
- Septuplets born and survive (1997)
- Octuplets born; seven survive (1998)
- Stem cell cloning (1998)
- Biologics and follow-on biologics (2004)

With the catastrophe of September 11, 2001, the need to immunize people for smallpox and countless other public health issues emerged, as did the need for emergency preparedness.

Biologics are complex medicines that are manufactured with the use of living organisms. The increasing use of biologics and new follow-on biologics are the cutting edge of pharmaceutical therapies. The biogeneric market is about $2 billion. The Biotechnology Industry Organization (BIO) has stated that "the safety and effectiveness of a chemical drug can be established by the specification of its active ingredient, but the safety and effectiveness of a biotech product is determined by the manner in which it is made" (Samalonis, 2004). In other words, the consequences of this pioneering medicine will be expensive iatrogenic problems.

Grave concern is being expressed regarding the high costs of health care, the fact that between 16.1% and 17.5% of the population under 65 has no health insurance, that the costs of durable medical supplies and medications continue to rise, and so on. On one hand, we are seeking to ever expand therapeutic miracles; on the other hand, there is shock and dismay at the ever-increasing costs of health care. Box 7–1 lists recent examples of the impact that the insurance/no insurance and health care costs is having on families.

Box 7–1

Health Care Costs Create a Significant Barrier to Getting Health Care for Many Americans

According to the research conducted by the Kaiser Family, Harvard School of Public Health, reported in August 2005: "Health care costs are more than a barrier to access to care. Recent findings show that medical bills create a significant challenge for many American families, including those with insurance, impacting their lives in a variety of ways. . . ."

- Nearly one-quarter of Americans have had problems paying medical bills in the past year.
- More than 6 in 10 (61%) adults who report problems paying medical bills are covered by health insurance. Those who had problems paying medical bills report that the bills were for basic care, as doctor bills (85%), lab fees (62%), and prescription drugs (56%).
- More than 1 in 5 (21%) Americans currently has an overdue medical bill, and almost 2 in 10 (19%) report experiencing serious financial consequences in the past 5 years due to medical bills:
  - Fifteen percent report being contacted by a collection agency because of medical bills.
  - Twelve percent have used "all or most" of their savings.
  - Eight percent report borrowing money or taking out another mortgage.
  - Three percent have declared bankruptcy.
- Almost 2 in 10 (18%) Americans say health care costs are their biggest monthly expense, excluding rent or mortgage payments.
- Nearly 3 in 10 (28%) adults report a time in the past year when they did not have enough money to pay for medical or health care, and 62% of these adults are insured.
- Nearly 3 in 10 (29%) adults report that they or someone in their household skipped medical treatment, cut pills, or did not fill a prescription in the past year because of the cost.

Source: Henry J. Kaiser Family Foundation (2005). The USA Today/Kaiser Family Foundation/Harvard School of Public Health—Health Care Costs Survey. Menlo Park, CA: Author. Retrieved March 2, 2008 from http://www.kff.org/, pp. 8–12.

■ Common Problems in Health Care Delivery

Many problems exist within today's health care delivery system. Some of these problems affect all of us, and others are specific to the poor and to emerging majority populations. It has been suggested that the health care delivery system fosters and maintains a childlike dependence and depersonalized condition for the consumer. The following sections describe problems experienced by most consumers of health care, as categorized by Ehrenreich and Ehrenreich (1971, pp. 4–12). It is interesting to note that this historical framework was developed in 1971, yet it holds as a framework today.

Finding Where the Appropriate Care Is Offered at a Reasonable Price

It may be difficult for even a knowledgeable consumer to receive adequate care. One summer, I was on vacation with my 11-year-old daughter. She complained of a sore throat for 2 days, and, when she did not improve on the third day, I decided to take her to a pediatrician and have a throat culture taken. She was running a low-grade fever, and I suspected a strep infection. I phoned the emergency room of a local teaching hospital for the name of a pediatrician, but I was instructed to "bring her in." I questioned the practicality of using an emergency room, but the friendly voice on the other end of the line assured me: "If you have health insurance and the child has a sore throat, this is the best place to come." After a rather long wait, we were seen by an intern who was beginning his first day in pediatrics. To my dismay and chagrin, the young man appeared to have no idea of how to proceed. The resident entered and patiently demonstrated to the fledgling intern—using my daughter—how to go about doing a physical examination on a child. Since I had brought the child to the emergency room merely for a throat culture, I felt that what they were doing was unnecessary and said so. After much delay, the throat culture was taken; we were told we could leave and should call back in 48 hours for the report. As we left the cubicle, we had to pass another cubicle with an open curtain—where a woman was vomiting all over herself, the bed, and the equipment while another intern was attempting to insert a gastric tube. Needless to say, my daughter was distressed by the sight, which she could not help but witness. The reward for this trial was an inflated bill.

Two days later, I called back for the report. It could not be located. When it was finally "found," the result was negative. I took issue with this because it took 30 minutes for them to find the report. Perhaps this sounds a bit overstated; however, I had the feeling that they told me it was negative just to get me off the phone.

I related this personal experience to bring out two major points. First, it is not easy to obtain what I, as a health care provider, consider to be a rather minor procedure. Second—and perhaps more important—it was expensive!

The average health care consumer in such a circumstance may very well have no idea of what is really going on. When health care is sought, one should have access to professionally performed examinations and treatment. When one is seeking the results of a laboratory test, the results should be available immediately at the agreed-on time and place instead of being lost in a jungle of bureaucracy.

Finding One's Way Amidst the Many Available Types of Medical Care

A friend's experience illustrates how hard it may be to find appropriate medical care. She had minor gastric problems from time to time and initially sought help from a family physician. He was unable to treat the problem adequately; therefore, she decided to go elsewhere. However, for many reasons—including anger, embarrassment, and fear of reprisal—she chose not to tell the family physician that she was dissatisfied with his care, nor did she request a referral. She was essentially on her own in terms of securing an appointment with either a gastroenterologist or a surgeon. She very quickly discovered that no physician who was a specialist in gastroenterology would see her on a self-referral. In order to get an appointment, she had to ask her own general practitioner for a referral or else seek initial help from another general practitioner or internist. Since she had little money to spend on a variety of physicians, she decided to wait to see what would happen. In this instance, she was fortunate and has had few further problems.

As a teaching and learning experience, I ask students to describe how they go about selecting a physician and where they go for health care. The younger students in the class generally seek the services of their families' physicians. The older or married students often have doctors other than those with whom they "grew up." These latter students generally are quite willing to share the trials and tribulations they have experienced. When given the freedom to express their actions and reactions, most admit to having a great deal of difficulty in getting what they perceive to be good health care. A number of the older students state that they select a physician on the staff of the institution where they are employed. They have had an opportunity to see him or her at work and can judge, firsthand, whether he or she is "good" or "bad." One mother stated that she worked in pediatrics during her pregnancy solely to discover who was the best pediatrician. A newly married student stated that she planned to work in the delivery room to see which obstetrician delivered a baby with the greatest amount of concern for both the mother and the child.

That is an ideal situation for members of the nursing profession, but what about the average layperson who does not have access to this resource? This question alerts the students to the specialness of their personal situations and exposes them to the immensity of the problem that the average person experiences. After individual experiences are shared, the class can move on to work through a case study such as the following.

Ms. B. is a new resident in this city. She discovers a lump in her breast and does not know where to turn. How does she go about finding a doctor? Where does she go?

One initial course of action is to call the American Cancer Society for advice. From there, she is instructed to call the County Medical Society, since the American Cancer Society is not allowed to give out physicians' names. During a phone call to the County Medical Society, she is given the names of three physicians in her part of the city. From there, she is on her own in attempting to get an appointment with one of them. It is not uncommon for a stranger to call a physician's office and be told (1) "The doctor is no longer seeing any additional new patients," (2) "There is a 6-month wait," or (3) "He sees no one without a proper referral."

The woman, of course, has another choice: She can go to an emergency room or a clinic, but then she discovers that the wait in the emergency room is intolerable for her. She may rationalize that because a "lump" is not really an "emergency," she should choose another route. She may then try to secure a clinic appointment, and once again she may experience a great deal of difficulty in getting an appointment at a convenient time. She may finally get one and then discover that the wait in the clinic is unduly long, which may cause her to miss a day of work.

Figuring Out What the Physician Is Doing

It is not always easy for members of the health professions to understand what is happening to them when they are ill. What must it be like for the average person who has little or no knowledge of health care routines and practices?

Pretend that you are a layperson who has just been relieved of all your clothes and given a paper dress to put on. You are lying on a table with strange eyes peering down at you. A sheet is thrown over you, and you are given terse directions—"breathe," "cough," "don't breathe," "turn," "lift your legs." You may feel without warning a cold disk on your chest or a cold hand on your back. As the physical examination process continues, you may feel a few taps on the ribs, see a bright light shining in your eye, feel a cold tube in your ear, and gag on a stick probing the inside of your mouth. What is going on? The jargon you hear is unfamiliar. You are being poked, pushed, prodded, peered at and into, and jabbed, and you do not know why. If you are female and going for your first pelvic examination, you may have no idea what to expect. Perhaps you have heard only hushed whisperings, and your level of fear and discomfort is high. Insult is added to injury when you experience the penetration of a cold, unyielding speculum: "What is the doctor doing now and why?"

These hypothetical situations are typical of the usual physical examinations that you may encounter routinely in a clinic or private physician's office. Suppose you have a more complex problem, such as a neurological condition, for which the diagnostic procedures may indeed be painful and complicated. Have you ever had a CT scan? A magnetic resonance image (MRI)? An angioplasty? Quite often, those who deliver care have not experienced the vast number of procedures that are performed in diagnostic workups and in treatment. They have little awareness of what the patient is thinking, feeling, and experiencing. Similarly, because the names and the purposes of the procedures are familiar to health care workers—don't forget, this is their culture—they may take their own understanding of the procedures for granted and have difficulty appreciating why the patient cannot understand what is happening.

Finding Out What Went Wrong

What did you do the last time a patient asked to read the chart? Traditionally, you uttered an authoritative "tsk," turned abruptly on white-heeled shoes, and walked briskly away. Who ever heard of such nerve? A patient asking to read a chart! In recent years, a "patient's bill of rights" has evolved. One of its mandates is that the patient has the right to read his or her own medical record. Experience, however, demonstrates that this right is still not always granted. Suppose one enters the hospital for what is deemed to be a simple medical or surgical problem. All is well if everything goes according to routine. However, what happens when complications develop? The more determined the patient is to discover what the problem is or why there are complications, the more he or she believes that the health care providers are trying to hide something. The cycle perpetuates itself, and a tremendous schism develops between provider and consumer. Quite often, "the conspiracy of silence" tends to grow as more questions are asked. This unpleasant situation may continue until the patient is locked inside his or her subjective world. It is rare for a person truly to understand unforeseen complications. Nurses all too often enter into this collusion and play the role of a silent partner with the physician and the institution.

Overcoming the Built-in Racism and Male Chauvinism of Doctors and Hospitals

Students tend to have little difficulty in describing many incidents of racism and male chauvinism: That they are mostly women suffices and that they are nurses adds meaning to the problem. Classroom discussion helps identify subtle incidents of racism. For example, students may realize that Black patients may be the last to receive morning or evening care, meal trays, and so forth. If this is a normal occurrence on a floor, it is an indictment in itself. Racism may take another tack. Is it an accident that the Black person is the last patient to receive routine care or has he or she consciously been made to wait? Does the fact that the Black person may have to wait longest for water or a pill demonstrate racism on a conscious level, or is it subliminal?

Nurses recognize the subtle patronization of both themselves and female patients. Once the situation is probed and spelled out, the students adopt a much more realistic attitude toward the insensitivity of those who choose a racist or chauvinistic style of giving care. Students have noted that, when they are aware of what is happening, they are better able to take steps to block future occurrences. Some have written letters to me after they have begun or returned to the practice of nursing, stating that knowing the phenomenon is common helps them project a stronger image in their determination to work for change.

▨ Pathways to Health Services

When a health problem occurs, there is an established system whereby health care services are obtained. The classical theoretical work that was developed in the mid-1960s and the 1970s continues to establish a viable framework for describing sources of patient problems. Suchman (1965) contends that the family is usually the first resource. It is in the domain of the family that the person seeks validation that what he or she is experiencing is indeed an illness. Once the belief is validated, health care outside of the home is sought. It is not unusual for a family to be receiving care from many different providers, with limited or no communication among the attending caregivers. Problems and complications erupt when a provider is not aware that other providers are caring for a patient. Let us not forget that, in rural and remote areas, comprehensive health care is difficult to obtain. For patients who are forced to use the clinics of a hospital, there is certainly no continuity of care because intern and resident physicians come and go each year. This is known as the level of first contact, or the entrance into the health care system.

The second level of care, if needed, is found at the specialist's level: in clinics, private practice, or hospitals. Obstetricians, gynecologists, surgeons, neurologists, and other specialists make up a large percentage of those who practice in medicine. Recently, hospitalists have been added.

The third level of care is delivered within hospitals that provide inpatient care and services. Care is determined by need, whether long-term (as in a psychiatric setting or rehabilitation institute) or short-term (as in the acute care setting and community hospitals).

An in-depth discussion of the different kinds of hospitals—voluntary or profit-making and nonprofit institutions—is more appropriate to a book dealing solely with the delivery of health care (see the Bibliography at the end of this book). In our present context, the issue is "what does the patient know about such settings, and what kind of care can he or she expect to receive?"

To many students, the health care delivery problems of a given hospital unit are far removed from the scope of practice they know from nursing school and from what they ordinarily see in a work setting (unless they choose to work in a city or county public hospital). Many students assume that the care they observe and deliver in a suburban or community private hospital is the universal norm. This is a fundamental error in experience and understanding, which can be corrected if students are assigned to visit first the emergency room of a city hospital and then the emergency room of a suburban hospital in order to compare the two milieus. Unless students visit each setting, they fail to gain an appreciation of the major differences—how vastly such facilities differ in the scope of patients' treatment. Students typically report that, in the suburban emergency room, the patients are called by name, their families wait with them, and every effort is made to hasten their visit. The contrast with people in urban emergency rooms—who have waited for extended periods of time, are sometimes not addressed by name, and are not allowed to have family members come with them while they are examined—is astounding. The noise and confusion are also factors that confront and dismay students when they are exposed to big-city emergency rooms.

Figure 7–4 illustrates the maze of health care and the variety of obstacles a patient must deal with in attempting to navigate this complex system. Indeed, the patient not only needs to navigate an internal system of a given hospital but also needs to understand all the types of care available. Just to complicate matters more deeply, many people are given information that contradicts itself—as with the diagnosis and treatment of breast cancer or the use of estrogen replacement therapy—and then the patient is asked to make the choices.

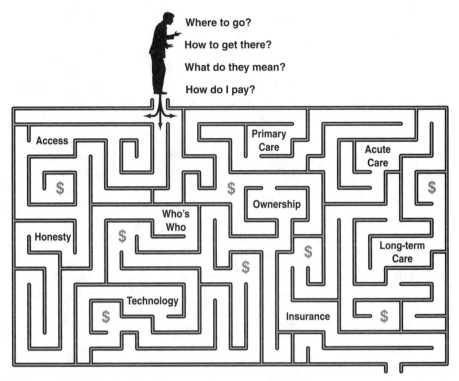

Figure 7-4 Navigating the amazing maze of health care.

■ Barriers to Health Care

There are countless factors, or barriers, in addition to financial that thwart a person's or family's ability to use the health care system to its greatest potential. The following are some examples:

Access	A person is unable to enter into the system because he or she lacks money, health insurance, or the ability to get to a center where health care is delivered. Another access factor is that primary care physicians are leaving their practices, either to retire or to limit the scope of their practices to "concierge" services.
Age	The person is too young or too old to enter into the system and is unaware of ways to overcome this.

(continued)

Class	A person may be from a class that is not part of the dominant culture, limiting their ability to determine the need for health care and to understand the subtleties involved in making health care system choices.
Education	A person may not know how to read and write English and may not read and write in his or her native tongue.
Gender	Existing services may be limited to a specific gender or the person may be unwilling or unable to access a system that does not deliver gender-specific care.
Geography	A person may not reside near a health care facility, and the costs of traveling to a facility may be unaffordable.
Homelessness	A person may be homeless in a place where health care is not provided to people who are homeless and the person does not know the ways to access the system.
Insurance	A person may not have health insurance or it may be inadequate to cover the scope of the person's needs.
Language	A person may not speak or understand English and adequate interpreter services may not be available.
Manners	A person's manners or expectations of the provider's manners may not be congruent.
Philosophy	The philosophy of an institution may not be congruent with a person's religious or personal philosophy.
Prejudice	The person seeking health care may sense the prejudice that the providers and institution exhibit.
Race	There may be residuals of racial prejudice as part of the institution's philosophy.
Racism	The institution may have specific barriers in place to not treat people from other races than the race of the owners of the facility.
Religion	A patient may not desire to be treated in an institution that is not derived from his or her religious background and there may be manifest prejudice on both sides—patient and institution.

SES (socio economic status)	The 2 extremes of socioeconomic status, poverty or great wealth, poverty can limit access to care and wealth may prevent people from seeking care in institutions where they prefer to not go because of the patient population served there.
Technology	A person may not be able to afford or want the plethora of diagnostic tests and therapies offered to him or her.
Transportation	There may be no public transportation available from where the patient resides to the institution.

■ Medicine as an Institution of Social Control

The people of today's youth-oriented, cure expected, death-denying, society have unusually high expectations of the healers of our time. We expect a cure (or if not a cure, then the prolongation of life) as the normal outcome of illness. The technology of modern health care dominates our expectations of treatment, and our primary focus is on the curative aspects of medicine, not on prevention.

As control over the behavior of a person has shifted from the family and church to a physician, "be good" has shifted to "take your medicine." The role that physicians play within society in terms of social control is ever-growing, so that conflict frequently arises between medicine and the law over definitions of accepted codes of behavior and the relative status of the two professions in governing American life. Zola (1966, 1972) uses the following examples to illustrate the "medicalization" of society.

Through the Expansion of What in Life Is Deemed Relevant to the Good Practice of Medicine

This factor is exemplified by the change from a specific etiological model of disease to a multicausal one. The "partners" in this new model include greater acceptance of comprehensive medicine, the use of the computer, and the practice of preventive medicine. In preventive medicine, however, the medical person must get to the layperson before the disease occurs: Clients must be sought out. Thus, forms of social control emerge in an attempt to prevent disease: eating a low-cholesterol diet, avoiding stress, stopping smoking, and getting proper and adequate exercise.

Through the Retention of Absolute Control over Certain Technical Procedures

This step is, in essence, the right to perform surgery and the right to prescribe drugs. In the life span of human beings, modern medicine can often determine life or death from the time of conception to old age through genetic counseling;

abortion; surgery; and technological devices, such as computers, respirators, and life-support systems. Medicine has at its command drugs that can cure or kill—from antibiotics to the chemotherapeutic agents used to combat cancer. There are drugs to cause sleep or wakefulness, to increase or decrease the appetite, to increase or decrease levels of energy. There are drugs to relieve depression and stimulate interest. (In the United States, those mood-altering drugs are consumed at a rate higher than the medications prescribed and used to treat specific diseases.) In addition, medicine can control what medications are available for legal consumption.

Through the Expansion of What in Medicine Is Deemed Relevant to the Good Practice of Life

This expansion is illustrated by the use of medical jargon to describe a state of being—such as the *health* of the nation or the *health* of the economy. Any political or economic proposal or objective that enhances the "health" of those concerned wins approval.

There are numerous areas in which medicine, religion, and law overlap. For example, public health practice, law, and medicine overlap in the creation of laws that establish quarantine and the need for immunization. As another example, a child is unable to enter school without proof of having received certain inoculations. Medicine and law also merge in areas of sanitation and rodent and insect control. A legal-medical dispute can arise over the guilt or innocence of a criminal as determined by his or her "mental state" at the time of a crime.

Some diseases carry a social stigma: One must be screened for tuberculosis before employment, a history of typhoid fever permanently prevents a person from commercially handling food, venereal disease must be reported and treated, and even the ancient disease of leprosy continues to carry a stigma.

Abortion represents an area replete with conflict that involves politics, law, religion, and medicine. Those in favor of abortion rights believe that it is a woman's right to have an abortion and that the matter is confidential between the patient and her physician. Opponents argue on religious and moral grounds that abortion is murder. At present, the law sanctions abortion. In many states, however, Medicaid will no longer pay for an abortion unless the mother's life is in danger, a policy that makes it increasingly difficult for the poor to obtain these services.

Another highly charged area of conflict involves the practice of euthanasia. With the burgeoning of technological improvements, the definition of *death* has changed in recent years. It sometimes takes a major court battle to "pull the plug," such as in the Nancy Cruzan case. The battles with Dr. Jack Kevorkian have stretched these issues even further.

Finally, although many daily practical activities are undertaken in the name of health—taking vitamins, practicing hygiene, using birth control, engaging in dietary or exercise programs—the "diseases of the rich" (cancer, heart disease, and stroke) tend to capture more public attention and funding than the diseases of the poor (malnutrition, high maternal and infant death rates, sickle-cell anemia, and lead poisoning).

In this chapter, we have explored, in a very limited way, the culture and characteristics inherent in the socialization into the health care professions; many of the issues surrounding the American health care delivery system by examining the history and trends that led to its present character; the experiences a person may have in attempting to obtain care; and how medicine is now an institution of social control. Table 7–6 brings closure to this chapter by comparing medical care and CULTURALCARE.

Table 7–6 Comparison: Medical Care and CULTURALCARE

	Medical Care	CULTURALCARE
Definition	"The art and science of the diagnosis and treatment of disease and the maintenance of health"	Professional health care that is culturally sensitive, culturally appropriate, and culturally competent
Goals	Prevention of disease and injury and promotion and maintenance of health Relief of pain and suffering caused by maladies Care and CURE of those with a malady and care of those who cannot be cured Avoidance of premature death and pursuit of a peaceful death	Provision of care that is *Culturally sensitive*—the provider possesses some basic knowledge of and constructive attitudes toward the health traditions observed among the diverse cultural groups found in the setting in which he or she is practicing *Culturally appropriate*—the provider applies the underlying background knowledge that must be possessed to provide a patient with the best possible health care *Culturally competent*—within the delivered care the provider understands and attends to the total context of the patient's situation and it is a complex combination of knowledge, attitudes, and skills Assistance to patient/family in pursuit of HEALTH and HEALING
Philosophy	Allopathic—body and mind "With enough money, energy, and scientific zeal, there are no diseases or maladies that it cannot cure or remedy"	Holistic care predicated on HEALTH traditions and patient/family/community articulated needs and situation

(continued)

Table 7-6 *Continued*

Challenges	Should life support be used far beyond the natural trajectory of a given episode? Should disease and death ever be accepted? Should such controversial issues such as physician-assisted suicide and euthanasia be accepted as part of medical practice? Ever-rising costs and iatrogenic problems	Disparagement and nonacceptance of HEALTH, ILLNESS, and HEALING traditions
Sources of stress	Former success Rise in chronic illness	Nonrecognition by modern providers of the meanings of HEALTH, ILLNESS, and HEALING traditions
Scientific and technological developments	Sophisticated, costly technology Experimental treatments Follow-on biologics	Steeped in ethnocultural HEALTH-related traditions
Cultural pressures	"Scientific progress" High quality = best available in diagnosis and treatment Assumption = better to come	Antithetical at times to allopathic practice Patient may be seen as "noncomplier" or to not appreciate provider efforts
Medicalization of life	Apply medical model and technologies to problems historically not thought of as medical in nature	Apply knowledge to entire sociocultural and HEALTH context of patients
Medicine and society	Fed by large amounts of money—public and private; influenced by social mores, values, and economics; and a substrate of dominant culture	Many traditions neither recognized nor known within the dominant culture Many beliefs and practices hidden
Define *health*	*Health* = "the experience of well-being and integrity of mind and body"	HEALTH = "the balance of the person, both within one's being—physical, mental, and spiritual—and in the outside world—natural, communal, and metaphysical, is a complex, interrelated phenomenon"
Define *illness*	Malady, disease, illness, and sickness—loss of freedom or opportunity, or the loss of pleasure	ILLNESS = "the imbalance of one's beings—physical, mental, and spiritual—and in the outside world—natural, communal, and metaphysical"

Table 7-6 *Continued*

Causes of illness	Viruses, bacteria, stress, etc.	Evil eye, or spirits; God's punishment; internal imbalance; jealousy; envy?
Maintain health	Health promotion—activities to stay well	Daily health practices, such as following dietary taboos, special clothing, and prayer
Protect health	Immunization	Protective items worn, carried, or hung in the home
Restore health	Technology Human experimentation Radical measures "Hope" at all costs	Traditional remedies—herbs, prayer, pilgrimages to shrines—both religious and secular
Birth practices	Medicalization Hospitalization In vitro fertilization	Use of midwife when possible Traditional rituals Prayer
Death practices	"Everything done to prevent" Long-term use of life support Experimental therapies	Prayer, vigils, acceptance
Attitudes toward other health care systems	Skeptical and sometimes contemptuous of "alternative medicine" Seen as a danger	May see modern medicine as an alternative to ethnocultural or religious traditions

Source: Adapted from: Hanson, M. J., & Callahan, D. (Eds.). (1999). *The goals of medicine.* Washington, DC: Georgetown Press.

The struggles continue as we attempt to find a balance between the high technology of the 21st century and primary preventive care and a strong public health care system. There must also be a balance between the forces of modern medical care and CULTURALCARE.

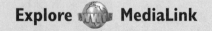

Explore MediaLink

Go to the Companion Website at www.prenhall.com/spector for chapter-related review questions, case studies, and activities. Contents of the CulturalCare Guide and CulturalCare Museum can also be found on the Companion Website. Click on Chapter 7 to select the activities for this chapter.

■ Internet Sources

Agency for Health Care—Florida. (2003). FloridaHealthFinder.gov. State of Florida Author. Retrieved July 2, 2007 from http://www.floridahealthfinder.gov/about-ahca/about-ahca.shtml

California Health Care Foundation. (2006). California Employer Health Benefits Survey, 2006. Oakland, CA: California HealthCare Foundation, Retrieved from http://www.chcf.org/topics/healthinsurance/index.cfm, March 2, 2008.

Henry J. Kaiser Family Foundation. (2005). The USA Today/Kaiser Family Foundation/Harvard School of Public Health—Health Care Costs Survey. Menlo Park, CA: Author. pub. #7371. Retrieved March 2, 2008 from http://www.kff.org/

Henry J. Kaiser Family Foundation (2007). Key Information on Health Care Costs and Their Impact. Menlo Park, CA: Author. Retrieved March 2, 2008 from http://www.kff.org/.

Samalonis, L.B. (2004). Follow-on biologies: The next frontier. Retrieved June 27, 2007 from http://www.drugtopics.com/drugtopics/article/articleDetail.jsp?id=115886

National Coalition on Health Care. (2008). Health Insurance Cost. Washington, DC: Author. Retrieved on March 2, 2008 from http://www.nchc.org/facts/cost.shtml

■ References

Abelson, R. (2007, June 14). In health care, cost isn't proof of high quality. *New York Times*, p. A-1.

Allen, S. (2007, May 20). Backlash on bipolar diagnoses in children, *Boston Globe*, p. A-1.

Dembner, A. (2007, June 18). Countdown to coverage. *Boston Globe*, p. C-1.

Ehrenreich, B., & Ehrenreich, J. (1971). *The American health empire: Power, profits, and politics*. New York: Random House, Vintage Books. (The headings that follow this reference in the text are quoted from this book.)

Harris, G., Carey, B., & Roberts, J. (2007, May 10). Psychiatrists, troubled children, and drug industry's role. *New York Times*, p. A1.

Kassirer, J. P. (2005). *On the take*. New York: Oxford University Press.

Knowles, J. (1970, January). It's time to operate. *Fortune*, p. 79.

Kowalczyk, L. (2007a, March 25). At the ER, the stay can reach 8 hours. *Boston Globe*, p. A-1.

Kowalczyk, L. (2007b, April 21). Five hospitals release data on inspections. *Boston Globe*, p. A-1.

Kowalczyk, L. (2007c, September 17). Many Mass. hospitals will pay for errors. *Boston Globe*, p. A-1.

Meier, B. (2007, May 11). Narcotic maker guilty of deceit over marketing. *New York Times*, p. A1.

National Center for Health Statistics [NCHS]. (2006). *Health, United States, 2006 with chartbook on trends in the health of Americans*. Hyattsville, MD: Author.

National Center for Health Statistics. (2007). *Health, United States, 2007 with chartbook on trends in the health of Americans*. Hyattsville, MD: Author.

Saltus, R. (1999, February 18). Managed, yes, but couple wonders, is care? *Boston Globe*, p. A-1.

Saul, S. (2007, July 22). Drug safety crusader gets results, criticism. *Boston Globe*, p. A-6.

Smith, S. (2007, July 20). Tests of ER trainees find signs of race bias in care. *Boston Globe*, p. A-1.

Suchman, E. A. (1964). Sociomedical variations among ethnic groups. *American Journal of Sociology, 70,* 319–331.

Suchman, E. A. (1965). Social patterns of illness and medical care. *Journal of Health and Human Behavior, 6,* 2–16.

Torrens, P. R. (1988). Historical evolution and overview of health services in the United States. In S. J. Williams & P. R. Torrens (Eds.), *Introduction to health services* (3rd ed.). New York: John Wiley & Sons.

USA Today/Kaiser Family/Harvard School of Public Health. (2005, August). Menlo Park, CA: Henry J. Kaiser Family Foundation.

Zitner, A. (1999, March 14). Demographers caught looking on US trends. *Boston Sunday Globe,* A1.

Zola, I. K. (1996 October). Culture and symptoms: An analysis of patients presenting complaints. *American Sociological Review, 31,* 615–630.

Zola, I. K. (1972, November). Medicine as an institution of social control. *Sociological Review, 20*(4), 487–504. (The headings that follow this reference in the text are quoted from this article.)

Unit

III

HEALTH and ILLNESS Panoramas

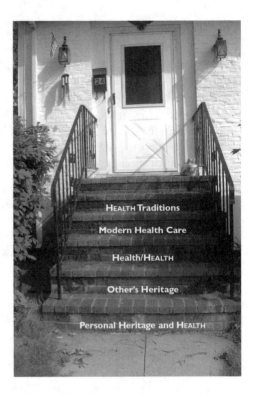

HEALTH Traditions

Modern Health Care

Health/HEALTH

Other's Heritage

Personal Heritage and HEALTH

Thus far, this book has discussed four of the six steps to CULTURALCOMPETENCY. The first six chapters presented the underlying theoretical rationale that is the foundation for CULTURALCOMPETENCY and brought you to the transparent door depicted in the introduction, to "observe" the various "bricks" philosophies, concepts, and situations involved in the theoretical development of CULTURALCOMPETENCY.

- Chapter 1 set the theoretical foundation of what was the first step, *know your personal heritage*, as it reviewed the sociological components of heritage.
- Chapter 2 developed the background necessary to understand the role that the changing demographics of the larger communities have had in society in general and specifically in the delivery of health care—this is the second step.
- Chapters 3, 4, and 5 explored the dynamics involved in health/HEALTH, illness/ILLNESS, and curing/HEALING—the third step.
- Chapter 6 provided the opportunity to look intensely inside this door from your personal experience and presented information regarding the exciting and challenging intricacies of exploring *your* heritage and your family's health/HEALTH and illness/ILLNESS beliefs and practices. As

201

stated, this completes the first and most important step in becoming CULTURALLY COMPETENT.

- ■ Chapter 7 examined the "culture" of health care providers and that of the health care delivery system as it introduced arguments relevant to the trends in the development of the health care system, common problems in the delivery of health care, pathways to health services, and medicine as an institution of social control and compared modern and traditional philosophies of health care delivery. This content relates to steps 3 and 4.

The five chapters in this unit embrace the fifth step—traditional HEALTH care—and will provide a framework for learning about the communities you may be practicing in. It presents examples of the *traditional* HEALTH, ILLNESS, and HEALING beliefs and practices of selected populations. Each chapter introduces the

- ■ Background of the population
- ■ *Traditional* definitions of HEALTH/ILLNESS/HEALING
- ■ *Traditional* methods of HEALTH maintenance and protection
- ■ *Traditional* methods of HEALTH restoration
- ■ Current health problems
- ■ Health disparities in morbidity and mortality rates and in manpower

These are areas that can be applied in researching information regarding the populations you are caring for and working with. The World Wide Web is extremely helpful in gathering the demographic and modern health-related data applicable to a given population.

The need for historical, pertinent, and compelling information was recently driven home when I was discussing New Year's Day with a cohort of fifteen 21-year-old college senior students. The students did not know that New Year's Day—January 1—is a religious holiday; they believed it was a secular holiday. The conversation that resulted from this incident revealed a "thirst" for knowledge regarding *tradition*. They were eager to learn about the HEALTH traditions and other cultural events from their own ethnocultural heritage, from the heritages of peers, and the heritages of other people. Thus, an effort has been exerted to maintain the integrity of older references and the primary data that have been gathered regarding HEALTH beliefs and practices over the 30 years I have developed this text. In the race to modernity, science, technology, and "scholarly" endeavors, the HEALTH traditions of family and others may well be lost—as the saying goes, the baby was "thrown away with the bath water," to this generation.

The chapters in Unit III will present an overview of relevant historical and contemporary theoretical content that will help you

1. Develop a level of awareness of the background and health/HEALTH problems of both the emerging majority and White ethnic populations.
2. Understand and describe selected *traditional* HEALTH beliefs and practices.
3. Understand the *traditional* pathways to HEALTH care and the relationship between these pathways and the American health care system.

4. Understand certain manpower problems of each of the communities discussed.

5. Be more familiar with the available literature regarding each of the communities.

The following exercises are appropriate to all chapters in Unit III:

1. Familiarize yourself with some literature of the given community—that is, read literature, poetry, or a biography of a member of each of the communities.

2. Familiarize yourself with the history and sociopolitical background of each of the communities.

The questions that follow should be thoughtfully considered:

1. What are the traditional definitions of *HEALTH* and *ILLNESS* in each of the communities? Are they alike or different?

2. What are the traditional methods of maintaining HEALTH?

3. What are the traditional ways of protecting HEALTH?

4. What are the traditional ways of restoring HEALTH?

5. Who are the traditional HEALERS? What functions do they perform?

This is an extraordinary way to build connections between communities and to see how much different ethnocultural and religious communities have in common. Since HEALTH is the metaphor for this text, it brings to the forefront a way to analyze and understand some of the variability in health care.

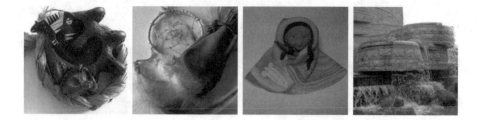

Chapter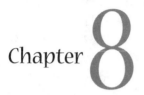

HEALTH and ILLNESS in the American Indian and Alaska Native Population

Everything on the earth has a purpose, every disease an herb to cure it, and every person a mission. This is the Indian theory of existence.

—*Morning Dove (Christine Quintasket) (1888–1936) Salish*

■ Objectives

1. Discuss the background of the American Indian and Alaska Native population.
2. Discuss the demographic profile of the American Indian and Alaska Native population.
3. Describe the traditional definitions of HEALTH and ILLNESS of the American Indian and Alaska Native population.
4. Describe the traditional methods of HEALING of the American Indian and Alaska native population.
5. Describe the practice of a traditional healer.
6. Describe current health care problems of the American Indian and Alaska Native population.
7. Describe the services rendered by the Indian Health Service.
8. Describe demographic disparity as it is seen in health manpower distribution of the American Indian and Alaska Native population as represented in the health care delivery system.

The images opening this chapter portray items that may be used or places visited by people of a North American Indian heritage. The bear and bear claw represent sacred symbols of an animal that is revered and sacred to many people. The bear is symbolic of the power of nature. The drawstring bag is symbolic of the tobacco bag one may carry; tobacco is a sacred plant. The sweet grass surrounding the claw is from the American Indian Sioux Nation. It is burned, the flame is blown out, and the smoke is used to purify a room or home. The dreamcatcher in the second image is from the Cherokee Nation in Carolina. Traditional lore says that, if you keep this dreamcatcher near you, it will filter out ILLNESS and keep you well. The medicine bag from the Acama Pueblo in New Mexico holds herbs used in restoring HEALTH. The figure in the third image is a Cherokee house minder. It is the spirit of the little people, who are mischievous and enjoy playing tricks on the people who live in the home. They protect the home while the residents are away. The last image is a corner of the National Museum of the American Indian, which is a part of the Smithsonian Institution in Washington, DC. The exhibits change frequently and present images of American Indian life and culture. If you have not visited this museum, or the ones in New York City or Maryland, visit the Web site for a preview of the outstanding exhibits.

■ Background

The descendants of the original inhabitants of the North American continent and Alaska numbered 4.1 million people, or 1.5% of the total population of the United States in 2000. This number included 2.5 million people, or 0.9%, who reported only American Indian and Alaska Native, in addition to 1.6 million people, or 0.6%, who reported American Indian and Alaska Native as well as one or more other races (Census 2000). When compared to "U.S. All Races," the American Indian/Alaska Native (AI/AN) population lags behind in several areas, including lower educational levels and higher unemployment rates. The AI/AN population is a young population. The median age of the population is 28.0 years, compared with 35.3 years for all races in the United States. The American Indian population served by the Indian Health Service is living longer than it did 30 or even 20 years ago. Statistics on age at death show that, during 1972–1974, life expectancy at birth for the AI/AN population was 63.6 years; as of 1999–2001, it had increased to 74.5 years. However, according to an article by E. Nieves in the *New York Times*, (2007), the young American Indians at the Rosebud and Pine Ridge Reservations are committing, or attempting, suicide in record numbers. Health services are underfunded and Congress has failed to reauthorize a law that would increase aid. In addition, the American Indian and Alaska Native (AI/AN) population has larger families, less health insurance, and a poverty level over two times that of the rest of the population.

The first time that American Indians were counted as a separate group was in the 1860 census, and the 1890 census was the first to count American Indians throughout the country. The counting of American Indians before 1890 was limited to those living in the general population of the various states;

the American Indians residing in American Indian Territory and on American Indian reservations were not included. Alaska Natives, in Alaska, have been counted since 1880, but until 1940 they were generally reported in the "American Indian" racial category. The people were enumerated separately (as Eskimo and Aleut) in 1940 in Alaska. It was not until the 1970 census that separate response categories were used to collect data on the Eskimo and Aleut population, and then only in Alaska.

The West has the largest American Indian population, as well as the highest proportion of American Indians in its total population. States with the largest American Indian population are California, Oklahoma, Arizona, Texas, New Mexico, New York, Washington, North Carolina, Michigan, and Alaska. The largest American cities with the largest American Indian and Alaska Native population are New York; Los Angeles, California; Phoenix, Arizona; Tulsa, Oklahoma; Oklahoma City, Oklahoma; Anchorage, Alaska; Albuquerque, New Mexico; Tucson, Arizona; Chicago, Illinois; San Diego, California; and Houston, Texas. Other cities with a population of 100,000 or more with the highest percentage of American Indians and Alaska Natives include Green Bay, Wisconsin; Tacoma, Washington; Minneapolis, Minnesota; Spokane, Washington; and Sacramento, California.

The American Indian Nations that were the largest in 2000, as illustrated in Figure 8–1 were Cherokee, Navajo, Latin American Indian, Choctaw, Sioux, and Chippewa. The largest Alaska Native group was Eskimo (Ogunwole, 2002, pp. 1–4, 6, 8–10).

To realize the plight of today's American Indian, it is necessary to journey back in time to the years when Whites settled in this land. Before the arrival of Europeans, this country had no name but was inhabited by groups of people who called themselves nations. The people were strong both in their knowledge of the land and in their might as warriors. The Vikings reached the shores of this country about A.D. 1010. They were unable to settle on the land and left after a decade of frustration. Much later, another group of settlers, since termed the "Lost Colonies," were repulsed. More people came to these shores, however, and the land was taken over by Europeans.

As the settlers expanded westward, they signed "treaties of peace" or "treaties of land cession" with the American Indians. These treaties were similar to those struck between nations, although in this case the agreement was imposed by the "big" nation onto the "small" nation. One reason for treaties was to legitimize the takeover of the land that the Europeans had "discovered." Once the land was "discovered," it was divided among the Europeans, who set out to create a "legal" claim to it. The American Indians signed the resultant treaties, ceding small amounts of their land to the settlers and keeping the rest for themselves. As time passed, the number of Whites rapidly grew, and the number of Indians diminished because of wars and disease. As these events occurred, the treaties began to lose their meaning; the Europeans disregarded them. They decided that these "natives" had no real claim to the land and shifted them around like cargo from one reservation to another. Although the American Indians tried to seek just settlements through the American court

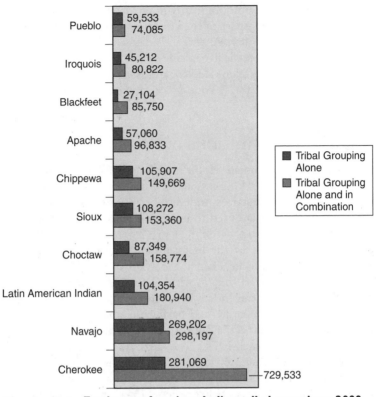

Figure 8–1   Ten largest American Indian tribal groupings: 2000.
Source: Orgunwole, S. H. (2002). The American Indian and Alaska Native Population: 2000. U.S.
Department of Commerce, U.S. Census Bureau, p. 10.

system, they failed to win back the land that had been taken from them through misrepresentation. For example, in 1831, the Cherokees were fighting in the courts to keep their nation in Georgia. They lost their legal battle, however, and, like other American Indian nations after the time of the early European settlers, were forced to move westward. During this forced westward movement, many died, and all suffered. Today, many nations are seeking to reclaim their land through the courts (Brown, 1970; Deloria 1969, 1974; Fortney, 1977). Several claims, such as those of the Penobscot and Passamaquody tribes in Maine, have been successful. The number of federally recognized tribes has increased from just over 100 as recently ago as the 1980s to 561 presently (IHS, 2007).

As the American Indians migrated westward, they carried with them the fragments of their culture. Their lives were disrupted, their land was lost, and many of their leaders and teachers perished, yet much of their history and culture somehow remained. Today, more and more American Indians are seeking to know their history. The story of the colonization and settlement of the United States is being retold with a different emphasis.

American Indians live predominantly in 26 states (including Alaska), with most residing in the western part of the country as a result of the forced westward migration. Although many American Indians remain on reservations and in rural areas, just as many people live in cities, especially on the West Coast. Oklahoma, Arizona, California, New Mexico, and Alaska have the largest numbers of American Indians (IHS, 2007). Today, more and more people are claiming to have American Indian roots.

■ Traditional Definitions of HEALTH and ILLNESS

Although each American Indian nation or tribe had its own history and belief system regarding HEALTH and ILLNESS and the traditional treatment of ILLNESS, some general beliefs and practices underlie the more specific tribal ideas. The terms HEALTH and ILLNESS are used to indicate that, among traditional people, the connotations are holistic, as defined in Chapter 4. The data—collected through an ongoing review of the literature and from interviews granted by members of the groups—come from the Navajo Nation, Hopis, Cherokees, Shoshones, and New England Indians with whom I have worked closely.

The traditional American Indian belief about HEALTH is that it reflects living in "total harmony with nature and having the ability to survive under exceedingly difficult circumstances" (Zuckoff, 1995). Humankind has an intimate relationship with nature (Boyd, 1974). The Earth is considered to be a living organism—the body of a higher individual, with a will and a desire to be well. The Earth is periodically HEALTHY and less HEALTHY, just as human beings are. According to the American Indian belief system, a person should treat his or her body with respect, just as the Earth should be treated with respect. When the Earth is harmed, humankind, is itself harmed and, conversely, when humans harm themselves, they harm the Earth. The Earth gives food, shelter, and medicine to humankind; for this reason, all things of the Earth belong to human beings and nature. "The land belongs to life, life belongs to the land, and the land belongs to itself." In order to maintain HEALTH, Indians must maintain their relationship with nature. "Mother Earth" is the friend of the American Indian, and the land belongs to the American Indian (Boyd, 1974).

According to American Indian belief, as explained by a medicine man, Rolling Thunder, the human body is divided into two halves, which are seen as plus and minus (yet another version of the concept that every whole is made of two opposite halves). There are also—in every whole—two energy poles: positive and negative. The energy of the body can be controlled by spiritual means. It is further believed that every being has a purpose and an identity. Every being has the power to control him- or herself and, from this force and the belief in its potency, the spiritual power of a person is kindled (Boyd, 1974).

In all American Indian cultures, disease is associated with the religious aspect of society as supernatural powers are associated with the causing and curing of disease. Disease is conceived of in a wide variety of ways. It is believed to occur due to a lack of prevention, which is given by wearing or using charms; the presence of some material object that has intruded into the body via sorcery; or the absence of the free soul from the body (Lyon, 1996, pp. 60–61). One example of an amulet is *Duklij*, turquoise or green malachite that is believed to contain supernatural qualities that ward off the evil spirits and bring rain (Lyon, 1996, p. 68).

Many American Indians with traditional orientations believe there is a reason for every sickness or pain. They believe that ILLNESS is the price to be paid either for something that happened in the past or for something that will happen in the future. In spite of this conviction, a sick person must still be cared for. Everything is seen as being the result of something else, and this cause-and-effect relationship creates an eternal chain. American Indians do not generally subscribe to the germ theory of modern medicine. ILLNESS is something that must be. Even the person who is experiencing the ILLNESS may not realize the reason for its occurrence, but it may, in fact, be the best possible price to pay for the past or future event(s) (Boyd, 1974).

The Hopi Indians associate ILLNESS with evil spirits. The evil spirit responsible for an ILLNESS is identified by the medicine man, and the remedy for the malady resides in the treatment of the evil spirit (Leek, 1975, p. 16).

According to legend, the Navajo people originally emerged from the depths of the Earth—fully formed as human beings. Before the beginning of time, they existed with holy people, supernatural beings with supernatural powers, in a series of 12 underworlds. The creation of all elements took place in these underworlds, and there all things were made to interact in constant harmony. A number of ceremonies and rituals were created at this time for "maintaining, renewing, and mending this state of harmony" (Bilagody, 1969, p. 21).

When the Navajo people emerged from the underworlds, one female was missing. She was subsequently found by a search party in the same hole from which they had initially emerged. She told the people that she had chosen to remain there and wait for their return. She became known as death, sickness, and witchcraft. Because her hair was unraveled and her body was covered with dry red ochre, the Navajos today continue to unravel the hair of their dead and to cover their bodies with red ochre. Members of the Navajo Nation believe that "witchcraft exists and that certain humans, known as witches, are able to interact with the evil spirits. These people can bring sickness and other unhappiness to the people who annoy them" (Bilagody, 1969, p. 36).

Traditionally, the Navajos see ILLNESS, disharmony, and sadness as the result of one or more combinations of the following actions: "(1) displeasing the holy people; (2) annoying the elements; (3) disturbing animal and plant life; (4) neglecting the celestial bodies; (5) misuse of a sacred Indian ceremony; or (6) tampering with witches and witchcraft" (Bilagody, 1969, p. 57). If disharmony exists, disease can occur. The Navajos distinguish between two types of disease: (1) contagious diseases, such as measles, smallpox, diphtheria, syphilis, and gonorrhea, and (2) more generalized ILLNESSES, such as "body fever" and "body ache." The notion that ILLNESS is caused by a microbe or another physiological agent is alien to the Navajos. The cause of disease, of injury to people or to their property, or of continued misfortune of any kind must be traced back to an action that should not have been performed. Examples of such infractions are breaking a taboo and contacting a ghost or witch. To the Navajos, the treatment of an ILLNESS, therefore, must be concerned with the external causative factor(s), not with the ILLNESS or injury itself (Kluckhohn & Leighton, 1962, pp. 192–193).

■ Traditional Methods of HEALING

Traditional HEALERS

The traditional HEALER of Native America is the medicine man or woman, and American Indians, by and large, have maintained their faith in him or her over the ages. The medicine men and women are wise in the ways of the land and of nature. They know well the interrelationships of human beings, the Earth, and the universe. They know the ways of the plants and animals, the sun, the moon, and the stars. Medicine men and women take time to determine first the cause of an ILLNESS and then the proper treatment. To determine the cause and treatment of an ILLNESS, they perform special ceremonies, which may take up to several days.

A medicine man or woman is also known among many people as a *Kusiut,* a "learned one." The acquisition of full shamanic powers takes many years, often as many as 30 years of training before one has the ability to cure illness. The shaman's power is accumulated through solitary vision quests and fasts repeated over the years. The purification rituals include scrubbing oneself in freezing cold water and ingesting emetics (Lyon, 1996, p. 141).

As a specific example, Boyd describes the medicine man, Rolling Thunder—the spiritual leader, philosopher, and acknowledged spokesman of the Cherokee and Shoshone tribes—as being able to determine the cause of ILLNESS when the ILL person does not know it. The "diagnostic" phase of the treatment may take as long as 3 days. There are numerous causes of ILLNESS and a great number of reasons—good or bad—for having become ILL. These causes are of a spiritual nature. When modern physicians see a sick person, they recognize and diagnose only the physical illness. Medicine men and women, in contrast, look for the spiritual cause of the problem. To the American Indian, "every physical thing in nature has a spiritual nature because the whole is viewed as being essentially spiritual in nature." The agents of nature, herbs, are seen as spiritual helpers, and the characteristics of plants must be known and understood. Rolling Thunder states that "we are born with a purpose in life and we have to fulfill that purpose" (Boyd, 1974, pp. 124, 263). The purpose of the medicine man or woman is to cure, and their power is not dying out.

The medicine man or woman of the Hopis uses meditation in determining the cause of an ILLNESS and sometimes even uses a crystal ball as the focal point for meditation. At other times, the medicine man or woman chews on the root of jimsonweed, a powerful herb that produces a trance. The Hopis claim that this herb gives the medicine man or woman a vision of the evil that has caused a sickness. Once the meditation is concluded, the medicine man or woman is able to prescribe the proper herbal treatment. For example, fever is cured by a plant that smells like lightning; the Hopi phrase for fever is "lightning sickness" (Leek, 1975, p. 16).

The Navajo Indians consider disease to be the result of breaking a taboo or the attack of a witch. The exact cause is diagnosed by divination, as is the ritual of treatment. There are three types of divination: motion in the hand (the most common form and often practiced by women), stargazing, and listening. The function of the diagnostician is first to determine the cause of the ILLNESS and then to recommend the treatment—that is, the type of chant that will be effective and the medicine man or woman who can best do it. A medicine man or woman may be called on to treat obvious symptoms, whereas the diagnostician is called on to ascertain the cause of the ILLNESS. (A person is considered wise if the diagnostician is called first.) Often, the same medicine man or woman can practice both divination (diagnosis) and the singing (treatment). When any form of divination is used in making the diagnosis, the diagnostician meets with the family, discusses the patient's condition, and determines the fee.

The practice of motion in the hand includes the following rituals. Pollen or sand is sprinkled around the sick person, during which time the diagnostician sits with closed eyes and face turned from the patient. The HEALER's hand begins to move during a song. While the hand is moving, the diagnostician thinks of various diseases and various causes. When the arm begins to move in a certain way, the diagnostician knows that the right disease and its cause have been discovered. He or she is then able to prescribe the proper treatment (Wyman, 1966, pp. 8–14). The ceremony of motion in the hand also may incorporate the use of sand paintings. (These paintings are a well-known form of art.) Four basic colors are used—white, blue, yellow, and black—and each color has a symbolic meaning. Chanting is performed as the painting is produced, and the shape of the painting determines the cause and treatment of the ILLNESS. The chants may continue for an extended time (Kluckhohn & Leighton, 1962, p. 230), depending on the family's ability to pay and the capabilities of the singer. The process of motion in the hand can be neither inherited nor learned. It comes to a person suddenly, as a gift. It is said that people able to diagnose their own ILLNESSES are able to practice motion in the hand (Wyman, 1966, p. 14).

Unlike motion in the hand, stargazing can and must be learned. Sand paintings are often but not always made during stargazing. If they are not made, it is either because the sick person cannot afford to have one done or because there is not enough time to make one. The stargazer prays the star prayer to the star spirit, asking it to show the cause of the ILLNESS. During stargazing, singing begins and the star throws a ray of light that determines the cause of the patient's ILLNESS. If the ray of light is white or yellow, the patient will recover; if it is red, the ILLNESS is serious. If a white light falls on the patient's home, the person will recover; if the home is dark, the patient will die (Wyman, 1966, p. 15).

Listening, the third type of divination, is somewhat similar to stargazing, except that something is heard rather than seen. In this instance, the cause of the ILLNESS is determined by the sound that is heard. If someone is heard to be crying, the patient will die (Wyman, 1966, p. 16).

The traditional Navajos continue to use medicine men and women when an ILLNESS occurs. They use this service because, in many instances, the treatment they receive from the traditional HEALERS is better than the treatment they receive from the health care establishment. Treatments used by singers include massage and heat treatment, the sweatbath, and use of the yucca root—approaches similar to those common in physiotherapy (Kluckhohn & Leighton, 1962, p. 230).

The main effects of the singer are psychological. During the chant, the patient feels cared for in a deeply personal way as the center of the singer's attention, since the patient's problem is the reason for the singer's presence. When the singer tells the patient recovery will occur and the reason for the ILLNESS, the patient has faith in what is heard. The singer is regarded as a distinguished authority and as a person of eminence with the gift of learning from the holy people. He or she is considered to be more than a mere mortal. The ceremony—surrounded by such high levels of prestige, mysticism, and power—takes the sick person into its circle, ultimately becoming one with the holy people by participating in the sing that is held on the patient's behalf. The patient once again comes into harmony with the universe and subsequently becomes free of all ILLS and evil (Kluckhohn & Leighton, 1962, p. 232).

The religion of the Navajos is one of good hope when they are sick or suffer other misfortunes. Their system of beliefs and practices helps them through the crises of life and death. The stories that are told during ceremonies give the people a glimpse of a world that has gone by, which promotes a feeling of security because they see that they are links in the unbroken chain of countless generations (Kluckhohn & Leighton, 1962, p. 233).

Many Navajos believe in witchcraft, and, when it is considered to be the cause of an ILLNESS, special ceremonies are employed to rid the individual of the evil caused by witches. Numerous methods are used to manipulate the supernatural. Although many of these activities may meet with strong social disapproval, Navajos recognize the usefulness of blaming witches for ILLNESS and misfortune. Tales abound concerning witchcraft and how the witches work. Not all Navajos believe in witchcraft but, for those who do, it provides a mechanism for laying blame for the overwhelming hardships and anxieties of life.

Such events as going into a trance can be ascribed to the work of witches. The way to cure a "witched" person is through the use of complicated prayer ceremonies that are attended by, friends and relatives, who lend help and express sympathy. The victim of a witch is in no way responsible for being sick and is, therefore, free of any punitive action by the community if the ILLNESS causes the victim to behave in strange ways. However, if an incurably "witched" person is affected so that alterations in the person's established role severely disrupt the community, the victim may be abandoned (Kluckhohn & Leighton, 1962, p. 244). Box 8–1 presents selected beliefs of a traditional Cherokee medicine man.

Box 8–1

Hawk Littlejohn, 1941–2000

I had the privilege of working with Hawk Littlejohn, a traditional medicine man, in 1979 at the Boston (Massachusetts) Indian Council. Thomas Crowe wrote in his obituary that Hawk Littlejohn "embraced tradition in the modern world. He was a native of Western North Carolina and a member of the Eastern Band of the Chero-kee nation. He was unique both in his skills in the traditional methods of natural and psychological healing and in his sensitivity and concern for his fellow man." I in-terviewed him in June 1979. Here are several of his thoughts in his own words:

- A medicine man sees himself in my tribe as a person who is many, many things. Not just as a HEALER or not just as a priest. We like to see ourselves like the fingers on a hand. They are separated and work independently of the hand if requested to, but they're still part of the whole. And each one of these fingers can do different things. It's like when I go to visit a home and there is a child there who is suffering from malnutrition but in our medicine we're more interested in the cause not the symptom. So, I've left my role as a HEALER and a priest to a role that might turn out to be social or political to find out why the child is hungry, why this child is feeling this way. And that might be dealing with the tribal government or some kind of social situation. We elect to see ourselves as representatives of our people's needs.

- The medicine man or HEALER in my tribe is considered to be chosen by the Great Spirit. For a couple of years the medicine men check all children for unusual marks, it is not any particular mark on the body but something they consider very unusual as a sign. The unusual marks that were on me were Simian Creases, the line that goes across my hand. I'm told it is unusual to have one of these but to have two, one on each hand, is very unusual. I was perhaps two or three years old when I was chosen.

- As a child I was taught that there are three parts of us and the most obvi-ous part is the physical aspect, then the second part is the intellectual part, and the third part is the spiritual aspect of a person. The physical is the tan-gible, the one we can see and touch and be with all the time. We go through acceptance of our physical being. This is what I have to walk the path of life with and I accept it for what it is. The intellectual aspect is the part that in-terprets things for you—dreams, visions, feelings, and what the spirit is say-ing to you. The spiritual aspect of a person of is the slowest and the last in most cases to mature. The spiritual aspect is kept in harmony and in balance by the awareness that it is part of everything else. We believe that all life forms have a spirit and the relationship of man to all other beings that are alive is a spiritual one. When all three aspects are working together it is called balance and harmony, or the center of the earth.

- Let's say a student, for example, puts a lot of emphasis on the intellect and neg-lects the physical and the spiritual aspect of him, we believe that there are nat-ural forces which always try to seek a balance. For instance, if you get a cut, you heal because it is natural to try to seek balance. We believe that there are

(continued)

many subtle things the Great Spirit made and very obvious things that the Great Spirit made like creatures like elephants, whales, and the obvious. And then much more subtle creatures like what you call germs and viruses and when we believe that when the Great Spirit created life, he created laws to govern life, that the wolf wouldn't eat the deer in one day, that there would be laws to govern these kinds of things. One of the laws was what we call a *"skilly."* It is a being or a creature and it has no good or bad. When a person neglects the spiritual and physical part for the intellect, and does not seek balance, the *skilly* comes in and one of the effects of the *skilly* is sickness and disease.

- One of the ways to treat people is indirectly. When I go to see people we talk about their corn and their lives and they talk about my corn and my life and then we get down to the reason why I am there. They don't tell me their physical symptoms. One of the things we've realized is that sickness isolates people from other people and the sickness has separated the person from the community and from his family. So we automatically try to make him or bring him back out of that isolation and one of the ways we do that is to include the family and friends in the HEALING process.
- In my tribe we have knowledge of about 500 different plants and use about 350 of them on a pretty regular basis. We see the plants as other life forms, but the commonality between all life forms is this spiritual aspect. We believe that each thing that is alive has a spirit and its spirit has a personality, so I use the spirit of the plant to cure another spirit—when the spirit of the sickness is not compatible with the spirit of the plant, the disease dissipates. We call the plants, plant people. My people's medicine started off as a trial and error, like most medicine did, using the plants. If you had a sickness that reminded them of a rabbit, for example, a plant that reminded them of a fox would be used to treat it.
- I think the solution to Indian problems is for Indian people to start identifying themselves. I see as a traditional person that one of the steps on this long journey is to gain pride and dignity in oneself. Naturally, I believe it is in traditionalism. Traditionalism is a philosophy, a way of life and living, a holistic sort of thing that we're a part of.

Traditional Remedies

American Indians practice an act of purification in order to maintain their harmony with nature and to cleanse the body and spirit. This is done by total immersion in water in addition to the use of sweatlodges, herbal medicines, and special rituals. Purification is seen as the first step in the control of consciousness, a ritual that awakens the body and the senses and prepares a person for meditation. The participants view it as a new beginning (Boyd, 1974, pp. 97–100).

The basis of therapy lies in nature, hence the use of herbal remedies. Specific rituals are to be followed when herbs are gathered. Each plant is picked to be dried for later use. No plant is picked unless it is the proper one, and only enough plants are picked to meet the needs of the gatherers. Timing is crucial, and the procedures are followed meticulously. So deep is their belief in the harmony of human beings and nature that the herb gatherers exercise great care not to disturb any of the other plants and animals in the environment (Boyd, 1974, pp. 101–136).

One plant of interest, the common dandelion, contains a milky juice in its stem and is said to increase the flow of milk from the breasts of nursing mothers. Another plant, the thistle, is said to contain a substance that relieves the prickling sensation in the throats of people who live in the desert. The medicine used to hasten the birth of a baby is called "weasel medicine" because the weasel is clever at digging through and out of difficult territory (Leek, 1975, p. 17).

The following is a list of common ailments and herbal treatments used by the Hopi Indians (Leek, 1975, pp. 17–26):

1. Cuts and wounds are treated with globe mallow. The root of this plant is chewed to help mend broken bones.

2. To keep air from cuts, piñon gum is applied to the wound. It is used also in an amulet to protect a person from witchcraft.

3. Cliff rose is used to wash wounds.

4. Boils are brought to a head with the use of sand sagebrush.

5. Spider bites are treated with sunflower. The person bathes in water in which the flowers have been soaked.

6. Snakebites are treated with the bladder pod. The bitter root of this plant is chewed and then placed on the bite.

7. Lichens are used to treat the gums. They are ground to a powder and then rubbed on the affected areas.

8. Fleabane is used to treat headaches. The entire herb is either bound to the head or infused and drunk as a tea.

9. Digestive disorders are treated with blue gillia. The leaves are boiled in water and drunk to relieve indigestion.

10. The stem of the yucca plant is used as a laxative. The purple flower of the thistle is used to expel worms.

11. Blanket flower is the diuretic used to provide relief from painful urination.

12. A tea is made from painted cup and drunk to relieve the pain of menstruation.

13. Winter fat provides a tea from the leaves and roots and is drunk if the uterus fails to contract properly during labor.

The use of American Indian cures and herbal remedies continues to be popular. Among the Oneida Indians, the following remedies are used (Knox & Adams, 1988):

Illness	Remedy
Colds	Witch hazel, sweet flag
Sore throat	Comfrey
Diarrhea	Elderberry flowers
Headache	Tansy and sage
Ear infection	Skunk oil
Mouth sores	Dried raspberry leaves

Among the Micmac Indians of Canada, the following remedies have been reported to be used (Basque and Young, 1984):

Illness	Remedy
Warts	Juice from milkweed plant
Obesity	Spruce bark and water
Rheumatism	Juniper berries
Diabetes	Combination of blueberries and huckleberries
Insomnia	A head of lettuce a day
Diarrhea	Tea from wild strawberry

Drums are another source of treatment. HEALING ceremonies are accompanied by drumming, rattles, and singing. The noise consists of sounds that interfere with the negative work of the spirits of the disease. The rhythm of the drumming plays a role in altering human consciousness (Lyon, 1996, p. 67). "Drumming is essential in helping the shaman make the transition from an ordinary state of consciousness to the shamanistic state of consciousness" (p. 68). Quiet HEALING ceremonies are unheard of.

Table 8–1 summarizes the cultural phenomena affecting American Indians, Aleuts, and Eskimos.

Table 8–1   Examples of Cultural Phenomena Affecting Health Care Among the American Indian and Alaska Native Population

Nations of origin	Five hundred sixty-one American Indian Nations indigenous to North America; Aleuts and Eskimos in Alaska
Environmental control	Traditional HEALTH and ILLNESS beliefs may continue to be observed by "traditional" people Natural and magico-religious folk medicine tradition Traditional HEALER—medicine man or woman
Biological variations	Accidents Heart disease Cirrhosis of the liver Diabetes mellitus
Social organization	Extremely family-oriented to both biological and extended families Children taught to respect traditions Community social organizations
Communication	Tribal languages Use of silence and body language
Space	Space is very important and has no boundaries
Time orientation	Present

Source: Spector, R. (1992). Culture, ethnicity, and nursing. In P. Potter & A. Perry (Eds.), *Fundamentals of nursing* (3rd ed.). St. Louis, MO: Mosby-Year Book. Reprinted with permission.

■ Current Health Care Problems

Today, American Indians are faced with a number of health-related problems and health disparities. Many of the old ways of diagnosing and treating illness have not survived the migrations and changing ways of life of the people. Because these skills often have been lost and because modern health care facilities are not always available, American Indian people are frequently caught in limbo when it comes to obtaining adequate health care. At least one third of American Indians exist in a state of abject poverty. With this destitution come poor living conditions and attendant problems, as well as diseases of the poor—including malnutrition, tuberculosis, and high maternal and infant death rates. Poverty and isolated living serve as further barriers that keep American Indians from using limited health care facilities even when they are available. Many of the illnesses that are familiar among White patients may manifest themselves differently in American Indian patients. As alluded to at the beginning of this chapter, suicide rates among the young are high—a rate that is more than three times that of the general population (Nieves, 2007, p. A-9). The traumas that the American Indians in the Plains States experienced over the past 175 years, such as the massacre at Wounded Knee, are part of the problem, as is the decimation of the land and culture.

Morbidity and Mortality

The American Indian and Alaska Native people have long experienced lower health status when compared with other Americans. Lower life expectancy and the disproportionate disease burden exist perhaps because of inadequate education, disproportionate poverty, discrimination in the delivery of health services, and cultural differences. These are broad quality-of-life issues rooted in economic adversity and poor social conditions.

American Indians and Alaska Natives born today have a life expectancy that is 2.4 years less than the U.S. population of all races (74.5 years to 76.9 years, respectively, American Indian and Alaska Native infants die at a rate of nearly 10 per every 1,000 live births, as compared to 7 per 1,000 for the U.S. population (2001–2003 rates). Given the higher health status enjoyed by most Americans, the lingering health disparities of American Indians and Alaska Natives are troubling. In trying to account for the disparities, health care experts, policymakers, and tribal leaders are looking at many factors that impact the health of Indian people, including the adequacy of funding for the American Indian health care delivery system (Indian Health Service [2007] Fact Sheet. Retrieved February 23, 2008, from http://www.INS.gov).

The American Indian and Alaska Native population has several characteristics different from the U.S. population that would impact assessing the cost for providing similar health services enjoyed by most Americans. The American Indian population is younger, because of higher mortality, than all other U.S. races. The IHS service population is predominately rural, which should suggest lower costs; however, the disproportionate incidence of

Table 8-2   Comparison of Selected Health Status Indicators—All Races and American Indians and Alaska Natives: 1999/2004

Health Indicator	All Races 1999/2004	American Indians and Alaska Natives 1999/2004
Crude birth rate per 1,000 population by race of mother	14.5/14.0	16.8/14.0
Percentage of live births of women receiving prenatal care first trimester	83.2/83.9	69.5/69.9
Percentage of live births of women receiving third-trimester or no prenatal care	3.8/3.6	8.2/7.9
Percentage of live births to teenage childbearing women—under 18	4.4/3.4	7.9/6.4
Percentage of low birth weight per live births >2,500 grams, 1997–1999	7.57/8.3	7.15/8.7
Infant mortality per 1,000 live births 1996–1998/2003	7.2/6.8	9.3/8.7
Cancer—all sites per 100,000 population, 1997/2003	384.5/447.1	148.6/298.5(2002)
Lung cancer incidence per 100,000 population, 1997/2003	Men: 65.4/73.0 Women: 40.7/48.7	Men[a] Women[a]
Breast cancer incidence per 100,000, 1997	113.1/121.1	28.7
Prostate cancer incidence per 100,000 1997	136.0/160.4	41.2
Male death rates from suicide, all ages, age adjusted per 100,000 resident population, 1999/2003	18.1/10.8	19.1/16.6
Male death rates from homicide, all ages, age adjusted per 100,000 resident population, 1999/2003	9.3/9.4	15.4/10.5

Source: National Center for Health Statistics. (2006). *Health, United States, 2006 with chartbook on trends in the health of Americans* (pp. 135, 140, 144, 149, 160, 227, 230, 244). Hyattsville, MD: Author.

[a] Data not available.

disease and medical conditions experienced by the American Indian population raises the costs, which almost obliterates the lower cost offsets. Table 8–2 compares selected health status indicators for all races and American Indians. As can be seen in Table 8–2, the crude birth rate among American Indians/Alaska Natives is higher than that of the general population; the infant mortality rate is higher, although it did drop in 2004 as compared to 1999; and the male suicide and homicide rates in 2004 are higher than in the general population. The incidence of both breast cancer and prostate cancer is lower.

The bold areas in Table 8–3 illustrate the greatest areas of disparity between American Indians and all other races in the United States. Diabetes, homicide, infant deaths, and so forth are notably higher.

Table 8-3 **Mortality Disparities Rates Between American Indians and Alaska Natives (AI/AN) in the IHS Service Area 1996–1998 to 2001–2003 and U.S. All Races 1997 and 2002 Age-Adjusted Rates per 100,000 Population**

	AI/AN Rate 2001–2003	U.S. All Races Rate— 2002	Ratio: AI/AN to U.S. All Races	AI/AN Rate 1996–1998	U.S. All Races Rates— 1997	Ratio: AI/AN to U.S. All Races
All Causes	1042.2	845.3	1.2	1070.8	888.5	1.2
Alcohol-induced	43.6	6.7	6.5	45.0	7.3	6.2
Breast cancer	15.4	25.6	0.6	19.8	28.9	0.7
Cerebrovascular	54.7	56.2	1.0	62.8	65.6	1.0
Cervical cancer	4.4	2.6	1.7	5.2	3.2	1.6
Diabetes	**75.2**	**25.4**	**3.0**	**77.8**	**24.2**	**3.2**
Heart disease	234.5	240.8	1.0	272.4	278.1	1.0
HIV infection	3.2	4.9	0.7	3.3	6.5	0.5
Homicide (assault)	**12.7**	**6.1**	**2.1**	**12.9**	**7.3**	**1.8**
Infant deaths[a]	**9.8**	**7.0**	**1.4**	**8.9**	**7.2**	**1.2**
Malignant neoplasm	181.8	193.5	0.9	187.5	207.9	0.9
Maternal deaths	**12.7**	**8.9**	**1.4**	**7.8**	**8.4**	**0.9**
Motor vehicle	**51.1**	**15.7**	**3.3**	**43.1**	**13.9**	**3.1**
Pneumonia/ influenza	**33.3**	**22.6**	**1.5**	**31.3**	**23.5**	**1.3**
Suicide	**17.1**	**10.9**	**1.6**	**18.0**	**11.4**	**1.6**
Tuberculosis	**1.8**	**0.3**	**6.0**	**2.0**	**0.4**	**5.0**
Unintentional injuries	**93.8**	**36.9**	**2.5**	**98.7**	**37.3**	**2.6**

Source: U.S. Department of Health and Human Services, Indian Health Service. (2007). *Facts on health disparities.* Retrieved from http://info.ihs.gov/

[a]Infant deaths per 1,000 live births.

Note: Rates are adjusted to compensate for misreporting of American Indian and Alaska Native race on state death certificates. American Indian and Alaska Native death rate columns present data for the 3-year period specified. U.S. All Races columns present data for a 1-year period. ICD-10 codes were introduced in 1999; therefore, comparability ratios were applied to deaths for years 1996–1998. Rates are based on American Indian and Alaska Native alone; 2000 census with bridged-race categories.

Mental Illness

The family in this population is often a nuclear family, with strong biological and large extended family networks. Children are taught to respect traditions, and community organizations are growing in strength and numbers. Many American Indians tend to use traditional medicines and HEALERS and are knowledgeable about these resources. People may frequently be treated by a traditional medicine man or woman. The sweatlodge and herbs are frequently used to treat

Table 8–4   Comparison: the 10 Leading Causes of Death for American Indians and Alaska Natives and for All Persons, 2004

American Indians and Alaska Natives	All Persons
1. Diseases of heart	Diseases of heart
2. Malignant neoplasms	Malignant neoplasms
3. Unintentional injuries	Cerebrovascular diseases
4. Diabetes mellitus	Chronic lower respiratory diseases
5. Cerebrovascular diseases	Unintentional injuries
6. Chronic liver disease and cirrhosis	Diabetes mellitus
7. Chronic lower respiratory diseases	Alzheimer's disease
8. Suicide	Influenza and pneumonia
9. Influenza and pneumonia	Nephritis, nephrotic syndrome, and
10. Nephritis, nephrotic syndrome, and	nephrosis
nephrosis	Septicemia

Source: National Center for Health Statistics. (2007). *Health, United States, 2007 with chartbook on trends in the health of Americans* (pp. 186–187). Hyattsville, MD: Author.

mental symptoms. Several diagnostic techniques include the use of divination, conjuring, and stargazing.

"Ghost sickness" affects some American Indians. This mental health problem involves a preoccupation with death and the deceased and is associated with witchcraft. Symptoms include bad dreams, weakness, feelings of danger, loss of appetite, and confusion. *Pibloktoq* is a malady that afflicts some members of arctic and subarctic Eskimo communities. It is characterized by abrupt dissociative episodes, accompanied by extreme excitement, followed by convulsive seizures and coma (American Psychiatric Association, 1994).

Alcoholism is a major mental health problem among American Indians. A comparison of the 10 leading causes of death among American Indians/Alaska Natives and the general population reveals that unintentional injuries (#3), chronic liver disease and cirrhosis (#6), and suicide (#8) rank higher as causes of death than for the population at large. Each of these causes of death is related to mental health problems, including alcoholism.

Table 8–4 compares the 10 leading causes of death between all persons and American Indians and Alaska Natives.

Fetal Alcohol Syndrome

"My son will forever travel through a moonless night with only the roar of the wind for company" (Dorris, 1989, p. 264). This quote reflects on the tragedy of fetal alcohol syndrome, an affliction that affects countless American Indian children. A new study from the Substance Abuse and Mental Health Services Administration (SAMHSA) shows that American Indians and Alaska Natives continue to have higher rates of alcohol use and illicit drug use disorders than other racial groups.

The markings of fetal alcohol syndrome include

■ Abnormal growth in height, weight, and/or head circumference, including microcephaly

■ Central nervous system in behavioral and/or mental health problems, including learning disabilities and abnormal sleeping and eating patterns

■ Appearance with a specific pattern of recognizable deformities, such as the three key facial features a smooth philtrum, a thin vermillion border, and small palpebral fissures (Bertrand, Floyd, & Weber, 2005, p. 3)

An estimated 70,000 fetal alcohol children are born each year in the United States, many of whom are American Indians. The worldwide numbers vary, with a range of 0.2–1.5 cases per 1,000 live births being most frequently reported (Bertrand et al, 2005, p. 3). Dorris (1989, p. 231) further points out that the son of an alcoholic biological father is three times more likely to become an abusive drinker.

This problem has grown over time and the impact increases with each generation. Mortality and morbidity rates for American Indians are directly affected by alcohol abuse. Alcohol abuse is the most widespread and severe problem in the American Indian community. It is extremely costly to the people and underlies many of their physical, mental, social, and economic problems, and the problem is growing worse. Hawk Littlejohn, the medicine man of the Cherokee Nation, Eastern band, attributes this problem, from a traditional point of view, to the fact that American Indians have lost the opportunity to make choices. They can no longer choose how they live or how they practice their medicine and religion. He believes that, once people return to a sense of identification within themselves, they begin to rid themselves of this problem of alcoholism. Whatever the solution may be, the problem is indeed immense (Littlejohn, 1979 Interview).

Domestic Violence

Another problem related to alcohol abuse in the American Indian people is domestic violence, sexual abuse, and the battering of women. A battered woman is one who is physically assaulted by her husband, boyfriend, or another significant other. The assault may consist of a push; severe, even permanent injury; sexual abuse; child abuse; or neglect. Once the pattern of abuse is established, subsequent episodes tend to get worse. This abuse is not traditional in American Indian life but has evolved. True American Indian love is based on a tradition of mutual respect and the belief that men and women are part of an ordered universe the people should live in peace. In the traditional American Indian home, children were raised to respect their parents, and they were not corporally punished. Violence toward women was not practiced. In modern times, however, the sanctions and protections against domestic violence have decreased, and the women are far more vulnerable. Many women are reluctant to admit that they are victims of abuse because they believe that they will be blamed for the assault. Hence, the beatings continue. A number of services are available to women who are victims, such as safe houses and support groups. It is believed that the long-range solution to this problem lies in teaching children to love—to nurture children and give them self-esteem, to teach boys to love and respect women, and to give girls a sense of worth. Amnesty International calls sexual abuse against American Indian women a "Maze of Injustice." It is "the failure to protect Indigenous women from sexual violence in the USA." The disproportionate impact on American Indian women is derived from disparate communities that vary with respect to law enforcement, jurisdiction, and health care and support services (Grenier & Lockjer, 2007, p. 3).

Domestic violence has a profound effect on the community and on the family. A pattern of abuse is easily established. It begins with tension: The female attempts to keep peace but the male cannot contain himself, a fight erupts, and then the crisis arrives. The couple may make up, only to fight again. Attempts to help must be initiated, or the cycle escalates. The problem is extremely complex. Some of the services available to a household experiencing domestic violence include

1. Tribal health: direct services for physical and mental health
2. Law enforcement: police protection may be necessary
3. Legal assistance: assistance for immediate shelter and emergency food and transportation

Urban Problems

More than 50% of American Indians live in urban areas; for example, in Seattle, Washington, there are over 15,000 American Indians. Although this population is not particularly dense, its rates of diphtheria, tuberculosis, otitis media with subsequent hearing defects, alcohol abuse, inadequate immunization, iron-deficiency anemia, childhood developmental lags, mental health problems (including depression, anxiety, and coping difficulties), and caries and other dental problems are high. As in all dysfunctional families, problems arise that are related to marital difficulties and financial strain, which usually are brought about by unemployment and the lack of education or knowledge of special skills. The tension often is compounded further by alcoholism.

Between 5,000 and 6,000 American Indians live in Boston. They experience the same problems as American Indians in other cities, yet there is an additional problem. Few non-Indian residents are even aware that there is an American Indian community in that city or that it is in desperate need of adequate health and social services.

Health Care Provider Services

Some historical differences in health care relate to geographic locations. American Indians living in the eastern part of this country and in most urban areas are not covered by the services of the Indian Health Service, services that are available to American Indians living on reservations in the West. In 1923, tribal government—under the control of the Bureau of Indian Affairs—was begun by the Navajos, who established treaties with the U.S. government, but in the areas of health and education the United States did not honor these treaties. Health services on the reservations were inadequate. Consequently, the people were sent to outside institutions for the treatment of illnesses, such as tuberculosis and mental health problems. As recently as 1930, the vast Navajo lands had only seven hospitals with 25 beds each. Not until 1955 were American Indians finally offered concentrated services with modern physicians. Only since 1965 have more comprehensive services been available to the Navajos.

■ The Indian Health Service

The Indian Health Service (IHS) is an agency within the U.S. Department of Health and Human Services. It is responsible for providing federal health services to American Indians and Alaska Natives. The provision of health services to members of federally recognized tribes grew out of the special government-to-government relationship between the federal government and Indian tribes. This relationship was established in 1787. It is based on Article I, Section 8, of the Constitution and has been given form and substance by numerous treaties, laws, Supreme Court decisions, and executive orders. The IHS is the principal federal health care provider and health advocate for American Indian people. Its goal is to raise their health status to the highest possible level.

Between 1990 and 2007, the U.S. AI/AN population increased by 65% from 2.0 to 3.3 million people. The Indian Health Service (IHS) service area population comprises approximately 56% of the U.S. Indian population, and increases at a rate of approximately 1.9% per year. The Indian Health system is challenged to meet even 65% of the health needs of Indian country. The increase in the IHS service population is the result of natural increase (births minus deaths) and the expansion of the IHS service delivery area, as the result of the federal recognition of Tribes. It must be noted that 43% of the Indian population resides in rural areas (Indian Health Service 2007. Indian Population Trends, 2007 p. 1. Retrieved February 24, 2008 from http://info.ihs.gov/). The principal legislation authorizing federal funds for health services to recognized Indian tribes is the Snyder Act of 1921. It authorized funds for the relief of distress and conservation of health . . . [and] for the employment of . . . physicians . . . for Indian tribes throughout the United States." Congress passed the Indian Self-Determination and Education Assistance Act (Public Law 93-638, as amended) to provide tribes the option of either assuming from the IHS the administration and operation of health services and programs in their communities or remaining within the IHS-administered direct health system. Congress subsequently passed the Indian Health Care Improvement Act (P.L. 94-437), which is a health-specific law that supports the options of P.L. 93-638. The goal of P.L. 94-437 is to provide the quantity and quality of health services necessary to elevate the health status of American Indians and Alaska Natives to the highest possible level and to encourage the maximum participation of tribes in the planning and management of health services.

The IHS provides a comprehensive health services delivery system for American Indians and Alaska Natives with an opportunity for maximum tribal involvement in developing and managing programs to meet health needs. The IHS goal is to ensure that comprehensive, culturally acceptable personal and public health services are available and accessible to all American Indian people.

In order to carry out its mission, attain its goal, and uphold its foundation, the IHS

1. Assists tribes in developing their health programs through activities such as health management training, technical assistance, and human resource development
2. Assists tribes in coordinating health planning, in obtaining and using health resources available through federal, state, and local programs, and in operating comprehensive health care services and health programs

Preventive measures involving environmental, educational, and outreach activities are combined with therapeutic measures into a single national health system. Within these broad categories are special initiatives in traditional medicine, elder care, women's health, the care of children and adolescents, injury prevention, domestic violence and child abuse, health care financing, state health care, sanitation facilities, and oral health. Most IHS funds are appropriated for American Indians who live on or near reservations. Congress also has authorized programs that provide some access to care for American Indians who live in urban areas.

IHS services are provided directly and through tribally contracted and operated health programs. Health services also include health care purchased from private providers. The federal system consists of 33 hospitals, 54 health centers, and 38 health stations. In addition, 34 urban Indian health projects provide a variety of health and referral services.

Through P.L. 93-638 self-determination contracts, American Indian tribes and Alaska Native corporations administer 15 hospitals, 229 health centers, 116 health stations, and 162 Alaska village clinics (*Indian Health Service Fact Sheet,* 2007).

The IHS headquarters is located in Rockville, Maryland. Some headquarter's functions are conducted in IHS offices in Phoenix and Tucson, Arizona, and in Albuquerque, New Mexico. IHS regional administrative units, called area offices, are located in the following cities (as shown on the map—Figure 8–2):

Aberdeen, South Dakota	605-226-7581
Anchorage, Alaska	907-729-3686
Albuquerque, New Mexico	505-248-4500
Bemidji, Minnesota	218-444-0451
Billings, Montana	406-247-7107
Nashville, Tennessee	615-467-1505
Oklahoma City, Oklahoma	405-951-3716
Phoenix, Arizona	602-364-4123
Portland, Oregon	503-326-2020
Sacramento, California	916-930-3927
Tucson, Arizona	520-295-2406
Window Rock, Arizona	928-871-5811

(http://www.ihs.gov, 2007)

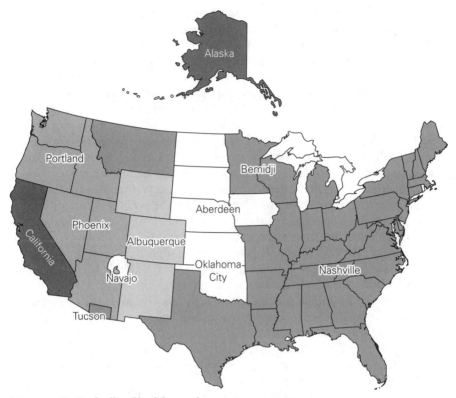

Figure 8-2   Indian Health service areas.
Source: Indian Health Service, 2007. Fact Sheet, author, Retrieved July, 2007 from http://www.ihs.gov

The ineligibility of American Indians living on the East Coast to secure such services has caused numerous difficulties for needy American Indians. Health care providers generally seem to think that American Indians should receive health services from the Indian Health Service and try to send them there. Unfortunately, there simply is no Indian Health Service on the East Coast, so American Indians tend to be shifted around among the regional health care resources that are available.

Many providers of health care and social services are not aware that many of the American Indians on the East Coast have dual citizenship as a result of the Jay Treaty of 1794, which allows for international citizenship between the United States and Canada, a fact that raises questions about whether American Indians can freely cross the border between the United States and Canada and whether those who live in the United States are eligible for welfare or Medicaid.

Cultural and Communication Problems

A factor that inhibits the American Indian use of White-dominated health services is a deep, cultural problem: American Indians suffer disease when they come into contact with White health care providers. American Indians feel uneasy because for too many years they have been the victim of haphazard care and disrespectful treatment. All too often, conflict arises between what the American Indians perceive their illness to be and what the physicians diagnose. American Indians, like most people, do not enjoy long waits in clinics; separation from their families; the unfamiliar, regimented environment of the hospital; or the unfamiliar behavior of the nurses and physicians, who often display demeaning and demanding attitudes. Their response to this treatment varies. Sometimes they remain silent; other times they leave and do not return. Many American Indians request that, if the ailment is not an emergency, they be allowed to see the medicine man or woman first and then receive treatment from a physician. Often, when a sick person is afraid of receiving the care of a physician, the medicine man or woman encourages the person to go to the hospital.

Health care providers must be aware of several factors when they communicate with American Indians. One is recognition of the importance of nonverbal communication. Often, American Indians observe providers and say very little. A patient may expect a provider to deduce the problem through instinct rather than by the extensive use of questions during history taking. In part, this derives from the belief that direct quoting is intrusive on individual privacy. When examining an American Indian with an obvious cough, a provider might be well advised to use a declarative statement—"You have a cough that keeps you awake at night"—and then allow time for the patient to respond to the statement.

It is American Indian practice to converse in a very low tone of voice. It is expected that the listener will pay attention and listen carefully in order to hear what is being said. It is considered impolite to say, "Huh?" or "I beg your pardon" or to give any indication that the communication was not heard. Therefore, an effort should be made to speak with patients in a quiet setting, where they will be heard more easily.

Note taking is taboo. Indian history has been passed through generations by means of verbal storytelling. American Indians are sensitive about note taking while they are speaking. When one is taking a history or interviewing, it may be preferable to use memory skills rather than to record notes. This more conversational approach may encourage greater openness between the patient and the provider.

Another factor to be considered is differing perceptions of time between the American Indian patient and the provider. Life on the reservation is not governed by the clock but by the dictates of need. When an American Indian moves from the reservation to an urban area, this cultural conflict concerning time often exhibits itself as lateness for appointments. One solution is the use of walk-in clinics.

American Indian Health Care Manpower

The number of American Indians enrolled in most health programs in selected health professions is low; when compared to the population percentages in Census 2000, demographic disparity is found in each of the professions. Tables 8–5 and 8–6 give the relative enrollment compared with total program enrollment and non-Hispanic White enrollment.

Recent nursing data are missing from the overall health professions enrollment data in Tables 8–5 and 8–6. However, the National Sample Survey of Registered Nurses 2004 prepared by the Bureau of Health Professions of the Health Resources Administration estimates that the registered nurse population in the

Table 8-5 American Indian Enrollment in Selected Health Profession Schools: 2004–2005

	Total Program Enrollment	American Indian Enrollment
Dentistry	18,315	93
Allopathic medicine	66,821	578
Osteopathic medicine	12,525	90
Nursing—registered[a]		
Optometry	5,377	29
Pharmacy	43,908	210
Podiatry	1,584	9

Source: National Center for Health Statistics. (2007). *Health, United States, 2007 with chartbook on trends in the health of Americans* (pp. 361–362). Hyattsville, MD: Author.

[a]The National League for Nursing changed the way it collects these data in 1991 and subsequently discontinued the practice, and enrollment data are not available after 1991.

United States in 2004 was 2,909,357. Of this number, 81.8% were White non-Hispanic and 0.2% were American Indian/Alaska Native (non-Hispanic) (HRSA/BHPr and the National Sample Survey of Registered Nurses). Given that in 2005 American Indian/Alaska Native (non-Hispanic) people comprised 0.9% of the resident population, this is a clear indication that there is no demographic parity in the percentage of American Indian/Alaska Native (non-Hispanic) people in nursing. This demographic picture and the percentages in the tables demonstrate a situation that is an ongoing concern. Somnath and Shipman, who reviewed a total of 55 studies, found that minority patients tend to receive better interpersonal care from practitioners of their own race or ethnicity, particularly in primary care and mental health settings, and that non–English speaking patients experience better interpersonal care, greater medical comprehension, and greater likelihood of keeping follow-up appointments when they see a language-concordant practitioner.

Table 8-6 Percentage of American Indians Enrolled in Selected Health Profession Schools, Compared with Non-Hispanic Whites: 2004–2005

	Non-Hispanic White (%)	American Indian (%)
Dentistry	66%	0.5
Allopathic medicine	63.3	0.9
Osteopathic medicine	73.5	0.7
Nursing—registered	[a]	[a]
Optometry	63.2	0.5
Pharmacy	59.7	0.5
Podiatry	60.4	0.6

Source: National Center for Health Statistics. (2007). *Health, United States, 2007 with chartbook on trends in the health of Americans* (pp. 361–362). Hyattsville, MD: Author.

[a]The National League for Nursing changed the way it collects these data in 1991 and subsequently discontinued the practice, and enrollment data are not available after 1991.

They concluded their study by stating that "the findings indicated greater health professions diversity will likely lead to improved public health by increasing access to care for underserved populations, and by increasing opportunities for minority patients to see practitioners with whom they share a common race, ethnicity or language." They also stated that "race, ethnicity, and language concordance, which is associated with better patient-practitioner relationships and communication, may increase patients' likelihood of receiving and accepting appropriate medical care" (Somnath & Shipman, 2006, p. 17). The Research on Culture box illustrates an example of research conducted in American Indian communities.

RESEARCH ON CULTURE

An infinite amount of research has been conducted among members of the American Indian and Alaska Native population. The following study is one example:

Dodgson, J. E., Struthers, R. (2005, October). Indigenous women's voices: Marginalization and health. Journal of Transcultural Nursing, 16(4), 339–346.

This study examines the ways that marginalization affects health care as experienced by 57 indigenous women. Marginalization is seen as a larger issue than cultural differences, as it includes exclusionary and isolating facets. The history of indigenous people is replete with examples of marginalization, and indigenous women have been particularly marginalized. A secondary analysis of qualitative data collected over 5 years was conducted with the goal of analyzing participants' experiences. The indigenous women participating in this study were urban and rural Ojibwe, Cree, Winnebago, and Lakota people residing in the northern Midwest region of the United States. The ages ranged from 18 to 65 years; most were employed outside the home; and their education ranged from less than high school to graduate education. The following three themes emerged:

1. **Historical trauma as lived marginalization.** The women spoke of the historical events that affected the current welfare of their families. They believed that current illnesses common among the people are due to lifestyle changes forced on their ancestors by the European colonists. Many participants spoke of the fact that their traditional culture was destroyed by the Christian church and others who were seeking their resources.

2. **Biculturalism experienced as marginalization.** The difficulties experienced when trying to negotiate mainstream culture and yet maintain their traditional perspectives. Some people choose to stay to themselves; others go out to the larger culture and tell of the traditional ways. All of the participants referred to biculturalism as a source of alienation.

3. **Interacting with complex health care system.** Family and community elders usually consulted before accessing mainstream health care services. A Cree medicine woman stated that "there is a need for non-aboriginal health professionals to understand what traditional healing is and to respect it."

The authors concluded by stating that this study provided insight into the misunderstandings that occur between health care providers and indigenous people.

Explore 🌐 MediaLink

Go to the Companion Website at www.prenhall.com/spector for chapter-related review questions, case studies, and activities. Contents of the CulturalCare Guide and CulturalCare Museum can also be found on the Companion Website. Click on Chapter 8 to select the activities for this chapter.

Internet Sources

Crowe, T. (2001). "Hawk Littlejohn embraced the traditional ways in the modern world." Smokey Mountain News. Retrieved from http://www.smokymountainnews.com/issues/1_01/1_17_01/front_littlejohn.shtml, July 21, 2007.

Grenier, D., and Lockjer, R. (2007). Domestic violence. http://www.ihs.gov/MedicalPrograms/MCH/M/obgyn0607_Feat.cfm#dv.

National Museum of the American Indian. (2008). Home Page. Washington, DC: Smithsonian http://www.nmai.si.edu/

Somnath, S., and Shipman, S. (2006). The rationale for diversity in the health professions: A review of the evidence. Washington, DC: U.S. Department of Health and Human Services Health Resources and Services Administration Bureau of Health Professions. http://www.hrsa.gov/

United States Department of Commerce, U.S. Census Bureau. Census 2000. (2002). Retrieved July 21, 2007 from http://www.census.gov/

United States Department of Health and Human Services, Health Resources and Services. (2004). The National Survey of Registered Nurses 2004 Documentation for the General Public Use File, 2006, Bureau of Health Professions Health Resources and Services Administration. HRSA/BHPr and the National Sample Survey of Registered Nurses. http://www.hrsa.gov/

United States Department of Health and Human Services, Indian Health Service, IHS. (2007). Fact Sheets Indian Population Trends, Indian Health Service Trends. Retrieved July, 2007 and February, 2008 from http://info.ihs.gov/

References

American Psychiatric Association. (1994). *Diagnostic and statistical manual of mental disorders* (4th ed.). Washington, DC: Author.

Basque, E. and Young, P. (1984). Personal Interviews, Boston Indian Council.

Bertrand, J., Floyd, R. L., Weber, M. K. (2005). Guidelines for identifying and referring persons with fetal alcohol syndrome. MMWR. V.54/RR-11.

Bilagody, H. (1969). An American Indian looks at health care. In R. Feldman & D. Buch (Eds.), *The Ninth Annual Training Institute for Psychiatrist-Teachers of Practicing Physicians*. Boulder, CO: WICHE, No. 3A30.

Boyd, D. (1974). *Rolling Thunder*. New York: Random House.

Brown, D. (1970). *Bury my heart at Wounded Knee*. New York: Holt.

Deloria, V., Jr. (1969). *Custer died for your sins*. New York: Avon Books.

Deloria, V., Jr. (1974). *Behind the trail of broken treaties*. New York: Delacorte.

Dorris, M. (1989). *The broken cord*. New York: Harper & Row.

Fortney, A. J. (1977, January 23). Has White man's lease expired? *Boston Sunday Globe*, pp. 8–30.

Kluckhohn, C., & Leighton, D. (1962). *The Navaho* (Rev. ed.). Garden City, NY: Doubleday.

Knox, M. E., & Adams, L. (1988). *Traditional health practices of the Oneida Indian*. Oshkosh: University of Wisconsin, College of Nursing.

Leek, S. (1975). *Herbs: Medicine and mysticism*. Chicago: Henry Regnery.

Littlejohn, Hawk. (1979). Personal Interview. Boston MA.

Lyon, W. S. (1996). *Encyclopedia of Native American healing*. New York: Norton.

National Center for Health Statistics. (2006). *Health, United States, 2006 with chartbook on trends in the health of Americans* (pp. 135, 140, 144, 149, 160, 244, 230, 227). Hyattsville, MD: Author.

National Center for Health Statistics. (2007). *Health, United States, 2007 with chartbook on trends in the health of Americans*. Hyattsville, MD: Author.

Nieves, E. (2007, June 9). *Indian reservation reeling in weave of youth suicides and attempts. New York Times*, p. A-9.

Ogunwole, S. H. (2002). *The American Indian and Alaska Native population: 2000. U.S. Census 2000*. Washington, DC: U.S. Department of Commerce.

Spector, R. (1992). Culture, ethnicity, and nursing. In P. Potter & A. Perry (Eds.), *Fundamentals of nursing* (3rd ed.). St. Louis: Mosby-Year Book.

Wyman, L. C. (1966). Navaho diagnosticians. In W. R. Scott & E. H. Volkhart (Eds.), *Medical care*. New York: John Wiley & Sons.

Zuckoff, M. (1995, April 18). More and more claiming American Indian heritage. *Boston Globe*, A8.

■ Additional Readings

Bear, S., & Bear, W. (1996). *The medicine wheel*. New York: Fireside.

Catlin, G. (1993). *North American Indian portfolio*. Washington, DC: Library of Congress.

Neihardt, J. G. (1991—original 1951). *When the tree flowered*. Lincoln: University of Nebraska Press.

Neihardt, N. (1993). *The sacred hoop*. Tekamah, NE: Neihardt.

Neihardt, J. G. (1998—original 1961). *Black Elk speaks*. Lincoln: University of Nebraska Press.

Noble, M. (1997). *Sweet Grass: Lives of contemporary Native women of the Northeast*. Mashpee, MA: C. J. Mills.

Peltier, L. (1999). *Prison writings: My life is my sun dance*. New York: St Martin's Press.

Senier, S. (2001). *Voices of American Indian assimilation and resistance*. Norman: University of Oklahoma Press.

Wiebe, R., & Johnson, Y. (1998). *Stolen life—The journey of a Cree woman*. Athens: Ohio University Press.

Wolfson, E. (1993). *From the Earth to the sky*. Boston: Houghton Mifflin.

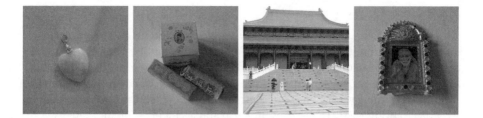

Chapter 9

HEALTH and ILLNESS in the Asian Populations

But when she arrived in the new country, the immigration officials pulled her swan away from her leaving the woman fluttering her arms and with only one swan feather for a memory.

—*Amy Tan*

■ Objectives

1. Discuss the background of the selected communities of the Asian populations.
2. Discuss the demographic profile of selected communities of the Asian populations.
3. Describe the traditional definitions of HEALTH and ILLNESS of selected communities of the Asian populations.
4. Describe the traditional methods of HEALTH maintenance and protection of selected communities of the Asian populations.
5. Describe the traditional methods of HEALING within selected communities of the Asian populations.
6. Describe the practice of a traditional healer.
7. Describe current health care problems of members of selected communities of the Asian populations.

The images opening this chapter depict objects, substances, places, and people that people of Asian origins may use, visit, or beseech to protect, maintain, and/or restore HEALTH. Jade, from China, is believed to be the most precious of all stones. It is the giver of children, health, immortality, and wisdom. Jade charms are worn to bring HEALTH—to prevent harm and accidents—and in these ways to protect HEALTH. The two small boxes in the second section contain minute pills made of herbs used for stomach ailments and the larger box contains a large wax ball with a preparation of *Jen Shen Lu Jung Wan* (Ginseng antler pills) in it. These pills are used as a general tonic to strengthen the body and to improve digestion. The image in the third section is that of the *Hsi Lai* Buddhist Temple in Hacienda Heights, California. The massive temple was built in order to be a cultural and spiritual center and is the ideal of its founder, Venerable Master *Hsing Yun* to promote Humanistic Buddhism. The fourth section contains an icon with the image of the *Sai Baba*. He was a healer in India who continues to have a following of many people. A further discussion of his activities is in this chapter on page 250.

■ Background

The nearly 12 million people who constitute the Asian communities are the United States' third largest emerging majority group. This number included 10.2 million people, or 3.6% of total population, who reported only Asian and 1.7 million people, or 0.6%, who reported Asian as well as one or more other races. The term *Asian* refers to people having origins in any of the original peoples of the Far East, Southeast Asia, or the Indian subcontinent (for example, Cambodia, China, India, Japan, Korea, Malaysia, Pakistan, the Philippine Islands, Thailand, and Vietnam). The Asian groups are not limited to nationalities but are characterized by their diversity: More than 30 different languages are spoken and there is a similar number of cultures (Martin, 1995) and many different religions, including, but not limited to, Buddhism, Confucianism, Hinduism, Islam, and Taoism. The Asian population increased faster than the total population of the United States between 1990 and 2000. About one half (49%) of the Asian population lived in the West, 20% lived in the Northeast, 19% lived in the South, and 12% lived in the Midwest. Over half of all people who reported Asian lived in just three states: Hawaii, California, and Washington. The cities with the largest Asian populations are New York, Los Angeles, San Jose, San Francisco, and Honolulu (Barnes & Bennett, 2002, pp. 1–3, 7). Table 9–1 illustrates selected variables from the demographic profiles of people born in Asia, China, and India who entered the United States before 2000. There have been 8,226,255 people admitted from Asia since before 1980, 50.8% of whom have been naturalized; 1,192,435 people admitted from China, 50% of whom have been naturalized; and 1,022,550 people admitted from India, 38% of whom have been naturalized (U.S. Census Bureau, 2002).

Census 2000 designated the Native Hawaiian and other Pacific Islanders as a separate category. However, because the population is small, health data are not reported for this group alone. Therefore, the data related to the population are nested within this chapter. The population of Native Hawaiian and Other Pacific Islanders numbers 874,000, or 0.3%, of the total U.S. population. The term

Table 9–1   Profile of Selected Demographic and Social Characteristics of People Entering the United States from Asia, China, and India: 1980–2000

Variable	Asia n = 8,226,255	China n = 1,192,435	India n = 1,022,550
Naturalized U.S. citizen	50.8%	50.0%	38.0%
Language other than English spoken at home (population 5 years and older)	90.7%	93.2%	90.8%
Speak English less than very well	48.5%	63.8%	27.2%
Median age	38.7 years	41.3 years	35.4 years
Marital status	65.6%	70.3%	74.8%
School enrollment—college or graduate school—population 3 years and over	57.0%	60.9%	57.8%
Educational attainment—bachelor's degree or higher—population 25 years and older	43.1%	42.7%	69.1%
Veteran status—civilian veterans	2.6%	1.7%	0.9%
Employment status—over 16 years of age employed	62.8%	61.0%	69.2%
Median household income	$50,554	$46,432	$69,076
Household income—$150,000 or more	7.7%	8.5%	13.3%
Median family income	$56,335	$52,579	$74,630
Per capita earnings	$26,222	$25,038	$36,937
Poverty status—families	11%	11.5%	5.4%

Source: U.S. Census Bureau, Census 2000. Special Tabulations. Profile of Selected Demographic and Social Characteristics: 2000 Asia, China, and India. Retrieved June 9, 2007 from http://factfinder.census.gov. http://www.census.gov/population/cen2000/stp-159/STP-159-Asia.pdf, http://www.census.gov/population/cen2000/stp-159/STP-159-China.pdf, http://www.census.gov/population/cen2000/stp-159/STP-159.india.pdf

refers to people having origins in any of the original peoples of Hawaii, Guam, Samoa, or other Pacific Islands. The people come from different cultures and speak many different languages (Grieco, 2001, pp. 1–2).

In Census 2000, the largest group of Asians was Chinese, with a total of 2.7 million people. Filipinos (2.4 million) and Asian Indians (1.9) were the next largest groups. Combined, Chinese, Filipinos, and Asian Indians account for 58% of the Asian population. Asian-born residents comprised 26% of the country's foreign-born population in 2000. Close to half of the nation's Asian-born population lived in one of three metropolitan areas—Los Angeles, New York, or San Francisco. Table 9–1 illustrates many of the demographic and social characteristics of the Asian, Chinese, and Indian people who have immigrated since 1980.

This chapter focuses on the traditional HEALTH and ILLNESS beliefs and practices of the Chinese and Indian Americans because those of many of the other Asians and Pacific Islanders are derived in part from the Chinese and Ayurvedic HEALTH traditions.

Chinese immigration to the United States began over 100 years ago. In 1850 there were only 1,000 Chinese inhabitants in this country; in 1880 there were well over 100,000. This rapid increase occurred in part because of the discovery of gold in California and in part because of the need for cheap labor to build the transcontinental railroads. The immigrants were laborers who met the needs of the dominant society. Like many early immigrant groups, they came here intending only to stay as temporary workers. Most of the immigrants were men, and they clung closely to their customs and beliefs and stayed together in their own communities. The hopes that many had for a better life when they came to the United States did not materialize. Subsequently, many of the workers and their kin returned to China before 1930. Part of the disharmony and disenchantment occurred because these immigrants were not White and did not have the same culture and habits as Whites. For these reasons, they were not welcomed, and many jobs were not open to them. For example, Chinese immigrant workers were excluded from many mining, construction, and other hard-labor jobs, even though the transcontinental railroad was constructed mainly by Chinese laborers. Between 1880 and 1930, the Chinese population declined by nearly 20%. One factor that helped perpetuate this decline in population was a series of exclusion acts halting further immigration. The people who remained behind were relegated to menial jobs, such as cooking and dishwashing. The Chinese workers first took these jobs in the West and later moved eastward throughout the United States. They tended to move to cities where they were allowed to let their entrepreneurial talents surface—their main pursuits included running small laundries, food shops, and restaurants.

The people settled in tightly knit groups in urban neighborhoods that took the name "Chinatown." Here they were able to maintain the ancient traditions of their homeland. They were hard workers and, in spite of the dull, menial jobs usually available to them, they were able to survive.

Both U.S. immigration laws and political problems in China have had an effect on the nature of today's Chinese population. When the exclusion acts were passed, many men were left alone in this country without the possibility that their families would join them. For this reason, a great majority of the men spent many years alone. In addition, the political oppression experienced by the Chinese in the United States was compounded—at a time when immigration laws were relaxed here after World War II, people were unable to return to or leave China because of that country's restrictive new regulations. By 1965, however, a large number of refugees who had relatives here were able to come to this country. They settled in the Chinatowns of America, causing the population of these areas to swell. The rate of increase since 1965 has been 10% per year.

■ Traditional Definitions of HEALTH and ILLNESS

Chinese medicine teaches that HEALTH is a state of spiritual and physical harmony with nature. In ancient China, the task of the physician was to prevent ILLNESS. A first-class physician not only cured an ILLNESS but could also prevent disease from occurring. A second-class physician had to wait for patients to become ill before they could be treated. The physician was paid by the patient while the patient was healthy. When illness occurred, payments stopped. Indeed, not only was the physician not paid for services when the patient became ill, but the physician also had to provide and pay for the needed medicine (Mann, 1972, p. 222).

To understand the Chinese philosophy of HEALTH and ILLNESS, it is necessary to look back at the age-old philosophies from which more current ideas have evolved. The foundation rests in the religion and philosophy of Taoism. Taoism originated with a man named Lao-Tzu, who is believed to have been born about 604 B.C. The word *Tao* has several meanings: way, path, or discourse. On the spiritual level, it is the way of ultimate reality. It is the way of all nature, the primeval law that regulates all heavenly and earthly matters. To live according to the Tao, one must adapt oneself to the order of nature. Chinese medical works revere the ancient sages who knew the way and "led their lives in Tao" (Smith, 1958, pp. 175–192).

The Chinese view the universe as a vast, indivisible entity, and each being has a definite function within it. No one thing can exist without the existence of the others. Each is linked in a chain that consists of concepts related to each other in harmonious balance. Violating this harmony is like hurling chaos, wars, and catastrophes on humankind—the end result of which is ILLNESS. Individuals must adjust themselves wholly within the environment. Five elements—wood, fire, earth, metal, and water—constitute the guiding principles of humankind's surroundings. These elements can both create and destroy each other. For example, "wood creates fire," "two pieces of wood rubbed together produce a spark," "wood destroys earth," "the tree sucks strength from the earth." The guiding principles arise from this "correspondences" theory of the cosmos (Wallnöfer & von Rottauscher, 1972, pp. 12–16, 19–21). Tables 9–2 and 9–3 highlight common elements of Asian/Pacific Island religions and give examples of phenomena affecting health care.

For a person to remain HEALTHY, his or her actions must conform to the mobile cycle of the correspondences. The exact directions for achieving this were written in such works as the *Lu Chih Ch'un Ch'iu* (*Spring and Autumn Annals*) written by Lu Pu Wei, who died circa 230 B.C.

The holistic concept, as explained by Dr. P. K. Chan (1988), is an important idea of traditional Chinese medicine in preventing and treating diseases. It has two main components:

1. A human body is regarded as an integral organism, with special emphasis on the harmonic and integral interrelationship between the viscera and the superficial structures in these close physiological connections, as well as their mutual pathological connection. In Chinese medicine, the local pathological changes always are considered in conjunction with other tissues and organs of the entire body, instead of considered alone.

2. Special attention is paid to the integration of the human body with the external environment. The onset, evolution, and change of disease are considered in conjunction with the geographic, social, and other environmental factors.

Table 9–2 Highlights of Common Elements of Asian Eastern Religions

The teachings of Asian religions, including Confucianism and Buddhism, are complementary and have played a major role in the shaping of the cultural values in Asia.

Buddhism teaches

- Harmony/nonconfrontation (silence as a virtue)
- Respect for life
- Moderation in behavior, self-discipline, patience, humility, modesty, friendliness, selflessness, dedication, and loyalty to others
- Individualism devalued

Confucianism teaches

- Achievement of harmony through observing the five basic relationships of society
  1. Ruler and ruled
  2. Father and son
  3. Husband and wife
  4. Older and younger brother
  5. Between friends
- Hierarchical roles, social class system, clearly defined behavioral code
- Importance of family
- Filial piety and respect for elders
- High regard for education and learning

Taoism teaches

- Harmony between humans and nature
- Nature is benign because *yin* (evil) and *yang* (good) are in balance and harmony
- Happiness and a long life
- Charity, simplicity, patience, avoidance of confrontation and an indirect approach to problems

Shamanism teaches

- Emphasis on nature
- Everything in nature is endowed with a spirit

Hinduism teaches

- "You can have what you want"
  1. Pleasure—through marriage and family
  2. Success—through vocation
  3. Duty—through civic participation
- The community is greater than ourselves
- The stages of life—student, householder, retirement, and *sannyasin*—"one who neither hates nor loves anything"
- Many paths to the same summit

Source: Romo, R. G. (1995, May 3). Hispanic health traditions and issues. Presented at the Minnesota Health Educators Conference. *Health education expanding our horizons.* Reprinted with permission; Smith, H. (1998). *The world's religions.* New York: HarperCollins.

Table 9–3   Examples of Cultural Phenomena Affecting Health Care Among Americans of Asian/Pacific Islander Heritage

Nations of Origin	China, Japan, Hawaii, the Philippines, Vietnam, Asian India, Bangladesh, and Pakistan, Korea, Samoa, Guam, and the remaining Asian/Pacific islands
Environmental Control	Traditional HEALTH and ILLNESS beliefs may continue to be observed by "traditional" people
Biological Variations	Hypertension
	Liver cancer
	Stomach cancer
	Coccidioidomycosis
	Lactose intolerance
	Thalassemia
Social Organization	Family—hierarchical structure, loyalty
	Large, extended family networks
	Devotion to tradition
	Many religions, including Taoism, Buddhism, Islam, and Hinduism
	Community social organizations
Communication	National language preference
	Dialects, written characters
	Use of silence
	Nonverbal and contextual cueing
Space	Noncontact people
Time Orientation	Present

Adapted from Spector, R. (1992). Culture ethnicity, and nursing. In P. Potter & A. Perry (Eds.), *Fundamentals of Nursing* (p. 101). St. Louis, MO: Mosby-Year Book. Reprinted with permission.

Four thousand years before the English physician William Harvey described the circulatory system in 1628, *Huang-ti Nei Ching* (*Yellow Emperor's Book of Internal Medicine*) was written. This is the first known volume that describes the circulation of blood. It described the oxygen-carrying powers of blood and defined the two basic world principles: *yin* and *yang*, powers that regulate the universe. *Yang* represents the male, positive energy that produces light, warmth, and fullness. *Yin* represents the female, negative energy—the force of darkness, cold, and emptiness. *Yin* and *yang* exert power not only over the universe but also over human beings.

Yin and *yang* were further explained by Dr. Chan as having been originally a philosophical theory in ancient China. Later, the theory was incorporated into Chinese medicine. The theory holds that "everything in the Universe contains two aspects—*yin* and *yang*, which are in opposition and also in unison. Hence, matters are impelled to develop and change." In traditional Chinese medicine, the phenomena are further explained as follows:

■ Matters that are dynamic, external, upward, ascending, and brilliant belong to *yang*.
■ Those that are static, internal, downward, descending, dull, regressive, and hypoactive are *yin*.

■ *Yin* flourishing and *yang* vivified steadily is the state of health. *Yin* and *yang* regulate themselves in the basic principle to promote the normal activities of life.

■ Illness is the disharmony of *yin* and *yang*, a disharmony that leads to pathological changes, with excesses of one and deficiencies of the other, disturbances of vital energy and blood, malfunctioning of the viscera, and so forth (Chan 1988).

The various parts of the human body correspond to the dualistic principles of *yin* and *yang*. The inside of the body is *yin*; the surface of the body is *yang*. The front part of the body is *yin*; the back is *yang*. The five *ts'ang* viscera—liver, heart, spleen, lungs, and kidney—are *yang*; the six *fu* structures—gallbladder, stomach, large intestine, small intestine, bladder, and "warmer"—are *yin*. (The "warmer" is now believed to be the lymph system.) The diseases of winter and spring are *yin*; those of summer and fall are *yang*. The pulses are controlled by *yin* and *yang*. If *yin* is too strong, the person is nervous and apprehensive and catches colds easily. If the individual does not balance *yin* and *yang* properly, his or her life will be short. Half of the *yin* forces are depleted by age 40, at 40 the body is sluggish, and at 60 the *yin* is totally depleted, at which time the body deteriorates. *Yin* stores the vital strength of life. *Yang* protects the body from outside forces, and it, too, must be carefully maintained. If *yang* is not cared for, the viscera are thrown into disorder, and circulation ceases. *Yin* and *yang* cannot be injured by evil influences. When *yin* and *yang* are sound, the person lives in peaceful interaction with mind and body in proper order (Wallnöfer & von Rottauscher, 1972).

Chinese medicine has a long history. The Emperor Shen Nung, who died in 2697 B.C., was known as the patron god of agriculture. He was given this title because of the 70 experiments he performed on himself by swallowing a different plant every day and studying the effects. During this period of self-experimentation, Nung discovered many poisonous herbs and rendered them harmless by the use of antidotes, which he also discovered. His patron element was fire, for which he was known as the Red Emperor. The Emperor Shen Nung was followed by Huang-ti, whose patron element was earth. Huang-ti was known as the Yellow Emperor and ruled from 2697 B.C. to 2595 B.C. The greater part of his life was devoted to the study of medicine. Many people ascribe to him the recording of the *Nei Ching*, the book that embraces the entire realm of Chinese medical knowledge. The treatments described in the *Nei Ching*—which became characteristic of Chinese medical practices—are almost totally aimed at reestablishing balances that are lost within the body when ILLNESS occurs. Disrupted harmonies are regarded as the sole cause of disease. Surgery was rarely resorted to; when it was, it was used primarily to remove malignant tumors. The *Nei Ching* is a dialogue between Huang-ti and his minister, Ch'i Po. It begins with the concept of the Tao and the cosmological patterns of the universe and goes on to describe the powers of the *yin* and *yang*. This learned treatise discusses in great detail the therapy of the pulses and how a diagnosis can be made on the basis of alterations in the pulse beat. It also describes various kinds of fevers and the use of acupuncture (Wallnöfer & von Rottauscher, 1972, pp. 26–28).

The Chinese view their bodies as a gift given to them by their parents and forebears. A person's body is not his or her personal property. It must be cared for and well maintained. Confucius taught that "only those shall be truly revered who at the end of their lives will return their physical bodies whole and sound."

The body is composed of five solid organs (*ts'ang*), which collect and store secretions, and five hollow organs (*fu*), which excrete. The heart and liver are regarded as the noble organs. The head is the storage chamber for knowledge, the back is the home of the chest, the loins store the kidneys, the knees store the muscles, and the bones store the marrow.

The Chinese view the functions of the various organs as comparable to the functions of persons in positions of power and responsibility in the government. For example, the heart is the ruler over all other civil servants, the lungs are the administrators, the liver is the general who initiates all the strategic actions, and the gallbladder is the decision maker.

The organs have a complex relationship, which maintains the balance and harmony of the body. Each organ is associated with a color. For example, the heart—which works in accordance with the pulse, controls the kidneys, and harmonizes with bitter flavors—is red. In addition, the organs have what is referred to as an "aura," the meaning of which, in the medical context, is HEALTH. The aura is determined by the color of the organ. In the balanced, healthy body, the colors look fresh and shiny.

Disease is caused by an upset in the balance of *yin* and *yang*. The weather, too, has an effect on the body's balance and the body's relationship to *yin* and *yang*. For example, heat can be injurious to the heart, and cold is injurious to the lungs. Overexertion is harmful to the body. Prolonged sitting is harmful to the flesh and spine, and prolonged lying in bed can be harmful to the lungs.

Disease is diagnosed by the Chinese physician through inspection and palpation. During inspection, the Chinese physician looks at the tongue (glossoscopy), listens and smells (osphretics), and asks questions (anamnesis). During palpation, the physician feels the pulse (sphygmopalpation).

The Chinese believe that there are many different pulse types, which are all grouped together and must be felt with the three middle fingers. The pulse is considered the storehouse of the blood, and a person with a strong, regular pulse is considered to be in good health. By the nature of the pulse, the physician is able to determine various illnesses. For example, if the pulse is weak and skips beats, the person may have a cardiac problem. If the pulse is too strong, the person's body is distended (Wallnöfer & von Rottauscher, 1972).

There are 6 different pulses, three in each hand. Each pulse is specifically related to various organs, and each pulse has its own characteristics. According to ancient Chinese sources, there are 15 ways of characterizing the pulses. Each of these descriptions accurately determines the diagnosis. There are 7 *piao* pulses (superficial) and eight *li* pulses (sunken). An example of an illness that manifests with a *piao* pulse is headache; anxiety manifests with a *li* pulse. The pulses also take on a specific nature with various conditions. For example, specific pulses are associated with epilepsy, pregnancy, and the time just before death.

The Chinese physician is aided in making a diagnosis by the appearance of the patient's tongue. More than 100 conditions can be determined by glossoscopic examination. The color of the tongue and the part of the tongue that does not appear normal are the essential clues to the diagnosis.

Breast cancer has been known to the Chinese since early times. "The disease begins with a knot in the breast, the size of a bean, and gradually swells to the size of an egg. After seven or eight months it perforates. When it has perforated, it is very difficult to cure" (Wallnöfer & von Rottauscher, 1972).

■ Traditional Methods of HEALTH Maintenance and Protection

There are countless ways by which HEALTH is maintained. One example is the practices involved in daily nutrition. Foods, such as thousand-year eggs, are ingested on a daily basis. There are strict rules governing food combinations and foods that must be eaten preceding and after life events, such as childbirth and surgery. Daily exercise is also important, and many people participate in formal exercise programs, such as tai chi.

The Chinese often prepare amulets to prevent evil spirits and protect HEALTH. These amulets consist of a charm with an idol or a Chinese character painted in red or black ink and written on a strip of yellow paper. These amulets are hung over a door or pasted on a curtain or wall, worn in the hair, or placed in a red bag and pinned on clothing. The paper may be burned and the ashes mixed in hot tea and swallowed to ward off evil. Jade is believed to be the most precious of all stones because it is seen as the giver of children, HEALTH immortality, wisdom, power, victory, growth, and food. Jade charms are worn to bring HEALTH and, should they turn dull or break, the wearer will surely meet misfortune. The charm prevents harm and accidents. Children are kept safe with jade charms, and adults are made pure, just, humane, and intelligent by wearing them (Morgan, 1942 [1972], pp. 133–134).

■ Traditional Methods of HEALTH Restoration

Just as there are countless methods used to maintain and protect HEALTH, there are countless ways to restore HEALTH. The following discussion describes traditional methods of restoring HEALTH.

Acupuncture

Acupuncture is an ancient Chinese practice of puncturing the body to cure disease or relieve pain. The body is punctured with special metal needles at points that are precisely predetermined for the treatment of specific symptoms. According to one source, the earliest use of this method was recorded between 106 B.C. and A.D. 200. According to other sources, however, it was used even earlier. This treatment modality stems from diagnostic procedures described earlier. The most important aspect of the practice of acupuncture is the acquired skill and ability to know precisely where to puncture the skin. Nine needles are used in acupuncture, each with a specific purpose. The following is a list of the needles and their purposes (Wallnöfer & von Rottauscher, 1972).

- Superficial pricking: arrowhead needle
- Massaging: round needle
- Knocking or pressing: blunt needle
- Venous pricking: sharp three-edged needle
- Evacuating pus: swordlike needle
- Rapid pricking: sharp, round needle
- Puncturing thick muscle: sharp, round needle
- Puncturing thick muscle: long needle
- Treating arthritis: large needle
- Most extensively used: filiform needle

The specific points of the body into which the needles are inserted are known as meridians. Acupuncture is based on the concept that certain meridians extend internally throughout the body in a fixed network. There are 365 points on the skin where these lines emerge. Since all the networks merge and have their outlets on the skin, the way to treat internal problems is to puncture the meridians, which are also categorically identified in terms of *yin* and *yang*, as are the diseases. The treatment goal is to restore the balance of *yin* and *yang* (Wallnöfer & von Rottauscher, 1972). The practice of this art is far too complex to explain in great detail in these pages.

Readers may find it interesting to visit acupuncture clinics in their area. After the therapist carefully explains the art and science of acupuncture, one may be able to grasp the fundamental concepts of this ancient treatment. The practice of acupuncture is based in antiquity, yet it took a long time for it to be accepted as a legitimate method of healing by practitioners of the Western medical system. Currently, numerous acupuncture clinics attract a fair number of non-Asians, and acupuncture is being used as a method of anesthesia in some hospitals.

Moxibustion, Cupping, Bleeding, and Tui Na

Moxibustion has been practiced for as long as acupuncture. Its purpose, too, is to restore the proper balance of *yin* and *yang*. Moxibustion is based on the therapeutic value of heat, whereas acupuncture is a cold treatment. Acupuncture is used mainly in diseases in which there is an excess of *yang*, and moxibustion is used in diseases in which there is an excess of *yin*. Moxibustion is performed by heating pulverized wormwood and passing this concoction above the skin, but not touching it, over certain specific meridians. Great caution must be used in this application because it cannot be applied to all the meridians that are used for acupuncture. Moxibustion is believed to be most useful during the period of labor and delivery, if applied properly.

Other important traditional HEALTH restoring practices are cupping, bleeding, and a form of traditional massage, *Tui Na*.

- Cupping, as seen in Figures 9–1A and 9–1B, involves creating a vacuum in a small glass by burning the oxygen out of it, then promptly placing

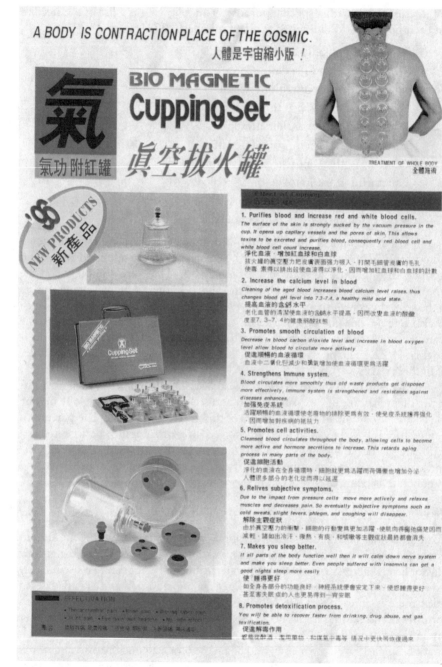

Figure 9-1a   Cupping.

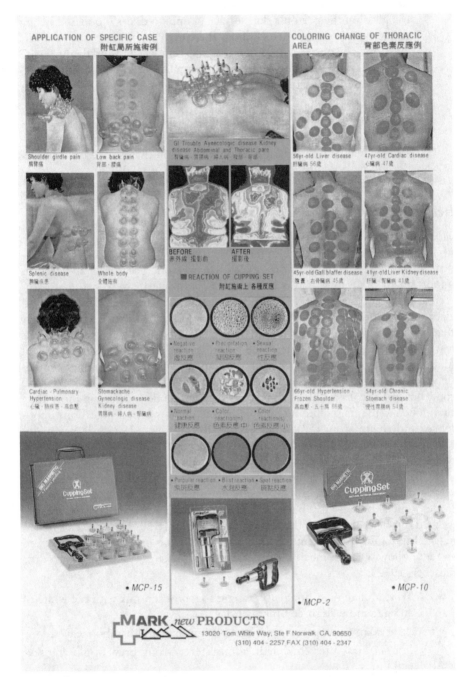

Figure 9–1b   Cupping.

the glass on the person's skin surface. Cupping draws blood and lymph to the body's surface that is under the cup. This increases the local circulation. The purpose for doing this is to remove cold and damp "evils" from the body and/or to assist blood circulation. The procedure is frequently used to treat lung congestion.

■ Bleeding, often done with the use of leeches, is performed to "remove heat from the body." Only small amounts of blood are removed.

■ Massage, *Tui Na*, "pushing and pulling," is a complex system of massage or manual acupuncture point stimulation that is used on orthopedic and neurological conditions (Ergil, 1996, pp. 208–209).

Herbal Remedies

Medicinal herbs were used widely in the practice of ancient Chinese healing. Many of these herbs are available and in use today.

Herbology is an interesting subject. The gathering season of an herb was important for its effect. It was believed that some herbs were better if gathered at night and that others were more effective if gathered at dawn. The ancient sages understood quite well the dynamics of growth. It is known today that a plant may not be effective if the dew has been allowed to dry on its leaves. The herbalist believes that the ginseng root must be harvested only at midnight in a full moon if it is to have therapeutic value. Ginseng's therapeutic value is due to its nonspecific action. The herb, which is derived from the root of a plant that resembles a person, is recommended for use in more than two dozen ailments, including anemia, colics, depression, indigestion, impotence, and rheumatism (Wallnöfer & von Rottauscher, 1972). It has maintained its reputation for centuries and continues to be a highly valued and widely used substance.

To release all the therapeutic properties of ginseng and to prepare it properly are of paramount importance. Ginseng must not be prepared in anything made of metal because it is believed that some of the necessary constituents are leeched out by the action of the metal. It must be stored in crockery. It is boiled in water until only a sediment remains. This sediment is pressed into a crock and stored. Following are some of the specific uses of ginseng (Wallnöfer & von Rottauscher, 1972):

■ To stimulate digestion: rub ginseng to a powder, mix with the white of an egg, and take three times per day.

■ As a sedative: prepare a light broth of ginseng and bamboo leaves.

■ For faintness after childbirth: administer a strong brew of ginseng several times a day.

■ As a restorative for frail children: give a dash of raw, minced ginseng several times per day.

There are many Chinese medicinal herbs, but none is as famous as ginseng.

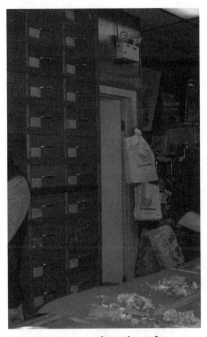

Figure 9-2a   Interior of a Chinese pharmacy.

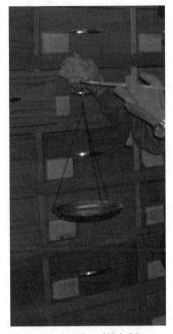

Figure 9-2b   Weighing herbs for a prescription.

I had the opportunity to visit, with one of my Asian American students, an import-export store in Boston's Chinatown where they sell Chinese herbs—if one has the proper prescriptions. The front of the store is a gift shop that attracts tourists. A room in the back is separated from the rest of the store. We were allowed to enter this room when the student explained to the proprietor, in Chinese, that I was her teacher and that she had brought me to the store to purchase herbs. We stayed there for quite a long time, observing the people who came in with prescriptions. The man carefully weighed different herbs, mixed them together, and dispensed them.

Figures 9–2A and 9–2B illustrate the interior of a Chinese pharmacy, the drawers containing herbs, and the method by which the herbs are weighed in the preparation of a prescription. The herbs necessary to fill the prescription are laid out on the paper in Figure 9–2A and the directions for preparing them are carefully given to the patient. In general, the herbs are wrapped in cheesecloth and placed in a determined amount of boiling water for a determined amount of time. The resulting liquid is then ingested in specific amounts, at specific times each day. The amount of time that the herbs are boiled determines the concentration of the medicine. Thus, the directions for preparation are carefully followed.

The Chinese doctor who practices in the pharmacy writes the prescription, and the cost of filling a prescription varies from nominal ($5.00) to quite expensive (several hundred dollars), depending on the herbs that are used.

We asked to purchase some of the herbs that he took from the drawers lining the entire wall behind him. He refused to sell us anything except some of the preparations that were on the counter because a prescription was necessary to purchase any of the herbal compounds that he prepared. Undaunted, we purchased a wide variety of herbs that could be used for indigestion, in addition to ointments and liniments used for sore muscles and sprains.

In addition to herbs and plants, the Chinese use other products with medicinal and healing properties. Some of these products were also used in ancient Europe and are still used today. For example, in China, boys' urine was used to cure lung diseases, soothe inflamed throats, and dissolve blood clots in pregnant women. In Europe, it was used during the two world wars as emergency treatment for open wounds. Urea is still used today as a treatment that promotes the healing of wounds. Other popular Chinese remedies include

■ Deer antlers—used to strengthen bones, increase a man's potency, and dispel nightmares

■ Lime calcium—used to clear excessive mucus

■ Quicksilver—used externally to treat venereal diseases

■ Rhinoceros horns—highly effective when applied to pus boils; an antitoxin for snakebites

■ Turtle shells—used to stimulate weak kidneys and to remove gallstones

■ Snake flesh—eaten as a delicacy to keep eyes healthy and vision clear

■ Seahorses—pulverized and used to treat gout

Traditional HEALERS

The physician was the primary HEALER in Chinese medicine. Physicians who had to treat women encountered numerous difficulties because men were not allowed to touch women directly who were not family members. Thus, a diagnosis might be made through a ribbon that was attached to the woman's wrist. As an alternative to demonstrating areas of pain or discomfort on a woman's body, an alabaster figure was substituted. The area of pain was pointed out on the figurine (Dolan, 1973, p. 30).

Not much is known about women doctors except that they did exist. Women were known to possess a large store of medical talent. There were also midwives and female shamans. The female shamans possessed gifts of prophecy. They danced themselves into ecstatic trances and had a profound effect on the people around them. As the knowledge that these women possessed was neither known nor understood by the general population, they were feared rather than respected. They were said to know all there was to know about life, death, and birth.

Chinese Pediatrics

Babies are generally breast-fed because neither cow's milk nor goat's milk is acceptable to the Chinese. Sometimes children are nursed for as long as 4 or 5 years. However, the practice is now varying as more women are working.

Since early time the Chinese have known about and practiced immunization against smallpox. A child was inoculated with the live virus from the crust of a pustule from a smallpox victim. The crust was ground into a powder, and this powder was subsequently blown into the nose of the healthy child through the lumen of a small tube. If the child was healthy, he or she did not generally develop a full-blown case of smallpox but, instead, acquired immunity to this dreaded disease (Wallnöfer & von Rottauscher, 1972).

Box 9–1 presents an overview of Ayurvedic Medicine.

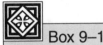

Box 9–1

Ayurvedic Medicine

Ayurveda is the science of life.
—Deepak Chopra, M.D.

Deepak Chopra introduced Ayurvedic medicine to the United States in 1984. He has emerged as one of the world's leading proponents of the innovative combination of Eastern and Western healing.

Ayurvedic medicine (also called Ayurveda) is one of the world's oldest, and many credit it with being the oldest, medical system. It originated in India and has evolved there over thousands of years. It developed from Hinduism, one of the world's oldest and largest religions and ancient Persian thoughts about HEALTH and HEALING. *Ayurveda* means "the science of life" and is built on theories of HEALTH and ILLNESS and on ways to prevent, manage, or treat HEALTH problems. It is holistic, as it integrates and balances the body, mind, and spirit. The balance is believed to lead to contentment and HEALTH and to help prevent ILLNESS, and it treats specific health problems, whether they are physical or mental. One goal of Ayurvedic practice is to cleanse the body of substances that can cause disease to reestablish harmony and balance (Fugh-Berman, 1996, pp. 36–38).

In the Ayurvedic philosophy, people, HEALTH, and the universe are said to be related, and HEALTH problems can result when the relationships are out of balance. Herbs, metals, massage, and other products and techniques are used with the intent of cleansing the body and restoring balance. Many of the Ayurvedic practices were handed down by word of mouth and were used before there were written records. Two ancient books, written in Sanskrit on palm leaves more than 2,000 years ago, are thought to be the first texts on Ayurveda: *Caraka Samhita* and *Susruta Samhita*. They cover many topics, including

- Pathology (the causes of illness)
- Diagnosis
- Treatment
- How to care for children
- Advice for practitioners, including ethics

(continued)

Ayurveda is the main system of health care in India, and variations of it have been practiced for centuries in Pakistan, Nepal, Bangladesh, Sri Lanka, and Tibet. About 70% of India's population lives in rural areas and about two thirds of rural people still use Ayurveda and medicinal plants to meet their primary health care needs. In addition, most major Indian cities have an Ayurvedic college and hospital.

The following is a summary of major beliefs in Ayurveda that pertain to HEALTH and disease.

- All things in the universe (both living and nonliving) are joined together.
- Every human being contains elements that can be found in the universe.
- All people are born in a state of balance within themselves and in relation to the universe.
- Disease arises when a person is out of harmony with the universe.

Traditional Definitions of HEALTH and ILLNESS

Basic HEALTH and ILLNESS beliefs include the following.

The constitution, or HEALTH, is called the *prakriti*. The *prakriti* is thought to be a unique combination of physical and psychological characteristics and the way the body functions. It is influenced by such factors as digestion and how the body deals with waste products. The *prakriti* is believed to be unchanged over a person's lifetime.

Three qualities, called *doshas*, form important characteristics of the constitution and control the activities of the body. Practitioners of Ayurveda call the *doshas* by their original Sanskrit names: *vata, pitta*, and *kapha*. It is also believed that

1. Each *dosha* is made up of one or two of the five basic elements: space, air, fire, water, and earth.
2. Each *dosha* has a particular relationship to body functions and can be upset for different reasons.
3. A person has his or her own balance of the three *doshas*, although one *dosha* usually is prominent. *Doshas* are constantly being formed and reformed by food, activity, and bodily processes.

The *vata dosha* is thought to be a combination of the elements space and air, and it controls very basic body processes, such as cell division, the heart, breathing, and the mind. *Vata* can be thrown out of balance by, for example, staying up late at night, eating dry fruit, or eating before the previous meal is digested. People with *vata* as their main *dosha* are thought to be especially susceptible to skin, neurological, and mental diseases.

The *pitta dosha* represents the elements fire and water. *Pitta* is said to control hormones and the digestive system. When *pitta* is out of balance, a person may experience negative emotions (such as hostility and jealousy) and have physical symptoms (such as heartburn within 2 or 3 hours of eating). *Pitta* is upset by, for example, eating spicy or sour food; being angry, tired, or fearful; or spending too much time in the sun. People with a predominantly *pitta* constitution are thought to be susceptible to heart disease and arthritis.

The *kapha dosha* combines the elements water and earth. *Kapha* is thought to help keep up strength and immunity and to control growth. An imbalance in the *kapha dosha* may cause nausea immediately after eating. *Kapha* is aggravated by, for example, sleeping during the daytime, eating too many sweet foods, eating

(continued)

after one is full, and eating and drinking foods and beverages with too much salt and water (especially in the springtime). Those with a predominant *kapha dosha* are thought to be vulnerable to diabetes, gallbladder problems, stomach ulcers, and respiratory illnesses, such as asthma (Roy, 1999, pp. 96–97).

Traditional Methods of HEALTH Restoration
In diagnosing a patient, the practitioner will

- Ask about diet, behavior, lifestyle practices, and the reasons for the most recent illness and symptoms the patient had
- Carefully observe such physical characteristics as teeth, skin, eyes, and weight
- Take a person's pulse, because each *dosha* is thought to make a particular kind of pulse

In addition to questioning, Ayurvedic practitioners use observation, touch, therapies, and advising. During an examination, the practitioner checks the patient's urine, stool, tongue, bodily sounds, eyes, skin, and overall appearance. The practitioner will also consider the person's digestion, diet, personal habits, and resilience (ability to recover quickly from illness or setbacks). As part of the effort to find out what is wrong, the practitioner may prescribe some type of treatment. The treatment is generally intended to restore the balance of a particular *dosha*.

The practitioner will develop a treatment plan and may work with people who know the patient well and can help. This helps the patient feel emotionally supported and comforted, which is considered important.

Patients are expected to be active participants in their treatment, because many Ayurvedic treatments require changes in diet, lifestyle, and habits. In general, treatments use several approaches, often more than one at a time. The following are the goals of treatment:

- *Eliminate impurities.* A process called *panchakarma* is intended to be cleansing; it focuses on the digestive tract and the respiratory system. For the digestive tract, cleansing may be done through enemas, fasting, or special diets. Some patients receive medicated oils through a nasal spray or an inhaler. This part of treatment is believed to eliminate worms or other agents thought to cause disease.
- *Reduce symptoms.* The practitioner may suggest various options, including yoga exercises, stretching, breathing exercises, meditation, and exposure to the sun. The patient may take herbs (usually several), often with honey, with the intent to improve digestion, reduce fever, and treat diarrhea. Sometimes foods such as lentil beans or special diets are also prescribed. Very small amounts of metal and mineral preparations also may be given, such as gold or iron. Careful control of these materials is intended to protect the patient from harm.
- *Reduce worry and increase harmony in the patient's life.* The patient may be advised to seek nurturing and peacefulness through yoga, meditation, exercise, or other techniques.
- *Help eliminate both physical and psychological problems.* Vital points therapy and/or massage may be used to reduce pain, lessen fatigue, or improve circulation. Ayurveda proposes that there are 107 "vital points" in the body where life energy is stored, and these points may be massaged to improve health. Other types of Ayurvedic massage use medicinal oils.

(continued)

In Ayurveda, the distinction between food and medicine is not as clear as in Western medicine. Food and diet are important components of Ayurvedic practice, so there is a heavy reliance on treatments based on herbs and plants, oils (such as sesame oil), common spices (such as turmeric), and other naturally occurring substances.

Currently, some 5,000 products are included in the "pharmacy" of Ayurvedic treatments. The following are a few examples of how some botanicals (plants and their products) have been or are currently used in treatment. In some cases, these may be mixed with metals.

- The spice turmeric has been used for various diseases and conditions, including rheumatoid arthritis, Alzheimer's disease, and wound healing.
- A mixture (*Arogyawardhini*) of sulfur, iron, powdered dried fruits, tree root, and other substances has been used to treat problems of the liver.
- An extract from the resin of a tropical shrub (*Commiphora mukul*, or guggul) has been used for a variety of illnesses. In recent years, there has been research interest in its possible use to lower cholesterol.

Traditional HEALERS

One example of a traditional Indian HEALER was *Sai Baba*, known as the God that descended to earth. *Sri Sai Baba*, who left his mortal body in 1918, is the living spiritual force that is drawing people from all walks of life, from all parts of the world, into his fold. It is believed that he came to serve humankind and to free them from the clutches of fear. He lived his message through the "Essence of His Being." His life and relationship with the common people was his teaching. He lived with the common people as a penniless *fakir*, wearing a torn *kafni*, sleeping over a mat while resting his head on a brick, and begging for his food. He radiated a mysterious smile and a deep, inward look, of a peace that was all-understanding. One story about him was that he saved a child from drowning. One report has it that word had spread that the 3-year-old daughter of a poor man called Babu Kirwandikar had fallen into a well and had drowned. When the villagers rushed to the well, they saw the child suspended in midair, as if some invisible hand was holding her up! She was quickly pulled out. *Sai Baba* was fond of that child, who was often heard to say, "I am *Baba's* sister!" After this incident, the villagers took her at her word. "It is all *Baba's Leela*," the people would say philosophically. It is from stories such as this that the people who believe in *Sri Sai Baba* gather strength.

Source: Sai Movement. (2002). *Shri SaiBaba of Shirdi* the Perfect Master of the Age. Shirdi, India: Shri SaiBaba Trust. Retrieved August 27, 2007 from http://www.shrisaibabasansthan.org/

■ Current Health Problems

In many instances, people who were born in the United States into families established here for generations are largely indistinguishable from the general population in their health care beliefs. Other groups, however, especially new immigrants, differ from the general population on many social and health-related issues. Table 9–4 compares selected health indicators in the Asian/Pacific Islander population with people of all races. In each of the selected categories, the rates for the Asian/Pacific Islander population are lower than those for the general population.

Table 9-4   Comparison of Selected Health Status Indicators, All Races and Asian/Pacific Islanders: 1999/2004

Health Indicator	All Races 1999/2004	Asian/Pacific Islanders 1999/2004
Crude birth rate per 1,000 population by race of mother	14.5/14.0	16.7/16.8
Percentage of live births of women receiving prenatal care first trimester	83.2/83.9	83.7/85.6
Percentage of live births of women receiving third-trimester or no prenatal care	3.8/3.6	3.5/3.0
Percentage of live births to teenage childbearing women—under 18	4.4/3.4	1.8/1.1
Percentage of low-birth-weight per live births <2,500 grams, 1997–1999/2003	7.57/8.3	7.37/7.7
Infant mortality per 1,000 live births 1996–1998/2003	7.2/6.8	5.2/4.8
Cancer—all sites per 100,000 population, 1997/2003	384.5/447.1	279.9/314.7
Lung cancer incidence per 100,000 population, 1997/2003	Men: 65.4/73.0 Women: 40.7/48.0	Men: 49.8/[a] Women: 22.1/[a]
Breast cancer incidence per 100,000, 1997/2003	113.1/121.1	85.6/87.4
Prostate cancer incidence per 100,000, 1997/2003	136.0/160.4	74.3/97.9
Male death rates from suicide, all ages, age adjusted per 100,000 resident population, 1999/2003	18.1/10.8	9.7/8.5
Male death rates from homicide, all ages, age adjusted per 100,000 resident population, 1999/2003	9.3/9.4	4.3/4.2

Source: National Center for Health Statistics. (2006). *Health, United States, 2006 with chartbook on trends in the health of Americans* (pp. 135, 140, 144, 149, 160, 227, 230, 244). Hyattsville, MD: Author.

[a]Data not available.

Poor health, however, continues to be found among the residents of Chinatowns partly because of poor working and crowded living conditions. Many people work long hours in restaurants and laundries and receive the lowest possible wages for their hard work. Many cannot afford even minimal, let alone preventive, health care. Americans of Asian and Pacific Island heritage frequently experience unique barriers, including linguistic and cultural differences, when they try to access the unfamiliar health care system.

Language difficulties and adherence to native Chinese culture compound problems already associated with poverty, crowding, and poor health. Many people still prefer the traditional forms of Chinese medicine and seek help from Chinatown "physicians" who treat them with traditional herbs and other methods.

Often, Asian people do not seek help from the Western system at all. Others use Chinese methods in conjunction with Western methods of health care, although the Chinese find many aspects of Western medicine distasteful. For example, they cannot understand why so many diagnostic tests, some of which are painful, are necessary. They do, however, accept the practice of immunization and the use of x-rays. An example of a modern health care practice that may cause a problem is the drawing of blood.

Chinese people cannot understand why the often frequent taking of blood samples, considered routine in Western medicine, is necessary. Blood is seen as the source of life for the entire body, and it is believed that blood is not regenerated. The Asian reluctance to have blood drawn for diagnostic tests may have its roots in the revered teachings of Confucius. The Chinese people also believe that a good physician should be able to make a diagnosis simply by examining a person. Consequently, they do not react well to the often painful procedures used in Western diagnostic workups. Some people—because of their distaste for the drawing of blood—leave the Western system rather than tolerate the pain. The Chinese have deep respect for their bodies and believe that it is best to die with their bodies intact. For this reason, many people refuse surgery or consent to it only under the most dire circumstances. This reluctance to undergo intrusive surgical procedures has deep implications for those concerned with providing health care to Asian Americans.

The hospital is an alien place to the Asian people. Not only are the customs and practices strange but also the patients often are isolated from the rest of their people, which enhances the language barrier and feelings of helplessness. Something as basic as food creates another problem. Hospital food is strange to Asian patients and is served in an unfamiliar manner. The typical Chinese patient rarely complains about what bothers him or her. Often the only indication that there may be a problem is an untouched food tray and the silent withdrawal of the patient. Unfortunately, the silence may be regarded by the nurses as reflecting good, complacent behavior, and the health care team exerts little energy to go beyond the assumption. The Chinese patient who says little and complies with all treatment is seen as stoic, and there is little awareness that deep problems may underlie this "exemplary" behavior. Ignorance on the part of health care workers may cause the patient a great deal of suffering.

Much action has been taken in recent years to make Western health care more available and appealing to the Chinese. In Boston, for example, there is a health clinic staffed primarily by Chinese dialects–speaking nurses and physicians who work as paid employees and as volunteers. Most of the common health-related pamphlets have been translated into Chinese languages and into Vietnamese, Cambodian, and Laotian, and they are distributed to the patients. Booklets on such topics as breast self-examination and smoking cessation are available. Since the languages spoken in the clinic are Mandarin Chinese and other dialects, the problem of interpreters has been largely eliminated. The care is personal, and the patients are made to feel comfortable. Unnecessary and painful tests are avoided as much as possible. In addition, the clinic, which is open for long hours, provides social services and employment placements and is

Table 9-5   Comparison of the 10 Leading Causes of Death for Asian/Pacific Islanders American and for All Persons: 2004

Asian/Pacific Islanders American	All Persons
1. Malignant neoplasms	Diseases of heart
2. Diseases of heart	Malignant neoplasms
3. Cerebrovascular diseases	Cerebrovascular diseases
4. Unintentional injuries	Chronic lower respiratory diseases
5. Diabetes mellitus	Unintentional injuries
6. Influenza and pneumonia	Diabetes mellitus
7. Chronic lower respiratory diseases	Alzheimer's disease
8. Suicide	Influenza and pneumonia
9. Nephritis, nephrotic syndrome, and nephrosis	Nephritis, nephrotic syndrome, and nephrosis
10. Alzheimer's disease	Septicemia

Source: National Center for Health Statistics. (2007). *Health, United States, 2007 with chartbook on trends in the health of Americans* (pp.186–187). Hyattsville, MD: Author.

quite popular with the community. Although it began as a part-time, storefront operation, the clinic is now housed in its own building.

Table 9-5 compares the 10 leading causes of death among Asian/Pacific Islanders with those of the general population.

The following is a synopsis of cultural beliefs regarding mental health and illness, possible causes of mental illness, and methods of preventing mental illness among people of Asian/Pacific Island origin. Lack of knowledge or skills in mental health therapy is seen in the Asian communities, as mental illness is much ignored in medical classics. Two points must be noted: the importance placed on the family in caring for the mentally ill and the tendency to identify mental illness in somatic terms. There is a tremendous amount of stigma attached to mental illness. Asian patients tend to come to the attention of mental health workers late in the course of their illness, and they come with a feeling of hopelessness (Lin, 1982, pp. 69–73).

One example of cross-cultural therapy is the Japanese practice of Morita therapy. This 70-year-old treatment originated from a treatment for shinkeishitsu, a form of compulsive neurosis with aspects of neurasthenia. The patient is separated from the family for 1 to 2 weeks and taught that one's feelings are the same as the Japanese sky and instantly changeable. One cannot be responsible for how one feels, only for what one does. At the end of therapy, the patient focuses on what is being done and less on his or her inner feelings, symptoms, concerns, or obsessive thoughts (Yamamoto, 1982, p. 50). In addition, there are countless culture-bound mental HEALTH syndromes that may be identified in the Asian communities:

■ Korea—*Hwa-byung*—a syndrome attributed to the suppression of anger is known as "anger syndrome"; symptoms include insomnia, indigestion, and dyspnea

■ China—*Koro*—the occurrence of sudden, intense anxiety when a man believes his penis is folding into his body

■ Japan—*Taijin kyofusho*—intense anxiety about possibly offending others (Fontaine, 2003, p. 119)

Asian American Health Care Manpower

Asian Americans, a group that constituted 4.7% of the resident U.S. population in the 2005 census, are for the most part well represented in the health professions, as illustrated in Tables 9–6 and 9–7. Today, persons who desire to be physicians in China have the option of studying either Chinese or Western medicine. If they select Western medicine, a limited amount of Chinese medicine is also taught. As Chinese traditional medicine is becoming better recognized and better understood in the United States, more doors are being opened to those who prefer or understand this mode of treatment.

Table 9–6 Asian Enrollment in Selected Health Professions Schools: 2004–2005

	Total Program Enrollment	Asian Enrollment
Dentistry	18,315	4,053
Allopathic medicine	66,821	13,811
Osteopathic medicine	12,525	1,961
Nursing—Registered[a]	a	a
Optometry	5,377	1,266
Pharmacy	43,908	9,103
Podiatry	1,584	176

Source: National Center for Health Statistics. (2007). *Health, United States: 2007* with chartbook on trends in the health of Americans (pp. 361–362). Hyattsville, MD: Author.

[a]no data available

Table 9–7 Percentage of Asian Enrolled in Selected Health Professions Schools Compared with Non-Hispanic Whites: 2004–2005

	Non-Hispanic Whites (%)	Asians (%)
Dentistry	66.1	22.1
Allopathic medicine	63.3	20.7
Osteopathic medicine	73.5	15.7
Nursing—Registered[a]	a	a
Optometry	63.2	23.5
Pharmacy	59.7	20.7
Podiatry	60.4	11.1

Source: National Center for Health Statistics. (2007). *Health, United States, 2007* with chartbook on trends in the health of Americans (pp. 361–362). Hyattsville, MD: Author.

[a]The National League for Nursing changed the way it collects these data in 1991 and subsequently discontinued the practice; enrollment data are not available after 1991.

The National Sample Survey of Registered Nurses 2004, prepared by the Bureau of Health Professions of the Health Resources Administration, estimates that the registered nurse population in the United States in 2004 numbered 2,909,357. Of this number, 81.8% were White non-Hispanic and 3.1% were Asian (non-Hispanic) and Native Hawaiian/Pacific Islander (non-Hispanic). Given that in 2005 people of Asian (non-Hispanic) and Native Hawaiian/ Pacific Islander (non-Hispanic) comprised 4.70% of the resident population (see Table 2–2 from Chapter 2) and (http://factfinder.census.gov September 18, 2007), this is a clear indication that there is not demographic parity in the percentage of Asian (non-Hispanic) and Native Hawaiian/Pacific Islander (non-Hispanic) people in nursing. One consequence of this factor may well be that there are insufficient numbers of nurses to work within the community and to serve as cultural advocates for community members, especially the new immigrants who may not speak English (see Table 9–1). See the discussion related to this issue in Chapter 8.

This demographic picture and the percentages in Tables 11–10 and 11–11 demonstrate a situation that is an ongoing concern. The findings of Somnath and Shipman who reviewed a total of 55 studies and found that minority patients tend to receive better interpersonal care from practitioners of their own race or ethnicity, particularly in primary care and mental health settings and that non-English speaking patients experience better interpersonal care, greater medical comprehension, and greater likelihood of keeping follow-up appointments when they see a language-concordant practitioner.

They concluded their study by stating that "the findings indicated greater health professions diversity will likely lead to improved public health by increasing access to care for underserved populations, and by increasing opportunities for minority patients to see practitioners with whom they share a common race, ethnicity or language." They also stated that "race, ethnicity, and language concordance, which is associated with better patient-practitioner relationships and communication, may increase patients' likelihood of receiving and accepting appropriate medical care" (Somnath & Shipman, 2006, p.17).

This chapter has presented an introductory overview of selected cultural phenomena, HEALTH traditions, and health issues of people from Asian heritages. Needless to say, a bigger picture of the phenomenon could fill many books. However, given the significant number of new Asians immigrants, especially from China and India, this beginning discussion is very necessary.

RESEARCH ON CULTURE

A large amount of research has been conducted among members of the Asian American populations. The study described in the following article is one example:

> Chou, F., Dodd, M., Abrams, D., & Padilla, G. (2007). Symptoms, self-care, and quality of life of Chinese American patients with cancer. Oncology Nursing Forum, 34(6), 1162–1167.

(continued)

This descriptive study explored the cancer symptoms, self-care strategies, and quality-of-life issues among a cohort of 25 Chinese-speaking patients in an urban clinical setting. The participants were first-generation immigrants, with low levels of acculturation; 88% could not read English; 64% had an annual household income of less than $20,000. The methods used included the Suinn-Lew Acculturation Scale, the Memorial Symptom Assessment Scale, and the Short Form 36 Health Survey. The study instruments were translated into Chinese. The participants reported experiencing an average of 14 symptoms weekly, including lack of energy, loss of hair, dry mouth, sleep difficulty, and loss of appetite. About 20% of the cohort reported the use of Chinese medicines as a part of the self-care methods.

The authors concluded that the use of translated tools can be a feasible method of data collection in studies with non-English-speaking patients and that it is important to have data collectors who are bilingual and well trained. The authors recommend that more attention to long-care cancer self-management in minority patients is needed. The implication is that further research with larger samples, more efficient community-based recruitment strategies, and the testing of culturally sensitive instruments is also needed.

Explore ▓▓▓ MediaLink

Go to the Companion Website at www.prenhall.com/spector for chapter-related review questions, case studies, and activities. Contents of the CulturalCare Guide and CulturalCare Museum can also be found on the Companion Website. Click on Chapter 9 to select the activities for this chapter.

■ Internet Sources

Hay, V. (1994). An Interview with Deepak Chopra. A Magazine of People and Possibilities online http://www.intouchmag.com/chopra.html

National Center for Alternative and Complimentary Medicine. (2007). Backgrounder: What is Ayurvedic Medicine? Bethesda, Maryland: Author. Retrieved July 2, 2007, from http://nccam.nih.gov/health/ayurveda/

Sai Movement. (2002). *Shri SaiBaba of Shirdi* the Perfect Master of the Age. Shirdi, India: *Shri SaiBaba* Trust. Retrieved August 27, 2007 from http://www.shrisaibabasansthan.org/

Somnath, S., and Shipman, S. (2006). The rationale for diversity in the health professions: A review of the evidence (Washington, DC: U.S. Department of Health and Human Services, Health Resources and Services Administration Bureau of Health Professions. http://www.hrsa.gov/

U.S. Census Bureau, Census 2000. Special Tabulations. Profile of Selected Demographic and Social Characteristics: 2000 Asia, China, and India. Retrieved June 9, 2007 from http://factfinder.census.gov, http://www.census.gov/population/cen2000/stp-159/STP-159-Asia.pdf, http://www.census.gov/population/cen2000/stp-159/STP-159-China.pdf, http://www.census.gov/population/cen2000/stp-159/STP-159India.pdf

United States Department of Commerce, U.S. Census Bureau. Census 2000. (2002). Retrieved July 21, 2007 from http://www.census.gov/

United States Department of Health and Human Services, Health Resources and Services. (2004). The National Survey of Registered Nurses 2004 Documentation for the General Public Use File, 2006, Bureau of Health Professions Health Resources and Services Administration. HRSA/BHPr and the National Sample Survey of Registered Nurses. http://www.hrsa.gov/

References

Barnes, J. S., & Bennett, C. E. (2002). *The Asian population: 2000*. Washington, DC: U.S. Department of Commerce.

Chan, P. K. (1988, August 3). Herb specialist, interview by author. New York City. Dr. Chan prepared a supplemental written statement in Chinese and English for inclusion in this text.

Dolan, J. (1973). *Nursing in society: A historical perspective*. Philadelphia: W. B. Saunders. National Center for Health Statistics.

Ergil, K. V. (1996). China's traditional medicine. In M. S. Micozzi (Ed.), *Fundamentals of complementary and alternative medicine*, New York: Churchill Livingstone.

Fontaine, K. L. (2003). *Mental health nursing* (5th ed.). Upper Saddle River, NJ: Prentice Hall.

Fugh-Berman, A. (1996). *Alternative medicine: What works*. Tucson, AZ: Odonian Press.

Grieco, E. M. (2001). *The Native Hawaiian and other Pacific Islander population: 2000*. Washington, DC: U.S. Department of Commerce.

Lin, K. M. (1982). Cultural aspects in mental health for Asian Americans. In A. Gaw (Ed.), *Cross-cultural psychiatry*. Boston: John Wright.

Mann, F. (1972). *Acupuncture*. New York: Vintage Books.

Martin, J. A. (1995). Birth characteristics for Asian or Pacific Islander subgroups, 1992. *Monthly Vital Statistics Report, 43*(10), 1.

Morgan, H. T. (1942 [1972]). *Chinese symbols and superstitions*. Detroit, MI: Gale Research. Reprint, S. Pasadena, CA: Ione Perkins.

National Center for Health Statistics. (2006). *Health, United States, 2006 with chartbook on trends in the health of Americans*. Hyattsville, MD: Author.

National Center for Health Statistics. (2007). *Health, United States, 2007 with chartbook on trends in the health of Americans*. Hyattsville, MD: Author.

Romo, R. G. (1995, May 3). *Hispanic health traditions and issues*. Paper presented at the Minnesota Health Educators Conference.

Roy, C. (1999). *Nurse's handbook of alternative and complementary therapies*. Springhouse, PAS: Springhouse.

Smith, H. (1958). *The religions of man*. New York: Harper & Row.

Spector, R. (1992). Culture, ethnicity, and nursing. In P. Potter & A. Perry (Eds.), *Fundamentals of nursing*. St. Louis: Mosby-Year Book.

U.S. Census Bureau. (2002). *A profile of the nation's foreign-born population from Asia*. Washington, DC: U.S. Department of Commerce.

Wallnöfer, H., & von Rottauscher, A. (1972). *Chinese folk medicine*. M. Palmedo (Trans.), New York: American Library.

Yamamoto, J. (1982). Japanese Americans. In A. Gaw (Ed.), *Cross-cultural psychiatry*. Boston: John Wright.

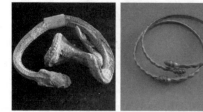 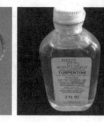 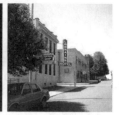

Chapter 10

HEALTH and ILLNESS in the Black Population

Who are we? We are the embodiment of the American dream, the architects of rock and roll, the builders of the cities, and the artisans on the assembly line. We are deep and real.

—*Bass & Pugh (2001)*

■ Objectives

1. Discuss the background of members of the Black population.
2. Discuss the demographic and new immigrant profiles of members of the Black population.
3. Describe the traditional definitions of HEALTH and ILLNESS of members of the Black population.
4. Describe the traditional methods of HEALTH maintenance and protection of selected communities of the Black population.
5. Describe the traditional methods of HEALING of selected communities of the Black population.
6. Describe current health care problems of members of the Black population.
7. Describe demographic disparity as it is seen in health manpower distribution of the Black population as represented in the health care delivery system.

258

The opening photos depict HEALTH-related items that may be used by people of Black, or African American, heritage to protect, maintain, and/or restore their HEALTH. The dried garden snake is ground up and brewed as a tea, and the liquid may be used to treat skin blemishes. Silver bangle bracelets from Saint Thomas, the Virgin Islands, are open to let out evil yet closed to prevent evil from entering the body. They are said to tarnish when the person wearing them is vulnerable to ILLNESS; this alerts the person to take better care of him- or herself. They are worn from birth, and many people believe that they will die if they remove them. Often, many bracelets are worn together, and the bell-like sound that they make when they touch is said to scare the evil spirits away. These are worn to protect HEALTH. Rectified turpentine with sugar is used to treat a cough. Nine drops of turpentine 9 days after intercourse may act as a contraceptive. Sugar and turpentine may also be used to get rid of intestinal worms. The last segment is the Lorraine Hotel in Memphis, Tennessee, the site of the assassination of Dr. Martin Luther King, Jr., in 1968.

■ Background

"Black or African American" refers to people having origins in any of the Black race groups of Africa (McKinnon, 2001, p. 1). Blacks or African Americans are the largest emerging majority population in the United States, constituting an estimated 12.3% of the U.S. population in 2000 (Dalaku, 2001, p. 1) and 12.8% of the U.S. population of the United States in 2005.

"Black" is used in this chapter's text to refer to the Black or African American population, but "Black or African American" is used in tables and figures. This follows the pattern used in Census 2000. Most members of the present Black American community have their roots in Africa, and the majority descend from people who were brought here as slaves from the west coast of Africa (Bullough & Bullough, 1972, pp. 39–41). The largest importation of slaves occurred during the 17th century, which means that Black people have been living in the United States for many generations. Today, a number of Blacks have immigrated to the United States voluntarily—from African countries, the West Indian islands, the Dominican Republic, Haiti, and Jamaica.

Black Americans live in all regions of the country. In 2000, the majority of the Black population, 54.8%, lived in the South. About three fifths of all people who reported their racial identity as Black lived in the following 10 states: New York (3.2 million), California (2.5 million), Texas (2.5 million), Florida (2.5 million), Georgia (2.4 million), Illinois, North Carolina, Maryland, Michigan, and Louisiana. The cities with the largest numbers of Blacks were New York, Chicago, Detroit, Memphis, and Houston.

Blacks are represented in every socioeconomic group; however, 22.1% of the group lived in poverty in 2000 and in 2005 the percentage was 24.9. Blacks have remained disproportionately poor (Dalaku, 2001, p. 1). Furthermore, over half of Black Americans live in urban areas surrounded by the symptoms of poverty—crowded and inadequate housing, poor schools, and high crime rates.

For example, Kotlowitz (1991) described the Henry Horner Homes in Chicago as "16 high-rise buildings which stretch over eight blocks and at last census count housed 6,000 people, 4,000 of whom are children." The degree of social and economic change between 1990 and 2000 has been minimal. He presented two facts about public housing: "Public housing served as a bulwark to segregation and as a kind of anchor for impoverished neighborhoods" and "It was built on the cheap—the walls are a naked cinder block with heating pipes snaking through the apartment; instead of closets, there are eight-inch indentations in the walls without doors; and the heating system so storms out of control in the winter that it is 85 degrees." Situations similar to this prevail presently. The Black population is also young, 54.5% of the Black population in combination with one or more races are under 18 (Dalaku, 2001, p. 9), and the mean age in 2005 was 32.4 years.

There are now a growing number of people arriving from Africa as new immigrants. The total population of people born in Africa and who have entered the United States since before 1980 and 2000 is 881,300; from Nigeria 134,940; from Somalia 36,760; and from Sudan 19,790 (U.S. Census Bureau). The rates of naturalization, learning English, and educational achievement are low as of this writing. This is demonstrated in Table 10–1.

According to some sources, the first Black people to enter this country arrived a year earlier than the Pilgrims, in 1619. Other sources claim that Blacks arrived with Columbus in the 15th century (Bullough & Bullough, 1972, pp. 39–41). In any event, the first Blacks who came to the North American continent did not come as slaves, but, between 1619 and 1860, more than 4 million people were transported here as slaves. One need read only a sampling of the many accounts of slavery to appreciate the tremendous hardships that the captured and enslaved people experienced during that time. Not only was the daily life of the slave very difficult, but the experience of being captured, shackled, and transported in steerage was devastating. Many of those captured in Africa died before they arrived here. The strongest and healthiest people were snatched from their homes by slave dealers and transported en masse in the holds of ships to the North American continent. In general, Black captives were not taken care of or recognized as human beings and treated accordingly. Once here, they were sold and placed on plantations and in homes all over the country—it was only later that the practice was confined to the South. Families were separated; children were wrenched from their parents and sold to other buyers. Some slave owners bred their slaves much as farmers breed cattle today, purchasing men to serve as studs, and judging women based on whether they would produce the desired stock with a particular man (Haley, 1976). However, in the midst of all this inhuman and inhumane treatment, the Black family grew and survived. Gutman (1976), in his careful documentation of plantation and family records, traces the history of the Black family from 1750 to 1925 and points out the existence of families and family or kinship ties before and after the Civil War, dispelling many of the myths about the Black family and its structure. Despite overwhelming hardships and enforced separations, the people managed in most circumstances to maintain both a family and community awareness.

Table 10-1 **Profile of Selected Demographic and Social Characteristics of People Entering the United States from Africa, Nigeria, Somalia, and Sudan: 2000**

Variable	Africa $n = 881,300$	Nigeria $n = 134,940$	Somalia $n = 36,760$	Sudan $n = 19,790$
Naturalized U.S. citizens	36.1%	37.1%	14.3%	21.4%
Language other than English spoken at home	78.5%	78.0%	96.4%	92.5%
Speak English less than very well	26.8%	11.8%	61.3%	43.8%
Median age	36.1 years	38.1 years	26.1 years	30.2 years
Marital status—married	57.2%	61.9%	43.4%	52.8%
School enrollment—college or graduate school	57.2%	65.4%	25.0%	36.6%
Educational attainment—bachelor's degree or higher—population 25 years and older	57.2%	28.3%	16.6%	40.2%
Veteran status—civilian veterans	2.0%	2.0%	1.0%	1.7%
Employment status—over 16 years of age employed	71.1%	78.0%	58.1%	66.5%
Median household income	$41,196	$45,072	$18,499	$29,437
Household income—$150,000 or more	5.6%	4.5%	1.0%	2.2%
Median family income	$48,305	$52,586	$19,255	$31,399
Per capita earnings	$25,836	$26,956	$10,135	$14,765
Poverty status—families below the poverty level	13.1%	9.8%	46.1%	27.9%

Sources: U.S. Census Bureau, Census 2000 Special Tabulations. Profile of Selected Demographic and Social Characteristics: 2000 Africa, Nigeria, Somalia, and Sudan. Retrieved July 25, 2007 from http://www.census.gov/population/cen2000/stp-159/STP-159-Africaica.pdf, http://www.census.gov/population/cen2000/stp-159/STP-159-Nigeria.pdf, http://www.census.gov/population/cen2000/stp-159/STP-159-Somalia.pdf and http://www.census.gov/population/cen2000/stp-159/STP-159-Sudan.pdf

The people who came to America from West Africa brought a rich variety of traditional beliefs and practices and came from religious traditions that respected the spiritual power of ancestors. They worshiped a diverse pantheon of gods, who oversaw all aspects of daily life, such as the changes of the seasons, the fertility of nature, physical and spiritual personal health, and communal success. Initiation rites and naming rituals, folktales, and healing practices, dance, song, and drumming were a part of the religious heritage. Many aspects of today's Christian religious practices are believed to have originated in these practices. In addition, it has been estimated that between 10% and 30% of the slaves brought to America between 1711 and 1808 were Muslim. The people brought their prayer practices, fasting and dietary practices, and their knowledge of the Qur'an (Eck, 1994).

Box 10–1

Highlights of the Civil Rights Movement

1954	*Brown v. Board of Education*—segregation in public schools found to be illegal by the landmark Supreme Court ruling
1955	Rosa Parks refuses to give up her seat on a bus in Montgomery, Alabama, and the bus boycott in Alabama begins
	Emmett Till murdered in Mississippi
1957	Central High School, Little Rock, Arkansas, integrated by the "Little Rock Nine"
1959	Sit-ins at lunch counters
1961	Segregation of interstate bus terminals ruled unconstitutional
	Freedom Riders attacked
	James Meredith is the first Black student to enroll in the University of Mississippi
1962	Civil Rights Movement formally organized
1963	Martin Luther King, Jr., writes the seminal "Letter from Birmingham Jail," in which he argues that people have the moral duty to disobey unjust laws
	March on Washington led by Dr. Martin Luther King, Jr.
1964	Killing of Charles Moore and Henry Dee
	Civil Rights Act passed
1965	Malcolm X assassinated
1965–1968	Over 100 race riots in American cities
1968	Dr. Martin Luther King, Jr., assassinated
1991	Beating of Rodney King
1992	Major race riots in Los Angeles
1995	Million Man March
2007	*Parents v. Seattle Schools* and *Meredith v. Jefferson Schools*
	Jena, Louisiana—Black students held for beating a White student and tried as adults
	James Ford Seale convicted and sentenced to three life prison terms for his role in the Moore/Dee murders in 1964

Source: Brunner, B. and Haney, E. (2007). Civil Rights Timeline: Milestones in the modern civil rights movement. Upper Saddle River, NJ: Pearson Education. Retrieved June 9, 2007 from http://www.infoplease.com/spot/civilrightstimeline1.html

Ostensibly, the Civil War ended slavery, but in many ways it did not emancipate Blacks. Daily life after the war was fraught with tremendous difficulty, and Black people—according to custom—were stripped of their civil rights. In the South, Black people were overtly segregated, most living in conditions of extreme hardship and poverty. Those who migrated to the North over the years were subject to all the problems of fragmented urban life: poverty, racism, and covert segregation (Bullough & Bullough, 1972, p. 43; Kain, 1969, pp. 1–30).

The historic problems of the Black community need to be appreciated by the health care provider who attempts to juxtapose modern practices and traditional health and illness beliefs. In addition, health care providers must be aware of the ongoing and historical events in the struggle for civil rights that affect people's lives. Box 10–1 highlights several events in the early history of this struggle. In 2007 the Supreme Court ruled in *Parents v. Seattle Schools* and *Meredith v. Jefferson Schools* that public schools can't consider race when making student school assignments. This may be viewed as an effort to strike down *Brown v. Board of Education*, the landmark ruling of 1956. Also, in 2007, James Ford Seale, a Mississippi Klansman was sentenced to three life terms in prison for the Moore/Dee murder of 1964.

It is hard to believe that a half-century has passed since the teenage students known today as the "Little Rock Nine" integrated Central High School in Little Rock, Arkansas (Figure 10–1). I vividly remember the scenes on television of nine brave teenagers, my age at the time, trying to enter the school, the cadre of hostile, angry White people spitting at them and hollering epitaphs, and the heavily armed soldiers protecting the teens. These images seared my consciousness and left an indelible imprint on my life. The activities that I accomplished each day—getting up in the morning, walking to school, attending classes, being with my friends, and so forth—were completely disrupted for the students. I remember thinking that this was not Europe; this was not Armenia or Spain, or Russia, or Germany; this was happening in "my backyard," in the United States. People who could be my neighbors violated everything that I had been taught about human dignity and respect. Two years later, my "little sister" in

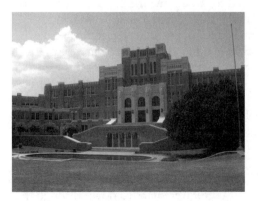

Figure 10-1 Central High School, Little Rock, Arkansas.

nursing school was one of the Little Rock Nine—I learned firsthand the damage this event wrought on her life and I believe on the lives of all of us. Central High School had acquired a most personal meaning. As I write this chapter in 2007, celebrations are being held nationally to recognize and honor the integration of Central High School and the Little Rock Nine. Ostensibly, Central High School and many other schools were integrated, the practices of separate water fountains and "back of the bus" were over and life moved on. However, on the other hand, there has been the recent (2007) event in Jena, Louisiana. How can it be that racial tensions continue to simmer?

■ Traditional Definitions of HEALTH and ILLNESS

According to Jacques (1976), the traditional definition of HEALTH stems from the African belief about life and the nature of being. To the African, life was a process rather than a state. The nature of a person was viewed in terms of energy force rather than matter. All things, whether living or dead, were believed to influence one another. Therefore, one had the power to influence one's destiny and that of others through the use of behavior, whether proper or otherwise, as well as through knowledge of the person and the world. When one possessed HEALTH, one was in harmony with nature; ILLNESS was a state of disharmony. Traditional Black belief regarding HEALTH did not separate the mind, body, and spirit.

Disharmony—that is, ILLNESS—was attributed to a number of sources, primarily demons and evil spirits. These spirits were generally believed to act of their own accord, and the goal of treatment was to remove them from the body of the ILL person. Several methods were employed to attain this result, in addition to voodoo, which is discussed in the next section. The traditional healers, usually women, possessed extensive knowledge of the use of herbs and roots in the treatment of ILLNESS. Apparently, an early form of smallpox immunization was used by slaves. Women practiced inoculation by scraping a piece of cowpox crust into a place on a child's arm. These children appeared to have a far lower incidence of smallpox than those who did not receive the immunization.

The old and the young were cared for by all members of the community. The elderly were held in high esteem because African people believed that the living of a long life indicated that a person had the opportunity to acquire much wisdom and knowledge. Death was described as the passing from one realm of life to another (Jacques, 1976, p. 117) or as a passage from the evils of this world to another state. The funeral was often celebrated as a joyous occasion, with a party after the burial. Children were passed over the body of the deceased, so that the dead person could carry any potential illness of the child away with him or her.

Many of the preventive and treatment practices of Black people have their roots in Africa but have been merged with the approaches of Native Americans, to whom the Blacks were exposed, and with the attitudes of Whites among whom they lived and served. Then, as today, ILLNESS was treated in a combination of ways. Methods found to be most useful were handed down through the generations.

■ Traditional Methods of HEALTH Maintenance and Protection

The following sections present examples of practices employed presently or in earlier generations to maintain and protect HEALTH and to treat various types of maladies to restore HEALTH. This discussion cannot encompass all the types of care given to and by the members of the Black community but instead presents a sample of the richness of the traditional HEALTH practices that have survived over the years.

Essentially, HEALTH is maintained with proper diet—that is, eating three nutritious meals a day, including a hot breakfast. Rest and a clean environment also are important. Laxatives were and are used to keep the system "running" or "open."

Asafetida—rotten flesh that looks like a dried-out sponge—is worn around the neck to prevent the contraction of contagious diseases. Cod liver oil is taken to prevent colds. A sulfur and molasses preparation is used in the spring because it is believed that at the start of a new season people are more susceptible to illness. This preparation is rubbed up and down the back, not taken internally. A physician is not consulted routinely and is not generally regarded as the person to whom one goes for the prevention of disease.

Copper or silver bracelets may be worn around the wrist from the time a woman is a baby or young child. These bracelets are believed to protect the wearer as she grows. If for any reason these bracelets are removed, harm befalls the owner. In addition to granting protection, these bracelets indicate when the wearer is about to become ill: the skin around the bracelet turns black, alerting the woman to take precautions against the impending illness. These precautions consist of getting extra rest, praying more frequently, and eating a more nutritious diet.

■ Traditional Methods of HEALTH Restoration

The most common method of treating ILLNESS is prayer. The laying on of hands is described quite frequently. Rooting, a practice derived from voodoo, also is mentioned by many people. In rooting, a person (usually a woman who is known as a "root-worker)" is consulted as to the source of a given ILLNESS, and she then prescribes the appropriate treatment. Magic rituals often are employed (Davis, 1998).

The following home remedies have been reported by some Black people as being successful in the treatment of disease.

1. Sugar and turpentine are mixed together and taken by mouth to get rid of worms. This combination can also be used to cure a backache when rubbed on the skin from the navel to the back.

2. Numerous types of poultices are employed to fight infection and inflammation. The poultices are placed on the part of the body that is painful or infected to draw out the cause of the affliction. One type of poultice is made of potatoes. The potatoes are sliced or grated and placed in a bag, which is placed on the affected area of the body. The

potatoes turn black; as this occurs, the disease goes away. It is believed that, as these potatoes spoil, they produce a penicillin mold that is able to destroy the infectious organism. Another type of poultice is prepared from cornmeal and peach leaves, which are cooked together and placed either in a bag or in a piece of flannel cloth. The cornmeal ferments and combines with an enzyme in the peach leaves to produce an antiseptic that destroys the bacteria and hastens the healing process. A third poultice, made with onions, is used to heal infections, and a flaxseed poultice is used to treat earaches.

3. Herbs from the woods are used in many ways. Herb teas are prepared—for example, from goldenrod root—to treat pain and reduce fevers. Sassafrass tea frequently is used to treat colds. Another herb boiled to make a tea is the root or leaf of rabbit tobacco.

4. Bluestone, a mineral found in the ground, is used as medicine for open wounds. The stone is crushed into a powder and sprinkled on the affected area. It prevents inflammation and is used to treat poison ivy.

5. To treat a "crick" in the neck, two pieces of silverware are crossed over the painful area in the form of an X.

6. Nine drops of turpentine 9 days after intercourse act as a contraceptive.

7. Cuts and wounds can be treated with sour or spoiled milk that is placed on stale bread, wrapped in a cloth, and placed on the wound.

8. Salt and pork (salt pork) placed on a rag can be used to treat cuts and wounds.

9. A sprained ankle can be treated by placing clay in a dark leaf and wrapping it around the ankle.

10. A remedy for treating colds is hot lemon water with honey.

11. When congestion is present in the chest and the person is coughing, the chest is rubbed with hot camphorated oil and wrapped with warm flannel.

12. An expectorant for colds consists of chopped raw garlic, chopped onion, fresh parsley, and a little water, all mixed in a blender.

13. Hot toddies are used to treat colds and congestion. These drinks consist of hot tea with honey, lemon, peppermint, and a dash of brandy or whatever alcoholic beverage the person likes and is available. Vicks Vaporub also is swallowed.

14. A fever can be broken by placing raw onions on the feet and wrapping the feet in warm blankets.

15. Boils are treated by cracking a raw egg, peeling the white skin off the inside of the shell, and placing it on the boil. This brings the boil to a head.

16. Garlic can be placed on the ill person or in the room to remove the "evil spirits" that have caused the illness.

Folk Medicine

In the Black community, folk medicine previously practiced in Africa is still employed. The methods have been tried and tested and are still relied on. Healers or voodoo practitioners make no class or status distinctions among their patients, treating everyone fairly and honestly. This tradition of equality of care and perceived effectiveness accounts for the faith placed in the practices of the HEALER and in other methods. In fact, the home remedies used by some members of the Black community have been employed for many generations. Another reason for their ongoing use is that hospitals are distant from people who live in rural areas. By the time they might get to the hospital, they would be dead, yet many of the people who continue to use these remedies live in urban areas close to hospitals—sometimes even world-renowned hospitals. Nonetheless, the use of folk medicine persists, and many people avoid the local hospital except in extreme emergencies.

Traditional Methods of HEALING

Voodoo, or Voudou. Voodoo, or American voudou, is a belief system often alluded to but rarely described in any detail (Davis, 1998). At various times, patients may mention terms such as *fix, hex,* or *spell.* It is not clear whether voodoo is fully practiced today, but there is some evidence in the literature that there are people who still believe and practice it to some extent (Wintrob, 1972). It also has been reported that many Black people continue to fear voodoo and believe that when they become ILL they have been "fixed." Voodoo involves two forms of magic: white magic, described as harmless, and black magic, which is quite dangerous. Belief in magic is, of course, ancient (Hughes & Bontemps, 1958, pp. 184–185).

Voodoo came to this country about 1724, with the arrival of slaves from the West African coast, who had been sold initially in the West Indies. The people who brought voodoo with them were "snake worshippers." Vodu, the name of their god, with the passage of time became *voodoo* (also *hoodoo*), an all-embracing term that included the god, the sect, the members of the sect, the priests and priestesses, the rites and practices, and the teaching (Tallant, 1946, p. 19).

Tallant goes on to explain that the sect spread rapidly from the West Indies. In 1782, the governor of Louisiana prohibited the importation of slaves from Martinique because of their practice of voodoo. (Despite the fact that gatherings of slaves were forbidden in Louisiana, small groups persisted in practicing voodoo.) In 1803, the importation of slaves to Louisiana from the West Indies was finally allowed, and with them came the strong influence of voodoo. The practice entailed a large number of rituals and procedures. The ceremonies were held with large numbers of people, usually at night and in the open country. Sacrifice and the drinking of blood were integral parts of all the voodoo ceremonies. There were those who believed that this blood was from children. However, it was most commonly thought to be the blood of a cat or young goat. Such behavior evolved from primitive African rites, to which Christian rituals were added to form the ceremonies that exist today. Leaders of the voodoo sect tended to be women, and stories abound in New Orleans about the workings of the sect and the women who ruled it—such as Marie Laveau.

In 1850, the practice of voodoo reached its height in New Orleans. At that time, the beliefs and practices of voodoo were closely related to beliefs about health and illness. For example, many illnesses were attributed to a "fix" that was placed on one person out of anger. Gris-gris, the symbols of voodoo, were used to prevent illness or to give illness to others. Some examples of commonly used gris-gris follow (Tallant, 1946, p. 226):

1. **Good gris-gris:** powders and oils that are highly and pleasantly scented. The following are examples of good gris-gris: love powder, colored and scented with perfume; love oil, olive oil to which gardenia perfume has been added; luck water, ordinary water that is purchased in many shades (red is for success in love, yellow for success in money matters, blue for protection and friends).

2. **Bad gris-gris:** oils and powders that have a vile odor. The following are examples of bad gris-gris: anger powder, war powder, and moving powder, which are composed of soil, gunpowder, and black pepper, respectively.

3. **Flying devil oil:** olive oil that has red coloring and cayenne pepper added to it

4. **Black cat oil:** machine oil

In addition to these oils and powders, a variety of colored candles are used, the color of the candle symbolizing the intention. For example, white symbolizes peace; red, victory; pink, love; yellow, driving off enemies; brown, attracting money; and black, doing evil work and bringing bad luck (Tallant, 1946, p. 226).

The following story exhibits the profound influence that belief in voodoo can have on a person. It was reported in Baltimore, Maryland, in 1967.

> The patient was a young, married black woman who was admitted to the hospital for evaluation of chest pain, syncope, and dyspnea. Her past history was one of good health. However, she had gained over 50 pounds in the past year and was given to eating Argo starch. She began to have symptoms 1 month before she was admitted. Her condition grew worse once in the hospital, and she was treated for heart failure and also for pulmonary embolism. She revealed that she had a serious problem. She had been born on Friday, the thirteenth, in the Okefenokee Swamp and was delivered by a midwife who delivered three children that day. The midwife told the mothers that the children were hexed and that the first would die before her 16th birthday,

the second before her 21st birthday, and the third (the patient) before her 23rd birthday. The first girl was a passenger in a car involved in a fatal crash the day before her 16th birthday, the second girl was celebrating her 21st birthday in a saloon when a stray bullet hit and killed her. This patient also believed she was doomed. She, too, died—on August 12—a day before her 23rd birthday. (Webb, 1971, pp. 1–3)

There are a number of Catholic saints or relics to whom or to which the practitioners of voodoo attribute special powers. Portraits of Saint Michael, who makes possible the conquest of enemies; Saint Anthony de Padua, who brings luck; Saint Mary Magdalene, who is popular with women who are in love; the Virgin Mary, whose presence in the home prevents illness; and the Sacred Heart of Jesus, which cures organic illness, may be prominently displayed in the homes of people who believe in voodoo (Tallant, 1946, p. 228). These gris-gris are available today and can be purchased in stores in many American cities.

Other Practices.　Many Blacks believe in the power of some people to HEAL and help others, and there are many reports of numerous HEALERS among the communities. This reliance on HEALERS reflects the deep religious faith of the people. (Maya Angelou vividly describes this phenomenon in her book *I Know Why the Caged Bird Sings.*) For example, many Blacks followed the Pentecostal movement long before its present more general popularity. Similarly, people often went to tent meetings and had an all-consuming belief in the HEALING powers of religion.

Another practice takes on significance when one appreciates its historical background: the eating of Argo starch. "Geophagy," or eating clay and dirt, occurred among the slaves, who brought the practice to this country from Africa. In *Roots*, Haley mentions that pregnant women were given clay because it was believed to be beneficial to both the mother and the unborn child (Haley, 1976, p. 32). In fact, red clays are rich in iron. When clay was not available, dirt was substituted. In more modern times, when people were no longer living on farms and no longer had access to clay and dirt, Argo starch became the substitute (Dunstin, 1969). The following was reported by a former student:

> It was my fortune, or misfortune to be born into a family that practiced geophagy (earth eating) and pica (eating Argo laundry starch). Even before I became pregnant I showed an interest in eating starch. It was sweet and dry, and I could take it or leave it. After I became pregnant, I found I wanted not only starch, but bread, grits, and potatoes. I found I craved starchy substances. I stuck to starchy substances and dropped the Argo because it made me feel sluggish and heavy.

It is believed that anemia arose from this practice of substituting non–iron-rich clays or starch for red clays that contain iron. Table 10–2 illustrates examples

Table 10–2 Examples of Cultural Phenomena Affecting Health Care Among Black or African Americans

Nations of Origin	Many West African countries (as slaves) West Indian Islands Dominican Republic Haiti Jamaica
Environmental Control	Traditional HEALTH and ILLNESS beliefs may continue to be observed by "traditional" people
Biological Variations	Sickle-cell anemia Hypertension Cancer of the esophagus Stomach cancer Coccidioidomycosis Lactose intolerance
Social Organization	Family: many single-parent households headed by females Large, extended family networks Strong church affiliations within community Community social organizations
Communication	National languages Dialect: Pidgin French, Spanish, Creole
Space	Close personal space
Time Orientation	Present over future

Adapted from Spector, R. (1992). Culture, ethnicity, and nursing (p. 101). In P. Potter & A. Perry (Eds.), *Fundamentals of nursing* (3rd ed.). St. Louis, MO: Mosby-Year Book. Reprinted with permission.

of cultural phenomena that affect health care among Blacks. Many Black Americans and new immigrants from African countries are Muslims. Box 10–2 presents an overview of Islam and information that must be known in health care settings.

■ Current Health Problems

Health Differences between Black and White Populations

Morbidity.   Many people experience factors such as the lack of access to health services, low income, and a tendency to self-treat illness and to wait until symptoms are so severe that a doctor must be seen. When statistical adjustments are made for age, Blacks exceed Whites in the average number of days spent in acute care settings, on bed rest, and in restricted activity. In addition, Blacks have a greater incidence of tooth decay and periodontal disease than Whites (National Center for Health Statistics, 2006, pp. 278, 279). Adolescent pregnancy is a major concern with the population. The risk of infant mortality and low birth

Box 10–2

Black Muslims

Many members of the Black community are practicing Muslims. The religion of Islam is the acceptance of and obedience to the teachings of God, which He revealed to His last prophet, Muhammad. The Five Pillars of Islam are the framework of Muslim life. They are the testimony of faith, prayer, giving *zakat* (support of the needy), fasting during the month of Ramadan, and the pilgrimage to Mecca once in a lifetime for those who are able.

The people may be descendants of the earlier people who were Muslims and came to America as slaves, or they have chosen to convert to Islam. However, it is difficult to generalize in any way about American Muslims because the people come from all walks of life—converts, immigrants, factory workers, doctors, professionals, and so forth. In addition, there are many African immigrants from countries, such as the Sudan, who are practicing Muslims, and countless people from Islamic countries are seeking health care services in the United States. The community is unified by a common faith.

Religious beliefs are an important part of the Muslim lifestyle, and health care providers should be familiar with them:

- Muslims are taught that a "person is what he or she eats." Islamic dietary restrictions consist of eating a strictly Halal diet, and a newly admitted patient who refuses to eat should be asked if the hospital's ordinary diet interferes with his or her religious beliefs. The rules of a Halal diet include not eating pork or any pork products (such as nonbeef hamburger and ham). Islamic law teaches that certain foods affect the way a person thinks and acts. Therefore, one's diet should consist of food that has a clean, positive effect. Muslims do not drink alcohol because they feel that it dulls the senses and causes illness. Halal foods are produced using equipment that is cleansed according to Islamic law.
- Muslims pray five times a day. Each prayer does not take more than a few minutes and is offered at dawn, noon, mid-afternoon, sunset, and night in almost any setting, such as in fields, offices, factories, universities, or hospitals. Prayer in Islam is a direct link between the worshipper and God. Before a person prays, he or she must be clean and hands and feet are washed. Prayers are generally said in a prostrate position on a carpet on the floor.
- Muslims fast for a 30-day period during the year (fast of Ramadan). Ramadan is a special time—a month of prayer and repentance. Nothing is taken by mouth from just before sunrise until after sundown. Ill Muslims, small children, and pregnant women are exempt from this rule. When a person is following the fast, institutions must provide the environment for the safe observance of the practice.

There is also a practice of modesty, with women covering their heads with scarves, *jibabs,* and wearing long dresses, *hijabs.* The need for gender-specific care—that is, males caring for male patients and females caring for female patients, must be adhered to.

(continued)

The Muslim lifestyle is strictly regulated. According to those who have practiced the religion for many generations, this stems in part from the need for self-discipline, which many Black people have not had because of living conditions associated with urban decay and family disintegration. Muslims believe in self-help and assist in uplifting each other. The Muslim lifestyle is not so rigid that the people do not have good times. Good times, however, are tempered with the realization that too much indulgence in sport and play can present problems. To Muslims, life is precious: if a person needs a transfusion to live, it will be accepted. Because of the avoidance of pork or pork products, however, it is important to understand that a diabetic Muslim will refuse to take insulin that has a pork base. If the insulin is manufactured from the pancreas of a pig, it is considered unclean and will not be accepted. There are preparations of insulin and/or other products that can be prescribed.

Many Muslim communities differ in their practice and philosophy of Islam. Members of some communities dress in distinctive clothing—for example, the women wear long skirts and a covering on the head at all times. Other communities are less strict about dress. Some adherents do not follow the Halal diet and are allowed to drink alcoholic beverages in moderation.

Sources: Ibrahim, I. A. (2002). A Brief Illustrated Guide to Understanding Islam. Houston, Texas: Darussalam. Retrieved from http://www.islam-guide.com/frm-editors.htm, July 21, 2007, and Office of Dawah. (2006–2008). The Religion of Islam. Rawdah: Author. Retrieved Sept. 19, 2007 from http://www.islamreligion.com/

weight are also greater in the community, as is the rate of low-birth-weight babies. Table 10–3 compares selected health status indicators for Black and all races. It illustrates that the birth rate is higher, that the percentages of women not getting early prenatal care and third-trimester or no prenatal care are higher, and that the percentage of teenage births to women under 18 is nearly double, as is the infant mortality rate.

Sickle-Cell Anemia. The sickling of red blood cells is a genetically inherited trait that is hypothesized to have originally been an African adaptation to fight malaria. This condition occurs only in Blacks and causes the normal, disk-like red blood cell to assume a sickle shape. Sickling results in hemolysis and thrombosis of red blood cells because these deformed cells do not flow properly through the blood vessels. Sickle-cell disease comprises the following blood characteristics:

1. The presence of two hemoglobin-S genes (Hb SS)
2. The presence of the hemoglobin-S gene with another abnormal hemoglobin gene (Hb SC, Hb SD, etc.)
3. The presence of the hemoglobin-S gene with a different abnormality in hemoglobin synthesis

Some people (carriers) have the sickle-cell trait (HbSS, HbSC, or others) but do not experience symptoms of the disease.

The clinical manifestations of sickle-cell disease include hemolysis, anemia, and states of sickle-cell crises, in which severe pain occurs in the areas of the body

Table 10-3 Comparison of Selected Health Status Indicators—All Races and Black or African Americans: 1999/2004

Health Indicator	All Races	Black or African Americans
Crude birth rate per 1,000 population by race of mother	14.5/14.0	17.4/16.0
Percentage of live births of women receiving prenatal care first trimester	83.2/83.9	74.1/76.4
Percentage of live births of women receiving third-trimester prenatal care or no prenatal care	3.8/3.6	6.6/5.7
Percentage of live births to teenage childbearing women—under 18	4.4/3.4	8.2/6.4
Percentage of low birth weight per live births <2,500 grams, 1997–1999/2003	7.57/8.3	13.11/15.3
Infant mortality per 1,000 live births, 1996–1998/2003	7.2/6.8	13.9/13.5
Cancer—all sites per 100,000 population, 1997/2003	384.5/447.1	426.5/489.0
Lung cancer incidence per 100,000 population, 1997/2003	Men: 65.4/73.0 Women: 40.7/48.0	Men: 100.5/107.8 Women: 42.3/52.6
Breast cancer incidence per 100,000, 1997/2003	113.1/121.1	101.3/119.2
Prostate cancer incidence per 100,000, 1997/2003	136.0/160.4	207.9/237.5
Male death rates from suicide, all ages, age adjusted per 100,000 resident population, 1999/2003	18.1/10.8	10.6/9.2
Male death rates from homicide, all ages, age adjusted per 100,000 resident population, 1999/2003	9.3/9.4	38.4/36.7

Source: National Center for Health Statistics. (2006). *Health, United States, 2006 with chartbook on trends in the health of Americans* (pp. 135, 140, 144, 149, 160, 227, 230, 244). Hyattsville, MD: Author.

where the thrombosed red cells are located. The cells also tend to clump in abdominal organs, such as the liver and the spleen. At present, statistics indicate that only 50% of children with sickle-cell disease live to adulthood. Some children die before the age of 20, and some suffer chronic, irreversible complications during their lifetime.

It is possible to detect the sickle-cell trait in healthy adults and to provide genetic counseling about their risk of bearing children with the disease. However, for many people, this is not an option (Bullock & Jilly, 1975, pp. 234–272). The cost of genetic counseling, for example, may be prohibitive.

Table 10-4 Comparison of the 10 Leading Causes of Death for Black or African Americans and for All Persons: 2004

Black or African Americans	All Persons
1. Diseases of heart	Diseases of heart
2. Malignant neoplasms	Malignant neoplasms
3. Cerebrovascular diseases	Cerebrovascular diseases
4. Diabetes mellitus	Chronic lower respiratory diseases
5. Unintentional injuries	Unintentional injuries
6. Homicide	Diabetes mellitus
7. Nephritis, nephrotic syndrome, and nephrosis	Alzheimer's disease
8. Chronic lower respiratory diseases	Influenza and pneumonia
9. Human immunodeficiency virus (HIV) disease	Nephritis, nephrotic syndrome, and nephrosis
10. Septicemia	Septicemia

Source: National Center for Health Statistics. (2007). *Health, United States, 2007 with chartbook on trends in the health of Americans* (p. 188). Hyattsville, MD: Author.

Mortality. Blacks born in 2000 in the United States will live, on average, 5.7 fewer years than Whites. The life expectancy for Whites born in 2000 is 77.6 years; for Blacks, it is 71.9 years (National Center for Health Statistics, 2007, p. 175).

The leading chronic diseases that are causes of death for African Americans are the same as those for Whites, but the rates are greater:

- Blacks die from strokes at almost twice the rate of the White population. (National Center for Health Statistics, 2007, p. 204).
- Coronary heart disease death rates are higher for Blacks than for Whites.
- Black men experience a higher risk of cancer of the prostate than White men do.
- Homicide is the most frequent cause of death for Black American men between the ages of 25 and 34 the rate in 2004 was 81.6 per 100,000 resident population. (NCHS, 2007, p. 227)
- The rate of AIDS among Black American men generally is higher than that for White men and the mortality rate for both Black men, 29.2/100,000 and women, 13.0/100,000 resident population in 2004 is the highest rate. (NCHS, p. 219)

Table 10–4 lists the 10 leading causes of death for Black Americans and compares them with the causes of death for the general population in 2004.

Mental Health Traditions

The family often has a matriarchal structure, and there are many single-parent households headed by females but there are strong and large extended family networks. There are a continuation of tradition and a strong church affiliation within the families and community. Members of the community may be treated by a traditional voodoo priest, the "Old Lady" ("granny" or "Mrs. Markus"), or other traditional healers, and herbs are frequently used to treat mental symptoms. Several diagnostic techniques include the use of biblical phrases and/or material from old folk medical books, observation, and/or entering the spirit of the patient. The therapeutic measures include various rituals, such as the reading of bones, the wearing of special garments, or some rituals from voodoo (Spurlock, 1988, p. 173). In addition, there are countless culture-bound mental HEALTH syndromes that may be identified in the Black community:

- West Africa and Haiti—*Boufée delirante*—the sudden outburst of agitated and aggressive behavior, confusion, occasional hallucinations
- Southern United States and Caribbean groups—Falling-Out—sudden collapse without warning
- North African countries—Zar—person is possessed by a spirit and may shout, weep, laugh, hit his or her head against the wall, or sing
- West Africa—Brain Fog—physical and mental exhaustion, difficulty concentrating, memory loss, irritability, and sleeping and appetite problems (Fontaine, 2003, p. 119)

Blacks and the Health Care System

To some, receiving health care is all too often a degrading and humiliating experience. In many settings, Black patients continue to be viewed as beneath the White health care giver. Quite often, the insult is a subtle part of experiencing the health care system. The insult may be intentional or unintentional. An intentional insult is, of course, a blatant remark or mistreatment. An unintentional insult is more difficult to define. A health care provider may not intend to demean a person, yet an action or a tone of voice may be interpreted as insulting. The provider may have some covert, underlying fears or difficulties in relating to Blacks, but the patient quite often senses the difficulty. An unintentional insult may occur because the provider is not fully aware of the patient's background and is unable to comprehend many of the patient's beliefs and practices. The patient, for example, may be afraid of the impending medical procedures and the possibility of misdiagnosis or mistreatment. It is not a secret among the people of the Black community that those who receive care in public clinics and hospitals—and even in clinics of private institutions—are the "material" on whom students practice and on whom medical research is done.

Some Blacks fear or resent health clinics. When they have a clinic appointment, they usually lose a day's work because they have to be at the clinic at an early hour and often spend many hours waiting to be seen by a physician. They often receive inadequate care, are told what their problem is in incomprehensible medical jargon, and are not given an identity, being seen rather as a body segment ("the appendix in treatment room A"). Such an experience creates a tremendous feeling of powerlessness and alienation from the system.

In some parts of the country, segregation and racism are overt. There continue to be reports of hospitals that refuse admission to Black patients. In one case, a Black woman in labor was not admitted to a hospital because she had not "paid the bill from the last baby." There was not enough time to get her to another hospital, and she was forced to deliver in an ambulance. In light of this type of treatment, it is no wonder that some Black people prefer to use time-tested home remedies rather than be exposed to the humiliating experiences of hospitalization.

Another reason for the ongoing use of home remedies is poverty. Indigent people cannot afford the high costs of American health care. Quite often—even with the help of Medicaid and Medicare—the hidden costs of acquiring health services, such as absence from work, transportation, and/or child care, are a heavy burden. As a result, Blacks may stay away from clinics or outpatient departments or receive their care with passivity while appearing to the provider to be evasive. Some Black patients believe that they are being talked down to by health care providers and that the providers fail to listen to them. They choose, consequently, to "suffer in silence." Many of the problems that Blacks relate in dealing with the health care system can apply to anyone, but the inherent racism within the health system cannot be denied. Currently, efforts are being made to overcome these barriers.

Since the 1960s, health care services available to Blacks and other people of color have improved. A growing number of community health centers have emphasized health maintenance and promotion. Community residents serve on the boards.

Among the services provided by community health centers is an effort to discover children with high blood levels of lead in order to provide early diagnosis of and treatment for lead poisoning. Once a child is found to have lead poisoning, the law requires that the source of the lead be found and eradicated. Today, only apartments free of lead paint can be rented to families with young children. Apartments that are found to have lead paint must be stripped and repainted with nonlead paint. Another ongoing effort by the community health centers is to inform Blacks who are at risk of producing children with sickle-cell anemia that they are carriers of this genetic disease. This program is fraught with conflict because many people prefer not to be screened for the sickle-cell trait, fearing they may become labeled once the tendency is discovered.

Birth control is another problem that is recognized with mixed emotions. To some, especially women who want to space children or who do not want to have numerous children, birth control is a welcome development. People who believe in birth control prefer selecting the time when they will have children, how many children they will have, and when they will stop having children. To many other people, birth control is considered a form of "Black genocide" and a way of limiting the growth of the community. Health workers in the Black community must be aware of both sides of this issue and, if asked to make a decision, remain neutral. Such decisions must be made by the patients themselves.

Special Considerations for Health Care Providers

White health care providers know far too little about how to care for a Black person's skin or hair, or how to understand both Black nonverbal and verbal behavior.

Physiological Assessment. Examples of possible physiological problems include the following (in observing skin problems, it is important to note that skin assessment is best done in indirect sunlight) (Bloch & Hunter, 1981):

1. **Pallor.** There is an absence of underlying red tones; the skin of a brown-skinned person appears yellow-brown, and that of a black-skinned person appears ashen gray. Mucous membranes appear ashen, and the lips and nailbeds are similar.

2. **Erythema.** Inflammation must be detected by palpation; the skin is warmer in the area, tight, and edematous, and the deeper tissues are hard. Fingertips must be used for this assessment, as with rashes, since they are sensitive to the feeling of different textures of skin.

3. **Cyanosis.** Cyanosis is difficult to observe in dark-colored skin, but it can be seen by close inspection of the lips, tongue, conjunctiva, palms of the hands, and soles of the feet. One method of testing is pressing the palms. Slow blood return is an indication of cyanosis. Another sign is ashen gray lips and tongue.

4. **Ecchymosis.** History of trauma to a given area can be detected from a swelling of the skin surface.

5. **Jaundice.** The sclera are usually observed for yellow discoloration to reveal jaundice. This is not always a valid indication, however, since carotene deposits can also cause the sclera to appear yellow. The buccal mucosa and the palms of the hands and soles of the feet may appear yellow.

Several skin conditions are of importance in Black patients (Sykes & Kelly, 1979):

1. **Keloids.** Keloids are scars that form at the site of a wound and grow beyond the normal boundaries of the wound. They are sharply elevated and irregular and continue to enlarge.

2. **Pigmentary disorders.** Pigmentary disorders, areas of either postinflammatory hypopigmentation or hyperpigmentation, appear as dark or light spots.

3. **Pseudofolliculitis.** "Razor bumps" and "ingrown hairs" are caused by shaving too closely with an electric razor or straight razor. The sharp point of the hair, if shaved too close, enters the skin and induces an immune response as to a foreign body. The symptoms include papules, pustules, and sometimes even keloids.

4. **Melasma.** The "mask of pregnancy," melasma, is a patchy tan to dark brown discoloration of the face more prevalent in dark pregnant women.

Hair Care Needs. The care of the hair of Blacks is not complicated, but special consideration must be given to help maintain its healthy condition (Bloch & Hunter, 1981):

1. The hair's dryness or oiliness must be assessed, as well as its texture (straight or extra curly) and the patient's hairstyle preference.
2. The hair must be shampooed as needed and groomed according to the person's preference.
3. Hair must be combed well, with the appropriate tools, such as a "pic" or comb with big teeth, before drying to prevent tangles.
4. If the hair is dry and needs oiling, the preparations that the person generally uses for this purpose ought to be on hand.
5. Once dry, the hair is ready to be styled (curled, braided, or rolled) as the person desires.

Additional Considerations. The majority of the members of the health care profession are steeped in a middle-class White value system. In clinical settings, providers are being helped to become familiar with and to understand the value systems of other ethnic and socioeconomic groups. They are being taught to recognize the symptoms of illness in Blacks and to provide proper skin and hair care. The following are guidelines that a health care provider can follow in caring for members of the Black community.

1. The education of an ever-increasing number of Blacks in the health professions must continue to be encouraged.
2. The needs of the patient must be assessed realistically.
3. When a treatment or special diet is prescribed, every attempt must be made to ascertain whether it is consistent with the patient's physical needs, cultural background, income, and religious practices.
4. The patient's belief in and practice of folk medicine must be respected; the patient must not be criticized for these beliefs. Every effort should be made to assist the patient to combine folk treatment with standard Western treatment, as long as the two are not antagonistic. Most people who have a strong belief in folk remedies continue to use them with or without medical sanction.
5. Providers should be familiar with formal and informal sources of help in the Black community. The formal sources consist of churches, social clubs, and community groups. The informal ones include the women who provide care for members of their community in an informal way.
6. The beliefs and values of the health care provider should not be forced on the patient.
7. The treatment plan and the reasons for a given treatment must be shared with the patient.

Table 10-5   Black or African American Non-Hispanic Enrollment in Selected Health Professions Schools: 2004–2005

	Total Program Enrollment	Black Non-Hispanic Enrollment
Dentistry	18,315	1,059
Allopathic medicine	66,821	4,947
Osteopathic medicine	12,525	469
Nursing—registered	a	a
Optometry	5,377	189
Pharmacy	43,908	3,784
Podiatry	1,584	228

Source: National Center for Health Statistics (2007). Health, United States, 2007 with urban and rural health chartbook (pp. 361–362). Hyattsville, MD: National Center for Health Statistics.

a no data available

Table 10-6   Percentage of Non-Hispanic Blacks or African Americans Enrolled in Selected Health Professions Schools, Compared to Non-Hispanic Whites: 2004–2005

	Non-Hispanic Whites (%)	Non-Hispanic Blacks (%)
Dentistry	66.1	5.4
Allopathic medicine	63.3	7.4
Osteopathic medicine	73.5	3.7
Nursing—Registered	a	a
Optometry	63.2	3.5
Pharmacy	59.7	8.6
Podiatry	60.4	14.4

Source: National Center for Health Statistics. (2007). Health, United States, 2007, with urban and rural health chartbook (pp. 361–362). Hyattsville, MD: Author.

a The National League for Nursing changed the way it collects these data in 1991 and subsequently discontinued the practice; enrollment data are not available after 1991.

Black American Health Care Manpower

The number of Black Americans both enrolled in health programs and in practice in selected health professions is low, as illustrated in Tables 10–5 and 10–6. The National Sample Survey of Registered Nurses 2004, prepared by the Bureau of Health Professions of the Health Resources Administration, estimates that the registered nurse population in the United States in 2004 numbered 2,909,357. Of this number, 81.8% were White non-Hispanic and 4.2% were Black (non-Hispanic). Given that, in 2005, 12.8% of the resident population was Black (non-Hispanic) (see Table 2–2 in Chapter 2), this is a clear indication that there is not demographic parity in the percentage of Black (non-Hispanic) people in nursing. The findings of Somnath and Shipman (2006), who reviewed a total of 55 studies in 2006 found that minority patients tend to receive better interpersonal care from practitioners of their own race or ethnicity, particularly in primary care and mental health settings, and that non-English speaking patients experience better interpersonal care, greater medical comprehension, and greater likelihood of keeping follow-up appointments when they see a language-concordant practitioner.

Somnath and Shipman concluded their study by stating that "the findings indicated greater health professions diversity will likely lead to improved public health by increasing access to care for underserved populations, and by increasing opportunities for minority patients to see practitioners with whom they share a common race, ethnicity or language." They also stated that "race, ethnicity, and language concordance, which is associated with better patient-practitioner relationships and communication, may increase patients' likelihood of receiving and accepting appropriate medical care" (Somnath & Shipman, 2006, p. 17). The study presented in the Research on Culture box substantiates these findings. Efforts must be made to recruit and maintain more Blacks in the health professions.

RESEARCH ON CULTURE

A large amount of research has been conducted among members of the Black population. The study described in the following article is one example:

Wilson, D. W. (2007). *From their own voices: The lived experience of African American registered nurses.* Journal of Transcultural Nursing, 18(2), 142–149.

This phenomenological study describes the lived experiences of African American nurses who provide care to individuals, families, and communities in southeast Louisiana. The sample consisted of 13 nurses whose ages ranged from 40 to 62, with an average age of 49.53. Their nursing experience ranged from 8 to 39 years and they were educated in ad, diploma, and baccalaureate programs. Four of the informants had earned master's degrees in nursing. The essential themes found in the study were that the participants' experiences included connecting with the patients through the delivery of holistic nursing care and "proving yourself." Holistic care included respect for the patients' cultural backgrounds and the realization that in many ways they were vitally important in meeting the needs of the patients and families. They believed that they were also important in meeting the spiritual and religious needs of patients. The nurses also participated in patient teaching and advocacy. The incidental themes included fulfilling a dream, being invisible and voiceless, surviving and persevering, and mentoring and role modeling. The author recommends that, if the nursing profession is to promote nursing care that is congruent with the needs of culturally diverse patients, it must increase the representation of African American registered nurses.

Explore 🌐 MediaLink

Go to the Companion Website at www.prenhall.com/spector for chapter-related review questions, case studies, and activities. Contents of the CulturalCare Guide and CulturalCare Museum can also be found on the Companion Website. Click on Chapter 10 to select the activities for this chapter.

Internet Sources

Brunner, B., and Haney, E. (2007). Civil Rights Timeline: Milestones in the modern civil rights movement. Upper Saddle River, NJ: Pearson Education. Retrieved June 9, 2007 from http://www.infoplease.com/spot/civilrightstimeline1.html

Hogan, H., and Lamas, E. J. (2007). The American Community—Blacks: 2004. Washington, D.C.: U. S. Census Bureau. Retrieved from http://www.census.gov/population/www/socdemo/race.html, February 24, 2008

Ibrahim, I. A. (2002). A Brief Illustrated Guide to Understanding Islam. Houston, Texas: Darussalam. Retrieved from http://www.islam-guide.com/frm-editors.htm, July 21, 2007.

Office of Dawah. (2006–2008). The Religion of Islam. Rawdah: Author. Retrieved Sept. 19, 2007 from http://www.islamreligion.com/

Somnath, S., and Shipman, S. (2006). The rationale for diversity in the health professions: A review of the evidence (Washington, DC: U.S. Department of Health and Human Services, Health Resources and Services Administration Bureau of Health Professions. http://www.hrsa.gov/, January 5, 2008

United States Census Bureau, Census 2000 Special Tabulations. Profile of Selected Demographic and Social Characteristics: 2000 Africa, Nigeria, Somalia, and Sudan. Retrieved July 25, 2007 from http://www.census.gov/population/cen2000/stp-159/STP-159-Africaica.pdf, http://www.census.gov/population/cen2000/stp-159/STP-159-Nigeria.pdf, http://www.census.gov/population/cen2000/stp-159/STP-159-Somalia.pdf, and http://www.census.gov/population/cen2000/stp-159/STP-159-Sudan.pdf

United States Department of Health and Human Services. (2004). The Registered Nurse Population Findings from the March, 2004 National Sample of Registered Nurses. Washington DC: Author. Retrieved from ftp://ftp.hrsa.gov/bhpr/workforce/0306rnss.pdf, January 5, 2008

References

American Psychiatric Association. (1994). *Diagnostic and statistical manual of mental disorders* (4th ed.). Washington, DC: Author.

Bass, P. H., & Pugh, K. (2001). *In our own image—Treasured African-American traditions, journeys, and icons.* Philadelphia: Running Press.

Bloch, B., & Hunter, M. L. (1981, January–February). Teaching physiological assessment of Black persons. *Nurse Educator,* 26.

Bullock, W. H., & Jilly, P. N. (1975). Hematology. In R. A. Williams (Ed.), *Textbook of Black-related diseases.* New York: McGraw-Hill.

Bullough, B., & Bullough, V. L. (1972). *Poverty, ethnic identity, and health care.* New York: Appleton-Century-Crofts.

Dalaku, J. (2001). *Poverty in the United States: 2000.* U.S. Census Bureau Current Population Reports Series P60-214. Washington, DC: U.S. Government Printing Office.

Davis, R. (1998). *American voudou—Journey into a hidden world.* Denton: University of North Texas Press.

Dunstin, B. (1969). Pica during pregnancy. Chap. 26 in *Current concepts in clinical nursing.* St. Louis, MO: Mosby.

Eck, D. (1994). *African religion in America: On common ground.* New York: Columbia University Press.

Fontaine, K. L. (2003). *Mental health nursing* (5th ed.). Upper Saddle River, NJ: Prentice Hall.

Gutman, H. G. (1976). *The Black family in slavery and freedom, 1750–1925.* New York: Pantheon.

Haley, A. (1976). *Roots.* New York: Doubleday.

Hughes, L., & Bontemps, A. (Eds.), (1958). *The book of negro folklore.* New York: Dodd, Mead.

Jacques, G. (1976). Cultural health traditions: A Black perspective. In M. Branch & P. P. Paxton (Eds.), *Providing safe nursing care for ethnic people of color.* New York: Appleton-Century-Crofts.

Kain, J. F. (Ed.). (1969). *Race and poverty.* Englewood Cliffs, NJ: Prentice Hall.

Kotlowitz, A. (1991). *There are no children here: The story of two boys growing up in the other America.* New York: Doubleday.

Manderschied, R. W., & Sonnenschein, M. A. (Eds.). (1992). *Mental health, United States.* Washington, DC: Center for Mental Health Services and National Institute of Mental Health, DHHS Pub. No. (SMA) 92-1942, U.S. Government Printing Office.

McKinnon, J. (2001). *The Black population: 2000.* Washington, DC: U.S. Census Bureau.

National Center for Health Statistics. (2006). *Health, United States, 2006 with chartbook on trends in the health of Americans.* Hyattsville, MD: Author.

National Center for Health Statistics. (2007). *Health, United States, 2007 with chartbook on trends in the health of Americans.* Hyattsville, MD: Author.

Spector, R. (1992). Culture, ethnicity, and nursing. In P. Potter & A. Perry (Eds.), *Fundamentals of nursing* (3rd ed.). St. Louis: Mosby-Year Book.

Spurlock, J. (1988). Black Americans. In L. Comas-Diaz & E. E. H. Griffith (Eds.), *Cross-cultural mental health.* New York: John Wiley & Sons.

Sykes, J., & Kelly, A. P. (1979, June). Black skin problems. *American Journal of Nursing,* 1092–1094.

Tallant, R. (1946). *Voodoo in New Orleans* (7th printing). New York: Collier.

Webb, J. Y. (1971). Letter. Dr. J. R. Krevans to Y. Webb, 15 February 1967. Reported in *Superstitious influence—VooDoo in particular—Affecting health practices in a selected population in southern Louisiana.* Paper. New Orleans, LA.

Wintrob, R. (1972). Hexes, roots, snake eggs? M.D. vs. occults. *Medical Opinion,* *1*(7), 54–61.

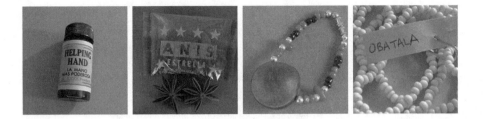

Chapter 11

HEALTH and ILLNESS in the Hispanic Populations

My heart is in the earth . . .

—*Greenhaw (2000)*

■ Objectives

1. Discuss the background of members of selected communities of the Hispanic populations.

2. Discuss the demographic profile of selected communities of the Hispanic populations.

3. Describe the traditional definitions of *HEALTH* and *ILLNESS* of selected communities of the Hispanic populations.

4. Describe the traditional methods of HEALTH maintenance and protection of selected communities of the Hispanic populations.

5. Describe the traditional methods of HEALING of selected communities of the Hispanic populations.

6. Describe current health care problems of the Hispanic populations.

7. Describe demographic disparity as it is seen in health manpower distribution of the Hispanic populations as represented in the health care delivery system.

The images opening this chapter are examples of the many remedies and objects a person may purchase to protect, maintain, and/or restore HEALTH. The first item is "helping hand oil"; it is applied to the body to protect the wearer from *mal ojo*, the evil eye. The second item is anise, licorice, a popular herbal remedy that is prepared as a tea and used to soothe the stomach. The third item is a "deer's eye" bracelet for a baby or child; it is used to ward off the evil eye and bring good luck. The last item represents the beads of *Santeria*. These beads are worn by a person whose patron, or *Orisha*, is *Obatala*. *Obatala* is the major Yoruba deity and father of the Yoruba gods. The discussion later in this chapter will provide an explanation of the *Orishas*, or gods of *Santeria*.

■ Background

The largest emerging majority group in the United States is composed of the Hispanic or Latino populations. The terms *Hispanic* and *Latino* are used inter-changeably in Census 2000 and will be used accordingly in this chapter. This is done to reflect the new terminology in the standards issued by the Office of Management and Budget in 1997, used in the reporting of Census 2000, and became official in 2003 (Therrien & Ramirez, 2001, p. 1). The term *Hispanic*, or *Latino, Americans* refers to people who were born in or whose predecessors came from (even generations ago) Mexico, Puerto Rico, Cuba, Central and South America, Spain, and other Spanish-speaking communities and who now live in the United States. Figure 11–1 and Table 11–1 display the population dis-tribution in 2002. The Hispanic people constituted 9% of the population in the 1990 census, grew to 12% in 2000, and reached 15% in 2005. They are the

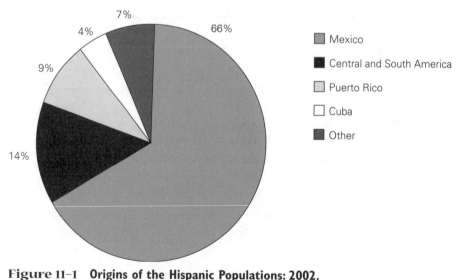

Figure 11-1 Origins of the Hispanic Populations: 2002.
Source: Ramirez, R., & de la Cruz, G. P. (2002, March). *The Hispanic population in the United States* (p. 1). Retrieved July 25, 2007 from http://www.census.gov/prod/2003pubs/p20-545.pdf

Table 11-1 Origins of the Hispanic Populations

Mexico	66.9%
Central and South America	14.3%
Puerto Rico	8.6%
Cuba	3.7%
Other Hispanic	6.5%

Source: Ramirez, R., & de la Cruz, G. P. (2002, March). *The Hispanic population in the United States.* Retrieved July 25, 2007 from http://www.census.gov/prod/2003pubs/p20-545.pdf

fastest growing and, with a mean age of 25.8 years and a median age of 24 years, the youngest population group.

The most recent analysis of demographic data, 2002, relevant to the Hispanic community showed

- Hispanics are more geographically concentrated than non-Hispanic Whites, with 44.2% living in the West and 34.8% living in the South.
- Hispanics are more likely than non-Hispanic Whites to be less than 18 years old, as 34.4% of Hispanics are younger than 5 and 22.8% of the non-Hispanic White population are younger than 5.
- Two in five Hispanics are foreign-born.
- Hispanics live in family households that are larger than those of non-Hispanic Whites.
- The percentage of Hispanics graduating from high school or attending some college was 45.9% in 2002 and having at least a high school diploma was 45.9% in 2002, as compared to non-Hispanic Whites, for whom the percentages were 59.3% graduating from high school or attending some college and 88.7% having at least a high school diploma.
- Hispanics were much more likely than non-Hispanic Whites to not have full-time year-round employment with annual earnings of $35,000 or more in 2001.
- Hispanics were more likely than non-Hispanic Whites to live in poverty—21.4% of the Hispanic population and 7.8% of the White alone population. (Ramirez & de la Cruz, 2003, pp. 1–6)

Table 11–2 illustrates selected variables from the demographic profiles of new immigrants, the people born in Latin America, with examples of people born in Guatemala and Mexico, who entered the United States since 1980. There have been 16,089,975 people legally admitted from Latin America; with 480,665 people from Guatemala, and 9,177,485 people from Mexico. The percentages of people who have been naturalized as citizens are low and one factor that is reported by community workers is money. In fact, the fee to apply for citizenship rose from $400 to $675 on July 30, 2007 (Ballou, 2007, p. B5).

Table 11-2   **Profile of Selected Demographic and Social Characteristics of People Entering the United States from Latin America, Guatemala, and Mexico: 2000**

Variable	Latin America	Guatemala	Mexico
Naturalized U. S. citizens	30.2%	23.2%	22.5%
Language other than English spoken at home	87.7%	94.9%	94.4%
Speak English less than very well	62.4%	70.2%	71.7%
Median age	34.2 years	32.1 years	31.5 years
Marital status—married	57.7%	51.7%	61.3%
School enrollment—college or graduate school	29.4%	29.1%	18.7%
Educational attainment—bachelor's degree or higher—population 25 years and older	9.6%	6.0%	4.3%
Veteran status—civilian veterans	2.0%	1.4%	1.5%
Employment status—over 18 years of age employed	61.2%	63.8%	60.1%
Median household income	$33,519	$33,353	$31,503
Household income—$150,000 or more	1.1%	1.6%	0.8%
Median family income	$33,421	$31,532	$30,686
Per capita earnings	$15,607	$14,3992	$13,020
Poverty status—families	20.7%	20.1%	24.4%

Source: U.S. Census Bureau, Census 2000 Special Tabulations. Profile of Selected Demographic and Social Characteristics: 2000 Latin America, Guatemala, Mexico. Retrieved July 25, 2007 from http://www.census.gov/ponulation/cen2000/stp-159/STP-159-LatinAmerica.pdf, http://www.census.gov/population/cen2000/stp-159/STP-159-Guatemala.pdf, and http://www.census.gov/population/cen2000/stp-159/STP-159-Mexico.pdf

This section has described the Hispanic, or Latino, populations as a whole; the next two sections describe the Mexican, or Mesoamerican, population and the Puerto Rican groups. The term *Mesoamerican* is inclusive in that it describes peoples with Mexican and Central and South American origins. (Carmack, R. M., Gasco, J., and Gossen, G. H., 1996, p. xvii). There is much confusion as to what their proper name is and, for the purposes of this chapter, overall government designations of *Hispanic* or *Latino* will be used for the aggregate populations and *Mexican* or *Mesoamerican* to refer to people who have a history and origins south of the United States/Mexico border and Spanish or Iberian origins.

■ Mexicans

The United States shares a 2,000-mile-long border with Mexico, which, in spite of walls and tightened security, remains easily crossed in both directions. The flow of people, goods, and ideas across it has a powerful impact on both countries.

Figure 11–2 is the fence, or wall, as it appears in Nogales, Arizona. It is an enormous structure that will eventually hug all 2,000 miles of the U.S./Mexico border. Here, you can see that it abuts the yards of families residing on the Mex-

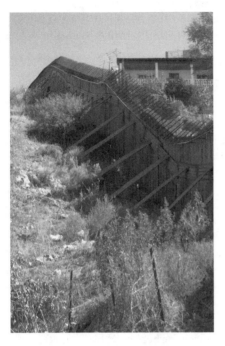

Figure 11-2 The fence along the United States/Mexico border; Mexico is on the right hand side.
Source: Author, Nogales, Arizona, November 4, 2007.

ican side of the border. The United States federal government is planning to complete building a wall such as this across the entire 2,000 miles of the United States/Mexico border.

Americans of Hispanic origin, according to the 2002 census, numbered at least 37.4 million people; of this number, 66.9% were of Mexican origin (Ramirez & de la Cruz, 2002, p. 1). The Mexicans have been in the United States for a long time, moving from Mexico and later intermarrying with Indians and Spanish people in the southwestern parts of what is now the United States. Santa Fe, New Mexico was settled in 1609. Most of the descendants of these early settlers now live in Arizona, California, Colorado, New Mexico, and Texas. A large number of Mexicans also live in Illinois, Indiana, Kansas, Michigan, Missouri, Nebraska, New York, Ohio, Utah, Washington, and Wisconsin, where most arrived as migrant farm workers. While located there as temporary farm workers, they found permanent jobs and stayed. Contrary to the popular views that Mexicans live in rural areas, most live in urban areas. Mexicans are employed in all types of jobs. Few, however, have high-paying or high-status jobs in labor or management. The majority work in factories, mines, and construction; others are employed in farm work and service areas. At present, only a small—though growing—number are employed in clerical and professional areas. The number of unemployed in this group is high (estimated to be between 25% and 30%), and the earnings of those employed are well below the national average. The education of Mexicans, like that of most minorities in the United States, lags behind that of most of the population. Many Mexicans fail to complete high school. In the past few years, this situation has begun to change, and Mexican children are being encouraged to stay in school, go on to college, and enter the professions.

Traditional Definitions of HEALTH and ILLNESS

There are conflicting reports about the traditional meaning of HEALTH among Mexicans. Some sources maintain that HEALTH is considered to be purely the result of "good luck" and that a person loses his or her health if that luck changes (Welch, Comer, & Steinman, 1973, p. 205). Some people describe HEALTH as a reward for good behavior. Seen in this context, HEALTH is a gift from God and should not be taken for granted. People are expected to maintain their own equilibrium in the universe by performing in the proper way, eating the proper foods, and working the proper amount of time. The protection of HEALTH is an accepted practice that is accomplished with prayer, the wearing of religious medals or amulets, and the keeping of relics in the home. Herbs and spices can be used to enhance this form of prevention, as can exemplary behavior (Lucero, 1975). ILLNESS is seen as an imbalance in an individual's body or as punishment meted out for wrongdoing. The causes of ILLNESS can be grouped into five major categories:

1. *The body's imbalance.* Imbalance may exist between "hot" and "cold" or "wet" and "dry." The theory of hot and cold was taken to Mexico by Spanish priests and was fused with Aztec beliefs. The concept actually dates to the early Hippocratic theory of disease and four body humors. The disrupted relationship among these humors is often mentioned by Mexicans as the cause of disease (Lucero, 1975).

   There are four body humors, or fluids: (1) blood, hot and wet; (2) yellow bile, hot and dry; (3) phlegm, cold and wet; and (4) black bile, cold and dry. When all four humors are balanced, the body is HEALTHY. When any imbalance occurs, an ILLNESS is manifested (Currier, 1966). These concepts, of course, provide one way of determining the remedy for a particular ILLNESS. For example, if an ILLNESS is classified as hot, it is treated with a cold substance. A cold disease, in turn, must be treated with a hot substance. Food, beverages, animals, and people possess the characteristics of hot and cold to various degrees. Hot foods cannot be combined; they are to be eaten with cold foods. There is no general agreement as to what is a hot disease or food and what is a cold disease or food. The classification varies from person to person, and what is hot to one person may be cold to another (Saunders, 1958, p. 13). Therefore, if a Mexican patient refuses to eat the meals in the hospital, it is wise to ask precisely what the person can eat and what combinations of foods he or she thinks would be helpful for the existing condition. It is important to note that *hot* and *cold* do not refer to temperature but are descriptive of a particular substance itself.

For example, after a woman delivers a baby, a hot experience, she cannot eat pork, which is considered a hot food. She must eat something cold to restore her balance. Penicillin is a hot medication; therefore, it may be believed that it cannot be used to treat a hot disease. The major problem for the health care provider is to know that the rules, so to speak, of hot and cold vary from person to person. If health care providers understand the general nature of the hot and cold imbalance, they will be able to help the patient reveal the nature of the problem from the patient's perspective and manage it accordingly.

2. *Dislocation of parts of the body.* Two examples of "dislocation" are *empacho* and *caida de la mollera* (Nall & Spielberg, 1967). *Empacho* is believed to be caused by a ball of food clinging to the wall of the stomach. Common symptoms of this illness are stomach pains and cramps. This ailment is treated by rubbing and gently pinching the spine. Prayers are recited throughout the treatment. Another, more common, cause of such illness is thought to be lying about the amount of food consumed. A 20-year-old Hispanic woman experienced the acute onset of sharp abdominal pain. She complained to her friend, and together they diagnosed the problem as *empacho* and treated it by massaging her stomach and waiting for the pain to dissipate. It did not, and they continued folk treatment for 48 hours. When the pain did not diminish, they sought help in a nearby hospital. The diagnosis was acute appendicitis. The young woman nearly died and was quite embarrassed when she was scolded by the physician for not seeking help sooner.

Caida de la mollera is a more serious illness. It occurs in infants and young children aged under 1 year who are dehydrated (usually because of diarrhea or severe vomiting) and whose anterior fontanelle is depressed below the contour of the skull (Dorsey & Jackson, 1976, p. 56). Much superstition and mystery surround this problem. Some of the poorly educated and rural people, in particular, may believe that it is caused by a nurse's or physician's having touched the baby's head. This can be understood if we take into account that (1) an infant's fontanelle becomes depressed if the infant is dehydrated and (2) when physicians or nurses measure an infant's head they touch this area. If a mother takes her baby to a physician for an examination and sees the physician touch the child's head, and if the baby gets sick thereafter with *caida de la mollera,* it might be very easy for the woman to believe it is the fault of the physician's or nurse's touch. Unfortunately, epidemics of diarrhea are common in the rural and urban areas of the Southwest, and a number of children tend to be affected. One case of severe dehydration that leads to *caida de la mollera* may create quite a stir among the people. The folk treatment of this illness has not been found to be effective. Unfortunately, babies are rarely taken to the hospital in time, and the mortality rate for this illness is high (Lucero, 1975).

3. *Magic or supernatural causes outside the body.* Witchcraft or possession is considered to be culturally patterned role-playing, a safe vehicle for restoring oneself. Witchcraft or possession legitimizes acting out bizarre behavior or engaging in incoherent speech. Hispanic tradition, especially in the Borderlands (the geographic area along the United States/Mexico border) blends the medieval heritage of medieval Castilian and English traditions with Mexican Indian folk beliefs (Kearney & Medrano, 2001, p. 119). *Brujas* (witches) use black, or malevolent, magic, while *curanderos* use white, or benevolent, magic. Spells may be cast to influence a lover or to get back at a rival, and cards are read to tell the future. *Herbrias* sell herbs, amulets, and talismans (Kearney & Medrano, p. 117).

A lesser disease that is caused from outside the body is *mal ojo.* *Mal ojo* means "bad eye," and it is believed to result from excessive admiration on the part of another. General malaise, sleepiness, fatigue, and severe headache are the symptoms of this condition. The folk treatment is to find the person who has caused the illness by casting the "bad eye" and having him or her care for the afflicted person (Nall & Spielberg, 1967). The belief in the evil eye, *mal de ojo,* can be traced back to the mid-1400s and Spain (Kearney & Medrano, 2001, p. 118). It has origins that go back even further in many parts of the world. This belief is common today.

4. *Strong emotional states. Susto* is described as an illness arising from fright. It afflicts many people—males and females, rich and poor, rural dwellers and urbanites. It involves soul loss: The soul is able to leave the body and wander freely. This can occur while a person is dreaming or when a person experiences a particularly traumatic event. The symptoms of the disease are (1) restlessness while sleeping; (2) listlessness, anorexia, and disinterest in personal appearance when awake, including disinterest in both clothing and personal hygiene; and (3) loss of strength, depression, and introversion. The person is treated by *curandero* (a folk healer, discussed above and in the section on *curanderismo*), who coaxes the soul back into the person's body. During the healing rites, the person is massaged and made to relax (Rubel, 1964).

5. *Envidia. Envidia,* or envy, also is considered to be a cause of illness and bad luck. Many people believe that to succeed is to fail. That is, when one's success provokes the envy of friends and neighbors, misfortune can befall the person and his or her family. For example, a successful farmer, just when he is able to purchase extra clothing and equipment, is stricken with a fatal illness. He may well attribute the cause of this illness to the envy of his peers. A number of social scientists have, after much research, concluded that the "low" economic and success rates of Mexicans can ostensibly be attributed to belief in *envidia* (Lucero, 1975).

Religious Rituals

Magico-religious practices are quite common among the Mexican population. The more severe an illness, the more likely these practices will be used. There are four types of practices:

1. **Making promises.** A *promesa* may be made to God or to a saint; for example, a person may promise to donate money to a cause if he or she recovers from an ILLNESS.

2. **Visiting shrines.** Many people make pilgrimages to shrines to offer prayers and gifts. This practice has origins in Jerusalem and later Spain with the visits to Santiago de Compestello starting in the 11th century (Kearney & Medrano, 2001, p. 110).

3. **Offering medals and candles**

4. **Offering prayers** (Nall & Spielberg, 1967)

It is not unusual for the Mexico people residing near the southern border of the continental United States to return home to Mexico on religious pilgrimages. The film mentioned in Chapter 5, *We Believe in Niño Fedencio,* demonstrates how these pilgrimages are conducted. The lighting of candles also is a frequently observed practice. Beautiful candles made of beeswax and tallow can be purchased in many stores, particularly grocery stores and pharmacies located in Mexican neighborhoods (Figures 11–3, 11–4A, and 11–4B). Many homes have shrines

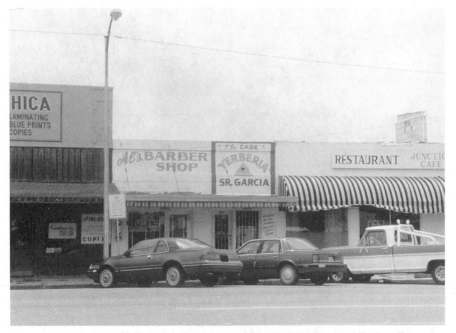

Figure 11-3   A traditional community resource *Yerberia* in Mission, Texas.

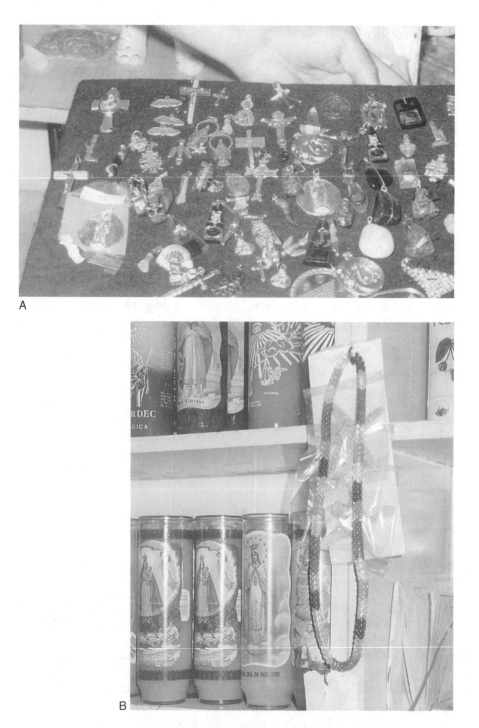

Figure 11-4   A and B Samples of amulets and candles sold in Sr. Garcia's
Yerberea.

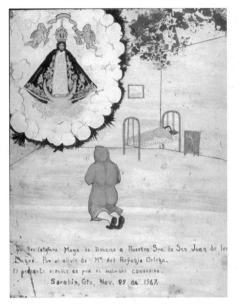

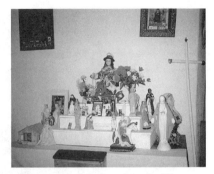

Figure 11-6   An altar in _El Santuario de Chimayo_, Chimayo, New Mexico..

Figure 11-5   A person giving thanks to the Virgin of San Juan de la Valle for the recovery of a loved one.

with statues and pictures of saints. The candles are lit here and prayers are recited. Some homes have altars with statues and pictures on them and are the focal point of the home. Some Mexicans are devoted to the Virgin de San Juan del Valle and make pilgrimages to the shrine in San Juan, Texas (Figure 11-5).

In Catholic churches in communities with Hispanic populations, such as San Antonio, Texas, or Chimayo, New Mexico (Figure 11-6), it is not unusual to see statues covered with flowers and votive figures, such as those in Figures 11-7 and 11-8. These miniature articles are known in Spanish as _milagros,_ meaning "miracles," _ex-votos,_ or _promesas._ They are offered to a saint in thanks for answering a person's prayers for HEALING, success, a good marriage, and so forth. The _milagros_ are made from wax, wood, bone, or a variety of metals and are an integral part of an ancient folk tradition found in many cultures (Egan, 1991, pp. 1–2). This practice, too, originated in Spain and even today one can see and purchase these objects in countless churches (Kearney & Medrano, 2001, p. 115).

Curanderismo

There are no specific rules for knowing who in the community uses the services of folk healers. Not all Mexicans do, and not all Mexicans believe in their precepts. Initially, it was thought that only the poor used a folk healer, or _curandero,_ because they were unable to get treatment from the larger, institutionalized health care establishments. It now appears, however, that the use of HEALERS occurs widely

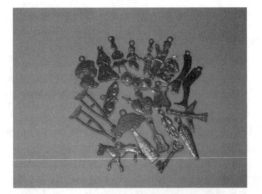

Figure 11-7 *Milagros.* This photograph is an example of the assortment of various miniature articles that may be purchased for the nominal cost of $1.00 in *botanicas* or in a marketplace from traditional people. In this image are crutches, a head, a woman, children and a baby, an arm, a leg, eyes, breasts, a torso, a heart, a car, a horse, a key, a whisky bottle, and others. When a person is experiencing a problem with one of these anatomical areas or objects, he or she may pray for recovery; make a *promesa* to a saint; and when the person's prayer is answered, take the *milagro* to a church and place it near the saint the person prayed to.

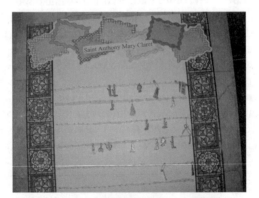

Figure 11-8 *Milagros* placed at the Shrine of Saint Anthony in the Church of the Sacred Heart of Mary in San Antonio, Texas.

throughout the Mexican population. Some people try to use HEALERS exclusively, whereas others use them along with institutionalized care. The HEALERS do not usually advertise, but they are well known throughout the population because of informal community and kinship networks.

Curanderismo is defined as a medical system (Maduro, 1976). It is a coherent view with historical roots that combine Aztec, Spanish, spiritualistic, homeopathic, and scientific elements. There are *curanderos* practicing in Spain, and there is an established community of *curanderos* in close proximity to Granada.

The *curandero(a)* is a holistic healer. The people who seek help from him or her do so for social, physical, and psychological purposes. The *curandero(a)* can be either a "specialist" or a "generalist," a full-time or part-time practitioner. Mexicans who believe in *curanderos* consider them to be religious figures.

A *curandero(a)* may receive the "gift of healing" through three means:

1. He or she may be "born" to heal. In this case, it is known from the moment of a *cuandero(a)'s* birth that something unique about this person means that he or she is destined to be a healer.

2. He or she may learn by apprenticeship—that is, the person is taught the ways of healing, especially the use of herbs.

3. He or she may receive a "calling" through a dream, trance, or vision by which contact is made with the supernatural by means of a "patron" (or "caller"), who may be a saint. The "call" comes either during adolescence or during the midlife crisis. This "call" is resisted at first. Later, the person becomes resigned to his or her fate and gives in to the demands of the "calling."

Other folk healers include the *materia,* or spirit channeler, and the *partera,* or lay midwife. Box 11–1 describes the scope of the *partera's* practice.

HEALTH *Restoration*

The most popular form of HEALTH restoration used by folk healers involves herbs, especially when used as teas. The *curandero* knows what specific herbs to use for a problem. This information is revealed in dreams, in which the "patron" gives suggestions.

Because the *curandero* has a religious orientation, much of the treatment includes elements of both the Catholic and Pentecostal rituals and artifacts: offerings of money, penance, confession, the lighting of candles, *milagros,* and the laying on of hands. Massage is used in illnesses such as *empacho.*

Cleanings, the removal of negative forces or spirits, or *limpias,* are done in two ways. The first is by passing an unbroken egg over the body of the ILL person. The second method entails passing herbs tied in a bunch over the body. The back of the neck, which is considered a vulnerable spot, is given particular attention.

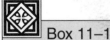

Box 11–1

Parteras

In Mexico and South Texas there is a long history of the use of midwives, or *parteras*. The practice of midwifery predates Cortes. The goddess Tlozoteotl was the goddess of childbirth, and the midwives were known as "Tlamatqui-Tuti." A *partera* is viewed as a HEALER by many members of the Mexican American and Mexican communities. She (most are women, although currently obstetricians from Mexico are providing this service in South Texas) is described as an individual who has the ability to HEAL and is outgoing, warm, gentle, caring, and cooperative. The *partera*'s duties include (1) giving advice to the pregnant woman, (2) giving physical aid, such as treating any illness the woman experiences during pregnancy, (3) guiding the woman through her pregnancy in terms of nutrition or activities she can and cannot do, and (4) being in attendance during labor and delivery.

Patients are most often referred to *parteras* by their friends or relatives, and a *partera* with a good reputation is always busy. Some *parteras* receive referrals from the health department with which they register, some advertise in the local newspaper or telephone book, and some have signs on their homes or clinics (Figure 11–9).

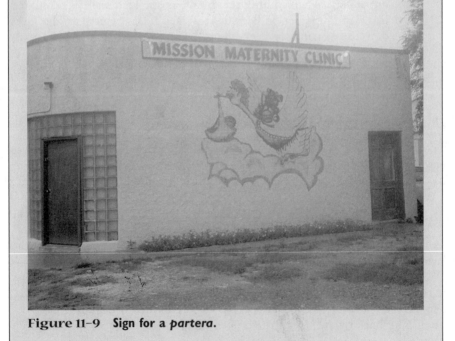

Figure 11-9   Sign for a *partera*.

The *parteras* avoid delivering women with high blood pressure, anemia, a history of diabetes, multiple babies, and transverse presentations. Some *parteras* also prefer to send women with breech presentations to the hospital. If an unfamiliar woman in labor appears at their door in the middle of the night who is very poor with no place to go to deliver, most claim they will take her in.

Most *parteras* keep records of their deliveries. Included in these records are such data as the name of the mother, date, time of admission, stage of labor, time in labor, contractions, time of delivery, presenting part, time of delivery and condition of the placenta, and physical condition of the mother and baby.

The amount of prenatal care the *parteras* deliver ranges from a lot to a little. In general, the mothers seek assistance during their third or fourth month of pregnancy. When the *partera*'s assistance is sought, the mother is sent either to the health department or to a doctor for routine blood work. The *partera* is able to follow the mother's case and gives her advice and massages. One important service that the *partera* performs is the repositioning of the fetus in the womb through massage.

A *partera* may give several forms of advice to the pregnant woman. For example, she may advise the woman who is experiencing pica (the craving for and ingestion of nonfood substances, such as clay and laundry starch) to purchase solid milk of magnesia in Mexico. The milk of magnesia tastes like clay, thereby satisfying the pica, and is not considered harmful. The mother with food cravings is advised to satisfy them. The mothers also are instructed:

1. not to lift heavy objects,
2. to take laxatives to prevent constipation,
3. to exercise often by walking frequently,
4. not to cross their legs and
5. not to bathe in hot water. The reason for the last two admonitions is the belief that crossing the legs and taking hot baths can cause the baby to assume the breech position.

If the *partera* knows the exact date of the mother's last period, she is able to estimate accurately when the woman is going to deliver by calculating eight lunar months and 27 days from the onset of the last period.

With the onset of labor, the mother contacts the *partera*. She goes to the birthing place—the home or clinic of the *partera*—or the *partera* goes to her home. The mother is examined vaginally to determine how far along in labor she is and the position of the baby. She is instructed to shower and to empty her bowels—with an enema, if necessary—and she is encouraged to walk and move around until the delivery is imminent. Once the mother is ready to deliver, she is put to bed. Most of the mothers are delivered lying down in bed. If the mother chooses to do so, however, she is delivered in a squatting or sitting position. Several home remedies may be used during labor, including comino (cumin seed) tea or canela (cinnamon) tea to stimulate labor.

The baby is stimulated if needed, and the mucus is removed from the mouth and nose as needed with the use of a bulb syringe. The cord is clamped, tied with cord ties, and cut with scissors that have been boiled and soaked in alcohol. The stump is then treated with merbromin (Mercurochrome), alcohol, or a combination of the two. The baby is weighed, and some time after the delivery

(continued)

it is bathed. Most *parteras* bind both the mother and the baby. The baby may be fed oregano or cumin tea right after birth or later to help it spit up the mucus. Eyedrops are instilled in the baby's eyes, in compliance with state laws (silver nitrate is used most frequently).

The *partera* stays at the mother's home for several hours after the delivery and then returns to check the mother and the baby the next day. If the mother delivers at the home of the *partera*, she generally stays 12 to 14 hours.

There are several ways of disposing of the placenta. It may just be placed in a plastic bag and thrown in the trash, or it may be buried in the yard. Some placentas are buried with a religious or folk ceremony. There are several folk reasons for the burial of the placenta. The placenta must be buried so that the animals will not eat it. If it is eaten by a dog, the mother will not be able to bear any more children. If it is thrown in the trash, the mother's womb may become "cold." If the baby is a girl, the placenta is buried near the home, so the daughter will not go far away. If it is a boy, it is buried far away from the home to ensure the child's independence.

The practice of the *partera* continues today. In 2004, the most recent year that statistics are available for the state of Texas, there were 381,441 births. Of this number, 360,120, or 94.4%, were delivered by physicians and 21,321, or 5.6%, by midwives and others. Of the 21,321 births, 2,743, or 12.9%, of the babies were delivered at home. In San Juan, Texas, a city in Hidalgo County in the Rio Grande Valley, there are 20 registered *parteras* who continue to practice in the traditional manner. They charge an average of $450–$1,000 for prenatal care and the delivery and practice under the supervision of the Department of Public Health. Generally, the mothers seek care from the *partera* in their sixth month of pregnancy but may not seek prenatal care until late in their ninth month when they must have prenatal blood work done (Ochoa, 2007). The practice of the *partera* in the Rio Grande Valley is the life of the past, the present, and the future: "a way of life *de ayer, hoy y mañana*" (Castillo, 1982).

Source: Adapted from Spector, R. (1996). *Cultural diversity in health and illness* (4th ed.) (pp. 305–325). Stamford, CT: Appleton & Lange.

In contrast to the depersonalized care Mexicans expect to receive in medical institutions, their relationship with and care by the *curandero* are uniquely personal, as described in Table 11–3. This special relationship between Mexicans and the *curanderos* may well account for folk healers' popularity. In addition to the close, personal relationship between patient and healer, other factors may explain the continuing belief in *curanderismo:*

1. The mind and body are inseparable.
2. The central problem of life is to maintain harmony, including social, physical, and psychological aspects of the person.
3. There must be harmony between the hot and cold, wet and dry. The treatment of ILLNESS should restore the body's harmony, which has been lost.

Table 11-3   Comparison Between *Curanderos, Parteras,* and Other Traditional Healers and Allopathic Health Care Providers

Curanderos, Parteras, and Other Traditional Healers	Allopathic Health Care Providers
1. Maintain informal, friendly, affective relationship with entire family	1. Businesslike, formal relationship; deal only with the patient
2. Make house calls day or night	2. Patient must go to physician's office or clinic, and only during the day; may have to wait for hours to be seen; home visits are rarely made
3. For diagnosis, consult with head of house, create a mood of awe, talk to all family members, are not authoritarian, have social rapport, build expectation of cure	3. Rest of family is usually ignored; deal solely with the ill person, and may deal only with the sick part of the patient; authoritarian manner creates fear
4. Are generally less expensive than physicians	4. More expensive than *curanderos*
5. Have ties to the "world of the sacred"; have rapport with the symbolic, spiritual, creative, or holy force	5. Secular; pay little attention to the religious beliefs or meaning of an illness
6. Share the world view of the patient— that is, speak the same language, live in the same neighborhood or in some similar socioeconomic conditions, may know the same people, understand the patient's lifestyle	6. Generally do not share the world view of the patient—that is, may not speak the same language, do not live in the same neighborhood, do not understand the patient's socioeconomic conditions or lifestyle

4. The patient is the passive recipient of disease when the disease is caused by an external force. This external force disrupts the natural order of the internal person, and the treatment must be designed to restore this order. The causes of disharmony are evil and witches.

5. A person is related to the spirit world. When the body and soul are separated, soul loss can occur. This loss is sometimes caused by *susto,* a disease or illness resulting from fright, which may afflict individuals from all socioeconomic levels and lifestyles.

6. The responsibility for recovery is shared by the ILL person, the family, and the *curandero(a).*

7. The natural world is not clearly distinguished from the supernatural world. Thus, the *curandero(a)* can coerce, curse, and appease the spirits. The *curandero(a)* places more emphasis on his or her connections with the sacred and the gift of healing than on personal properties. (Such personal properties might include social status, a large home, and expensive material goods.)

Several types of emotional illnesses are found among the traditional people from Hispanic communities. These are further divided into **mental illness** (in which the illness is not judged) and **moral illness** (in which others can judge the victim). The causes of mental illness and examples of the illness they cause are as follows:

- Heredity—epilepsy (*epilepsia*)
- Hex—evil eye (*mal ojo*)
- Worry—anxiety (*tirisia*)
- Fright—hysteria (*histeria*)
- Blow to the head—craziness (*locura*)

The causes of moral illness and examples of the illness they cause are as follows:

- Vice—use of drugs (*drogadicto*)
- Character weakness—alcoholism (*alcoholismo*)
- Emotions—jealousy (*celos*) and/or rage (*coraje*) (Spencer, Nichols, Lipkin, et al., 1993, p. 133)

Ethnopharmacologic teas may be used to treat these maladies and amulets may be worn or religious rituals followed to prevent or treat them. The following are examples of herbs that may be purchased in grocery stores, markets, and *botanicas* and are used as teas to treat the listed maladies:

- Camomile tea, *Manzanilla,* used to cure fright
- Spearmint tea, *Yerb Buena,* used to treat nervousness
- Orange leaves, *Te de narranjo,* used as a sedative to treat nervousness
- Sweet basil, *Albacar,* used to treat fright and to ward off evil spirits (p. 133)

The HEALTH beliefs and practices discussed here are prevalent today (2008). I recently spoke with an immigrant from a small village in Mexico and inquired about *curanderismo*. He was excited to know that I was familiar with the practice and was proud to share his knowledge and experiences.

Puerto Ricans

Puerto Rican migrants to the United States mainland are American citizens, albeit with a different language and culture. They are neither immigrants nor aliens. According to the 2000 census, 9% of the Hispanic population are Puerto Ricans. Most live on the East Coast, with the greatest number living in New York City and metropolitan New Jersey. Most Puerto Ricans migrate to search for a better life or because relatives, particularly spouses and parents, have migrated previously. Life on the island of Puerto Rico is difficult because there is a high level of unemployment. Puerto Ricans are not well known or understood by the majority of people in the continental United States. Little is known about their cultural identity. Mainlanders tend to forget that Puerto Rico is, for the most part, a poor island whose people have many problems. When many Puerto Ricans migrate to the mainland, they bring many of their problems—especially those with poor health and social circumstance (Cohen, 1972).

Puerto Ricans, along with Cubans, constitute the most recent major immigration group to these shores. They cover the spectrum of racial differences and have practiced racial intermarriage. Many are Catholic, but some belong to Protestant sects.

Many people from Puerto Rico perceive HEALTH and ILLNESS and use folk healers and remedies in ways similar to those used by other Hispanics, whereas others practice *santeria*. Most studies on health and illness beliefs and healing have been conducted on Mexicans. It is not easy to find information about the beliefs of Puerto Ricans. Much of the information presented here was gleaned from students and patients. Both groups feel that their beliefs should be known by health care deliverers. One student, whose mother is a healer and is teaching her daughter the art, corroborated much of the following material.

Common Folk Diseases and Their Treatment

Table 11–4 lists a number of folk diseases and the usual source and type of treatment as reported to me by several Puerto Ricans. Many of these diseases or disharmonies were mentioned in the section on Mexican approaches. Nonetheless, there are subtle differences in the ways folk diseases are perceived by Mexicans and Puerto Ricans. For example, although diseases are classified as hot and

Table 11–4   Folk Diseases

Name	Description	Treatment	Source of Treatment
Susto	Sudden fright, causing shock	Relaxation	Relative or friend
Fatigue	Asthmalike symptoms	Oxygen; medications	Western health care system
Pasmo	Paralysis-like symptoms, face or limbs	Prevention; massage	Folk
Empacho	Food forms into a ball and clings to the stomach, causing pain and cramps	Strong massage over the stomach; medication; gently pinching and rubbing the spine	Folk
Mal ojo	Sudden, unexplained illness in a usually well child or person	Prevention; babies wear a special charm	Depends on the severity of the symptoms: usually home or folk
Ataque	Screaming; falling to ground; wildly moving arms and legs; hysterical crying	None—ends spontaneously	

Table 11-5   The Hot-Cold Classification Among Puerto Ricans

	Frio (Cold)	*Fresco* (Cool)	*Caliente* (Hot)
Illness or bodily conditions	Arthritis Menstrual period Joint pains	Colds	Constipation Diarrhea Pregnancy Rashes Ulcers
Medicine and herbs		Bicarbonate of soda Linden flowers Milk of magnesia Nightshade Orange flower water Sage Tobacco	Anise Aspirin Castor oil Cinnamon Cod-liver oil Iron tablets Penicillin Vitamins
Foods	Avocado Banana Coconut Lima beans Sugar cane White beans	Barley water Whole milk Chicken Fruits Honey Raisins Salt cod Watercress Onions Peas	Alcoholic beverages Chili peppers Chocolate Coffee Corn meal Evaporated milk Garlic Kidney beans

Source: Schilling, B., & Brannon, E. (1986, September). Health-related dietary practices, in *Cross-cultural counseling—A guide for nutrition and health counselors* (p. 5). Alexandra, VA: U.S. Department of Agriculture, U.S. Department of Health and Human Services. Nutrition and Technical Services Division. Reprinted with permission.

cold, treatments—that is, food and medications—are categorized as hot (*caliente*), cold (*frio*), and cool (*fresco*). Cold illnesses are treated with hot remedies; hot diseases are treated with cold or cool remedies. Table 11–5 lists the major illnesses, foods, and medicines and herbs associated with the hot-cold system as it is applied among Puerto Ricans in the United States.

A number of activities are carried out to maintain the proper hot-cold balance in the body.

Examples are as follows:

1. *Pasmo,* a form of paralysis, usually is caused by an upset in the hot-cold balance. For example, if a woman is ironing (hot) and then steps out into the rain (cold), she may get facial or other paralysis.

2. A person who is hot cannot sit under a mango tree (cold) because he or she can get a kidney infection or "back problems."

3. A baby should not be fed a formula (hot), as it may cause rashes; whole milk (cold) is acceptable.

4. A man who has been working (hot) must not go into the coffee fields (cold), or he could contract a respiratory illness.
5. A hot person must not drink cold water, as it could cause colic.

There is often a considerable time lag between disregarding these precautions and the occurrence of illness. A patient who had injured himself while lifting heavy cartons in a factory revealed that the "true" reason he was now experiencing prolonged back problems was because as a child he often sat under a mango tree when he was "hot" after running. This childhood habit had significantly damaged his back, so that, as an adult, he was unable to lift heavy objects without causing injury. Table 11–5 provides additional examples of this phenomenon.

The following are examples of selected behaviors a patient may manifest with an illness thought to be caused by an imbalance of hot and cold:

■ During pregnancy a woman may avoid hot-classified foods and medicines and take cool-classified medicines.
■ During the postpartum period or during menstruation a woman may avoid cool-classified foods and medicines.
■ Infant formulas containing evaporated milk, which are hot-classified, may be avoided as the baby is fed cold-classified whole milk.
■ Penicillin, a hot-classified prescription, may not be taken for diarrhea, constipation, or a rash, as these are hot-classified symptoms.
■ When a diuretic is prescribed that needs to be supplemented with cold-classified bananas or raisins, the bananas or raisins may not be eaten when the disease is a cold-classified condition.

These examples illustrate the use of foods or medicines to restore a sense of balance (Harwood, 1971).

Puerto Ricans also share with others of Hispanic origin a number of beliefs in spirits and spiritualism. They believe that mental illness is caused primarily by evil spirits and forces. People with such disorders are preferably treated by a "spiritualist medium" (Cohen, 1972). The psychiatric clinic is known as the place where locos, mentally ill people, go. This attitude is exemplified in the Puerto Rican approach to visions and the like. The social and cultural environment encourages the acceptance of having visions and hearing voices. In the dominant culture of the continental United States, when one has visions or hears voices, one is encouraged to see a psychiatrist. When a Puerto Rican regards this experience as a problem, he or she may seek help through *Santeria* (Mumford, 1973).

Santeria is the form of Latin American magic that had its birth in Nigeria, the country of origin of the Yoruba people, who were brought to the New World as slaves over 400 years ago. The *Santeria*, or *santero*, may use storytelling as a way of helping people cope with day-to-day difficulties (Flores-Pena, 1991). They brought with them their traditional religion, which was in time synthesized with Catholic images. The believers continue to worship in the traditional way, especially in Puerto Rico, Cuba, and Brazil. The Yorubas identified their gods—*Orishas*—with

Table 11-6 Selected *Orishas*, the Corresponding Saints, and Related Health Problems

Orisha	Saint	Health Problem
Obatala	Crucified Christ	Bronchitis
Chango	Saint Barbara	Violent death
Babalu-Aye	Saint Lazarus	Sickness
Bacoso	Saint Christopher	Infections
Ibeyi	Saints Cosmos and Damian	Infant illnesses
Ifa	Saint Anthony	Fertility
Yemaya	Our Lady of Regla	Maternity

Sources: Gonzalez-Wippler, M. (1987). *Santeria— African magic in Latin America.* Bronx, New York: Original Publications, pp. 1–30 and Riva, A. (1990). *Devotions to the saints.* Los Angeles: International Imports, pp. 91–93.

the Christian saints and invested in these saints the same supernatural powers of gods. The *orishas*/saints related to health situations are listed in Table 11–6.

Santeria is a structured system consisting of *espiritismo* (spiritualism), which is practiced by gypsies and mediums who claim to have *facultades* (sacred abilities). These special *facultades* provide them with the "license" to practice. The status or positions of the practitioners form a hierarchy: The head is the *babalow*, a male; second is the *presidente*, the head medium; and third are the *santeros*. Novices are the "believers." The *facultades* are given to the healer from protective Catholic saints, who have African names and are known as *protecciones*. *Santeria* can be practiced in storefronts, basements, homes, and even college dormitories. *Santeros* dress in white robes for ceremonies and wear special beaded bracelets as a sign of their identity.

Puerto Ricans are able to accept much of what Anglos may judge to be idiosyncratic behavior. In fact, behavioral disturbances are seen as symptoms of illness that are to be treated, not judged. Puerto Ricans make a sharp distinction between "nervous" behavior and being *loco*. To be *loco* is to be bad, dangerous, evil. It also means losing all one's social status. Puerto Ricans who seek standard American treatment for mental illness are castigated by the community. They understandably prefer to get help for the symptoms of mental illness from the *santero*, who accepts the symptoms and attributes the cause of the illness to spirits outside the body. Puerto Ricans have great faith in this system of care and maintain a high level of hope for recovery.

The *santero* is an important person, respecting the patient and not gossiping about either the patient or his or her problems. Anyone can pour his or her heart out with no worry of being labeled or judged. The *santero* is able to tell a person what the problem is, prescribe the proper treatment, and tell the person what to do, how to do it, and when to do it. A study in New York found that 73% of the Puerto Rican patients in an outpatient mental health clinic reported having visited a *santero*. Often, a sick person is taken to a psychiatrist by his or her family to be "calmed down" and prepared for treatment by a *santero*. Fam-

Table 11-7 Examples of Cultural Phenomena Affecting Health and Health Care Among Hispanic Americans

Nations of Origin	Hispanic countries: Spain, Cuba, Mexico, Central and South America, Puerto Rico
Environmental Control	Traditional health and illness beliefs may continue to be observed by "traditional" people Folk medicine tradition Traditional healers: *Curanderoa, espiritista, partera, senoria*
Biological Variations	Diabetes mellitus Parasites Coccidiodomycosis Lactose intolerance
Social Organization	Nuclear families Large, extended family networks *Compadrazzo* (godparents) Strong church affiliations within community Community social organizations
Communication	Primary language: Spanish or Portuguese
Space	Tactile relationships: touch, handshakes, embrace Value physical presence
Time Orientation	Present

Source: *Adapted from* Spector, R. Culture, ethnicity, and nursing. In P. Potter and A. Perry (Eds.), *Fundamentals of nursing* (3rd. ed.). St. Louis, MO: Mosby Yearbook, 1992. p. 101. Reprinted with permission.

ilies may become angry if the psychiatrist does not encourage belief in God and prayer during work with the patient. Because of cultural differences and beliefs, a psychiatrist may diagnose as illness what Puerto Ricans may define as health. Frequently, a spiritualist treats the "mental illness" of a patient as *facultades,* which makes the patient a "special person." Thus, esteem is granted to the patient as a form of treatment. I visited a *santero* in Los Angeles with the hope of his granting me an interview. Instead, he argued that if I wanted to know about his practice I should "sit," so I did. He proceeded to examine my head and palms, throw and read cowerie shells, tell me a story, and asked me to interpret it. Once this was accomplished, he recommended certain interventions. His manner was extremely calming and, when he interpreted the story with me, I discovered his uncanny ability to read habits and behavior (Flores-Pena, 1991). A number of cultural phenomena affect the health and health care of Hispanic Americans (Table 11–7) (Mumford, 1973).

Entry into Mainland Health Systems

Puerto Ricans living in New York City and other parts of the northern United States experience a high rate of illness and hospitalization during their first year on the mainland, as do other people of Hispanic origin. It is worthwhile considering the vast differences between living in New York and living in Puerto Rico. In Puerto Rico, there is no winter weather. The winters in the North can be bitterly cold, and adjustment to climate change in itself is extremely difficult. Migrant people may be forced to live in crowded living quarters with poor sanitation.

Puerto Ricans seeking health care may go to a physician, a folk practitioner, or both. The general progression of seeking care is as follows:

1. The person seeks advice from a daughter, mother, grandmother, or neighbor woman. These sources are consulted because the women of this culture are the primary healers and dispensers of medicine on the family level.

2. If the advice is not sufficient, the person may seek help from a *senoria* (a woman who is especially knowledgeable about the causes and treatment of illness).

3. If the *senoria* is unable to help, the person goes to a more sophisticated folk practitioner, an *espiritista* or a *curandera*. If the problem is "psychiatric," a *santero* may be consulted. These names describe similar people—those who obtain their knowledge from spirits and treat illness according to the instructions of the spirits. Herbs, lotions, creams, and massage often are used.

4. If the person is still not satisfied, he or she may go to a physician.

5. If the results are not satisfactory, the person may return to a folk practitioner. He or she may seek medical help sooner than step 4 or may go back and forth between the two systems.

Not all people from Puerto Rico use the folk system. Health care providers should remember that people who appear to have delayed seeking health care have most likely counted on curing their illness through the culturally known and well-understood folk process. Often when people disappear (or "elope") from the established health system, they may have elected to return to the folk system. Those who elope from the larger, institutionalized medical system may visit a *botanica* (Figures 11–10 and 11–11). In these small *botanicas,* one can purchase herbs, potents, Florida water, ointments, and incense prescribed by spiritualists. Some of these *botanicas* are so busy that each customer is given a number and is assisted only after the number is called (Mumford, 1973). There are countless *botanicas* located in one small area of New York City. A Spanish-speaking colleague and I visited a *botanica* in Boston that was similar to a pharmacy. The owner explained the various remedies that were for sale. We were allowed to purchase only a few items because we did not have a spiritualist's prescription for herbs. The store also sold amulets, candles, religious statues, cards, medals, and relics.

A limited number of *santeros* place advertisements in local Spanish daily newspapers. Some of the more industrious ones distribute flyers in the New York City subways. Others maintain a low profile, and patients visit them because of their well-established reputations.

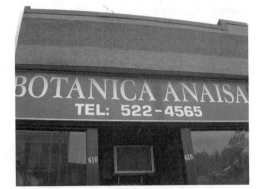

Figure 11–10 A *botanica* in Boston, Massachusetts. There are several *botanicas* in the Boston's metropolitan area. The *botanicas* are visited primarily by people from Puerto Rico, the Dominican Republic, Mexico, and other Hispanics residing in the area. They sell numerous herbs and herbal preparations, amulets of all sorts, *milagros,* and statues of saints. A *santera* works in this *botanica,* and she is available to people to give advice and sell herbal remedies.

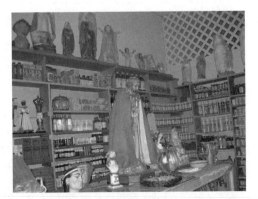

Figure 11–11 Interior of a *botanica* in Boston, Massachusetts.

Table 11-8 **Comparison of Selected Health Status Indicators—All Races and Hispanic or Latino: 1999/2004**

Health Indicator	All Races 1999/2004	Hispanic or Latino 1999/2004
Crude birth rate per 1,000 population by race of mother	14.5/14.0	24.4/22.9
Percentage of live births of women receiving prenatal care first trimester	83.2/83.9	74.4/77.5
Percentage of live births of women receiving third-trimester or no prenatal care	3.8/3.6	6.3/5.4
Percentage of live births to teenage childbearing women—under 18	4.4/3.4	6.7/5.4
Percentage of low-birth-weight per live births <2,500 grams, 1997–1999/2003	7.57/8.3	6.38/6.2
Infant mortality per 1,000 live births, 1996–1998/2003	7.2/6.8	5.9/5.6
Cancer—all sites per 100,000 population, 1997/2003	384.5/447.1	249/323.5
Lung cancer incidence per 100,000 population, 1997/2003	Men: 65.4/73.0 Women: 40.7/48.0	Men: 32.8/41.3 Women: 17.5/20.8
Breast cancer incidence per 100,000, 1997/2003	113.1/121.1	65.5/79.6
Prostate cancer incidence per 100,000, 1997/2003	136.0/160.4	91.9/127.3
Male death rates from suicide, all ages, age adjusted per 100,000 resident population, 1999/2003	18.1/10.8	10.7/9.7
Male death rates from homicide, all ages, age adjusted per 100,000 resident population, 1999/2003	9.3/9.4	13.8/12.1

Sources: National Center for Health Statistics. (2006). *Health, United States, 2006 with chartbook on trends in the health of Americans* (pp. 135, 140, 144, 149, 160, 227, 230, 244). Hyattsville, MD: Author.

Current Health Problems

The Hispanic health profile is marked by diversity, and people of the Hispanic community experience perhaps the most varied set of health issues encountered by any of the emerging majority populations. The diversity in health problems is intertwined with the effects of socioeconomic status, as well as with geographic and cultural differences. The most important health issues for Hispanics are related to these demographic facts: The population is young and has a high birth rate.

Table 11–8 compares selected health status indicators between all races and Hispanics. The leading causes of death among Hispanic Americans illustrate differences between their health experiences and those of the total population, as can be seen in Table 11–9.

Table 11–9   Comparison of the 10 Leading Causes of Death for Hispanic or Latino Americans and for All Persons: 2004

Hispanic or Latino Americans	All Persons
1. Diseases of heart	Diseases of heart
2. Malignant neoplasms	Malignant neoplasms
3. Unintentional injuries	Cerebrovascular diseases
4. Cerebrovascular diseases	Chronic lower respiratory diseases
5. Diabetes mellitus	Unintentional injuries
6. Chronic liver disease and cirrhosis	Diabetes mellitus
7. Homicide	Alzheimer's disease
8. Chronic lower respiratory diseases	Influenza and pneumonia
9. Influenza and pneumonia	Nephritis, nephrotic syndrome, and
10. Certain conditions originating in the	nephrosis
perinatal period	Septicemia

Source: National Center for Health Statistics. (2007). *Health, United States, 2007, with chartbook on trends in the health of Americans* (p. 188). Hyattsville, MD: Author.

Hispanics experience a number of barriers when seeking health care. The most obvious one is language. In spite of the fact that Spanish-speaking people constitute one of the largest minority groups in this country, very few health care deliverers speak Spanish. This is especially true in communities in which the number of Spanish-speaking people is relatively small. Hispanics who live in these areas experience tremendous frustration because of the language barrier. Even in large cities, there are far too many occasions when a sick person has to rely on a young child to act not only as a translator but also as an interpreter. One way of sensitizing young nursing students to the pain of this situation is to ask them to present a health problem to a person who does not speak or understand a word of English. Needless to say, this is extremely difficult; it is also embarrassing. People who try this rapidly comprehend and appreciate the feelings of patients who are unable to speak or understand English. (After this experience, two of my students decided to take a foreign-language elective.) Language will continue to be a problem until (1) there are more physicians, nurses, and social workers from the Spanish-speaking communities and (2) more of the present deliverers of health care learn to speak Spanish.

A second crucial barrier that Hispanic people encounter is poverty. The diseases of the poor—for example, tuberculosis, malnutrition, and lead poisoning—all have high incidences among Spanish-speaking populations.

A final barrier to adequate health care is the time orientation of Hispanic Americans. To Hispanics, time is a relative phenomenon. Little attention is given to the exact time of day. The frame of reference is wider, and the issue is whether it is day or night. The American health care system, on the other hand, places great emphasis on promptness. Health care providers demand that clients arrive at the exact time of the appointment—despite the fact that clients are often kept waiting. Health system workers stress the client's promptness rather than their own. In fact, they tend to deny responsibility for the waiting periods by blaming them on the "system." Many facilities commonly schedule all appointments for 9:00 A.M. when it is clearly known and understood by the staff members that the doctor will not even arrive until 11:00 A.M. or later. The Hispanic person frequently responds to this practice by arriving late for appointments or failing to go at all. They prefer to attend walk-in clinics, where the waits are shorter. They also much prefer going to traditional healers.

Hispanic American Health Care Manpower

The number of Americans of Hispanic origin who are enrolled in selected health professions schools is low, as illustrated in Tables 11–10 and 11–11. The percentage of Hispanics in the total United States population is now 14%, yet, in each of these health care–related educational programs, the percentage of Hispanic students is less than 8%. Efforts must be made to recruit and maintain countless more Hispanics in the health professions.

The National Sample Survey of Registered Nurses 2004, prepared by the Bureau of Health Professions of the Health Resources Admimstration, estimates that the registered nurse population in the United States in 2004 numbered 2,909,357 nurses. Of this number of nurses, 81.8% were White non-Hispanic and there were 1.7% Hispanic/Latino (of any race) nurses. Given that, in 2005 Hispanic/Latino people of any race comprised 15% of the resident population (see Table 2–2 in Chapter 1) this is a clear indication that there is not a demographic parity in the percentage of Hispanic/Latino people in nursing.

This demographic picture and the percentages in Tables 11–10 and 11–11 demonstrate a situation that is an ongoing concern. The findings of Somnath and Shipman (2006), who reviewed a total of 55 studies found that minority patients tend to receive better interpersonal care from practitioners of their own race or ethnicity, particularly in primary care and mental health settings. In addition, non-English speaking patients experience better interpersonal care,

Table 11-10 Hispanic Enrollment in Selected Health Professions Schools: 2003–2005

	Total Program Enrollment	Hispanic Enrollment
Dentistry	18,315	1,059
Allopathic medicine	66,821	4,947
Osteopathic medicine	12,525	472
Nursing—Registered[a]		
Optometry	5,377	273
Pharmacy	43,908	1,691
Podiatry	1,584	122

Source: National Center for Health Statistics. (2007). *Health, United States, 2007, with chartbook on trends in the health of Americans* (pp. 361–362). Hyattsville, MD: Author.

[a]The National League for Nursing changed the way it collects these data in 1991 and subsequently discontinued the practice; enrollment data are not available after 1991.

Table 11–11 Percentage of Hispanics Enrolled in Selected Health Professions Schools Compared with Non-Hispanic Whites: 2003–2005

	Non-Hispanic Whites (%)	Hispanics (%)
Dentistry	66.1	5.8
Allopathic medicine	63.3	6.7
Osteopathic medicine	73.5	3.8
Nursing—Registered	a	a
Optometry	63.2	5.1
Pharmacy	59.7	3.9
Podiatry	60.4	11.1

aThe National League for Nursing changed the way it collects these data in 1991 and subsequently discontinued the practice; enrollment data are not available after 1991.

Source: National Center for Health Statistics. (2007). Health, United States, 2007, with chartbook on trends in the health of Americans (pp. 361–362). Hyattsville, MD: Author.

greater medical comprehension, and greater likelihood of keeping follow-up appointments when they see a language-concordant practitioner.

Somnath and Shipman concluded their study by stating that "the findings indicated greater health professions diversity will likely lead to improved public health by increasing access to care for underserved populations, and by increasing opportunities for minority patients to see practitioners with whom they share a common race, ethnicity or language." They also stated that "race, ethnicity, and language concordance, which is associated with better patient-practitioner relationships and communication, may increase patients' likelihood of receiving and accepting appropriate medical care" (Somnath & Shipman, 2006, p. 17). The study in the Research in Culture box corroborates these findings.

RESEARCH ON CULTURE

Much research has been conducted among members of the Hispanic American population. The following article describes one such study:

Whittemore, R. (2007). Culturally competent interventions for Hispanic adults with type 2 diabetes: A systemic review. Journal of Transcultural Nursing, 18 (2), 157–166.

Significant research has been conducted in the past several decades with the goal of reducing health disparities in Hispanic adults with type 2 diabetes. The purpose of this study was to describe and synthesize the research on culturally competent interventions aimed at improving outcomes in the target population. The author used an integrative review method to describe the intervention components of culturally competent interventions; the efficacy of interventions in terms of clinical outcomes, behavioral outcomes, and knowledge; cultural strategies of interventions; and factors associated with attendance and attrition of interventions. She analyzed 11 studies

(continued)

conducted between 1994 and 2005 on this topic and found that most culturally competent interventions were efficacious. The culturally competent interventions included community-based education in the language—Spanish—understood by the patients. Other strategies included family involvement, translation as needed, bilingual professional staff, emphasis on types of food, and support groups.

Other interventions that were examined included the following:

- *Clinical outcomes.* Improvements in glycemic control with education were documented.
- *Behavioral outcomes.* Evaluation of dietary and exercise behaviors and significant improvements were found.
- *Diabetes-related knowledge.* A significant increase in diabetes-related knowledge was reported for participants who received culturally competent interventions.

The author notes that the development of culturally competent interventions requires attention to countless cultural factors, is complex, and requires a multidisciplinary and multifaceted approach.

Explore 🌐 MediaLink

Go to the Companion Website at www.prenhall.com/spector for chapter-related review questions, case studies, and activities. Contents of the CulturalCare Guide and CulturalCare Museum can also be found on the Companion Website. Click on Chapter 11 to select the activities for this chapter.

■ Internet Sources

Grieco, E., and Cassidy, R. C. (2001). Overview of Race and Hispanic Origin. Census Brief. Washington, DC: Census Bureau. Retrieved from http://www.census.gov/prod/2001pubs/c2kbr01-1.pdf July 25, 2007

Ramirez, R., and de la Cruz, G. P. (2002). *The Hispanic population in the United States:* March 2002, Current Population Reports, P20–54, U.S. Census Bureau, Washington, D.C. Retrieved July 25, 2007 from http://www.census.gov/prod/2003pubs/p20–545.pdf.

Somnath, S., and Shipman, S. (2006). The rationale for diversity in the health professions: A review of the evidence (Washington, DC: U.S. Department of Health and Human Services, Health Resources and Services Administration Bureau of Health Professions. http://www.hrsa.gov/ January 5, 2008

U.S. Census Bureau, Census 2000 Special Tabulations. Profile of Selected Demographic and Social Characteristics: 2000 Latin America, Guatemala, Mexico. Retrieved July 25, 2007 from http://www.census.gov/population/cen2000/stp-159/STP-159-LatinAmerica.pdf, http://www.census.gov/population/cen2000/stp-159/STP-159-Guatemala.pdf, and http://www.census.gov/population/cen2000/stp-159/STP-159-Mexico.pdf

United States Department of Health and Human Services. (2004). The Registered Nurse Population Findings from the March, 2004 National Sample of Registered Nurses. Washington DC: Author. Retrieved from ftp://ftp.hrsa.gov/bhpr/workforce/0306rnss.pdf, January 5, 2008

References

Ballou, B. (2007, July 22). *Boston Sunday Globe*, p. B-5.

Carmack, R. M., Gasco, J., & Gossen, G. H. (1996). *The legacy of Mesoamerica.* Upper Saddle River, NJ: Prentice Hall.

Cohen, R. E. (1972, June). Principles of preventive mental health programs for ethnic minority populations: The acculturation of Puerto Ricans to the United States. *American Journal of Psychiatry, 128*(12), 79.

Currier, R. L. (1966, March). The hot-cold syndrome and symbolic balance in Mexican and Spanish-American folk medicine. *Ethnology, 5,* 251–263.

Dorsey, P. R., & Jackson, H. Q. (1976). Cultural health traditions: The Latino/Mexican perspective. In M. F. Branch & P. P. Paxton (Eds.), *Providing safe nursing care for ethnic people of color.* New York: Appleton-Century-Crofts.

Egan, M. (1991). *Milagros.* Santa Fe: Museum of New Mexico Press.

Flores-Pena, Y. & Evanchuk, R. J. (1994). *Santeria garments and alters.* Jackson: University of Mississippi Press.

Flores-Pena, Y. (1991). Personal interview. Los Angeles, CA.

Gonzalez-Wippler, M. (1987). *Santeria—African magic in Latin America.* New York: Original.

Greenhaw, W. (2000). *My heart is in the earth.* Montgomery, AL: River City.

Harwood, A. (1971). The hot-cold theory of disease: Implications for treatment of Puerto Rican patients. *Journal of the American Medical Association, 216,* 1154–1155.

Kearney, M., & Medrano, M. (2001). *Medieval culture and the Mexican American borderlands.* College Station: Texas A & M University Press.

Lucero, G. (1975, March). *Health and illness in the Mexican community.* Lecture given at Boston College School of Nursing.

Maduro, R. J. (1976, January). *Curanderismo: Latin American folk healing.* Conference, San Francisco.

Mumford, E. (1973, November–December). Puerto Rican perspectives on mental illness. *Mount Sinai Journal of Medicine, 40*(6), 771–773.

Nall, F. C., II, & Spielberg, J. (1967). Social and cultural factors in the responses of Mexican-Americans to medical treatment. *Journal of Health and Social Behavior, 8,* 302.

National Center for Health Statistics. (2001). *Health, United States, 2001, with urban and rural health chartbook.* Hyattville, MD: Author.

National Center for Health Statistics. (2006). *Health, United States, 2006 with chartbook on trends in the health of Americans.* Hyattville, MD: Author.

National Center for Health Statistics. (2007). *Health, United States, 2007 with chartbook on trends in the health of Americans.* Hyattville, MD: Author.

Ochoa, C. (December 15, 2007). Personal Telephone Interview. Mission, Texas.

Riva, A. (1990). *Devotions to the saints.* Los Angeles: International Imports.

Rubel, A. J. (1964, July). The epidemiology of a folk illness: Susto in Hispanic America. *Ethnology, 3*(3), 270–271.

Saunders, L. (1958). Healing ways in the Spanish southwest. In E. G., Jaco (Ed.), *Patients, physicians, and illness*. Glencoe, IL: Free Press.

Schilling, B., & Brannon, E. (1986). Health-related dietary practices. In *Cross-cultural counseling: A guide for nutrition and health counselors*. Alexandria, VA: U.S: Department of Health and Human Services.

Spector, R. (1996). *Cultural diversity in health and illness* (4th ed.). Stamford, CT: Appleton & Lange.

Spencer, R. T., Nichols, L. W., Lipkin, G. B., et al. (1993). *Clinical pharmacology and nursing management* (4th ed.). Philadelphia: Lippincott.

Therrien, M., & Ramirez, R. R. (2001). *Hispanic population in the United States, 2000*. Washington, DC: U.S. Census Bureau.

Welch, S., Comer, J., & Steinman, M. (1973, September). Some social and attitudinal correlates of health care among Mexican Americans. *Journal of Health and Social Behavior, 14*, 205.

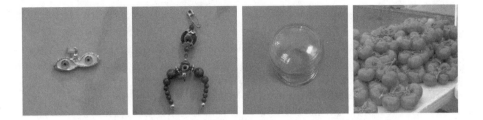

Chapter 12

HEALTH and ILLNESS in the White Populations

Grand Contested Election for the Presidency of the United States.
BLOODY BATTLE IN AFGHANISTAN

—*H. Melville*, Moby Dick *(1851)*

■ Objectives

1. Discuss the background of the White populations.
2. Discuss the demographic profile of the White populations.
3. Describe the traditional definitions of *HEALTH* and *ILLNESS* of the White populations.
4. Describe the traditional methods of HEALTH maintenance and protection of selected communities of the White populations.
5. Describe the traditional methods of HEALING of the White populations.
6. Describe health problems of the White populations.

The opening images for this chapter are symbolic of traditional health-related objects that people of White European heritage may use to protect, maintain, and/or restore their HEALTH. The eyes represent the eyes of Saint Lucy, the patron saint of eye diseases and are worn to prevent blindness. The bead and horseshoe, from Armenia, may be pinned on a baby or child for protection from the evil eye. *Bankes*, from Russia and other Eastern European countries, are small, bulb-shaped, thick-glass jars that may be used to create negative pressure to break the congestion that occurs with bronchitis or pneumonia. (*Directions:* Place cotton saturated with alcohol in the jar and light it. Place grease on the skin in the area where you will place the jar. Turn the jar upside down on the skin. The flame goes out. Leave it for 5 minutes and then gently remove the jar. Go to bed and keep warm for several hours.) The *bankes* were commonly used a generation ago and is still used in many places today. The succulent tomatoes are reminders of the nutritional adage to eat "fresh foods" common among Italian gardeners—here is a selection of the early autumn harvest.

■ Background

Members of White European American communities have been immigrating to this country since the very first settlers came to the shores of New England. The White population has diverse and multiple origins. The recent literature in the area of ethnicity and health/HEALTH has focused on people of color, and little has been written about the HEALTH traditions of the White ethnic communities. In this chapter, an overview of the differences in traditional HEALTH beliefs and practices, by ethnicity, is presented. Given that we are talking about 68% of the American population, the enormity of the task of attempting to describe each difference is readily apparent. Instead, this chapter presents an overview of the relevant demographics of the White population, highlights some of the basic beliefs of selected groups (those groups with which I have had the greatest exposure), and presents a comparison of the health status of Whites to the whole population as well as the census cohorts. The overview includes not only library research but also firsthand interviews and observations of people in their daily experiences with the health care delivery system, both as inpatients and as community residents receiving home care.

The major groups migrating to this country between 1820 and 1990 included people from Germany, Italy, the United Kingdom, Ireland, Austria-Hungary, Canada, and Russia; this was a majority of the total immigrant population. However, in 1970, the numbers of immigrants from Europe began to decrease and in 2003 the percentage of foreign-born people from Europe was 13.7% (Larsen, 2004). Chapter 2 explores immigration in greater detail. The 1980 census was the first to include a question about ancestry. The U.S. Census Bureau uses the term **ancestry** to refer to a person's ethnic origin or descent, roots, heritage, or the place of birth of the person or the person's parents or ancestors before their arrival in the United States. Some ethnic identities, such as "German" can be traced to geographic areas outside the United States, while other ethnicities, such as "Pennsylvania Dutch" or "Cajun," evolved in the United States.

The responses to the question of ancestry were a reflection of the ethnic group(s) with which persons identified, and they were able to indicate their ethnic group regardless of how many generations they were removed from it. The following list shows the most common European ancestries in the U.S. population in 2000 (Brittingham, A., and de la Cruz, G. P., 2004 p. 3).

Ancestry	Numbers Identifying Themselves as This Ancestry (Millions)	Percent
German	42.8	15.2
Irish	30.5	10.8
English	24.5	8.7
Italian	15.6	5.6
Polish	9.0	3.2
French (except Basque)	8.3	3.0
Scottish	4.9	1.7

Table 12–1 illustrates selected variables from the demographic profiles of people born in Europe who entered the United States from 1980 to 2000. There have been 4,915,555 people admitted from Europe; 706,705 from Germany, 473,340 from Italy, and 466,740 Poland.

The discussion in Chapter 2 referred to age in general; in this chapter, it is important to examine the age of the White populations more specifically. The median age of Whites alone is 38 years, the oldest of each population group. In addition, it is important to note that the percentage of people over 65 in the total population is 12.4, whereas for Whites alone the number is 14.4%, and the percentage of the total population under 18 is 25.7% and for Whites alone it is 23.5% (Meyer, 2001, p. 5).

An additional facet to note is that in many cities the White alone population is now a minority. These cities include New York, Los Angeles, Chicago, Houston, Detroit and Philadelphia. Table 12–2 lists the top 10 cities in the United States and the percentage of White alone.

The following discussion focuses on several white ethnic groups and attempts to describe some of the history of their migration to America, the areas where they now live, the common beliefs regarding health and illness, some kernels of information regarding family and social life, and problems that members from a given group may have in interacting with health care providers. The intention is not to create a vehicle for stereotyping but to whet the reader's appetite to search out more information about the people in their care, given the

Table 12-1 Profile of Selected Demographic and Social Characteristics of People Entering the United States from Europe, Germany, Italy, and Poland: 2000

Variable	Europe	Germany	Italy	Poland
Naturalized U.S. citizen	55.9%	65.3%	74.8%	54.4%
Language other than English spoken at home	67.6%	57.4%	77.0%	85.5%
Speak English less than very well	29.4%	11.1%	39.6%	50.3%
Median age	50 years	54.6 years	59.8 years	47.0 years
Marital status—married	63.4%	61.2%	68.0%	62.1%
School enrollment—college or graduate school	46.8%	50.7%	61.8%	46.7%
Educational attainment— bachelor's degree or higher— population 25 years and older	29.2%	26.8%	13.8%	21.9%
Veteran status—civilian veterans	6.2%	10.7%	8.4%	4.4%
Employment status—over 16 years of age employed	54.2%	51.7%	44.4%	56.4%
Median household income	$42,763	$41,181	$42,090	$41,452
Household income—$150,000 or more	3.4%	3.4%	5.4%	4.4%
Median family income	$54,823	$56,806	$53,885	$51,373
Per capita earnings	$29,747	$31,179	$29,446	$25,806
Poverty status—families below the poverty level	7.0%	5.3%	5.1%	5.0%

Source: U.S. Census Bureau, Census 2000 Special Tabulations. Profile of Selected Demographic and Social Characteristics: 2000 United States, Germany, Italy, and Poland. Retrieved from http://factfinder.census.gov., http://www.census.gov/population/cen2000/stp-159/STP-159-Europe.pdf, http://www.census.gov/population/cen2000/stp-159/STP-159-Germany.pdf, http://www.census.gov/population/cen2000/stp-159/STP-159-Italy.pdf, http://www.census.gov/population/cen2000/stp-159/STP-159-Poland.pdf, retrieved February 23, 2008.

Table 12-2 The Largest Cities in Total Population and Percentage of White Alone Population: 2000

Place	Rank	Percentage of White Alone Population
New York	1	44.7%
Los Angeles	2	46.9%
Chicago	3	42.0%
Houston	4	49.3%
Philadelphia	5	45.0%
Phoenix	6	71.1%
San Diego	7	60.2%
Dallas	8	50.8%
San Antonio	9	67.7%
Detroit	10	12.3%

Source: Grieco, E. M. (2001). The White Population: 2000. Washington, DC: U.S. Census Bureau, pp. 1–2. Retrieved from https://ask.census.gov/cgibin/askcensus.ctg, retrieved February 23, 2003.

Table 12-3   Examples of Cultural Phenomena Affecting Health Care Among European (White) Americans

Nations of Origin	Germany, England, Italy, Ireland, former Soviet Union, and all other European countries
Environmental Control	Primary reliance on "modern, Western" health care delivery system
	Remaining traditional HEALTH and ILLNESS beliefs and practices may be observed
	Some remaining traditional folk medicine
	Homeopathic medicine resurgent
Biological Variations	Breast cancer
	Heart disease
	Diabetes mellitus
	Thalassemia
Social Organization	Nuclear families
	Extended families
	Judeo-Christian religions
	Community and social organizations
Communication	National languages
	Many learned English rapidly as immigrants
	Verbal, rather than nonverbal
Space	Noncontact people—aloof, distant
	Southern countries—closer contact and touch
Time Orientation	Future over present

Adapted from Spector, R. (1992). Culture, ethnicity, and nursing. In P. Potter and A. Perry (Eds.), *Fundamentals of nursing* (3rd ed.) (p. 101). St. Louis, MO: Mosby-Year Book. Reprinted with permission.

vast differences among Whites. There are countless cultural phenomena affecting health care; Table 12–3 suggests a few.

■ German Americans

The following material, relating to both the German American and Polish American communities, was obtained from research conducted in southeastern Texas in May 1982 and updated over time. It is by no means indicative of the HEALTH and ILLNESS beliefs of the entire German American and Polish American communities. It is included here to demonstrate the type of data that can be gleaned using an "emic" (a description of behavior dependent on the person's categorization of the action) approach to collecting data. It cannot be generalized, but it allows the reader to grasp the diversity of beliefs that surround us (Lefcowitz, 1990, p. 6).

Since 1830 more than 7 million Germans have immigrated to the United States. There are presently 42.8 million Americans who claim German ancestry. Over 57.4% of the people 5 years and older speak German at home and 11.1% speak English less than very well. Thirty-nine percent of people of German ancestry reside in the Northeast and 39% reside in the South (U.S.

Bureau of the Census, 2001, p. 46). The Germans represent a cross section of German society and have come from all social strata and walks of life. Some people have come to escape poverty, others have come for religious or political reasons, and still others have come to take advantage of the opportunity to open up the new lands. Many were recruited to come here, as were the Germans who settled in the German enclaves in Texas. The immigrants represented all religions, including primarily Lutherans, Catholics, and Jews. They represented the rich and the poor, the educated and the ignorant, and were of all ages. Present-day descendants are farmers, educators, and artists. The Germans brought to the United States the cultural diversity and folkways they observed in Germany. The festivals of Corpus Christi, Kinderfeste (children's feast), and Sangerfeste (singing festival) all originated in Germany (Conzen, 1980, pp. 405–425).

The Germans began to migrate to the United States in the 17th century and have contributed 15.2% of the total immigration population. They are the least visible ethnic group in the United States, and people often are surprised to discover that there is such a large Germanic influence in this country. In some places, the German communities maintain strong identification with their German heritage. For example, the city of Fredericksberg, Texas, maintains an ambience of German culture and identity. Some people born there who are fourth-generation and more continue to learn German as their first spoken language (Spector, 1983).

The German ethnic community is the second largest in the state of Texas and is exceeded only by the Mexican community. Germans have been immigrating to Texas since 1840 and continue to arrive. They are predominantly Catholic, Lutheran, and Methodist. Many of these people have maintained their German identity. The major German communities in Texas are Victoria, Cuero, Gonzales, New Braunfels, and Fredericksberg.

During the European freedom revolutions of 1830 and 1848, Texas was quite popular, especially in Germany, and was seen as a "wild and fabulous land." For tradition-bound German families, however, the abandonment of the homeland was difficult. They were enticed, however, by the hopes of economic and social improvement and political idealism. An additional reason for the mass migration was the overpopulation of Germany and the immigrants' desire to escape an imminent European catastrophe. By the 1840s, several thousand northern Germans had come to Texas, and another large migration occurred in 1890. This second cluster of people came because there was a severe crop failure in Russian-occupied Germany, and the Russian language had become a required subject in German schools. Other German migrations occurred from 1903 to 1905.

The Germans found pleasure in the small things of everyday life. They were tied together by the German language because it bound them to the past, entertaining them with games, riddles, folk songs and literature, and folk wisdom. The greatest amusement was singing and dancing. Religion for the Lutherans, Catholics, and Methodists was a part of everyday life. The year was measured by the church calendar; observance of church ritual paced the milestones of the life cycle. The Germans believed that each individual was a "part of the fabric of humanity," that "history was a continued process," and "everything had a purpose as mankind strove to something better" (Lich, 1982, pp. 33–72).

The Germans had a penchant for forming societies and clubs, the longest-lasting of which are the singing societies. The first was organized in 1850 and exists still today. The Germans brought with them their customs and traditions; their cures, curses, and recipes; and their tools and ways of building (Lich, 1982).

HEALTH *and* ILLNESS

Among the Germans, health is described as more than not being ill but as a state of well-being—physically and emotionally—the ability to do your duty, positive energy to do things, and the ability to do, think, and act the way you would like, to go and congregate, to enjoy life. Illness may be described as the absence of well-being: pain, malfunction of body organs, not being able to do what you want, a blessing from God to suffer, and a disorder of body, imbalance.

Causes of ILLNESS

Most German Americans believe in the germ theory of infection and in stress-related theories. Other causes of illness are identified, however, such as drafts, environmental changes, and belief in the evil eye and punishment from God.

The methods of maintaining health include the requirement of dressing properly for the season, proper nutrition, and the wearing of shawls to protect oneself from drafts—also, the taking of cod-liver oil, exercise, and hard work. Methods for preventing illness include wearing an asafetida bag around the neck in the winter to prevent colds, scapulars, religious practices, sleeping with the windows open, and cleanliness.

The use of home remedies to treat illness continues to be practiced. Table 12–4 gives examples of commonly used home remedies.

Current Health Problems

There do not appear to be any unusual health problems particular to German Americans.

■ Italian Americans

The Italian American community is made up of immigrants who came here from mainland Italy and from Sicily, Sardinia, and other Mediterranean islands that are part of Italy. The number of Americans claiming Italian ancestry is over 14.6 million. Over 77% of the people 5 years and older speak Italian at home and 39.6% speak English less than very well. Fifty-one percent of people of Italian ancestry reside in the Northeast (U.S. Bureau of the Census, 2001, p. 46).

Table 12-4 ILLNESS **Symptoms and Remedies Among German Americans**

Gastrointestinal Problems	
Symptom	**Remedy**
Constipation	Castor oil
	Black draught
Diarrhea or vomiting	Do not eat for 24 hours
	Chicken soup
Stomachache	Peppermint tea
	Tea and toast
	Berries, elderberries

Respiratory Problems	
Symptom	**Remedy**
Cold	Wet compress around throat—cover with wool
	Lemon juice and whiskey
	Chopped onions in a sack applied to the soles of the feet
	Olbas oil (made in Germany)
Cough	Goose fat—rub on chest
	Honey and milk
	Tausend Gülden Krout (thousand golden cabbage)—rum
Earache	Warm oil in ear
	Warm towels
	Bitter geranium leaves
Sore throat	Camphor on a wet rag—wrap around the throat
	Gargle with salt water
	Onion compress
	Chicken soup
	Liniments

Physical Injuries	
Symptom	**Remedy**
Bumps	Hard knife (cold metal), place on bump
Cuts	Iodine—clean well
Puncture wounds (nail)	Soak in kerosene
Wounds	Clean well with water—apply iodine

Miscellaneous Problems	
Symptom	**Remedy**
Aches and pains	Kytle's liniment
	Olbas oil
	Volcanic oil
	Salves and liniments

Table 12–4 *Continued*

Arthritis	Warm-water soaks
	Honey, vinegar, and water soaks
Boils	"Capital water"—sulfur water—drink this (this is available at the Texas capital)
Clean body after winter	Kur (similar to hot springs) drink
Fever	Cold compress on head—fluids
Headache	Iced cloth on head
Menstrual cramps	Cardui
Rheumatism	Aloe vera—rub on sore area
	Cod-liver oil—massage
	Apply fig juice
Ringworm	Camomile tea compress
Stye	One half of hard-boiled egg—apply warm white on eye
Toothache	Cloves
	Salbec tea
	Olbas oil
Warts	Apply fig juice and fig leaf milk

Source: Spector, R. E. (1983). A description of the impact of Medicare on health-illness beliefs and practices of White ethnic senior citizens in Central Texas. Ph.D. diss. University of Texas at Austin School of Nursing. Ann Arbor, MI: University Microfilms International. Reprinted with permission.

Italian Americans indeed have a proud heritage in the United States, for America was "founded" by an Italian—Christopher Columbus; named for an Italian—Amerigo Vespucci; and explored by several Italian explorers, including Verrazano, Cabot, and Tonti (Bernardo, 1981, p. 26).

History of Migration

Between 1820 and 1990, over 5 million people from Italy immigrated to the United States (Lefcowitz, 1990, p. 6). The peak years were from 1901 to 1920, and only a small number of people continue to come today. Italians came to this country to escape poverty and to search for a better life in a country where they expected to reap rewards for their hard labor. The early years were not easy, but people chose to remain in this country and not return to Italy. Italians tended to live in neighborhood enclaves, and these neighborhoods, such as the North End in Boston and Little Italy in New York, still exist as Italian neighborhoods. Although the younger generation may have moved out, they still return home to maintain family, community, and ethnic ties (Nelli, 1980, pp. 545–560).

The family has served as the main tie keeping Italian Americans together because it provides its members with the strength to cope with the surrounding world and produces a sense of continuity in all situations. The family is the primary focus of the Italian's concern, and Italians take pride in the family and the home. Italians are resilient, yet fatalistic, and they take advantage of the present. Many upwardly mobile third- and fourth-generation Italian Americans often experience conflict between familial solidarity and society's emphasis on individualization and autonomy (Giordano & McGoldrick, 1996, p. 571). As mentioned, the home is a source of great pride, and it is a symbol of the family, not a status symbol per se. The church also is an important focus for the life of the Italian. Many of the festivals and observances continue to exist today, and in the summer, the North End of Boston is alive each weekend with the celebration of a different saint (Figure 12–1).

The father traditionally has been the head of the Italian household, and the mother is said to be the heart of the household.

Italian Americans have tended to attain low levels of education in the United States, but their incomes are comparable to or higher than those of other groups.

The Italian population falls into four generational groups: (1) the elderly, living in Italian enclaves; (2) a second generation, living both within the neighborhoods and in the suburbs; (3) a younger, well-educated group, living mainly in the suburbs; and (4) new immigrants (Ragucci, 1981, p. 216). More than 80% of Italian Americans marry people from a different ethnic group (Giordano & McGoldrick, 1996).

70th GRAND RELIGIOUS FEAST
IN HONOR OF THE PROTECTRESS
SAINT AGRIPPINA DI MINEO

THE THREE-DAY FEAST IS IN HONOR AND PRAISE OF SAINT AGRIPPINA, THE PROTECTRESS AND PATRON SAINT OF THE IMMIGRANTS FROM THE SMALL TOWN OF MINEO IN SICILY AND THEIR DESCENDANTS.

EACH YEAR FOR THE PAST 69 YEARS THIS GROUP OF DEVOTED 'PAESANI', NOW SCATTERED THROUGHOUT THE STATE, COME TOGETHER IN THE NORTH END SECTION TO PROCLAIM ANEW THEIR FAITH, AS WAS THE CUSTOM IN THEIR LAND OF ORIGIN. EACH YEAR EVERYONE IS INVITED TO PARTICIPATE AND WITNESS THE HONOR AND GLORY THAT IS BESTOWED TO THIS MARTYRED SAINT.

Advisory Consultant - Peter Tardo
Maestro di Banda - Gaetano Giaraffo
Capo di Banda - Stanley Pugliese

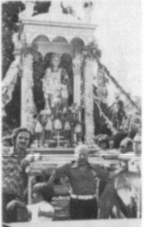

SANT'AGRIPPINA DI MINEO

A beautiful blonde maiden Saint'Agrippina was a princess by birth. This beautiful virgin martyr who was unmercifully scorged and tortured to death by the Emperor Valerion (256 AD). After her death, her relics were taken from Rome to Mineo by Saints Agatha Bassa and Paula.

The Greeks honor her in a lesser degree and claim to have relics of her. Also, in the city of Constantinople, they claim to have her body.

Saint Agrippina is the Patron Saint of thunderstorms, leprosy and evil spirits.

ST. AGRIPPINA PRAY FOR OUR DECEASED MEMBERS

A Tug of War will take place when the procession is over. The Saint is being carried by 20 men, namely Sicilians against the Romans.

Figure 12–1 Announcement of a North End (Boston) festival.

Health and Illness

Italians tend to present their symptoms to their fullest point and to expect immediate treatment for ailments. In terms of traditional beliefs, they may view the cause of illness to be one of the following: (1) winds and currents that bear diseases, (2) contagion or contamination, (3) heredity, (4) supernatural or human causes, and (5) psychosomatic interactions.

One such traditional Italian belief contends that moving air, in the form of drafts, causes irritation and then a cold that can lead to pneumonia. A belief an elderly person may express in terms of cancer surgery is that it is not a good idea to have surgery because surgery exposes the inner body to the air, and if the cancer is exposed to the air the person is going to die quicker. Just as drafts are considered to be a cause of illness, fresh air is considered to be vital for the maintenance of health. Homes and the workplace must be well ventilated to prevent illness from occurring.

One sees a belief in contamination manifested in the reluctance of people to share food and objects with people who are considered unclean, and often in not entering the homes of those who are ill. Traditional Italian women have a strong sense of modesty and shame, resulting in an avoidance of discussions relating to sex and menstruation.

Blood is regarded by some, especially the elderly, to be a "plastic entity" that responds to fluids and food and is responsible for many variable conditions. Various adjectives, such as *high* and *low* and *good* and *bad,* are used to describe blood. Some of the "old superstitions" include the following beliefs:

1. Congenital abnormalities can be attributed to the unsatisfied desire for food during pregnancy.
2. If a pregnant woman is not given food that she smells, the fetus will move inside, and a miscarriage will result.
3. If a pregnant woman bends, turns, or moves in a certain way, the fetus may not develop normally.
4. A woman must not reach during pregnancy because reaching can harm the fetus.

Italians may also attribute the cause of illness to the evil eye (*malocchio*) or to curses (*castiga*). The difference between these two causes is that less serious illnesses, such as headaches, may be caused by *malocchio,* whereas more severe illness, which often can be fatal, may be attributed to more powerful *castiga.* Curses are sent either by God or by evil people. An example of a curse is the punishment from God for sins and bad behavior (Ragucci, 1981, p. 216).

Italians recognize that illness can be caused by the suppression of emotions, as well as stress from fear, grief, and anxiety. If one is unable to find an emotional outlet, one well may "burst." It is not considered healthy to bottle up emotions (Ragucci, 1981, p. 232).

Often, the care of the ill is managed in the home, with all members of the family sharing in the responsibilities. The use of home remedies ostensibly is decreasing, although several students have reported the continued use of rituals for the removal of the evil eye and the practice of leeching. One practice described for the removal of the evil eye was to take an egg and olive oil and to drip them into a pan of water, make the sign of the cross, and recite prayers. If the oil spreads over the water, the cause of the problem is the evil eye, and the illness should get better. Mineral waters are also used, and tonics are used to cleanse the blood. There is a strong religious influence among Italians, who believe that faith in God and the saints will see them through the illness. One woman whom I worked with had breast cancer. She had had surgery several years before and did not have a recurrence. She attributed her recovery to the fact that she attended mass every morning and that she had total faith in Saint Peregrine, whose medal she wore pinned to her bra by the site of the mastectomy. Italian people tend to take a fatalistic stance regarding terminal illness and death, believing that it is God's will. Death often is not discussed between the dying person and the family members. I recall when caring for an elderly Italian man at home that it was not possible to have the man and his wife discuss his impending death. Although both knew that he was dying and would talk with the nurse, to each other he "was going to recover," and everything possible was done to that end.

Italian families observe numerous religious traditions surrounding death, and funeral masses and anniversary masses are observed. It is the custom for the widow to wear black for some time after her husband's death (occasionally for the remainder of her life), although this is not as common with the younger generations.

Health-Related Problems

Two genetic diseases commonly seen among Italians are (1) favism, a severe hemolytic anemia caused by deficiency of the X-linked enzyme glucose-6-phosphate dehydrogenase and triggered by the eating of fava beans, and (2) the thalassemia syndromes, also hemolytic anemias that include Cooley's anemia (or beta-thalassemia) and alpha-thalassemia (Ragucci, 1981, p. 222).

Language problems frequently occur when elderly or new Italian immigrants are seeking care. Often, due to modesty, people are reluctant to answer the questions asked through interpreters, and gathering of pertinent data is very difficult.

Problems related to time also occur. Physicians tend to diagnose emotional problems more often for Italian patients than for other ethnic groups because of the Italian pattern of reporting more symptoms and reporting them more dramatically (Giordano & McGoldrick, 1996, p. 576).

In general, Italian Americans are motivated to seek explanations with respect to their health status and the care they are to receive. If instructions and explanations are well given, Italians tend to cooperate with health care providers. It is often necessary to provide directions in the greatest detail and then to provide written instructions to ensure compliance with necessary regimens.

■ Polish Americans

The first people immigrating to this country from Poland came with Germans in 1608 to Jamestown, Virginia, to help develop the timber industry. Since that time, Poland, too, has given America one of its largest ethnic groups, with over 9 million people claiming Polish ancestry. The peak year for Polish immigration was 1921, and well over 578,875 people immigrated here. Many of the people arriving before 1890 came for economic reasons. Those coming here since that time have come for both economic and political reasons and for religious freedom. Polish heroes include Casimir Pulaski and Thaddeus Kosciuszko, who were heroes in the American Revolution. The major influx of Poles to the United States began in 1870 and ended in 1913. The people who arrived were mainly peasants seeking food and release from the political oppression of three foreign governments in Poland. The immigrants who came both before and after this mass migration were better educated and not as poor. In the United States, Polish immigrants lived in poor conditions either because they had no choice or because that was the way they were able to meet their own priorities. They were seen by other Americans to live as animals and were often mocked and called stupid. Quite often, the Polish people spoke and understood several European languages but had difficulty learning English and were therefore scorned. Polish people shared the problem as a community and banded together in tight enclaves called "Polonia." They attempted to be as self-sufficient as possible. They worked at preserving their native culture, and voluntary Polish ghettos grew up in close proximity to the parish church (Green, 1980, pp. 787–803). Over 85.5% of those 5 years and older speak Polish at home and 50.3% speak English less than very well. Thirty-seven percent of people of Polish ancestry reside in the Northeast, as well as 37% in the Midwest (U.S. Bureau of the Census, 2001, p. 46).

An example of the Polish experience in the United States is that of the Polish immigrants in Texas. The first Poles came to Texas in the second half of the 19th century, and most of them settled in Victoria, San Antonio, Houston, and Bandera. The first Polish colonies in America were located in Texas, the oldest being Panna Maria (Virgin Mary) in Karnes County, 50 miles southeast of San Antonio. Unlike other Poles who wanted to return to Poland, the colonists who arrived in Texas after 1850 came to settle permanently and had no intention of returning to their homeland. Although these people came to Texas for economic, political, and religious reasons, severe poverty was their major reason for leaving Poland.

The first collective Polish immigration to America was in 1854, when 100 families came to Texas. They landed in Galveston, where a few in the party remained. The rest traveled in a procession northwestward, taking with them a few belongings, such as featherbeds, crude farm implements, and a cross from their parish church. Their dream was to live in the fertile lands of Texas and raise crops, speak their own language, educate their children, and worship God as they pleased. This dream did not materialize, and members of the band grew discouraged. Some of the immigrants remained in Victoria and others went to San Antonio.

The people who went to San Antonio continued to travel; on Christmas Eve, 1854, they stopped at the junction of the San Antonio and Cibolo Rivers; There, under a live oak tree, they celebrated mass and founded Panna Maria. In 1855, 1856, and 1857, others followed this small group in moving to this part of Texas.

These settlers were exposed to many dangers from nature, such as heat, drought, snakes, and insects. The Polish settlers were not accepted by the other settlers in the area because their language, customs, and culture were different, but the immigrants survived, and many moved to settle other areas near Panna

Maria. Today, the people of Panna Maria continue to live simple lives close to nature and God and speak mainly Polish.

Much of the history of the Polish people in Texas is written around the founding and the location of the various church parishes. For example, in 1873 the Parish of the Nativity of the Blessed Virgin Mary was begun in Cestohowa. Within this church above the main altar is a large picture of the Virgin Mary of Czestochowa. This picture was taken to the church from Panna Maria. It is a copy of the famous Black Madonna of Czestochowa, Poland, a city 65 miles east of where the immigrants to Texas originated. The Black Madonna is a beloved, miraculous image and a source of faith to the Polish people. The Shrine of Our Lady in Czestochowa, Poland, is one of the largest shrines in the world. Since the 14th century, that picture had been the object of veneration and devotion of Polish Catholics. It is claimed to have been painted by Saint Luke the Evangelist. Its origin is traced to the 5th or 6th century and is the oldest picture of the Virgin in the world. The scars on the face date from 1430, when bandits struck it with a sword. The history, traditions, and miracles of Czestochowa are the heritage of the Polish people (Dworaczyk, 1979). One woman I interviewed said she had been ill with a fatal disease. The entire time that she lay close to death she prayed to the Virgin. When she finally did recover, she made a pilgrimage back to her homeland in Poland and visited the shrine to give thanks to the Virgin. The woman was positive that this was the source of her recovery.

HEALTH and ILLNESS

The definitions of HEALTH among the Polish people I interviewed included "feeling okay—as a whole—body, spirit, everything a person cannot separate;" happy, until war, do not need doctor, do not need medicine; "active, able to work, feel good, do what I want to do;" and "good spirit, good to everybody, never cross." The definitions of ILLNESS may include "something wrong with body, mind, or spirit;" "one wrong affects them all;" "not capable of working, see the doctor often;" "not right, something ailing you;" "not active"; "feeling bad"; and "opposite of health, not doing what I want to do." The methods for maintaining HEALTH include maintaining a happy home, being kind and loving, eating healthy food, remaining pure, walking, exercising, wearing proper clothing (sweaters), eating a well-balanced diet, trying not to worry, having faith in God, being active, dressing warmly, going to bed early, and working hard. The methods for preventing ILLNESS include cleanliness, the wearing of scapulars, avoiding drafts, following the proper diet, not gossiping, keeping away from people with colds, and wearing medals because "God is with you all the time to protect you and take care of you." Other ideas about ILLNESS include the beliefs that ILLNESSES are caused by poor diets and that the evil eye may well exist as a causative factor. This belief was attributed to the older generations and is not regarded as prevalent among younger Polish Americans.

The home remedies listed in Table 12–5 were described by informants and are in common use among Polish Americans.

Table 12-5 ILLNESS Symptoms and Remedies Among Polish Americans

Gastrointestinal Problems	
Symptom	**Remedy**
Colic	Tea—peppermint or chamomile
	Sugar, water, vinegar, and soda; makes soda water
	Bess-plant tea
	Homemade sauerkraut
Constipation	Epsom salts—teaspoon in water—cleans out stomach
	Cascara
	Castor oil
	Senna-leaf tea
Cramps	Camomile tea
Diarrhea	Paregoric
	Cinnamon tea
	Dried blueberries
	Chew coffee beans
Gas	Drink soda water
Indigestion	Aloes vulgaris—juniper and elderberries
	Peppermint and spearmint teas
	Blackberries
Respiratory Problems	
Symptom	**Remedy**
Cold	Castor oil—mentholatum
	Flaxseed or mustard poultice on chest
	Dried raspberries and tea with wine
	Mustard plaster
	Oatmeal poultices—hot bricks to feet
	Cupping
	Camphor salve
	Oxidine
	Rub goose fat on chest
Cough	Honey and hot water; bedrest
	Hot lemonade with whiskey; honey
	Few drops of turpentine and sugar
	"Gugel Mugel"—warm milk with butter, whiskey, and honey
	Honey and warm milk
	Milk with butter and garlic
	Mustard plaster
	Linden tea
	Onion poultice
Croup	Few drops of kerosene and sugar
Sore throat	Honey
	Warm water, salt—gargle
	Goose grease around throat covered with dry rag
	Paint throat with kerosene
	Goose fat in milk

(continued)

Table 12–5 *Continued*

Physical Injury	
Symptom	**Remedy**
Burns	Aloe vera
Cuts	Vinegar, water, flour paste
	Clean with urine
	Carbolic salve
Puncture wounds (nail)	Turpentine and liniment
	Put salt pork on wound and soak in hot water
	Hunt's lightning oil
Frostbite	Put snow on frozen place
Scratches, sores	Liniment
	Moss
	Spider webs
Sprains	Liniments—Sloan's Volcanic

Miscellaneous Problems	
Symptom	**Remedy**
Earache	Hot-water-bottle to ear
	Camphor on cotton—place in ear
Fever	Camomile tea
Flu	Novak oil—rub on head
	Knorr's Green Drops
Headache	Vinegar on a cloth applied to head
	Steam kettle—cover head and inhale
High blood pressure	Cooked garlic
	Garlic oil
Lice	Cover head with kerosene
Toothache	Hot salt compress
Neuralgia	Bedrest
Pyorrhea	Yarrow tea
Rheumatism	Lemon juice—rub on sore places
Trouble urinating	Juice of pumpkin seeds made into a tea
	Swamp root medicine

Source: Spector, R. E. (1983). *A description of the impact of Medicare on health-illness beliefs and practices of White ethnic senior citizens in Central Texas.* Ph.D. diss. University of Texas at Austin School of Nursing. Ann Arbor, MI: University Microfilms International. Reprinted with permission.

Health Care Problems

The Polish community has not tended to have any major problems with health care deliverers. Language may be a barrier if members of the older generation do not speak English, and the taking of health histories is complicated when the providers cannot communicate directly with the informant. Again, problems may develop when there is difficulty finding someone who is conversant in Polish whom the informant can trust to reveal personal matters to and who can translate medical terms accurately.

In Poland, there is a shortage of medical supplies, so the people tend to use faith healers and believe in miracle workers. On the main street of Warsaw all sorts of folk medicine and miracle-worker paraphernalia are on sale: divining rods, cotton sacks filled with herbs to be worn over an ailing heart or liver, coils of copper wire to be placed under food to rid it of poisons, and pendulums (*Letter from Poland*, 1983).

Health Status of White Population

There are countless health status indicators wherein the White cohort of the population differs from the total population, each of the racial groups, and Hispanics as the populations were designated by Census 2000. In each of the preceding four chapters, there has been a table comparing the relevant group and all races. In this chapter it is appropriate to compare the White populations to all races (Table 12–6) and to specific populations (Table 12–7). In spite of the fact that only 13 health

Table 12-6 Comparison of Selected Health Status Indicators—All Races and White: 1999/2004

Health Indicator	All Races 1999/2004	White 1999/2004
Crude birth rate per 1,000 population by race of mother	14.5/14.0	13.9/13.5
Percentage of live births of women receiving prenatal care first trimester	83.2/83.9	85.1/85.4
Percentage of live births of women receiving third-trimester or no prenatal care	3.8/3.6	3.2/3.2
Percentage of live births to teenage childbearing women—under 18	4.4/3.4	3.7/3.0
Percentage of low-birth-weight per live births <2,500 grams, 1997–1999/2003	7.57/8.3	6.56/7.2
Infant mortality per 1,000 live births, 1996–1998/2003	7.2/6.8	6.0/5.7
Cancer—all sites per 100,000 population, 1997/2003	384.5/447.1	386.2/456.0
Lung cancer incidence per 100,000 population, 1997/2003	Men: 65.4/73.0 Women: 40.7/48.0	Men: 63.7/72 Women: 42.9/50.7
Breast cancer incidence per 100,000, 1997/2003	113.1/121.1	117.0/125.7
Prostate cancer incidence per 100,000, 1997/2003	136.0/160.4	129.6/154.9
Male death rates from suicide, all ages, age adjusted per 100,000 resident population, 1999/2003	18.1/10.8	19.3/19.6
Male death rates from homicide, all ages, age adjusted per 100,000 resident population, 1999/2003	9.3/9.4	5.5/5.3

Source: National Center for Health Statistics. (2006). *Health, United States, 2006 with chartbook on trends in the health of Americans* (pp. 135, 140, 144, 149, 160, 227, 230, 244). Hyattsville MD: Author.

Table 12–7 Comparison of Selected Health Status Indicators—All Races, American Indian and Alaska Natives, Asian/Pacific Islanders, Black or African Americans, Hispanics or Latinos, and Whites: 1999/2004

Health Indicator	All Races 1990/2004	American Indian and Alaska Natives	Asian/Pacific Islanders	Black or African American	Hispanics or Latinos	White
Crude birth rate per 1,000 population by race of mother	14.5/14.0	16.8/14.0	16.7/16.8	17.4/16.0	24.4/22.9	13.9/13.5
Percentage of live births of women receiving prenatal care first trimester	83.2/83.9	69.5/69.9	83.7/85.6	74.1/76.4	74.4/77.5	85.1/85.4
Percentage of live births of women receiving third-trimester or no prenatal care	3.8/3.6	8.2/7.9	3.5/3.0	6.6/5.7	6.3/5.4	3.2/3.2
Percentage of live births to teenage childbearing women—under 18	4.4/3.4	7.9/6.4	1.8/1.1	8.2/6.4	6.7/5.4	3.7/3.0
Percentage of low-birth-weight per live births <2,500 grams, 1997–1999/2003	7.57/8.3	7.15/8.7	7.37/7.7	13.11/15.3	6.38/6.2	6.56/7.2
Infant mortality per 1,000 live births 1996–1998	7.2/6.8	9.3/8.7	5.2/4.8	13.9/13.5	5.9/5.6	6.0/5.7

Table 12–7 *Continued*

Cancer—all sites per 100,000 population, 1997/2002	384.5/447.1	148.6/298.5	279.9/314.7	426.5/489.0	249/323.5	386.2/456.0
Lung cancer incidence per 100,000 population, 1997/2003	Men: 65.4/73.0 Women: 40.7/48.7	Men[a] Women[a]	Men: 49.8/[a] Women: 22.1/[a]	Men: 100.5/107.8 Women: 42.3/52.6	Men: 32.8/41.3 Women: 17.5/20.8	Men: 63.7/72 Women: 42.9/50.7
Breast cancer incidence per 100,000, 1997/2003	113.1/121.1	/28.7	85.6/87.4	101.3/119.2	65.5/79.6	117.0/125.7
Prostate cancer incidence per 100,000, 1997/2003	136.0/160.4	/41.2	74.3/97.9	207.9/237.5	91.9/127.3	129.6/154.9
Male death rates from suicide, all ages, age adjusted per 100,000 resident population, 1999/2003	18.1/10.8	19.1/16.6	9.7/8.5	10.6/9.2	10.7/9.7	19.3/19.6
Male death rates from homicide, all ages, age adjusted per 100,000 resident population, 1999/2003	9.3/9.4	15.4/10.5	4.3/4.2	38.4/36.7	13.8/12.1	5.5/5.3

Source: National Center for Health Statistics. (2006). *Health, United States, 2006 with chartbook on trends in the health of Americans* (pp. 135, 140, 144, 149, 160, 227, 230, 244). Hyattsville, MD: Author.

[a] No data available

Table 12-8   Comparison of the 10 Leading Causes of Death for White Americans and for All Persons: 2004

White Americans	All Persons
1. Diseases of heart	Diseases of heart
2. Malignant neoplasms	Malignant neoplasms
3. Cerebrovascular diseases	Cerebrovascular diseases
4. Chronic lower respiratory diseases	Chronic lower respiratory diseases
5. Unintentional injuries	Unintentional injuries
6. Alzheimer's disease	Diabetes mellitus
7. Diabetes mellitus	Alzheimer's disease
8. Influenza and pneumonia	Influenza and pneumonia
9. Nephritis, nephrotic syndrome, and nephrosis	Nephritis, nephrotic syndrome, and nephrosis
10. Suicide	Septicemia

Source: National Center for Health Statistics. (2007). *Health, United States, 2007 with chartbook on trends in the health of Americans* (p. 187). Hyattsville, MD: Author.

indicators are listed as examples in the tables, the health differences and disparities in the overall populations are readily apparent.

Table 12–8 lists the 10 leading causes of death for Whites and compares them with the causes of death for the general population in 2004.

In this chapter, as in this entire book, I have attempted to open the door to the enormous diversity in health and illness beliefs that exists in White (European American) communities specifically and in the entire American population in general. I have only opened the door and invited you to peek inside. There is a richness of knowledge to be gained. It is for you to acquire it as you care for all patients. Ask them what they believe about health/HEALTH and illness/ILLNESS and what their traditional beliefs, practices, and remedies are. The students whom I am working with find this to be a very enlightening experience.

RESEARCH IN CULTURE

A great amount of research has been conducted among members of the White American populations. The following article describes one such study:

> Hutson, S. P., Dorgan, K. A., Phillips, A. N., & Behringer, B. (2007, November). The mountains hold things in: The use of community research review work groups to address cancer disparities in Appalachia. *Oncology Nursing Forum, 34*(6), 1133–1139.

The purpose of this research study was to review regional findings about cancer disparities with grass-roots community leaders in Appalachia and to discover what makes the experience of cancer unique in that part of the country. The study was community-based and information was gathered from focus groups. Four major themes emerged from the focus groups:

1. *Cancer storytelling.* One theme was the ubiquitous nature of cancer and that the members of the community expect to get cancer. Many participants believed that "cancer was more a hereditary thing" because of family histories.
2. *Cancer collectiveness.* Rural families tend to rely on themselves.
3. *Health care challenges.* Participants were doubtful about their ability to navigate and trust the health care system. They also told of the state's history of overlooking the people in this community.
4. *Cancer expectations.* Some rural people may not embrace what are seen as basic patients' rights.

The key discoveries were that the cancer experience in Appalachia appears to be affected uniquely by cultural, economic, and geographic influences; that health care professionals and researchers must respect and partner with existing social and familial community networks; and the use of community research review work is a viable method to examine cancer disparities in a marginalized population. Suggestions from this study supported the need for patient navigators and advocate services to reach communities and bridge the gaps between the health care system and laypeople. Cancer information should be tailored to individual patients' attributes, such as education and literacy levels and cultural and familial beliefs.

Explore 🌐 MediaLink

Go to the Companion Website at www.prenhall.com/spector for chapter-related review questions, case studies, and activities. Contents of the CulturalCare Guide and CulturalCare Museum can also be found on the Companion Website. Click on Chapter 12 to select the activities for this chapter.

■ Internet Sources

Brittingham, A., and de la Cruz, G. P. Ancestry: 2000 Census Brief (2004). Washington: DC: United States Census Bureau, pp. 1–2. Retrieved from https://ask.census.gov/cgi-bin/askcensus.cfg. February 23, 2008.

Grieco, E. M. (2001). The White Population: 2000. Washington, DC: U.S. Census Bureau. P. 7 Retrieved from http://www.census.gov/population/www/cen2000/briefs.html, February 23, 2008.

Larsen, L. J. (2004). *The Foreign-Born Population in the United States: 2003.* Washington, DC: U.S. Census Bureau. p.1 Retrieved from http://www.census.gov/prod/2004pubs/p20–551.pdf, May 23, 2008.

U.S. Census Bureau, Census 2000 Special Tabulations. Profile of Selected Demographic and Social Characteristics: 2000 United States, Germany, Italy, and Poland. Retrieved from http://factfinder.census.gov, http://www.census.gov/population/cen2000/stp-159/STP-159-Europe.pdf, http://www.census.

gov/population/cen2000/stp-159/STP-159-Germany.pdf, http://www.census.gov/ population/cen2000/stp-159/STP-159Italy.pdf, http://www.census.gov/ population/cen2000/stp-159/STP-159-Poland.pdf, February 23, 2008.

References

Bernardo, S. (1981). *The ethnic almanac*. New York: Doubleday.

Conzen, K. N. (1980). Germans. In S. Thernstrom (Ed.), *Harvard encyclopedia of American ethnic groups* (pp. 405–425). Cambridge, MA: Harvard University Press.

Dworaczyk, E. J. (1979). *The first Polish colonies of America in Texas*. San Antonio, TX: Naylor.

Folwarski, J., & Marganoff, P. P. (1996). Polish families. In M. McGoldrick, J. Giordano, & J. K. Pearce (Eds.), *Ethnicity and family therapy* (2nd ed.). New York: Guilford.

Giordano, J., & McGoldrick, M. (1996). Italian families. In M. McGoldrick, J. Giordano, & J. K. Pearce (Eds.), *Ethnicity and family therapy* (2nd ed.). New York: Guilford.

Green, V. (1980). Poles. In S. Thernstrom (Ed.), *Harvard encyclopedia of American ethnic groups*. Cambridge, MA: Harvard University Press.

Lefcowitz, E. (1990). *The United States immigration history timeline*. New York: Terra Firma Press.

Letter from Poland—of faith healers and miracle workers. (1983, August 21). *Boston Globe*, p.

Lich, G. E. (1982). *The German Texan*. San Antonio: University of Texas Institute of Texan Cultures.

Lollock, L. (2000). *The foreign-born population in the United States*. Washington, DC: U.S. Bureau of the Census.

Meyer, J. (2001). *Age: 2000*. Washington, DC: U.S. Census Bureau.

National Center for Health Statistics, et al. (2001). *Health, United States, 2001 urban and rural health chartbook*. Hyattsville, MD: Author.

National Center for Health Statistics. (2006). *Health, United States, 2006 with chartbook on trends in the health of Americans*. Hyattsville, MD: Author.

Nelli, H. S. (1980). Italians. In S. Thernstrom (Ed.), *Harvard encyclopedia of American ethnic groups*. Cambridge, MA: Harvard University Press.

Ragucci, A. T. (1981). Italian Americans. In A. Harwood (Ed.), *Ethnicity and medical care*. Cambridge, MA: Harvard University Press.

Spector, R. E. (1983). *A description of the impact of Medicare on health-illness beliefs and practices of White ethnic senior citizens in Central Texas*. PhD. diss. University Texas at Austin School of Nursing, Ann Arbor, MI: University Microfilms International.

Spector, R. (1992). Culture, ethnicity, and nursing. In P. Potter & A. Perry (Eds.), *Fundamentals of nursing* (3rd ed.). St Louis: Mosby.

U.S. Bureau of the Census. (2001). *Statistical abstract of the United States: 2001*. Washington, DC: Author.

Winawer, H., & Wetzel, N. A. (1996). German families. In M. McGoldrick, J. Giordano, & J. K. Pearce (Eds.), *Ethnicity and family therapy* (2nd ed.). New York: Guilford.

Epilogue

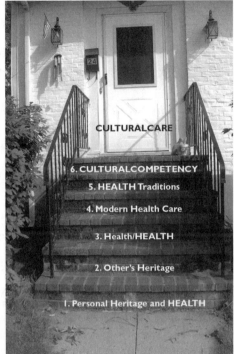

Why must health care deliverers—nurses, physicians, public health and social workers, and other health care professionals—study culture, ethnicity, religion, and become CULTURALLY COMPETENT? Why must they know the difference between *hot* and *cold* and *yin* and *yang*? Why must they be concerned with the patient's failure to practice what professionals believe to be good preventive medicine or with the patient's failure to follow a given treatment regimen or with the patient's failure to seek medical care during the initial phase of an illness? Is there a difference between curing and HEALING?

There is little disagreement that health care services in this country are unevenly distributed and that the poor and the emerging majority get the short end of the stick in terms of the care they receive (or do not receive). The apparent health disparities are a reality, as are the demographic and social disparities in areas of housing, employment, education, and opportunity. Just as there is the need to understand the people who constitute our multicultural society, there is also the need to understand new immigrants as more and more people flock to this country. However, it is often maintained that, when health care is provided, people fail to use it or use it inappropriately. Why is this seeming paradox so?

The major focus of this book has been on the provider's and the patient's differing perceptions of health/HEALTH and illness/ILLNESS. These differences may account for the health care provider's misconception that services are used inappropriately and that people do not care about their health/HEALTH. What to the casual observer appears to be "misuse" may represent our failure to understand and to meet the needs and expectations of the patient. This possibility may well be difficult for health care providers to face, but careful analysis of the available information seems to indicate that this may—at least in part—be the case. How, then, can we who are health care providers change our method of operations and provide both safe and effective care for the emerging majority and, at the same time, for the population at large? The answer to this question is not an easy one, and some researchers think we are not succeeding. A number of measures can and must be taken to ameliorate the current situation. CULTURALCARE and the educational preparation leading to this is a **process,** one that becomes a way of life and must be recognized as such. This is a philosophical issue. The changing of one's personal and professional philosophies, ideas, and stereotypes does *not* occur overnight, and the process, quite often, is neither direct nor easy. It is a multistep process, in which one must

- Explore one's own cultural identity and heritage and confront biases and stereotypes.
- Develop an awareness and understanding of the complexities of the modern health care delivery system—its philosophy and problems, biases, and stereotypes.
- Develop a keen awareness of the socialization process that brings the provider into this complex system.
- Develop the ability to "hear" things that transcend language and foster an understanding of the patient and his or her cultural heritage and the resilience found within the culture that supports family and community structures.

Given the processes of acculturation, assimilation, and modernism, this is often difficult and painful, yet, once the journey of exploring one's own cultural heritage and prejudices is undertaken, the awareness of the cultural needs of others becomes more subtle and understandable. This is well accomplished by using the umbrella of HEALTH traditions as the point of entry.

A student I once taught described the journey this way:

> I was born in 1973 to fourth-generation Japanese American parents. I understood Japanese culture and the way of thinking and did not question when my parents told me to eat noodles on New Year's Day to bring long life. Then I changed schools and went to the Caucasian school. I came to hate my heritage and wanted to scream that "I'm as white on the inside as you are." I was bitter and embarrassed by my heritage and blamed my family, who were proud of their ancestry. When my parents tried to teach me about Japanese American history, I was not interested. I came to know, understand, and hate racism. On the inside I felt as "white American" as everyone else but I soon realized what I felt inside was not what other people saw. I now acknowledge who I am and I accept myself.

The voice of this young student speaks for many. In the course of having to explore the family's traditional HEALTH beliefs and practices, the student began to see, think through, understand, and accept herself.

Although curricula in professional education are quite full, CULTURALCARE studies must be taken by all people who wish to deliver health care. In the wake of September 11, 2001, it is obvious that it is no longer sufficient to teach a student in the health professions to "accept patients for who they are." The question arises: Who is the patient? Introductory sociology and psychology courses fail to provide this information unless tailored to include cultural aspects of HEALTH and ILLNESS. It is learned best by meeting with the people themselves and letting them describe who they are from their own perspective. I have suggested two approaches to the problem. One is to have people who work as patient advocates or as nurses and physicians come to the class setting and explain how people of their ethnic group view health/HEALTH and illness/ILLNESS and describe the given community's HEALTH traditions. Another approach is to send students out into communities where they will have the opportunity to meet with people in their own settings. It is not necessary to memorize all the available lists of herbs, hot-cold imbalances, folk diseases, and so forth. The objective is to become more sensitive to the crucial fact that multiple factors underlie given patient behaviors. One, of course, is that the patient may well *perceive* and *understand* HEALTH from quite a different perspective than that of the health care provider. **Each person comes from a unique culture and a unique socialization process.**

The health care provider must be sensitive to his or her own perceptions of health/HEALTH and illness/ILLNESS and the practices he or she employs. Even though the perceptions of most health professionals are based on a middle-class and medical-model viewpoint, providers must realize that there are other ways of regarding health and illness. The early chapters of this book are devoted to consciousness raising about self-treatment. It is always an eye-opening experience to publicly scrutinize ourselves in this respect. Quite often, we are amazed to see how far we stray from the system's prescribed methods of keeping healthy. The dialogue confirms that we, too, delay in seeking health care and fail to comply with treatment regimens. Often, our ability to comply rests on quite pragmatic issues, such as "What is it doing for me?" and "Can I afford to miss work and stay in bed for 2 days?" As we gain insight into our own health-illness attitudes and behaviors, we tend to be much more sympathetic to and empathetic with the person who fails to come to the clinic, who hates to wait for the physician, or who delays in seeking health care.

The health care provider should be aware of the complex issues that surround the delivery of health care from the patient's viewpoint. Calling the medical society for the name of a physician (because a "family member has a health problem") and visiting and comparing the services rendered in an urban and a suburban emergency room are exercises that can enable us to better appreciate some of the difficulties that the poor, the emerging majority, and the population at large all too often experience when they attempt to obtain health care. Members of the health care team have a number of advantages in gaining access to the health care system. For example, they can choose a physician whom they know because they work with him or her or because someone they work with has recommended this physician. Health care providers must never forget, however, that most people do not have these advantages. It is indeed an unsettling, anxiety-provoking, and frustrating experience to be forced to select a physician from a list.

It is an even more frustrating experience to be a patient in an unfamiliar location—for example, an urban emergency room, where, quite literally, anything can happen. A recent film by Michael Moore, *Sicko*, paints a very painful picture of the modern health care system, yet all people entering the system ought to be familiar with it and the many issues mentioned, such as the costs of procedures and medications, as alluded to in Chapter 7.

Another barrier to adequate health care is the financial burden imposed by treatments and tests. There are other issues as well. For example, a Chinese patient—who traditionally does not believe that the body replaces the blood taken for testing purposes—should have as little blood work as necessary, and the reasons for the tests should be explained carefully. A Hispanic woman who believes that having a Pap smear is an intrusive procedure that will bring shame to her should have the procedure performed by a female physician or nurse. When this is not possible, she should have a female chaperone with her for the entire time that the male physician or nurse is in the room.

More members of the emerging majority must be represented in the health care professions. Multiple issues are related to the problem of demographic disparity. Many of the programs designed to increase the number of emerging majority students in the health care team have failed. Difficulties surrounding successful entrance into and completion of professional education programs are complex and numerous, having their roots in impoverished community structures and early educational deprivation. Although society is in some ways dealing with such issues—for example, initiating improvements in early education—we are faced with an *immediate* need to bring more emerging majority people into health care services.

One method would be the more extensive use of patient advocates and outreach workers from the given ethnic community who may be recognized there as HEALERS. These people can provide an overwhelmingly positive service to both the provider and the patient in that they can serve as the bridge in bringing health care services to the people. The patient advocate can speak to the patient in language that he or she understands and in a manner that is acceptable. Advocates also are able to coordinate medical, nursing, social, and even educational services to meet the patient's needs as the patient perceives them. In settings where advocates are employed, many problems are resolved to the convenience of both the health care member and, more importantly, the patient.

The nettlesome issue of language bursts forth with regularity. There is always a problem when a non–English-speaking person tries to seek help from the English-speaking majority. The more common languages, French, Italian, and Spanish, ideally should be spoken by at least some of the professional people who staff hospitals, clinics, neighborhood health care centers, and home health agencies. The use of an interpreter is always difficult because the interpreter generally "interprets" what he or she translates. To bring this thought home, the reader should recall the childhood game of "gossip": A message is passed around the room from person to person, and, by the time it gets back to the sender, its content is usually substantially changed. This game is not unlike trying to communicate through an interpreter, and the situation is even more frustrating when—as can often be the case in urban emergency rooms—the interpreter is a 6-year-old child. It is, obviously, far more satisfying and productive if the patient, nurse, and physician can all speak the same language. All institutions must follow the mandates of Title VI of the Civil Rights Law.

Health services must be made far more accessible and available to members of the emerging majority. I believe that one of the most important events in this modern era of health care delivery is the advent of neighborhood health centers. They are successful essentially because people who work in them know the people of the neighborhood. In addition, the people of the community can contribute to the decision making involved in governing and running the agency, so that services are tailored to meet the needs of the patients. Concerned members of the health care team have a moral obligation to support the increased use of health care centers and not their decreased use, as currently tends to occur because of cutbacks in response to allegations (frequently politically motivated) of too-high costs or the misuse of funds. These neighborhood health care centers provide greatly needed personal services in addition to relief from the widespread depersonalization that occurs in larger institutions. When health care providers who are genuinely concerned face this reality, perhaps they will be more willing to fight for the survival of these centers and strongly urge their increased funding rather than acquiesce in their demise. In rural areas, the problem is even greater, and far more comprehensive health planning is needed to meet patient needs.

The ascent to CULTURALCOMPETENCY is similar to driving on a road to anywhere. It takes time and thought and active participation. It is a learning experience wherein you discover countless facts (especially about yourself), a dynamic **process** in which you face a number of obstacles:

Collisions	Head on—meeting dense cultural conflicts and barriers— can be fatal
	Rear enders—they come at you from behind to sabotage efforts
	Fender benders—slips and blunders
	Side swipes—minor but hurtful frustrations
Conditions	Culture + climate—social/institutional attitudes
	Race/ethnicity/religion—Weather—rain, snow, fog, sun
Curves	The unknown—inability to anticipate the real responses, verbal vs. nonverbal
Destination	Physical, mental, spiritual—a realization of and respect for holistic HEALTH
Hills	The process of gaining CULTURALCOMPETENCY— content and experience—it is an up and down experience
Lights	Slow and control the progress

(continued)

No signs	Road twists and turns and there are no identifying markings
Open highway	Cruise along—but not too fast
Other drivers	Slow you down or speed you up on the destination of CULTURALCARE resistance/acceptance
Potholes	Frequent blocks to smooth movement, often unseen or covered with ice
Rush hour	Institutional and provider clogs
Ruts	When cruising along, the unexpected hits and it is often difficult to break free
Speed limits	Analogous to institutional and professional restraints—do not go too fast or too slowly—or you are in trouble and everyone is behind you
Tolls	Expensive—pay for books, travel, objects, admissions, tools
Unexpected events	Negative—radar, accidents, ice—anger, "isms"
	Positive—enduring friendships with people you may have never met
	Knowledge far deeper than ever anticipated
	Wisdom
	Deep love of life, people, and HEALTH

CULTURALCARE is the term I have coined to express all that is inherent in this text. Countless conflicts in the health care delivery arenas are predicated on cultural misunderstandings. Although many of these misunderstandings are related to universal situations, such as verbal and nonverbal language misunderstandings, the conventions of courtesy, sequencing of interactions, phasing of interactions, and objectivity, many cultural misunderstandings are unique to the delivery of health care. The need to provide CULTURALCARE—professional health care that is culturally sensitive, culturally appropriate, and culturally competent—is essential as we live in this millennium, and it demands that providers be able to assess and interpret a given patient's health/HEALTH beliefs and practices. CULTURALCARE alters the perspective of health care delivery as it enables the provider to understand, from a cultural perspective, the manifestations of the patient's HEALTH care beliefs and practices.

You'll know you are on the road to CulturalCompetency when you understand the following:

■ Even when you are a part of a group you are a person who has your own HERITAGE—your culture, ethnicity, and religion.
■ You have been socialized, first by your parents, then by schools/teachers, and later the society at large to be who you are.
■ You have your own HEALTH and ILLNESS beliefs and practices.

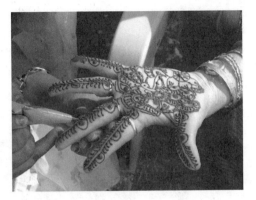

Figure E-1
Mehndi—The hena painting of a woman's hands before her wedding. The groom's hands may also be painted. It is often used for fertility and HEALTH protection in India.

■ There are countless ways to protect and maintain your HEALTH other than those prescribed by the dominant culture (Figure E–1).

■ Amulets are commonly used by people from many heritages. (Figure E–2).

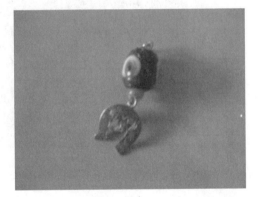

Figure E-2 Amulet for protection—may be found pinned on a person's clothing or hung in a home.

■ There are countless ways to restore your HEALTH other than those prescribed by the dominant culture's allopathic health care system (Figure E–3).

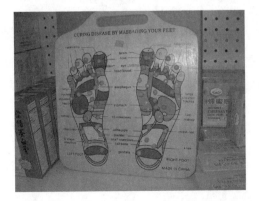

Figure E-3
Reflexology—a form of foot massage used to HEAL other parts of the body. These feet are a "map" of the corresponding places.

- Herbal remedies, teas, aromatherapy, and so on are used by people from countless traditional heritages.
- Religion plays a profound role in the HEALTH and HEALING beliefs and practices of traditional people from all walks of life (Figure E–4).

Figure E-4 Crutches at the altar of the Mission Church, Boston, Massachusetts—They are symbolic of the HEALINGS that have happened in the church.

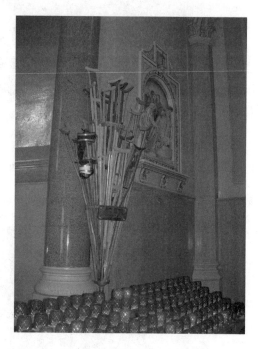

- Shrines, either secular or religious, are inherent in the HEALING process of countless people.

I should like to reiterate that this book was written with the hope that, by sharing the material I have learned and taught for over 35 years, some small changes will be made in the thinking of all health care providers who read it. There is nothing new in these pages. Perhaps it is simply a recombination of material with which the reader is familiar, but I hope it serves its purpose: the sharing of beliefs and attitudes and the stimulation of lots of consciousness raising concerning issues of vital concern to health care providers who must confront the needs of patients with diverse cultural backgrounds.

Appendix A

Selected Key Terms Related to Cultural Diversity in HEALTH and ILLNESS

The following terms have been defined to help you in the development of CULTURALCOMPETENCY. They are the "bricks" that comprise the steps that must be climbed. They are the language of CULTURALCARE.

Aberglaubish or *aberglobin*—The traditional German term for the "evil eye."

Access—Gaining entry into a system—the term used in this text refers to access into the modern health care system. *Access* also means entry into a profession, education, employment, housing, and so forth.

Acculturation—The process of adapting to another culture. To acquire the majority group's culture.

Acupuncture—The traditional Chinese medical way of restoring the balance of *yin* and *yang* that is based on the therapeutic value of cold. Cold is used in a disease where there is an excess of *yang*.

Alcoholismo—Alcoholism.

Alien—Every person applying for entry to the United States. Anyone who is not a U.S. citizen.

Allopathic—Health beliefs and practices that are derived from current scientific models and involve the use of technology and other modalities of present-day health care, such as immunization, proper nutrition, and resuscitation.

Allopathy—The treatment of a disease by using remedies that cause the opposite effects of the disease.

Alternative health system—A system of health care a person may use that is not predicated within his or her traditional culture but is not allopathic.

Amulet—An object with magical powers, such as a charm, worn on a string or chain around the neck, wrist, or waist to protect the wearer from both physical and psychic illness, harm, and misfortune.

Anamnesis—The traditional Chinese medical way of diagnosing a health problem by asking questions.

Apparel—Traditional clothing worn by people for cultural or religious beliefs on a daily basis, such as head coverings.

Aromatherapy—Ancient science that uses essential plant oils to produce strong physical and emotional effects in the body.

Assimilation—To become absorbed into another culture and to adopt its characteristics. To develop a new cultural identity.

Ataque de nervios—An attack of nerves or a nervous breakdown.

Average charge—Average amount of monetary charge in hospital bills for discharged patients.

Average length of stay—The typical number of days a patient stays in the hospital for a particular condition.

Ayurvedic—Four-thousand-year-old method of healing originating in India, the chief aim of which is longevity and quality of life. The most ancient existing medical system that uses diet, natural therapies, and herbs.

Bankes—Small, bell-shaped glass that is used to create a vacuum, placed on a person's chest, to loosen chest secretions.

Biofeedback—The use of an electronic machine to measure skin temperatures. The patient controls responses that are usually involuntary.

Biological variations—Biological differences that exist among races and ethnic groups in body structure, skin color, biochemical differences, susceptibility to disease, and nutritional differences.

Borders—Legal, geographic separations between nations.

Botanica—Traditional Hispanic pharmacy where amulets, herbal remedies, books, candles, and statues of saints may be purchased.

Bruja—A witch.

Caida de la mollera **(fallen fontanel)**—Traditional Hispanic belief that the fontanel falls if the baby's head is touched.

Calendar—Dates of religious holidays. Many of these dates of observance can change from year to year on the Julian calendar.

Care—Factors that assist, enable, support, or facilitate a person's needs to maintain, improve, or ease a health problem.

Celos—Jealousy.

Charm—Objects that combine the functions of both amulets and talismans but consist only of written words or symbols.

Chinese doctor—Physician educated in China who uses traditional herbs and other therapeutic modalities in the delivery of health care.

Chiropractic—A form of health care that believes in the use of "energy" to treat diseases.

Complementary medicine—Treatment modalities used to complement allopathic regimens.

Conjure—To effect magic.

Coraje—Rage.

Costs—The monetary price of an item or the consequences of ignoring social factors.

CULTURALCARE—A concept that describes holistic HEALTH care that is culturally sensitive, culturally appropriate, and culturally competent. CULTURALCARE is critical to meeting the complex nursing care needs of a person, family, and community. It is the provision of health care across cultural boundaries and takes into account the context in which the patient lives as well as the situations in which the patient's health problems arise.

Culturally appropriate—Implies that the health care provider applies the underlying background knowledge that must be possessed to provide a given patient with the best possible HEALTH care.

CULTURALLY COMPETENT—Implies that within the delivered care the health care provider understands and attends to the total context of the patient's situation. CULTURALCOMPETENCE is a complex combination of knowledge, attitudes, and skills.

Culturally sensitive—Implies that the health care providers possess some basic knowledge of and constructive attitudes toward the HEALTH traditions observed among the diverse cultural groups found in the setting in which they are practicing.

Culture—Nonphysical traits, such as values, beliefs, attitudes, and customs, that are shared by a group of people and passed from one generation to the next. A metacommunication system.

Culture shock—Disorder that occurs in response to transition from one cultural setting to another. Former behavior patterns are ineffective in such a setting, and basic cues for social behavior are absent.

Curandero—Traditional Hispanic holistic healer.

Curing*—Two-dimensional phenomenon that results in ridding the body or mind (or both) of a given disease.

Decoction—A simmered tea made from the bark, root, seed, or berry of a plant.

Demographic disparity—A variation below the percentages of the profile of the total population with a specific entity, such as poverty, or professional, such as nursing. Comparison with the demographic profile of the total population.

Demographic parity—An equal distribution of a given entity, such as registered nurses, and the demographic profile of the total population.

Demographics—The population profile of the nation, state, county, or local city or town.

Demography—The statistical study of populations, including statistical counts of people of various ages, sexes, and population densities for specific locations.

Determinism—Believing that life is under a person's control.

Diagnosis—The identifying of the nature or cause of something, especially a problem.

Disadvantaged background—Both educational and economic factors that act as barriers to an individual's participation in a health professions program.

Discrimination—Denying people equal opportunity by acting on a prejudice.

Divination—Traditional American Indian practice of calling on spirits or other forces to determine a diagnosis of a health problem.

Documentation—The papers necessary to prove one's citizenship or immigration status.

Duklij—A turquoise or green malachite amulet that may be used among American Indians to ward off evil spirits.

Dybbuk—Wandering, disembodied soul that enters another person's body and holds fast.

Emerging majority—People of color—Blacks; Asians/Pacific Islanders; American Indians, Eskimos, or Aleuts; and Hispanics—who are expected to constitute a majority of the American population by the year 2020.

Emic—Person's way of describing an action or event, an inside view.

Empacho—Traditional Hispanic belief that a ball of food is stuck in the stomach.

Envidia—Traditional Hispanic belief that the envy of others can be the cause of illness and bad luck.

Environmental control—Ability of a person from a given cultural group to actively control nature and to direct factors in the environment.

Epidemiology—The study of the distribution of disease.

Epilepsia—Epilepsy.

Ethnicity—Cultural group's sense of identification associated with the group's common social and cultural heritage.

Ethnocentrism—Tendency of members of one cultural group to view the members of other cultural groups in terms of the standards of behavior, attitudes, and values of their own group. The belief that one's own cultural, ethnic, professional, or social group is superior to that of others.

Ethnomedicine—Health beliefs and practices of indigenous cultural development. Not practiced in many of the tenets of modern medicine.

Etic—The interpretation of an event by someone who is not experiencing that event. An outside view.

Evil eye—Belief that someone can project harm by gazing or staring at another's property or person.

Excessism—Desiring to live with numerous possessions and material goods.

Exorcism—Ceremonious expulsion of an evil spirit from a person.

Faith—Strong beliefs in a religious or other spiritual philosophy.

Fatalism—Believing that life is not under a person's control.

Fatigue—Asthmalike symptoms.

Folklore—Body of preserved traditions, usually oral, consisting of beliefs, stories, and associated information of people.

Fundamentalism—Strict belief in the traditions of a heritage.

Geophagy—Eating of nonfood substances, such as starch.

Glossoscopy—Traditional Chinese medical way of diagnosing a health problem by examining the tongue.

Green card—Documentation that a person is a legally admitted immigrant and has permanent resident status in the United States.

Gris-gris—Symbols of voodoo. They may take numerous forms and be used either to protect a person or to harm that person.

Halal—A designation for meat from animals that has been slaughtered in the ritual way by Islamic law so that it is suitable to be eaten by traditional Islamic people and follows Islamic dietary laws.

Haragei—Japanese art of practice of using nonverbal communication.

HEALING*—Holistic, or three-dimensional, phenomenon that results in the restoration of balance, or harmony, to the body, mind, and spirit, or between the person and the environment.

HEALTH*—The balance of the person, both within one's being—physical, mental, and spiritual—and in the outside world—natural, communal, and metaphysical.

Herbrias—A person who sells herbs.

Heritage—The family culture, ethnicity, and/or religion that one is born into.

Heritage consistency—Observance of the beliefs and practices of one's traditional cultural belief system.

Heritage inconsistency—Observance of the beliefs and practices of one's acculturated belief system.

Hex—Evil spell, misfortune, or bad luck that one person can impose on another.

Histeria—Hysteria.

Homeopathic—Health beliefs and practices derived from traditional cultural knowledge to maintain health, prevent changes in health status, and restore health.

Homeopathic medicine—In the practice of homeopathic medicine, the person, not the disease, is treated.

Homeopathy—System of medicine based on the belief that a disease can be cured by minute doses of a substance, which, if given to a healthy person in large doses, would produce the same symptoms that the person being treated is experiencing.

Hoodoo—A form of conjuring and a term that refers to the magical practices of voodoo outside New Orleans.

Hydrotherapy—The use of water in the maintenance of health and treatment of disease.

Hypnotherapy—The use of hypnosis to stimulate emotions and control involuntary responses, such as blood pressure.

Iatrogenic—The unexpected symptom or illness that can result from the treatment of another illness.

ILLNESS*—State of imbalance among the body, mind, and spirit. A sense of disharmony both within the person and with the environment.

Immigrant—Alien entering the United States for permanent (or temporary) residence.

Indigenous—People native to an area.

Kineahora—Word spoken by traditional Jewish people to prevent the "evil eye."

Kosher—A designation for food that has been prepared so that it is suitable to be eaten by traditional Jewish people and follows Jewish dietary laws.

Kusiut—A reference term for an American Indian medicine man. A "learned one."

Lay midwife—A person who practices lay midwifery.

Lay midwifery—Assisting childbirth for compensation.

Legal Permanent Resident (LPR)—Green card recipient. A person who has been granted lawful permanent residence in the United States.

Limpia—Traditional Hispanic practice of cleansing a person.

Locura—Craziness.

Macrobiotics—Diet and lifestyle from the Far East adapted for the United States by Michio Kushif. The principles of this vegetarian diet consist of balancing *yin* and *yang* energies of food.

Magico-religious folk medicine—Use of charms, holy words, and holy actions to prevent and cure illness.

Mal ojo (**bad eye**)—Traditional Hispanic belief that excessive admiration by one person can bring harm to another person.

Massage therapy—Use of manipulative techniques to relieve pain and return energy to the body.

Materialism—Taking great pleasure from having more than is necessary.

Medically underserved community—Urban or rural population group that lacks adequate health care services.

Melting pot—The social blending of cultures.

Meridians—Specific points of the body into which needles are inserted in the traditional Chinese medical practice of acupuncture.

Mesmerism—Healing by touch.

Metacommunication system—Large system of communication that includes both verbal language and nonverbal signs and symbols.

Milagros—Small figures of body parts or other objects that are offered to Saints for thanksgiving.

Minimalism—Knowing how to live with few possessions and material goods.

Miracle—Supernatural, unexplained event.

Modern—Present-day health and illness beliefs and practices of the providers within the American, or Western, health care delivery system.

Modernism—Adherence to modern ways and a belief that other values no longer exist.

Motion in the hand—An example of a traditional American Indian practice of moving the diagnostician's hands in a ritual of divination.

Moxibustion—Traditional Chinese medical way of restoring the balance of *yin* and *yang* that is based on the therapeutic value of heat. Heat is used in a disease where there is an excess of *yin*.

Multicultural nursing—Pluralistic approach to understanding relationships between two or more cultures to create a nursing practice framework for broadening nurses' understanding of health-related beliefs, practices, and issues that are part of the experiences of people from diverse cultural backgrounds.

Mysticism—Aspect of spiritual healing and beliefs.

Natural folk medicine—Use of the natural environment and use of herbs, plants, minerals, and animal substances to prevent and treat illness.

Nonimmigrant—People who are allowed to enter the country temporarily under certain conditions, such as crewmen, students, and temporary workers.

Occult folk medicine—The use of charms, holy words, and holy actions to prevent and cure illness.

Orisha—Yoruba god or goddess.

Osphretics—Traditional Chinese medical way of diagnosing a health problem by listening and smelling.

Osteopathic medicine—School of medical practice that directs recuperative power of nature that is within the body to cure a disease.

Overheating therapy (hyperthermia)—Used since the time of the ancient Greeks. The natural immune system is stimulated with heat to kill pathogens.

Partera—A Mexican American or Mexican lay midwife.

Pasmo—Traditional Hispanic disease of paralysis, face or limbs.

Pluralistic society—A society comprising people of numerous ethnocultural backgrounds.

Poultice—A hot, soft, moist mass of herbs, flour, mustard, and other substances spread on muslin and placed on a sore body part.

Powwow—A form of traditional HEALING practiced by German Americans.

Prejudice—Negative beliefs or preferences that are generalized about a group and that leads to "prejudgment."

Promesa—A deep and serious promise.

Racism—The belief that members of one race are superior to those of other races.

Rational folk medicine—Use of the natural environment and use of herbs, plants, minerals, and animal substances to prevent and treat illness.

Raza-Latina—A popular term used as a reference group name for people of Latin American descent.

Reflexology—Natural science that manipulates the reflex points in the hands and feet that correspond to every organ in the body in order to clear the energy pathways and the flow of energy through the body.

Religion—Belief in a divine or superhuman power or powers to be obeyed and worshipped as the creator(s) and ruler(s) of the universe.

Remedies—Natural folk medicines that use the natural environment—herbs, plants, minerals, and animal substances to treat illnesses. Natural remedies have come to the United States from every corner of the world—the East and the West. They may be purchased in pharmacies, markets, and natural food stores.

Resident alien—A lawfully admitted alien.

Resiliency—The state of being strong and able to resist the consequences of an adverse event or emotional or physical danger.

Restoration—Process used by a person to return health.

Risk adjustment—Complex sets of data are put into terms whereby they are compared apples to apples.

Sacred objects—Objects, such as amulets and *milagros*, that have a spiritual purpose.

Sacred places—Places where people take petitions for favors or offer prayers of thanksgiving for the granting of a request.

Sacred practices—Religious practices, such as dietary taboos or lighting of candles, that a person is commanded to follow.

Santeria—A syncretic religion comprising both African and Catholic beliefs.

Santero(a)—Traditional priest and healer in the religion of *Santeria*.

Secular—Beliefs and practices that are not under the auspices of a religious body.

Self-denialism—Taking great pleasure from having less than is necessary.

Senoria—A woman who is knowledgeable about the causes and treatment of illness.

Sexism—Belief that members of one sex are superior to those of the other sex.

Shrine—A place—natural, secular, and/or affiliated with a religious tradition—where people make spiritual journeys or pilgrimages for the purposes of giving thanks or petitioning for favors. They are related to magico-religious folk medicine, and the use of charms, holy words, and holy actions, such as prayer, may be observed.

Singer—A type of traditional American Indian healer who is able to practice singing as a form of treating a health problem.

Skilly—An agent that is believed to cause disease by traditional Cherokee people.

Social organization—Patterns of cultural behavior related to life events, such as birth, death, childrearing, and health and illness, that are followed within a given social group.

Socialization—Process of being raised within a culture and acquiring the characteristics of the group.

Soul loss—Belief that a person's soul can leave the body, wander around, and then return.

Space—Area surrounding a person's body and the objects within that area.

Spell—A magical word or formula or a condition of evil or bad luck.

Sphygmopalpation—Traditional Chinese medical way of diagnosing a health problem by feeling pulses.

Spirit—The noncorporeal and nonmental dimension of a person that is the source of meaning and unity. The source of the experience of spirituality and every religion.

Spirit possession—Belief that a spirit can enter people, possess them, and control what they say and do.

Spiritual—Ideas, attitudes, concepts, beliefs, and behaviors that are the result of a person's experience of the spirit.

Spirituality—The experience of meaning and unity.

Stargazing—Example of a traditional American Indian practice of praying the star prayer to the star spirit as a method of divination.

Stereotype—Notion that all people from a given group are the same.

Superstition—Belief that performing an action, wearing a charm or an amulet, or eating something will have an influence on life events. These beliefs are upheld by magic and faith.

Susto (**soul loss**)—Traditional Hispanic belief that the soul is able to leave a person's body.

Szatan—The traditional Polish term for the "evil eye."

Taboo—A culture-bound ban that excludes certain behaviors from common use.

Talisman—Consecrated religious object that confers power of various kinds and protects people who wear, carry, or own them from harm and evil.

Tao—Way, path, or discourse. On the spiritual level, the way to ultimate reality.

Time—Duration, interval of time. Instances, points in time.

Tirisia—Anxiety.

Title VI—Under the provisions of Title VI of the Civil Rights Act of 1964, people with Limited English Proficiency (LEP) who are cared for in such health care settings as extended care facilities, public assistance programs, nursing homes, and hospitals and are eligible for Medicaid, other health care, or human services cannot be denied assistance because of their race, color, or national origin.

Traditional—Ancient, ethnocultural-religious beliefs and practices that have been handed down through the generations.

Traditional epidemiology—Belief in agents other than those of a scientific nature, causing disease. These could be such agents as "envy," "jealousy," and "hate."

Traditionalism—Belief in the traditional HEALTH, ILLNESS, and HEALING methods of a given cultural cohort.

Tui Na—A complex Chinese system of massage, "pushing and pulling," using meridian stimulation used to treat orthopedic and neurological problems.

Undocumented alien—Person of foreign origin who has entered the country unlawfully by bypassing inspection or who has overstayed the original terms of admission.

Universalism—Open beliefs in many domains that may not be part of a given personal heritage.

Unlocking—Steps taken to help break down and understand the definitions of the terms *health/HEALTH* and *illness/ILLNESS* in a living context. It consists of persistent questioning: What is health? No matter what the response, the question "What does that mean?" is asked. Initially, this causes much confusion, but as each term is analyzed the process makes sense.

Voodoo—A religion that is a combination of Christianity and African Yoruba religious beliefs.

Vulnerability—The state of being weak or prone to an adverse event or emotional or physical danger.

Witched—Example of a traditional American Indian belief that a person is harmed by witches.

Xenophobia—Morbid fear of strangers.

Yang—Male, positive energy that produces light, warmth, and fullness.

Yin—Female, negative energy. The force of darkness, cold, and emptiness.

Yoruba—The African tribe whose myths and rites are the basis of *Santeria*.

---

*These terms are defined with their traditional connotations, rather than with modern denotations (compiled over time by R. Spector).

Appendix B

Calendar: Religious Holidays That Change Dates

There are many Holy Days observed by people from many different religious heritages that do not fall on the same dates of the Julian calendar on an annual basis. Given the increasing amount of religious diversity in this country, it is imperative that consideration be given to this fact. Religious leaders of a given faith community must be contacted regarding the Julian dates of a given holiday and large meetings and other activities must not be scheduled at that time to cause conflict.

Heritage	Holiday	Approximate Date
Islam	Eid al-Fitr and Al Hisrah (New Year)	Varies
Chinese	Sending Off the Kitchen God Day	January
Islam	Laylat al-Qadr	January
Sikh	Guru Gobind Singh Ji's Birthday	January
Hindu	Makara Sakranti/Pongal	January
Chinese	New Year: Chinese, Korean, Tibetan, Vietnamese	February
Chinese	Lantern Festival	February
Baha'i	Intercalary Days	February or March
Hindu	Maha Shivaratri (Shiva's Night)	March
Christian	Shrove Monday	March
Christian	Shrove Tuesday	March
Christian	Ash Wednesday	March
Eastern Orthodox	Beginning of Lent, Eastern Orthodox Christian	March
Hindu	Holi	March
Iranian	Now Rouz	March
Chinese	Respect for Ancestors (Ch'ing-ming)	April
Islam	Muharram	April
Vietnamese	Thanh Minh (Respect for Ancestors Day)	April
Hindu	Ramanavami	April
Cambodian	New Year	April
Hindu	Vaisakhi (Solar New Year)	April
Sikh	Baisakhi (New Year)	April
Jain	Mahavir Jayanti	April
Christian	Palm Sunday	April
Jewish	Passover begins at sundown	April

Heritage	Holiday	Approximate Date
Jewish	Passover	April
Christian	Good Friday	April
Baha'i	Festival of Ridvan	April
Christian	Easter	April
Eastern Orthodox	Palm Sunday	April (a week after Christian Palm Sunday)
Christian	Easter Monday	April
Eastern Orthodox Christian	Good Friday	April (a week after Christian Good Friday)
Eastern Orthodox	Easter: Eastern Orthodox, also known as Pascha	April
Buddhist	Visakaha Day	May
Chinese	Dragon Boat Festival	June
Eastern Orthodox	Ascension Day	June
Jewish	Shavuoth begins at sundown	May or June
Christian	Pentecost	June
Islam	Maulid an-Nabi	June
Eastern Orthodox	Pentacost	June
Chinese	Seventh Night	August
Jewish	Tisha B' Av Fast Day	July or August
Hindu	Janmashtami	August
Korean	Chusok	September
Coptic Christian	Coptic New Year	September
Chinese	Midautumn Moon Festival—Chung-ch'iu	September
Jewish	Rosh Hashanah begins at sundown	September
Hindu	Durga Puja	October
Jewish	Yom Kippur begins at sundown	September or October
Jewish	Yom Kippur	October
Jewish	Sukkoth begins at sundown	October
Baha'i	Birthday of the Bab	October
Jewish	Shmini Atzeret begins at sundown	October
Jewish	Simchat Torah begins at sundown	October
Hindu	Diwali	October
Sikh	Nanak's Birthday	November
Baha'i	Birthday of Baha'u'llah	November
Islam	Ramadan	Varies

Source: Adapted from *Multicultural resource calendar.* (2000). Amherst, MA: Amherst Educational Publishing, 800-865-5549 or visit http://www.diversityresources.com. An annual calendar is available with the exact dates for the given holidays.

Appendix C

Suggested Course Outline

■ Capstone[1]: Holistic Living

Culture is the soul of life. It is what gives us roots, gives our lives meaning, and binds us to each other.

> —*Hillary Rodham Clinton, 12/5/98, Clinton Library,*
> *Little Rock, Arkansas*

The purposes of this course are to

1. Examine spirituality, community, personal and family relationships, and education through the lenses of cross-cultural holistic HEALTH[2] and HEALING practices.
2. Bring the student into a direct relationship with health care consumers from various cultural backgrounds—American Indian and Alaska Native, Asian/Pacific Islander, Black, Hispanic, and White populations.

Selected readings, films, and field visits will assist you to visualize the relationship of HEALTH to the holistic aspects of your life and that of the multicultural communities in which you will live and work. Through this study, the course will provide insight into the nature of health/HEALTH, the comparisons of health/HEALTH and healing/HEALING practices cross-culturally, and the consequences of health/ HEALTH–related choices.

---

[1]Capstone courses are university courses, coordinated in the Theology Department of Boston College and open to senior students throughout the university. A Capstone Seminar is an intensely personal experience for seniors and is just as intensely a shared experience with their peers and professor. The seminar is kept to about 15 students to promote that sharing. The format of the seminar combines a deep exploration of the self with a disciplined academic exercise in substantive reading, writing, and discussion. Each seminar prompts the student to look both backward and forward. It asks, "What have you made of your Boston College education? What has it made of you?" It also inquires, "How will you carry out the lifelong commitments you have begun to envision?" These questions go to the heart of the seniors' concerns. Thus, Capstone Seminars provide a place where students can ponder ultimate questions within a community of discourse.

[2]*HEALTH* used in this manner connotes the balance of the person, both within one's being—physical, mental, and spiritual—and in the outside environment—natural, familial and communal, and metaphysical.

357

The course content includes discussion of the following topics:

■ Cultural heritage and its contribution to health/HEALTH beliefs and practices
■ Diversity, demographic and economic, existing in contemporary society
■ Health care providers' and patients' ways of understanding the maintenance, protection, and restoration of health/HEALTH and illness/ILLNESS and related problems
■ Cultural and institutional factors that affect the patients' access to and use of health care resources

Course Purpose and Process

Capstone courses are designed to provide you with the opportunity to reflect upon and integrate your education and life experiences in preparation for your future life. This course aims at studying spirituality, the duties of citizenship, vocation/career, education, and personal relationships through the lenses of HEALTH and holistic living.

Two of the most significant tasks of your adult life will be

1. The development of CULTURALCOMPETENCY, given the dramatic demographic changes occurring in the United States and the globalization of the marketplace
2. Negotiating and advocating for comprehensive HEALTH care for
   a. Self and family
   b. Patients/clients from diverse cultural backgrounds

In fact, the development of an understanding of diversity within a HEALTH-centered focus leads to a broad understanding of and sensitivity to issues related to the larger issues of multiculturalism.

Ordinarily, a course dedicated to both HEALTH and holistic living would be structured to examine health practices and methods that may be employed to modify your health behaviors and choices. But, in this course, we will examine your HEALTH from a much deeper perspective and explore ways of expanding this concept to include social justice and work and the relationship that these concepts have to HEALTH. In each of the areas, we will use novels or films, guest speakers, and/or field trips to broaden your perspectives of HEALTH, holistic living, and cultural diversity. You will see the relationships of HEALTH to the holistic aspects of your life and that of the communities in which you will live and work.

Course Objectives

On completion of this course, the student will

1. Discuss the meanings of culture, ethnicity, religion, and socialization and their contribution to health/HEALTH beliefs and practices.
2. Discuss the diversity, demographic and economic, existing in contemporary society.

3. Discuss his or her ethnocultural heritage and socialization.
4. Analyze selected aspects of the modern health care delivery system.
5. Understand more fully the perception and meaning of health/HEALTH and illness among recipients of health care.
6. Deepen his or her understanding about self and reflect on what has been learned about personal HEALTH and cultural diversity.
7. Explore his or her existing knowledge about personal HEALTH care and holistic living.
8. Develop a long-term awareness about his or her role in citizenship, vocation/career, education, and personal relationships that is impacted on by both HEALTH and cultural diversity.
9. Develop an understanding and respect for the HEALTH traditions of people from many different cultural heritages.
10. Develop an understanding of the similarities and differences of culturally determined HEALTH traditions (beliefs and practices) and the relevance to overall cultural competency.

Texts

The following texts should be read in their entirety:

> Spector, R. E. (2009). *Cultural diversity in health and illness* (7th ed.). Upper Saddle River, NJ: Prentice Hall Health.
>
> Fadiman A. (1997). *The spirit catches you and you fall down*. New York: Farrar, Straus, Giroux.
>
> Kassirer, J. P. (2005). *On the take*. New York: Oxford University Press.

Course Content

   I. Culture, Diversity, and Heritage Consistency
  II. Perceptions of Health/HEALTH and Illness/ILLNESS
 III. Ethnocultural Familial Beliefs—Roots
  IV. Allopathic versus Homeopathic Philosophies
   V. Modern Health Care Delivery
  VI. Health/HEALTH and Illness/ILLNESS in Selected Populations

Teaching and Learning Methods

reading assignments	web assignments	field trips
discussion	films	seminars
academic project/paper		

Course Assignments

1. Class attendance and participation is mandatory.   25%
2. Weekly reflection & Web assignment   25%
3. Class presentation (with text)   Day of class   25%
4. Final integrating essay   Last class   25%

Films

Required:

> *Talk to Her*, Pedro Almodovar
> *Sicko*, Michael Moore

Class Schedule

The first 4 weeks set the stage with primary reflections on yourself and your family over time—what it was like as a child, in high school, and later, through the lenses of health/HEALTH.

Week 1—Introductions:
To each other, to Capstone, and to health/HEALTH and illness/ILLNESS and spirituality

Week 2—Culture, Ethnicity, Religion, and Diversity and their relationships to health/HEALTH and illness/ILLNESS
Readings: Spector, Chapters 1 and 2, Fadiman

Week 3—Americana—From Osteopathic Medicine, Homeopathic Medicine, and over-the-counter Medicines to New Age Spirituality
Readings & Activity: Spector, Chapters 3, 4, 5

Week 4—Health and HEALTH of our parents and ancestors
Chapter 6 & Discuss Ethnohealth Family Interviews

The second 4 weeks explore the dynamics of moving to the duties of citizenship, vocation/career, education, and personal relationships again through the lenses of health/HEALTH and illness/ILLNESS.

Weeks 5 & 6—The Western (Modern) Health Care System
Reading: Spector, Chapter 7, and *On the Take*
Film: *Sicko*

Week 7—Traditional (Homeopathic) Medicine and Spiritual HEALTH Care
Reading: Spector, Chapters 4 & 5

Week 8—Midterm Discussion: *The Spirit Catches You and You Fall Down* and Film—*Talk to Her*

The remainder of this class explores the spiritual aspects of HEALTH by examining spirituality as it is found in the HEALTH traditions of selected ethnocultural populations. The comparison to your own experiences of spirituality, primarily in respect to the notion of Holistic Living, will become the central focus of reflection.

Week 9—American Indian HEALTH Traditions
    Reading: Spector, Chapter 8; Film—*Dances with Wolves*
Week 10—Asian American HEALTH Traditions
    Reading: Spector, Chapter 9; Film—*The Joy Luck Club*
Week 11—Black American HEALTH Traditions
    Reading: Spector, Chapter 10; Film—*Boys in the Hood*
Week 12—Hispanic American HEALTH Traditions
    Reading: Spector, Chapter 11; Film—*El Norte*
Week 13—White or European American HEALTH Traditions
    Reading: Spector, Chapter 12; Film—*The Sorceress*
Week 14—Implications for Your Personal and Professional Future Life
    Reading—Spector, Epilogue
Week 15—HEALTHY HEALTH Traditions Cultural Banquet

EthnoHEALTH Family Interview

In preparation for the week 4 class, I am asking each of you to interview your *maternal* grandmother, your mother, or a *maternal* aunt. Please ask her for the following information:

1. Ethnic background

   Country of origin

   Religion

   Number of generations in U.S.

2. What does she do to *maintain HEALTH*? Also, if she can remember, what did her mother do?

3. What does she do to *protect HEALTH*? Also, if she can remember, what did her mother do?

4. What "home remedies" does she use to *restore HEALTH*? Also, if she can remember, what did her mother do?

5. How do her religious/spiritual beliefs define *birth*? What rituals accompany this event?

6. How do her religious/spiritual beliefs define *illness*? What rituals accompany this event?

7. How do her religious/spiritual beliefs define *healing*? What rituals accompany this event?

8. How do her religious/spiritual beliefs define *death*? What rituals accompany this event?

(Since I retired from the Boston College Connell School of Nursing in 2003, I have continued to teach this class at Boston College in the Theology Department to nursing, premed, and students from many other majors, including management, psychology, and political science. The course has been oversubscribed and well received by the students.)

Appendix D

Suggested Course Activity— Urban Hiking

We simply need that wild country available to us, even if we never do more than drive to its edge and look in. For it can be a means of reassuring ourselves of our sanity as creatures, a part of the geography of hope.

—*Wallace Stegner,*
plaque on Forest Service sign, Maroon Bells, Aspen, Colorado

Urban hiking—what is this? It is taking skills, knowledge, and curiosity applied to the great outdoors and applying it to peopled areas. It is an extraordinary way to tantalize your senses as you

1. See—the infrastructure of a new or familiar place, the housing stock, the stores and small businesses, the transportation system, the pharmacies, houses of worship, and so forth.
2. Hear—listen to the symphony of voices, traffic, and music.
3. Taste—new foods by eating in neighborhood restaurants.
4. Smell—food as it is prepared on the streets, in homes, or in restaurants.
5. Feel—the textures of different fabrics and objects.

It is a way to witness and learn about cultural diversity and the New America and to erase fears of the unknown social and cultural phenomena that may impede your ability to embrace the demographic changes occurring in the United States in 2008 and to embrace the vitality and excitement of change, for, as Stegner looks to the "wild country," one can look to the streets of a city or town and successfully realize that "this is a means of reassuring ourselves of our sanity as creatures," a part of the geography of American LIFE!

Needed are a good map, comfortable walking shoes, comfortable clothing, personal identification, and small amount of money for transportation, water, and food. There is no need to pack a lunch; restaurants are more than plentiful. And, of course, the greatest importance is a **good sense of humor and adventure.**

Indeed, the study of cultural diversity comes alive the moment you leave the confines of the classroom and go out into the community. One way to appreciate a given ethnoreligious community is to go into a community and observe firsthand what daily life is like for a member of the community. The following outline can serve as an assessment guide to the target community and facilitate the understanding of CULTURALCARE.

Demographic data
Total population size of entire city or town

Breakdown by areas—residential concentrations

Specific focus on demographics of the target community

Breakdown by ages

Other breakdowns

Education

Occupations

Income

Nations of origin of residents of the location and the target neighborhood

Traditional health/HEALTH and illness/ILLNESS beliefs and practices

- Definition of *health/HEALTH*
- Definition of *illness/ILLNESS*
- Overall health status

Traditional causes of illness/ILLNESS, such as

- Poor eating habits
- Wrong food combinations
- Punishment from God
- The evil eye
- Hexes, spells, or envy
- Witchcraft
- Environmental changes
- Exposure to drafts
- Grief and loss

Traditional methods of maintaining health/HEALTH

Traditional methods of protecting health/HEALTH

Traditional methods of restoring health/HEALTH

Home remedies

Visits to physicians, nurse practitioners, traditional healers, or other health care resources

Health care resources, such as neighborhood health centers

Traditional pharmacies, such as a *botanica*

Childbearing beliefs and practices

Childrearing beliefs and practices

Rituals and beliefs surrounding death and dying

Go on a "hike" through the community. Identify the various services that are available. If possible, visit a community health care provider, visit a church or community center within the neighborhood, visit grocery stores and pharmacies and point out differences in foods and over-the-counter remedies, and eat a meal in a neighborhood restaurant.

I have shared this experience with many groups of students over the years, and the experience has been well received.

Appendix E

Heritage Assessment Tool

This set of questions is to be used to describe a person's—or your own—ethnic, cultural, and religious background. In performing a *heritage assessment* it is helpful to determine how deeply a person identifies with his or her traditional heritage. This tool is very useful in setting the stage for assessing and understanding a person's traditional HEALTH and ILLNESS beliefs and practices and in helping determine the community resources that will be appropriate to target for support when necessary. The greater the number of positive responses, the greater the degree to which the person may identify with his or her traditional heritage. The one exception to positive answers is the question about whether a person's name was changed. The background rationale for the development of this tool is found in Chapter 1.

1. Where was your mother born? _____

2. Where was your father born? _____

3. Where were your grandparents born? _____

   A. Your mother's mother? _____

   B. Your mother's father? _____

   C. Your father's mother? _____

   D. Your father's father? _____

4. How many brothers _____ and sisters _____ do you have?

5. What setting did you grow up in? Urban _____ Rural _____

6. What country did your parents grow up in?

   Father _____

   Mother _____

7. How old were you when you came to the United States? _____

8. How old were your parents when they came to the United States?

   Mother _____

   Father _____

9. When you were growing up, who lived with you?_____

_____

10. Have you maintained contact with

    A. Aunts, uncles, cousins?   (1) Yes ____ (2) No ____
    B. Brothers and sisters?   (1) Yes ____ (2) No ____
    C. Parents?   (1) Yes ____ (2) No ____
    D. Your own children?   (1) Yes ____ (2) No ____

11. Did most of your aunts, uncles, and cousins live near your home?
    (1) Yes ____
    (2) No ____

12. Approximately how often did you visit family members who lived outside of your home?
    (1) Daily ____
    (2) Weekly ____
    (3) Monthly ____
    (4) Once a year or less ____
    (5) Never ____

13. Was your original family name changed?
    (1) Yes ____
    (2) No ____

14. What is your religious preference?
    (1) Catholic ____
    (2) Jewish ____
    (3) Protestant ____ Denomination ____
    (4) Other ____
    (5) None ____

15. Is your spouse the same religion as you?
    (1) Yes ____
    (2) No ____

16. Is your spouse the same ethnic background as you?
    (1) Yes ____
    (2) No ____

17. What kind of school did you go to?
    (1) Public ____
    (2) Private ____
    (3) Parochial ____

18. As an adult, do you live in a neighborhood where the neighbors are the same religion and ethnic background as you?
    (1) Yes ____
    (2) No ____

19. Do you belong to a religious institution?
    (1) Yes ____
    (2) No ____

20. Would you describe yourself as an active member?
    (1) Yes ____
    (2) No ____
21. How often do you attend your religious institution?
    (1) More than once a week ____
    (2) Weekly ____
    (3) Monthly ____
    (4) Special holidays only ____
    (5) Never ____
22. Do you practice your religion in your home?
    (1) Yes ____ (if yes, please specify)
    (2) No ____
    (3) Praying ____
    (4) Bible reading ____
    (5) Diet ____
    (6) Celebrating religious holidays ____
23. Do you prepare foods special to your ethnic background?
    (1) Yes ____
    (2) No ____
24. Do you participate in ethnic activities?
    (1) Yes ____ (if yes, please specify)
    (2) No ____
    (3) Singing ____
    (4) Holiday celebrations ____
    (5) Dancing ____
    (6) Festivals ____
    (7) Costumes ____
    (8) Other ____
25. Are your friends from the same religious background as you?
    (1) Yes ____
    (2) No ____
26. Are your friends from the same ethnic background as you?
    (1) Yes ____
    (2) No ____
27. What is your native language other than English? _____
28. Do you speak this language?
    (1) Prefer ____
    (2) Occasionally ____
    (3) Rarely ____
29. Do you read your native language?
    (1) Yes ____
    (2) No ____

Appendix F

Quick Guide for CULTURALCARE

Preparing

- Understand your own cultural values, biases, and traditional health/HEALTH beliefs and practices.
- Acquire basic knowledge of cultural values and health/HEALTH beliefs and practices for patient groups you serve.
- Be respectful of, interested in, and understanding of other cultures without being judgmental.

Enhancing Communication

- Determine the level of fluency in English and arrange for a competent interpreter, when needed.
- Ask how the patient prefers to be addressed.
- Allow the patient to choose seating for comfortable personal space and eye contact. If the patient prefers *not* to establish eye contact, do not become upset. In many cultures, it is considered polite to avoid eye contact.
- Avoid body language and gestures that may be offensive or misunderstood.
- Speak directly and quietly to the patient, whether an interpreter is present or not.
- Choose a speech rate and style that promotes understanding and demonstrates respect for the patient.
- Avoid slang, technical jargon, and complex sentences.
- Use open-ended questions or questions phrased in several ways to obtain information.
- Determine the patient's reading ability before using written materials in the teaching process.
- Provide reading material that is easily read in the patient's native language. Do not use cartoons and cartoon characters for illustrations.

Promoting Positive Change

- Build on cultural HEALTH practices, reinforcing those that are positive and promoting change only in those that are potentially harmful.
- Check for patient understanding and acceptance of recommendations.
- Remember: Not all seeds of knowledge fall into a fertile environment to produce change. Of those that do, some will take years to germinate. Be patient and provide CULTURALCARE nursing in a culturally appropriate environment to promote positive health/HEALTH behavior.

Source: (Adapted for nursing) Schilling, B., & Brannon, E. (1986). *Cross-cultural counseling—A guide for nutrition and health counselors.* Alexandria, VA: U.S. Department of Agriculture, U.S. Department of Health and Human Services, Nutrition and Technical Services Division. Adapted with permission.

Appendix G

Data Resources

Countless invaluable resources are available in both the public and private sectors.

1. The United States Census
2. United States Citizenship and Immigration Services
3. Office for Civil Rights
4. National Center for Health Statistics—*Healthy People 2010*
5. National Health Statistics
6. Health Resources and Services Administration (HRSA)
7. The Office of Minority Health
8. Complementary and alternative medicine
9. Specific health-related sites
10. Consumer information
11. Private sector

It is important to note that the URLs change; however, the new addresses are usually linked to the old site.

The United States Census

http://www.census.gov

This page provides links to census information at national, state, county, and local levels.

It also has statistics related to income, housing, and so forth.

Homeland Security

This agency has responsibility for information regarding immigration, commerce and trade, and emergency preparedness.

http://www.dhs.gov/index.shtm

United States Citizenship and Immigration Services

http://www.uscis.gov/portal/site/uscis

This site has information regarding citizenship application process.

http://www.usimmigrationsupport.org/?NS_cid=1

This site has helpful information for immigrants.

Office for Civil Rights

The Office for Civil Rights is located within the U.S. Department of Health and Human Services and is responsible for enforcing the nondiscrimination requirements of **Title VI of the Civil Rights Act of 1964.**

http://www.hhs.gov/ocr/discrimrace.html

National Center for Health Statistics—*Healthy People 2010*

The purpose of the National Center for Health Statistics is to monitor the nation's health. The goals have been set for health status for 2010 and the *Healthy People 2010 Mid-course Review* is now available online. This publication assesses progress toward achieving the *Healthy People 2010* goals and objectives through the first half of the decade.

http://www.cdc.gov/nchs/hphome.htm

National Health Statistics

The database Health, United States, is available from this source annually and has current information on a myriad of population- and health-related issues.

http://www.cdc.gov/nchs/Default.htm

Health Resources and Services Administration (HRSA)

This site has information regarding health professions and the health care system.

http://www.hrsa.gov

Other government health-related resources include the following:

U.S. Department of Health and Human Services

This agency's goal is "improving the health, safety, and well-being of America."

http://www.dhhs.gov

Center for Medicare & Medicaid Services

The mission of this agency is to ensure effective, up-to-date health care coverage and to promote quality care for beneficiaries.

http://www.cms.hhs.gov

Center for Disease Control and Prevention

This site provides links to countless credible health information resources.

http://www.cdc.gov

CDC's National Center for Chronic Disease Prevention and Health Promotion

http://www.cdc.gov/nccdphp/

National Information Center on Health Services Research and Health Care Technology (NICHSR)

The purpose of this agency is improving the collection, storage, analysis, retrieval, and dissemination of health services research.

http://www.nlm.nih.gov/nichsr

Healthfinder

Since 1997, healthfinder.gov has been recognized as a key resource for finding the best government and nonprofit health and human services information on the Internet. There are links to carefully selected information and Web sites from over 1,500 health-related organizations.

http://www.healthfinder.gov

The Office of Minority Health

National Center on Minority Health and Health Disparities

The mission of the National Center on Minority Health and Health Disparities (NCMHD) is to promote minority health and to lead, coordinate, support, and assess the NIH effort to reduce and ultimately eliminate health disparities. In this effort NCMHD will conduct and support basic, clinical, social, and behavioral research, promote research infrastructure and training, and foster emerging programs.

http://www.ncmhd.nih.gov

Complementary and Alternative Medicine

The National Center for Complementary and Alternative Medicine (NCCAM) is the federal government's lead agency for scientific research on complementary and alternative medicine (CAM). The mission of NCCAM is to

- Explore complementary and alternative healing practices in the context of rigorous science
- Train complementary and alternative medicine researchers
- Disseminate authoritative information to the public and professionals

http://nccam.nih.gov/

Specific Health-Related Sites—Public Resources

Aging

National Aging Information Center

The bibliographic database is managed by the Center for Communication and Consumer Services (CCCS). It contains references to program- and policy-related materials on aging not referenced in any other computer system or print resource. The database is intended to serve the State Units on Aging, Area Agencies on Aging, national aging organizations, aging services providers, legislators at all levels, policymakers, and the general public.

http://www.aoa.gov/naic

National Institute on Aging

http://www.nih.gov/nia/health

AIDS/HIV

AIDSinfo

AIDS*info* is a U.S. Department of Health and Human Services (DHHS) project that offers the latest federally approved information on HIV/AIDS clinical research, treatment and prevention, and medical practice guidelines for people living with HIV/AIDS, their families and friends, health care providers, scientists, and researchers.

http://www.hivatis.org

Diabetes

National Diabetes Surveillance System

The CDC Diabetes Surveillance System collects, analyzes, and disseminates data on diabetes and its complications. This public health surveillance (disease tracking) of diabetes is critical to

- Increase recognition of the disease
- Identify high-risk groups
- Develop strategies to reduce the economic and human cost of this disease
- Formulate health care policy
- Evaluate progress in disease prevention and control

The current Diabetes Surveillance System updates data from previous reports and will also contain new surveillance topics.

http://www.cdc.gov/diabetes/statistics/index.htm#prevalence

National Diabetes Education Program

http://ndep.nih.gov

Cancer

National Cancer Institute

This site contains links to a myriad of information regarding all aspects of cancer from diagnosis through various treatment modalities and options.

http://www.cancer.gov/

Heart Disease and Heart Health

National Heart, Lung, and Blood Institute (NHLBI) Health Information Center

The National Heart, Lung, and Blood Institute provides global leadership for a research, training, and education program to promote the prevention and treatment of heart, lung, and blood diseases and fulfilling lives.

http://www.nhlbi.nih.gov

Immunization

The National Immunization Program (NIP): Centers for Disease Control and Prevention

http://www.cdc.gov/vaccines

Injury Prevention

National Center for Injury Prevention and Control (NCIPC)

http://www.cdc.gov/ncipc

Lead Poisoning

National Lead Information Center

This site provides information about lead and lead hazards and provides some simple steps to protect the family.

http://www.epa.gov/lead/

Rural Health

Rural Information Center Health Service (RICHS)

Rural Health Funding Sources: National Foundations

This guide represents private and nonprofit foundations that fund programs related to rural health.

http://www.nal.usda.gov/ric/ricpubs/foundat.htm

San Francisco State University

Unnatural Causes: Is Inequality Making Us Sick?

An excellent film series about what are the sources of sickness in 2008.

http://www.pbs.org/unnaturalcauses/Or 1-877-7495.

Consumer Information Center

The Federal Citizen Information Center

USA.gov is the official portal to all government information, services, and transactions. This site pulls together more than 180 million federal, state, and local government Web pages. Here, citizens can get easy-to-understand information and services from the government 24 hours a day, 7 days a week. They can also use an e-mail form to send questions and comments in English and Spanish for a response within 2 business days.

http://www.usa.gov

Private Sector

There are countless agencies available in this sector, including numerous networks. The following Web page is a well-developed resource to link to the agencies.

http://www.healthpowerforminorities.org/resources/national.cfm

(The URLs of all sites listed have been checked and are current as of this publishing date.)

Johnson and Johnson Diabetes Institute

Addresses the shortage in diabetes specific training and offers training

http://www.jjdi.us/

Bibliography

Abraham, L. K. (1993). *Mama might be better off dead: The failure of health care in urban America*. Chicago: University of Chicago Press.

Abrahams, P. (1954). *Tell freedom: Memories of Africa*. New York: Knopf.

Achebe, C. (1987). *Anthills of Savannah*. New York: Anchor Press/Doubleday.

Achebe, C. (1959). *Things fall apart*. Greenwich, CT: Fawcett Crest.

Achterberg, J., Dossey, B., & Kolkmeier, L. (1994). *Rituals of healing: Using imagery for health and wellness*. New York: Bantam Books.

Aday, L. A. (1993). *At risk in America—The health and health care needs of vulnerable populations in the United States*. San Francisco: Jossey-Bass.

Aiken, L. G. (1981). *Health policy and nursing practice*. New York: McGraw-Hill.

Aiken, R. (1980). *Mexican folk tales from the borderland*. Dallas, TX: Southern Methodist University Press.

Albrecht, G. L., & Higgens, P. C. (Eds.). (1979). *Health, illness, and medicine*. Chicago: Rand McNally.

Alcott, W. A. (1839). *The house I live in; or the human body*. Boston, MA: George W. Light.

Allende, I. (1993). *The house of the spirits*. New York: Bantam Books.

Allison, D. (1992). *Bastard out of Carolina*. New York: Plume.

Allport, G. W. (1958). *The nature of prejudice* (abridged). Garden City, NY: Doubleday.

Alvarez, H. R. (1975). *Health without boundaries*. Mexico: United States–Mexico Border Public Health Association.

Alvarez, J. (1992). *How the Garcia girls lost their accents*. New York: Plume.

Ameer Ali, S. (1922, 1978). *The spirit of Islam*. Delhi, India: IDARAH-I-ADABIYAT-I-DELLI.

American Nurses' Association. (1979, June 9–10). *A strategy for change*. Papers presented at the conference of the Commission on Human Rights, Albuquerque, NM.

American Psychiatric Association. (1994). *Diagnostic and statistical manual of mental disorders* (4th ed.). Washington, DC: Author.

Anderson, D. M. (1995). *Maasai people of cattle*. San Francisco: Chronicle Books.

Anderson, E. T., & McFarlane, J. M. (1988). *Community as client*. Philadelphia, PA: J. B. Lippincott.

Anderson, J. Q. (1970). *Texas folk medicine*. Austin, TX: Encino Press.

Andrade, S. J. (1978). *Chicano mental health: The case of cristal*. Austin: Hogg Foundation for Mental Health.

Andrews, E. D. (1953). *The people called Shakers*. New York: Dover.

Andrews, M. M., & Boyle, J. S. (1995). *Transcultural concepts in nursing care* (2nd ed.). Philadelphia, PA: J. B. Lippincott.

Angelou, M. (1970). *I know why the caged bird sings*. New York: Random House.

Annas, G. J. (1975). *The rights of hospital patients*. New York: Avon.

Appelfeld, A. (1990). *The healer*. New York: Grove Weidenfeld.

Apple, D. (Ed.). (1960). *Sociological studies of health and sickness: A source book for the health professions*. New York: McGraw-Hill, Blakiston Division.

Archer, S. E., & Fleshman, R. P. (1985). *Community health nursing* (3rd ed.). Monterey, CA: Wadsworth.

Armstrong, D., & Armstrong, E. M. (1991). *The great American medicine show*. New York: Prentice Hall.

Arnold, M. G., & Rosenbaum, G. (1973). *The crime of poverty*. Skokie, IL: National Textbook Co.

Ashely, J. (1976). *Hospitals, paternalism, and the role of the nurse*. New York: Teachers College Press.

Aurand, A. M., Jr. (n.d.). *The realness of witchcraft in America*. Lancaster, PA: Aurand Press.

Ausubel, N. (1964). *The book of Jewish knowledge*. New York: Crown.

Bahti, T. (1974). *Southwestern Indian ceremonials*. Las Vegas: KC Publications.

Bahti, T. (1975). *Southwestern Indian tribes*. Las Vegas: KC Publications.

Bakan, D. (1968). *Disease, pain, and sacrifice: Toward a psychology of suffering*. Chicago: University of Chicago Press.

Baker, G. C. (1994). *Planning and organizing for multicultural instruction* (2nd ed.). Menlo Park, CA: Addison-Wesley.

Balch, J. F., & Balch, P. A. (1990). *Prescription for nutritional healing*. Garden City Park, NY: Avery.

Baldwin, R. (1986). *The healers*. Huntington, IN: Our Sunday Visitor.

Banks, J. A. (Ed.). (1973). *Teaching ethnic studies*. Washington, DC: National Council for Social Studies.

Bannerman, R. H., Burton, J., & Wen-Chieh, C. (1983). *Traditional medicine and health care coverage*. Geneva: World Health Organization.

Barden, T. E. (Ed.). (1991). *Virginia folk legends*. Charlottesville: University Press of Virginia.

Bauwens, E. F. (1979). *The anthropology of health*. St. Louis, MO: C. V. Mosby.

Bear, S., & Bear, W. (1996). *The medicine wheel*. New York: Fireside.

Beaudoin, T. (1998). *Virtual Faith: The irreverent spiritual quest of generation X*. San Francisco: Jossey Bass.

Becerra, R. M., & Shaw, D. (1984). *The elderly Hispanic: A research and reference guide*. Lanham, MD: University Press of America.

Becker, M. H. (1974). *The health belief model and personal health behavior*. Thorofare, NJ: Slack.

Beimler, R. R. (1991). *The days of the dead*. San Francisco: Collins Publishers.

Belgium, D. (Ed.). (1967). *Religion and medicine*. Ames: Iowa State University Press.

Ben-Amos, D., & Mintz, J. R. (1970). *In praise of the Baal Shem Tov*. New York: Shocken Books.

Benedict, R. (1946). *Patterns of culture*. New York: Penguin Books.

Benjamin, G. G. (1910, reprint 1974). *The Germans in Texas*. Austin: Jenkins.

Bennett, C. I. (1990). *Comprehensive multicultural education* (2nd ed.). Boston: Allyn and Bacon.

Benson, H. (1996). *Timeless healing*. New York: Scribner.

Berg, D. J. (Ed.). (1986). *Homestead hints*. Berkeley, CA: Ten Speed Press.

Berg, P. S. (Ed.). (1977). *An entrance to the tree of life*. Jerusalem, Israel: Research Center for Kabbalah.

Berman, E. (1976). *The solid gold stethoscope*. New York: Macmillan Co.

Bermann, E. (1973). *Scapegoat*. Ann Arbor: University of Michigan Press.

Bernardo, A. (n.d.). *Lourdes: Then and now*. Trans. Rand, P. T. Lourdes, France: Etablissements Estrade.

Bernardo, S. (1981). *The ethnic almanac*. Garden City, NY: Doubleday.

Berwick, D. M., Godfrey, A. B., & Roessner, J. (1990). *Curing health care*. San Francisco: Jossey-Bass.

Bienvenue, R. M., & Goldstein, J. E. (1979). *Ethnicity and ethnic relations in Canada* (2nd ed.). Toronto: Butterworths.

Birnbaum, P. (1988). *Encyclopedia of Jewish concepts.* New York: Hebrew.

Bishop, G. (1967). *Faith healing: God or fraud?* Los Angeles: Shervourne Press.

Bohannan, P. (1992). *We, the alien.* Prospect Heights, IL: Waveland Press, Inc.

Boney, W. (1939). *The French Canadians today.* London: J. M. Dent and Sons.

Bonfanti, L. (1974). *Biographies and legends of the New England Indians,* Vol. 4. Wakefield, MA: Pride.

Bonfanti, L. (1980). *Strange beliefs, customs, and superstitions of New England.* Wakefield, MA: Pride.

Bottomore, T. B. (1968). *Classes in modern society.* New York: Vintage Books.

Bowen, E. S. (1964). *Return to laughter.* Garden City, NY: Doubleday.

Bowker, J. (1991). *The meanings of death.* Cambridge: Cambridge University Press.

Boyd, D. (1974). *Rolling thunder.* New York: Random House.

Boyle, J. S., & Andrews, M. M. (1995). *Transcultural concepts in nursing care* (2nd ed.). Philadelphia, PA: J. B. Lippincott.

Bracq, J. C. (1924). *The evolution of French Canada.* New York: Macmillan.

Bradley, C. J. (1980). "Characteristics of Women and Infants Attended by Lay Midwives in Texas, 1971: A Case Comparison Study." Master's thesis, University of Texas Health Science Center at Houston, School of Public Health.

Branch, M. F., & Paxton, P. P. (1976). *Providing safe nursing care for ethnic people of color.* New York: Appleton-Century-Crofts.

Brand, J. (1978). *The life and death of Anna Mae Aquash.* Toronto: James Lorimer.

Brandon, G. (1997). *Santeria: From Africa to the New World.* Bloomington: University of Indiana Press.

Brink, J., & Keen, L. (1979). *Feverfew.* London: Century.

Brink, P. J. (Ed.). (1976). *Transcultural nursing: A book of readings.* Englewood Cliffs, NJ: Prentice Hall.

Brown, D. (1970). *Bury my heart at Wounded Knee.* New York: Holt, Rinehart & Winston.

Brown, D. (1980). *Creek Mary's blood.* New York: Holt, Rinehart & Winston.

Browne, G., Howard, J., & Pitts, M. (1985). *Culture and children.* Austin: University of Texas Press.

Browne, K., & Freeling, P. (1967). *The doctor–patient relationship.* Edinburgh: E & S Livingstone.

Brownlee, A. T. (1979). *Community, culture, and care: A cross cultural guide for healthworkers.* St. Louis, MO: C. V. Mosby.

Bruchac, J. (1985). *Iroquois stories heroes and heroines monsters and magic.* Freedom, CA: Crossing Press.

Bryant, C. A. (1985). *The cultural feast: An introduction to food and society.* St. Paul, MN: West.

Buchman, D. D. (1979). *Herbal medicine: The natural way to get well and stay well.* New York: Gramercy.

Budge, E. A. W. (1978). *Amulets and superstitions.* New York: Dover.

Bullough, B., & Bullough, V. L. (1972). *Poverty, ethnic identity, and health care.* New York: Appleton-Century-Crofts.

Bullough, V. L., & Bullough, B. (1982). *Health care for other Americans.* New York: Appleton-Century-Crofts.

Butler, H. (1967). *Doctor gringo.* New York: Rand McNally.

Buxton, J. (1973). *Religion and healing in Mandari.* Oxford: Clarendon Press.

Cafferty, P. S. J., Chiswick, B. R., Greeley, A. M., et al. (1983). *The dilemma of American immigration: Beyond the golden door.* New Brunswick, NJ: Transaction Books.

Cahill, R. E. (1990). *Olde New England's curious customs and cures.* Salem, MA: Old Saltbox Publishing House.

Cahill, R. E. (1990). *Strange superstitions.* Salem, MA: Old Saltbox Publishing House.

Calhoun, M. (1976). *Medicine show.* New York: Harper and Row.

Califano, J. (1994). *Radical surgery.* New York: Random House.

Campos, E. (1955). *Medicina popular: Supersticione credios e meizinhas* (2nd ed.). Rio de Janeiro: Livraria-Editora da Casa.

Candill, H. M. (1962). *Night comes to the Cumberlands.* Boston: Little, Brown.

Carnegie, M. E. (1987). *The path we tread: Blacks in nursing 1854–1984.* Philadelphia, PA: J. B. Lippincott.

Carson, V. B. (Ed.). (1989). *Spiritual dimensions of nursing practice.* Philadelphia, PA: W. B. Saunders.

Catlin, G. (1993). *North American Indian portfolios.* New York: Abbeville.

Chafets, Z. (1990). *Devil's night and other tales of Detroit.* New York: Vintage Books.

Chan, L. S., McCandless, R., Portnoy, B., et al. (1987). *Maternal and child health on the U.S.–Mexico border.* Austin: The University of Texas.

Chavira, L. (1975). *Curanderismo: An optional health-care system.* Edinburg, TX: Pan American University.

Chenault, L. R. (1938). *The Puerto Rican migrant in New York City.* New York: Columbia University Press.

Chiba, R. (1966). *The seven lucky gods of Japan.* Rutland, VT: Charles E. Tuttle Co.

Choron, J. (1964). *Death and modern man.* New York: Collier Books.

Chun, M. N. (1986). *Hawaiian medicine book.* Honolulu: Bess Press.

Chute, C. (1985). *The beans of Egypt, Maine.* New York: Ticknor & Fields.

Clark, A. (1978). *Culture, childbearing health professionals.* Philadelphia, PA: F. A. Davis.

Clark, A. L. (1981). *Culture and child rearing.* Philadelphia, PA: F. A. Davis.

Clark, M. (1959). *Health in the Mexican-American culture: A community study.* Berkeley: University of California Press.

Comas-Diaz, L., & Griffith, E. E. H. (1988). *Clinical guidelines in cross-cultural mental health.* New York: Wiley.

Committee on Medical Care Teaching (Eds.). (1958). *Readings in medical care.* Chapel Hill: University of North Carolina Press.

Conde, M. I. (1992). *Tituba, black witch of Salem.* New York: Ballantine Books.

Conway, M. (1974). *Rise gonna rise.* New York: Anchor Books.

Corish, J. L. (1923). *Health knowledge,* Vol. 1. New York: Domestic Health Society.

Cornacchia, H. J. (1976). *Consumer health.* St. Louis, MO: C. V. Mosby.

Corum, A. K. (1985). *Folk remedies from Hawai'i.* Honolulu: Bess Press.

Council of Churches. (1995). *Knowing my neighbor, religious beliefs and traditions at times of illness and death.* Springfield, MA: Visiting Nurse Hospice of Pioneer Valley.

Council on Cultural Diversity in Nursing Practice. (1994). *Proceedings of the Invitational Meeting on Multicultural Issues in the Nursing Workforce and Workplace.* Washington, DC: American Nurses Association.

Cowan, N. M., & Cowan, R. S. (1989). *Our parents' lives.* New York: Basic Books.

Cramer, M. E. (1923). *Divine science and healing*. Denver: Colorado College of Divine Science.

Crichton, M. (1970). *Five patients*. New York: Alfred A. Knopf.

Crispino, J. A. (1980). *Assimilation of ethnic groups: The Italian case*. Newark, NJ: New Jersey Center for Migration.

Cross, T. (1994). Understanding family resiliency from a relational worldview. In *Resiliency in families: Racial and ethnic minority families in America*. Madison: University of Wisconsin–Madison.

Crow Dog, L., & Erdoes, R. (1996). *Crow Dog*. San Francisco: Harper.

Culpeper, N. (1889). *Culpeper's complete herbal*. London: W. Foulsham.

Curry, M. A., project director. (1987). *Access to prenatal care: Key to preventing low birth weight*. Kansas City, MO: American Nurses Association.

Curtis, E. (1993). *Native American wisdom*. Philadelphia, PA: Running Press.

Cutter, C. (1850). *First book on anatomy, physiology, and hygiene, for grammar schools and families*. Boston, MA: Benjamin B. Mussey.

Danforth, L. M. (1982). *The death rituals of rural Greece*. Princeton, NJ: Princeton University Press.

Davis, F. (Ed.). (1966). *The nursing profession: Five sociological essays*. New York: Wiley.

Davis, R. (1998). *American voudou: Journey into a hidden world*. Denton, TX: University of North Texas Press.

DeBella, S., Martin, L., & Siddall, S. (1986). *Nurses' role in health care planning*. Norwalk, CT: Appleton-Century-Crofts.

De Castro, J. (1967). *The black book of hunger*. Boston, MA: Beacon Press.

Delaney, J., Lupton, M. J., & Toth, E. (1988). *The curse: A cultural history of menstruation*. Chicago: University of Chicago Press.

Deller, B., Hicks, D., & MacDonald, G., coordinators. (1979). *Stone boats and lone stars*. Hyde Park, Ontario: Middlesex County Board of Education.

Deloria, V. Jr. (1969). *Custer died for our sins: An Indian manifesto*. New York: Avon Books.

DeLys, C. (1948). *A treasury of American superstitions*. New York: Philosophical Library.

Densmore, F. (1974). *How Indians use wild plants for food, medicine, and crafts*. New York: Dover.

Deren, M. (1953). *Divine horseman: The living gods of Haiti*. New York: McPherson.

Dey, C. (1982). *The magic candle*. Bronx, NY: Original Publications.

Dickerson, J. (1998). *Dixie's dirty secret*. Armonk, NY: Sharpe.

Dickison, R. (Ed.). (1987). *Causes, cures, sense, and nonsense*. Sacramento, CA: Bishop Publishing Co.

Dinnerstein, L., & Reimers, D. M. (1988). *Ethnic Americans* (3rd ed.). New York: Harper & Row.

Dioszegi, V. (1996). *Folk beliefs and shamanistic practices in Siberia*. Budapest: Akademiai Kiado.

Doane, N. L. (1985). *Indian doctor book*. Charlotte, NC: Aerial.

Doka, K. J., & Morgan, J. D. (Eds.). (1993). *Death and spirituality*. Amityville, NY: Baywood.

Donegan, J. B. (1978). *Women and men midwives: Medicine, morality, and misogyny in early America*. Westport, CT: Greenwood Press.

Donin, H. H. (1972). *To be a Jew*. New York: Basic Books.

Dorris, M. (1989). *The broken cord*. New York: Harper & Row.

Dorson, R. H. D. (Ed.). (1972). *Folklore and folklife*. Chicago: University of Chicago Press.

Dossey, L. (1993). *Healing words*. San Francisco: Harper.

Dresser, N. (1993). Our Own Stories: *Cross-cultural communication practice*. White Plains, NY: Longman.

Dresser, N. (1999). *Multicultural celebrations*. New York: Three Rivers Press.

Dresser, N. (1996). *Multicultural manners*. New York: Wiley.

Dubos, R. (1968). *Man, medicine and environment*. New York: Mentor.

Dubos, R. (1961). *Mirage of health*. Garden City, NY: Anchor Books, Doubleday and Co.

Dubos, R. J. (1965). *Man adapting*. New Haven, CT: Yale University Press.

Dworaczyk, E. J. (1979). *The first Polish colonies of America in Texas*. San Antonio, TX: The Naylor Company.

Eck, D. L. (1998). *World religions in Boston* (2nd ed.). Cambridge: Harvard University Press.

Egan, M. (1991). *Milagros*. Santa Fe: Museum of New Mexico Press.

Ehrenreich, B., & Ehrenreich, J. (1970). *The American health empire: Power, profits, and politics*. New York: Random House, Vintage Books.

Ehrenreich, B., & English, D. (1973). *Witches, midwives, and nurses: A history of women healers* (2nd ed.). Old Westbury, NY: Feminist Press.

Ehrlich, P. R. (1979). *The golden door: International migration, Mexico and the United States*. New York: Wideview Books.

Eichler, L. (1923). *The customs of mankind*. Garden City, NY: Doubleday, Page.

Eisenberg, D. (1985). *Encounters with Qi*. New York: W. W. Norton.

Eisinger, P. K. (1998). *Toward an end to hunger in America*. Washington, DC: Brookings Institution.

Eliade, M., & Couliano, I. P. (1991). *The Eliade guide to world religions*. San Francisco: Harper.

Elling, R. H. (1977). *Socio-cultural influences on health and health care*. New York: Springer.

Elworthy, R. T. (1958). *The evil eye: The origins and practices of superstition*.

New York: Julian Press. (Originally published by John Murray, London, 1915.)

Epstein, C. (1974). *Effective interaction in contemporary nursing*. Englewood Cliffs, NJ: Prentice Hall.

Evans, E. F. (1881). *The divine law of cure*. Boston, MA: H. H. Carter.

Fadiman, A. (1997). *The spirit catches you and you fall down*. New York: Farrar, Straus and Giroux.

Farge, E. J. (1975). *La vida Chicana: Health care attitudes and behaviors of Houston Chicanos*. San Francisco: R and E Research Associates.

Feagin, J. R. (1975). *Subordinating the poor: Welfare and American beliefs*. Englewood Cliffs, NJ: Prentice Hall.

Feagin, J. R., & Feagin, C. B. (1978). *Discrimination American style*. Englewood Cliffs, NJ: Prentice Hall.

Feldman, D. M. (1986). *Health and medicine in the Jewish tradition*. New York: Crossroads.

Finney, J. C. (Ed.). (1969). *Culture change, mental health, and poverty*. New York: Simon and Schuster.

Fleming, A. S., chairman, U.S. Commission on Civil Rights. (1980). *The tarnished golden door: Civil rights issues on immigration*. Washington, DC: Government Printing Office.

Flores-Pena, Y., & Evanchuk, R. J. (1994). *Santeria garments and altars*. Jackson: University of Mississippi Press.

Fonseca, I. (1995). *Bury me standing: The gypsies and their journey*. New York: Vintage.

Forbes, T. R. (1966). *The midwife and the witch*. New Haven, CT: Yale University Press.

Ford, P. S. (1971). *The healing trinity: Prescriptions for body, mind, and spirit*. New York: Harper & Row.

Fox, M. (2001). *One river, many wells*. New York: Tarcher/Putnam.

Foy, F. A. (Ed.). (1980). *Catholic Almanac*. Huntington, IN: Our Sunday Visitor.

Francis, P., Jr. (1994). *Beads of the world*. Atglen, PA: Schiffer.

Frankel, E., & Teutsch, B. P. (1992). *The encyclopedia of Jewish symbols*. Northvale, NJ: Jason Aronson, Inc.

Frazer, J. G. (1923). *Folklore in the Old Testament*. New York: Tudor Publishing.

Freedman, L. (1969). *Public housing: The politics of poverty*. New York: Holt, Rinehart & Winston.

Freeman, H., Levine, S., & Reeder, L. G. (Eds.). (1972). *Handbook of medical sociology* (2nd ed.). Englewood Cliffs, NJ: Prentice Hall.

Freidson, E. (1971). *Profession of medicine*. New York: Dodd, Mead.

Freire, P. (1970). *Pedagogy of the oppressed*. Trans. M. B. Ramos. New York: Seabury Press.

Friedman, M., & Friedland, G. W. (1998). *Medicine's ten greatest discoveries*. New Haven, CT: Yale University Press.

Frost, M. (n.d.). *The Shaker story*. Canterbury, NH: Canterbury Shakers.

Fuentes, C. (1985). *The old gringo*. New York: Farrar, Straus and Giroux.

Fuller, J. G. (1974). *Arigo: Surgeon of the rusty knife*. New York: Pocket Books.

Galloway, M. R. U. (Ed.). (1990). *Aunt Mary, tell me a story*. Cherokee, NC: Cherokee Communications.

Gambino, R. (1974). *Blood of my blood: The dilemma of Italian-Americans*. Garden City, NY: Doubleday.

Gans, H. J. (1962). *The urban villagers*. New York: Free Press.

Garcia, C. (1992). *Dreaming in Cuban*. New York: Ballantine Books.

Garner, J. (1976). *Healing yourself* (6th ed.). Vashon, WA: Crossing Press.

Gaver, J. R. (1972). *Sickle cell disease*. New York: Lancer Books.

Gaw, A. (Ed.). (1982). *Cross-cultural psychiatry*. Boston, MA: John Wright.

Geissler, E. M. (1998). *Pocket guide cultural assessment* (2nd ed.). St. Louis, MO: Mosby.

Gelfond, D. E., & Kutzik, A. (Eds.). (1979). *Ethnicity and aging: Theory, research and policy*. New York: Springer.

Genovese, E. D. (1972). *Roll, Jordan, Roll*. New York: Vintage Books.

Gibbs, J. T., Huang, L. N., Nagata, D. K., et al. (1988). *Children of Color*. San Francisco: Jossey-Bass.

Gibbs, T. (1996). *A guide to ethnic health collections in the United States*. Westport, CT.: Greenwood.

Giger, J. N., & Davidhizar, R. E. (1995). *Transcultural nursing assessment and intervention* (2nd ed.). St. Louis: Mosby.

Giordano, J., & Giordano, G. P. (1977). *The Ethno-Cultural factor in mental health*. New York: New York Institute of Pluralism and Group Identity.

Glazer, N., & Moynihan, D. (Eds.). (1975). *Ethnicity: Theory and experience*. Cambridge: Harvard University Press.

Goldberg B. (1993). *Alternative medicine: The definitive guide*. Puyallup, WA: Future Medicine.

Gonzalez-Wippler, M. (1987). *Santeria: African magic in Latin America*. Bronx, NY: Original Publications.

Gonzalez-Wippler, M. (1985). *Tales of the Orishas*. New York: Original Publications.

Gonzalez-Wippler, M. (1982). *The Santeria experience*. Bronx, NY: Original Publications.

Gordon, A. F., & Kahan, L. (1976). *The tribal beads: A handbook of African trade beads*. New York: Tribal Arts Gallery.

Gordon, D. M. (1972). *Theories of poverty and underemployment*. Lexington, MA: D. C. Heath.

Gordon, F. (1966). *Role theory and illness*. New Haven, CT: College and University Press.

Goswami, S. D. (1983). *Prabhupada: He built a house in which the whole world can live*. Los Angeles: The Bhaktivedanta Book Trust.

Grant, G. (1994). *Obake: Ghost stories in Hawaii*. Honolulu: Mutual.

Gray, K. (1992). *Passport to understanding*. Denver: Center for Teaching International Relations.

Greeley, A. M. (1975). *The Irish Americans*. New York: Harper & Row.

Greeley, A. M. (1975). *Why can't they be like us? America's white ethnic groups*. New York: E. P. Dutton.

Grier, W. H., & Cobbs, P. M. (1968). *Black rage*. New York: Bantam Books.

Griffin, J. H. (1960). *Black like me*. New York: Signet.

Gruber R. (1987). *Rescue: The exodus of the Ethiopian Jews*. New York: Atheneum.

Gutman, H. G. (1976). *The black family in slavery and freedom, 1750–1925*. New York: Pantheon Books.

Gutmanis, J. (1994). *Kahuna La'au Lapa'au*. Aiea, Hawaii: Island Heritage Press.

Hailey, A. (1984). *Strong medicine*. Garden City, NY: Doubleday.

Hailey, A. (1976). *Roots*. Garden City, NY: Doubleday.

Hallam, E. (1994). *Saints*. New York: Simon & Schuster.

Hammerschlag, C. A. (1988). *The dancing healers*. San Francisco: Harper & Row.

Hand, W. D. (1973). *American folk medicine: A symposium*. Berkeley: University of California Press.

Hand, W. D. (1980). *Magical medicine*. Berkeley: University of California Press.

Harney, R. F., & Troper, H. (1975). *Immigrants: A portrait of urban experience 1890–1930*. Toronto: Van Nostrand Reinhold.

Harrington, C., & Estes, C. L. (1994). *Health policy and nursing*. Boston: Jones & Bartlett.

Harris, L. (1985). *Holy days: The world of a Hasidic family*. New York: Summit Books.

Harwood, A. (1971). "The Hot-Cold Theory of Disease: Implications for Treatment of Puerto Rican Patients," *Journal of the American Medical Asssociation, 216*, 1154–1155.

Harwood, A. (1981). (Ed.). *Ethnicity and medical care*. Cambridge, MA: Harvard University Press.

Haskins, J. (1978). *Voodoo and hoodoo*. Bronx, NY: Original Publications.

Hauptman, L. M., & Wherry, J. D. (1990). *The Pequots in southern New England: The fall and rise of an American Indian nation*. Norman: University of Oklahoma Press.

Hawkins, J. B. W., & Higgins, L. P. (1983). *Nursing and the health care delivery system*. New York: Tiresias Press.

Hecker, M. (1979). *Ethnic American, 1970–1977*. Dobbs Ferry, NY: Oceana.

Henderson, G., & Primeaux, M. (Eds.). (1981). *Transcultural health care*. Menlo Park, CA: Addison-Wesley.

Hennessee, O. M. (1989). *Aloe: Myth-magic medicine*. Lawton, OK: Universal Graphics.

Hernandez, C. A., Haug, M. J., & Wagner, N. N. (1976). *Chicanos' social and psychological perspectives*. St. Louis, MO: C. V. Mosby.

Herzlich, C. (1973). *Health and illness: A social psychological analysis*. Trans. D. Graham. New York: Academic Press.

Hiatt, H. H. (1987). *America's health in the balance: Choice or chance?* New York: Harper & Row.

Hickel, W. J. (1972). *Who owns America?* New York: Paperback Library.

Himmelstein, D. U., & Woolhandler, S. (1994). *The national health program book: A source guide for advocates*. Monroe, ME: Common Courage Press.

Hirsch, E. D. (1987). *Cultural literacy: What every American needs to know*. Boston, MA: Houghton Mifflin.

Hongo, F. M. (Gen. Ed.). (1985). *Japanese American journey: The story of a people.* San Mateo, CA: Japanese American Curriculum Project.

Honychurch, P. N. (1980). *Caribbean wild plants and their uses.* London: Macmillan.

Howard, M. (1980). *Candle burning* (2nd ed.). Weingborough, Northamptonshire, England: Aquarian Press.

Howe, I. (1976). *World of our fathers.* New York: Harcourt Brace Jovanovich.

Hufford, D. J. (1984). *American healing systems: An introduction and exploration.* Conference booklet. Philadelphia: University of Pennsylvania.

Hughes, H. S. (1953). *The United States and Italy.* Cambridge, MA: Harvard University Press.

Hughes, L., & Bontemps, A. (Eds.). (1958). *The Book of negro folklore.* New York: Dodd, Mead.

Hunter, J. D. (1994). *Before the shooting begins: Searching for democracy in America's culture war.* New York: Free Press.

Hunter, J. D. (1991). *Culture wars: The struggle to define America.* New York: Basic Books.

Hurmence, B. (Ed.). (1984). *My folks don't want me to talk about slavery.* Winston-Salem, NC: John F. Blair.

Hutchens, A. R. (1973). *Indian herbalogy of North America.* Windsor, Ontario: Meico.

Hutton, J. B. (1975). *The healing power.* London: Leslie Frewin.

Illich, I. (1975). *Medical nemesis: The expropriation of health.* London: Marion Bogars.

Illich, I., Zola, I. K., McKnight, J., et al. (1977). *Disabling professions.* Salem, NH: Boyars.

Iorizzo, L. J. (1980). *Italian immigration and the impact of the Padrone System.* New York: Arno Press.

Jackson, J. S., Chatters, L. M., & Taylor, R. J. (1993). *Aging in black America.* Newbury Park, CA: Sage.

Jaco, E. G. (Ed.). (1958). *Patients, physicians, and illness: Sourcebook in behavioral science and medicine.* Glencoe, IL: Free Press.

Jacobs, H. A. (1988). *Incidents in the life of a slave girl.* London: Oxford University Press.

Jacobs, L. (Ed.). (1990). *The Jewish mystics.* London: Kyle Cathie.

Jangl, A. M., & Jangl, J. F. (1987). *Ancient legends of healing herbs.* Coeur d'Alene, ID: Prisma Press.

Jarvis, D. C. (1958). *Folk medicine: A Vermont doctor's guide to good health.* New York: Henry Holt.

Jennings, P., & Brewater, T. (1998). *The twentieth century.* New York: Doubleday.

Jilek, W. G. (1992). *Indian healing: Shamanic ceremonialism in the Pacific Northwest today.* Blaine, WA: Hancock House.

Johnson, C. J., & McGee, M. G. (Eds.). (1991). *How different religions view death and afterlife.* Philadelphia, PA: Charles Press.

Johnson, C. L. (1985). *Growing up and growing old in Italian-American families.* New Brunswick, NJ: Rutgers University Press.

Johnson, E. A. (1976). *To the first Americans: The sixth report on the Indian health program of the U.S. Public Health Service.* Washington, DC: DHEW Publication (HSA) 77–1000.

Jonas, S., & Kovner, A. R. (Eds.). (1998). *Health care delivery in the United States.* New York: Springer.

Jordan, B., & Heardon, S. (1979). *Barbara Jordan: A self-portrait.* Garden City, NY: Doubleday.

Jung, C. G. (Ed.). (1964). *Man and his symbols.* Garden City, NY: Doubleday.

Kain, J. F. (Ed.). (1969). *Race and poverty: The economics of discrimination*. Englewood Cliffs, NJ: Prentice Hall.

Kanellos, N. (1997). *Hispanic firsts*. Detroit: Visible Ink.

Kaptchuk, T., & Croucher, M. (1987). *The healing arts*. New York: Summit Books.

Karolevitz, R. F. (1967). *Doctors of the old west*. New York: Bonanza Books.

Katz, J. H. (1978). *White awareness*. Norman: University of Oklahoma Press.

Kaufman, B. N., & Kaufman, S. L. (1982). *A land beyond tears*. Garden City, NY: Doubleday.

Kavanagh, K. H., & Kennedy, P. H. (1992). *Promoting cultural diversity: Strategies for health care professionals*. Newbury Park, CA: Sage.

Keith, J. (1982). *Old people as people: Social and cultural influences on aging and old age*. Boston, MA: Little, Brown.

Keith, J. (1982). *Old people, new lives*. Chicago: The University of Chicago Press.

Kekahbah, J., & Wood, R. (Eds.). (1980). *Life cycle of the American Indian family*. Norman, OK: AIANA Publishing Co.

Kelly, I. (1965). *Folk practice in North Mexico: Birth customs, folk medicine, and spiritualism in the Laguna Zone*. Austin: University of Texas Press.

Kelsey, M. T. (1973). *Healing and Christianity*. New York: Harper & Row.

Kennedy, E. M. (1972). *In critical condition: The crises in America's health care*. New York: Simon & Schuster.

Kennett, F. (1976). *Folk medicine, fact and fiction*. New York: Crescent Books.

Kiev, A. (1968). *Curanderismo: Mexican-American folk psychiatry*. New York: Free Press.

Kiev, A. (1964). *Magic, faith and healing: Studies in primitive psychiatry today*. New York: Free Press.

Killens, J. O. (1988). *The cotillion*. New York: Ballantine.

Kilner, W. J. (1965). *The human aura*. Secaucus, NJ: Citadel Press.

Kincaid, J. (1988). *A small place*. New York: Farrar, Straus and Giroux.

King, D. H. (1988). *Cherokee heritage*. Cherokee, NC: Cherokee Communications.

Kingston, M. H. (1989). *Tripmaster monkey: His fake book*. New York: Knopf.

Kirkland, J., Matthews, H. F. M., Sullivan, C. W., III, et al. (Eds.). (1992). *Herbal and magical medicine: Traditional healing today*. Durham, NC: Duke University Press.

Klein, A. M. (1991). *Sugarball, the American game, the Dominican dream*. New Haven, CT: Yale University Press.

Klein, J. W. (1980). *Jewish identity and self-esteem: Healing wounds through ethnotherapy*. New York: Institute on Pluralism and Group Identity.

Klein, M. (1998). *A time to be born: Customs and folklore of Jewish birth*. Philadelphia, PA: Jewish Publication Society.

Kluckhohn, C. (1944). *Navaho witchcraft*. Boston: Beacon Press.

Kluckhohn, C., & Leighton, D. (1962). *The Navaho* (rev. ed.). Garden City, NY: Doubleday and Co.

Kmit, A., Luciow, L. L., Luciow, J., et al. (1979). *Ukrainian Easter eggs and how we make them*. Minneapolis, MN: Ukrainian Gift Shop.

Knudtson, P., & Suzuki, D. (1992). *Wisdom of the elders*. Toronto: Stoddart.

Knutson, A. L. (1965). *The individual, society, and health behavior*. New York: Russell Sage Foundation.

Komisar, L. (1974). *Down and out in the USA: A history of social welfare*. New York: New Viewpoints.

Kordel, L. (1974). *Natural folk remedies*. New York: Putnam's.

Kosa, J., & Zola, I. K. (1976). *Poverty and health: A sociological analysis* (2nd ed.). Cambridge, MA: Harvard University Press.

Kotelchuck, D. (Ed.). (1976). *Prognosis negative*. New York: Vintage Books.

Kotz, N. (1971). *Let them eat promises*. Garden City, NY: Doubleday.

Kovner, A. (Ed.). (1990). *Health care delivery in the United States* (4th ed.). New York: Springer.

Kramer, R. M. (1969). *Participation of the poor*. Englewood Cliffs, NJ: Prentice Hall.

Kraut, A. M. (1994). *Silent travelers: Germs, genes, and the immigrant menace*. New York: Basic Books.

Kraybeill, D. B. (1989). *The riddle of Amish culture*. Baltimore: Johns Hopkins.

Kreiger, D. (1979). *The therapeutic touch*. Englewood Cliffs, NJ: Prentice Hall.

Krippner, S., & Villaldo, A. (1976). *The realms of healing*. Millbrae, CA: Celestial Arts.

Kronenfeld, J. J. (1993). *Controversial issues in health care policy*. Newbury Park, CA: Sage.

Kunitz, S. J., & Levy, J. E. (1991). *Navajo aging: The transition from family to institutional support*. Tucson: University of Arizona Press.

Lake, M. G. (1991). *Native healer initiation into an art*. Wheaton, IL: Quest Books.

Landmann, R. S. (Ed.). (1981). *The problem of the undocumented worker*. Albuquerque: Latin American Institute, University of New Mexico.

Lasker, R. D. (1997). *Medicine and public health*. New York: New York Academy of Medicine.

Lassiter, S. (1995). *Multicultural clients*. Westport, CT: Greenwood.

Last, J. M. (1987). *Public health and human ecology*. Norwalk, CT: Appleton.

Lau, T. (1979). *The handbook of Chinese horoscopes*. Philadelphia: Harper & Row.

Lavelle, R. (Ed.). (1995). *America's new war on poverty: A reader for action*. San Francisco: KQED Books.

Lawless, E. J. (1988). *God's peculiar people*. Lexington: University of Kentucky Press.

Lee, P. R., & Estes, C. L. (Eds.). (1994). *The nation's health* (4th ed.). Boston, MA: Jones & Bartlett.

Leek, S. (1975). *Herbs: Medicine and mysticism*. Chicago: Henry Regnery.

Leff, S., & Leff, V. (1957). *From witchcraft to world health*. New York: Macmillan.

Leininger, M. (1970). *Nursing and anthropology: Two worlds to blend*. New York: Wiley.

Leininger, M. (1978). *Transcultural nursing: Concepts, theories, and practices*. New York: Wiley.

Leong, L. (1974). *Acupuncture: A layman's view*. New York: Signet.

Lerner, M. (1994). *Choices in healing*. Cambridge: MIT Press.

Leslau, C., & Leslau, W. (1985). *African proverbs*. White Plains, NY: Peter Pauper Press.

Lesnoff-Caravaglia, G. (Ed.). (1987). *Realistic expectations for long life*. New York: Human Sciences Press.

Lewis, O. (1966). *A death in the Sanchez family*. New York: Random House.

Lewis, O. (1959). *Five families: Mexican case studies in the culture of poverty*. New York: New American Library Basic Books.

Lewis, O. (1966). *La vida: A Puerto Rican family in the culture of poverty—San Juan and New York*. New York: Random House.

Lewis, O. (1961). *The children of Sanchez: Autobiography of a Mexican family*. New York: Random House.

Lewis, T. H. (1990). *The medicine men: Oglala Sioux ceremony and healing*. Lincoln: University of Nebraska Press.

Lich, G. E. (1981). *The German Texans*. San Antonio, TX: The Institute of Texan Cultures.

Lieban, R. W. (1967). *Cebuano sorcery.* Berkeley: University of California Press.

Linck, E. S., & Roach J. G. (1989). *Eats: A Folkhistory of Texas foods.* Fort Worth: Texas Christian University Press.

Lipson, J. G., Dibble, S. L., & Minarik, P. A. (1996). *Culture and nursing care: A pocket guide.* San Francisco: UCSF Nursing Press.

Litoff, J. B. (1978). *American midwives 1860 to the present.* Westport, CT: Greenwood Press.

LittleDog, P. (1994). *Border healing woman: The story of Jewel Babb* (2nd ed.). Austin: University of Texas Press.

Livingston, I. L. (Ed.). (1994). *Handbook of black American health.* Westport, CT: Greenwood Press.

Logan, P. (1981). *Irish country cures.* Dublin: Talbot Press.

Louv, R. (1980). *Southwind: The Mexican migration.* San Diego: San Diego Union, 1980.

Lovering, A. T. (1923). *The household physician.* Vols. 1 & 2. Boston, MA: Woodruff.

Lum, D. (1992). *Social work practice and people of color: A process-stage approach* (2nd ed.). Pacific Grove, CA: Brooks/Cole.

Lynch, L. R. (Ed.). (1969). *The cross-cultural approach to health behavior.* Rutherford, NJ: Fairleigh Dickenson University Press.

Lyon, W. S. (1996). *Encyclopedia of Native American healing.* New York: Norton.

Mackintosh, J. (1836). *Principles of pathology and practice of physics* (3rd ed.) Vol. 1. Philadelphia, PA: Key & Biddle.

MacNutt, F. (1974). *Healing.* Notre Dame, IN: Ave Maria Press.

MacNutt, F. (1977). *The power to heal.* Notre Dame, IN: Ave Maria Press.

Magida, A. J. (Ed.). (1996). *How to be a perfect stranger,* Vol. 1. Woodstock, VT: Jewish Lights Publishing.

Malinowski, B. (1956). *Magic, science, and religion.* Garden City, NY: Doubleday.

Maloney, C. (Ed.). (1976). *The evil eye.* New York: Columbia University Press.

Malpezzi, F. M., & Clement, W. M. (1992). *Italian American folklore.* Little Rock, AR: August House Publishers.

Mandell, B. R. (Ed.). (1975). *Welfare in America: Controlling the "dangerous classes."* Englewood Cliffs, NJ: Prentice Hall.

Manderschied, R. W., & Sonnenschein, M. A. (Eds.). (1992). *Mental health, United States, 1992.* Washington, DC: Center for Mental Health Services and National Institute of Mental Health. Government Printing Office, DHHS Pub. No. (SMA) 92-1942, 1992.

Mann, F. (1972). Acupuncture: *The Ancient Chinese art of healing and how it works scientifically.* New York: Vintage Books.

Marquez, G. G. (1998). *Love in the time of cholera.* New York: Alfred A. Knopf.

Marsella, A. B., & Pedersens, P. B. (Eds.). 1982 *Cross cultural counseling and psychotherapy.* New York: Pergamon.

Marsella, A. J., & White, G. M. (Eds.). (1982). *Cultural conceptions of mental health therapy.* London: D. Reidel.

Martin, J., & Todnem, A. (1984). *Cream and bread.* Hastings, MN: Redbird Productions.

Martin, J. L., & Nelson, S. J. (1994). *They glorified Mary, we glorified rice.* Hastings, MN: Caragana Press.

Martin, J. L. (1995). *They had stories, we had chores.* Hastings, MN: Caragana Press.

Martin, L. C. (1984). *Wildflower folklore.* Charlotte, NC: East Woods Press.

Martinez, R. A. (Ed.). (1978). *Hispanic culture and health care.* St. Louis, MO: C. V. Mosby.

Matlins, S. M., & Magida, A. J. (Eds.). (1997). *How to be a perfect stranger*, Vol. 2. Woodstock, VT: Jewish Lights Publishing.

Matsumoto M. (1988). *The unspoken way*. Tokyo: Kodansha International.

Matthiessen, P. (1980). *In the spirit of Crazy Horse*. New York: Viking Press.

McBrid, I. R. (1975). *Practical folk medicine of Hawaii*. Hilo: Petroglyph Press.

McBride, J. (1996). *The color of water*. New York: Riverhead Books.

McCall, N. (1995). *Makes me wanna holler*. New York: Vintage Books.

McClain, M. (1988). *A feeling for life: Cultural identity, community, and the arts*. Chicago: Urban Traditions.

McCubbin, H. I., Thompson, E. A., Thompson, A. I., et al. (1994). *Resiliency in ethnic minority families*. Vol. 1, *Native and immigrant American families*. Madison: WI: University of Wisconsin.

McCubbin, H., Thompson, E. A., Thompson, A. I., et al. (1995). *Resiliency in ethnic minority families*. Vol. 2, *African-American families*. Madison: University of Wisconsin Center.

McCubbin, H. I., Thompson, E. A., Thompson, A. I., et al. (1994). *Sense of coherence and resiliency*. Madison: University of Wisconsin.

McGill, O. (1977). *The mysticism and magic of India*. South Brunswick, NJ, and New York: A. S. Baines.

McGoldrick, M., Giordano, J., & Pearce, J. K. (1996). *Ethnicity and family therapy* (2nd ed.). New York: Guilford Press.

McGregor, J. H. (1940). *The Wounded Knee massacre from the viewpoint of the Sioux*. Rapid City, SD: Fenwyn Press.

McLary, K. (1993). *Amish style*. Bloomington: Indiana Press.

McLemore, S. D. (1980). *Racial and ethnic relations in America*. Boston, MA: Allyn & Bacon.

Means, R. (1995). *Where white men fear to tread*. New York: St. Martin's Press.

Mechanic, D. (1968). *Medical sociology: A selective view*. New York: Free Press.

Melton, J. G. (2000). *American religions*. Santa Barbara, CA: A B C Clio.

Melville, H. (1851). *Moby Dick* (1967 edition). New York: Bantam Books.

Menchu, R. (1983). *I, Rigoberta Menchu*. Trans. A. Wright. London: Verso.

Merrill, F. E. (1962). *Society and culture*. Englewood Cliffs, NJ: Prentice Hall.

Metraux, A. (1972). *Voodoo in Haiti*. New York: Schocken Books.

Meyer, C. E. (1985). *American folk medicine*. Glenwood, IL: Meyerbooks.

Micozzi, M. S. (1996). *Fundamentals of complementary and alternative medicine*. New York: Churchill.

Milio, N. (1975). *The care of health in communities: Access for outcasts*. New York: Macmillan.

Millman, M. (1977). *The unkindest cut*. New York: William Morrow.

Mindel, C. H., & Habenstein, R. W. (Eds.). (1976). *Ethnic families in America*. New York: Elsevier.

Miner, H. (1939). *St. Denis, a French Canadian parish*. Chicago: University of Chicago Press.

Moldenke, H. N., & Moldenke, A. L. (1952). *Plants of the Bible*. New York: Dover Publications.

Montagu, A. (1971). *Touching*. New York: Harper & Row.

Montgomery, R. (1973). *Born to heal*. New York: Coward, McCann, and Geoghegan.

Moody, R. A. (1976). *Life after life*. New York: Bantam.

Mooney, J. (1982). *Myths of the Cherokee and sacred formulas of the Cherokees*. Nashville, TN: Charles and Randy Elder—Booksellers, and

Cherokee, NC: Museum of the Cherokee Indian.

Morgan, M. (1991). *Mutant message downunder.* Lees Summit, MO: MM CO.

Morgenstern, J. (1966). *Rites of birth, marriage, death, and kindred occasions among the Semites.* Chicago: Quadrangle Books.

Morley, P., & Wallis, R. (Eds.). (1978). *Culture and curing.* Pittsburgh: University of Pittsburgh Press.

Morrison, T. (1987). *Beloved.* New York: Knopf/Random House.

Morrison, T. (1981). *Tar baby.* New York: Alfred A. Knopf.

Morton, L. T., & Moore, R. J. (1998). *A chronology of medicine and related sciences.* Cambridge: University Press, 1998.

Murray, P. (1987). *Song in a weary throat: An American pilgrimage.* New York: Harper & Row.

Mushkin, S. V. (1974). *Consumer incentives for health care.* New York: Prodist.

National Center for Health Statistics. (1998). *Health United States 1998 with socioeconomic status and health chartbook.* Hyattsville, MD: Author.

Neihardt, J. G. (1991—original 1951). *When the tree flowered.* Lincoln: University of Nebraska Press.

Neihardt, J. G. (1998—original 1961). *Black Elk speaks.* Lincoln: University of Nebraska Press.

Neihardt, N. (1993). *The sacred hoop.* Tekamah, NE: Neihardt.

Nelli, H. S. (1983). *From immigrants to ethnics: The Italian Americans.* Oxford: Oxford University Press.

Nelson, D. (1985). *Food combining simplified.* Santa Cruz, CA: The Plan.

Nemetz-Robinson, G. L. (1988). *Crosscultural understanding.* New York: Prentice Hall.

Nerburn, K., & Mengelkoch, L. (Eds.). (1991). *Native American wisdom.* San Rafael, CA: New World Library.

Neugrossschel, J. (1991). *Great tales of Jewish occult and fantasy.* New York: Wings Books.

Newman, K. D. (1975). *Ethnic American short stories.* New York: Pocket Books.

Noble, M. (1997). *Sweet grass lives of contemporary Native women of the Northeast.* Mashpee, MA: C. J. Mills.

Norman, J. C. (Ed.). (1969). *Medicine in the ghetto.* New York: Appleton-Century-Crofts.

North, J. H., & Grodsky, S. J. (Comp.). (1979). *Immigration literature: Abstracts of demographic, economic, and policy studies.* Washington, DC: U.S. Department of Justice, Immigration & Naturalization Service.

Novak, M. (1972). *The rise of the unmeltable ethnics.* New York: Macmillan.

Null, G., & Stone, C. (1976). *The Italian-Americans.* Harrisburg, PA: Stackpole Books.

O'Berennan, J., & Smith, N. (1981). *The crystal icon.* Austin, TX: Galahad Press.

Oduyoye, M. (1996). *Words and meaning in Yoruba religion.* London: Karnak House.

Opler, M. K. (Ed.). (1959). *Culture and mental health.* New York: Macmillan.

Orlando, L. (1993). *The multicultural game book.* New York: Scholastic Professional Books.

Orque, M. S., Block, B., & Monrray, L. S. A. (1983). *Ethnic nursing care: A Multicultural approach.* St. Louis, MO: C. V. Mosby.

Osofsky, G. (1963). *Harlem: The making of a ghetto.* New York: Harper & Row.

Overfield, T. (1985). *Biologic variation in health and illness.* Menlo Park, CA: Addison-Wesley.

Ozaniec, N. (1997). *Little book of Egyptian wisdom.* Rockport, MA: Element.

Padilla, E. (1958). *Up from Puerto Rico.* New York: Columbia University Press.

Paley, V. G. (1979). *White teacher.* Cambridge, MA: Harvard University Press.

Palos, S. (1971). *The Chinese art of healing.* New York: Herter and Herter.

Pappworth, M. H. (1967). *Human guinea pigs: Experimentation on man.* Boston, MA: Beacon Press.

Parsons, T., & Clark, K. B. (1965). *The Negro American.* Boston, MA: Beacon Press.

Paul, B. (Ed.). (1955). *Health, culture, and community: Case studies of public reactions to health programs.* New York: Russell Sage Foundation.

Payer, L. (1988). *Medicine and culture.* New York: Penguin Books.

Pearsall, M. (1963). *Medical behavior science: A selected bibliography of cultural anthropology, social psychology, and sociology in medicine.* Louisville: University of Kentucky Press.

Peltier, L. (1999). *Prison writings: My life is my sun dance.* New York: St. Martin's Press.

Pelto, P. J., & Pelto, G. H. (1978). *Anthropological research: The structure of inquiry* (2nd ed.). Cambridge: Cambridge University Press.

Pelton, R. W. (1973). *Voodoo charms and talismans.* New York: Popular Library.

Perera, V. (1995). *The cross and the pear tree.* Berkeley: University of California Press.

Petry, A. (1985). *The street.* Boston: Beacon Press.

Philpott, L. L. (1979). "A Descriptive Study of Birth Practices and Midwifery in the Lower Rio Grande Valley of Texas." Ph.D. diss., University of Texas Health Science Center at Houston School of Public Health.

Pierce, R. V. (1983). *The people's common sense medical advisor in plain English, or medicine simplified* (12th ed.). Buffalo, NY: World's Dispensary.

Piven, F. F., & Cloward, R. A. (1971). *Regulating the poor: The functions of public welfare.* New York: Vintage Books.

Plotkin, M. J. (1993). *Tales of a shaman's apprentice.* New York: Viking.

Popenoe, C. (1977). *Wellness.* Washington, DC: YES!

Powell, C. A. (1938). *Bound feet.* Boston: Warren Press.

Power, S. (1994). *The grass dancer.* New York: Putnam.

Prabhupada, A. C. (1970). *Bhaktivedanta Swami. KRSNA: The supreme personality of godhead.* Vol. 1. Los Angeles: The Bhaktivedanta Book Trust.

Prose, F. (1977). *Marie Laveau.* New York: Berkeley.

Proulx, E. A. (1996). *Accordion crimes.* New York: Scribner.

Purnell, L. D., & Paulanka, B. J. (1988). *Transcultural health care.* Philadelphia: F. A. Davis.

Rand, C. *The Puerto Ricans.* (1958). New York: Oxford University Press.

Read, M. (1966). *Culture, Health, and Disease.* London: Javistock Publications, 1966.

Rector-Page, L. G. (1992). *Healthy healing: An alternative healing reference* (9th ed.). San Fransisco, CA: Healthy Healing Publications.

Redman, E. (1973). *The dance of legislation.* New York: Simon & Schuster.

Reichard, G. A. (1977). *Navajo medicine-man sandpaintings.* New York: Dover.

Reneaux, J. J. (1992). *Cajun folktales.* Little Rock, AR: August House Publishers.

Rist, R. C. (1979). *Desegregated schools: Appraisals of an American experiment.* New York: Academic Press.

Riva, A. (1990). *Devotions to the saints.* Los Angeles: International Imports.

Riva, A. (1985). *Magic with incense and powders.* N. Hollywood, CA: International Imports, 1985.

Riva, A. (1974). *The modern herbal spellbook.* N. Hollywood, CA: International Imports.

Rivera, J. R. (1977). *Puerto Rican tales.* Mayaquez, Puerto Rico: Ediciones Libero.

Roby, P. (Ed.). (1974). *The poverty establishment.* Englewood Cliffs, NJ: Prentice Hall.

Rodriquez, C. E. (1991). *Puerto Ricans born in the U.S.A.* Boulder, CO: Westview Press.

Roemer, M. I. (1990). *An introduction to the U.S. health care system* (2nd ed.). New York: Springer.

Rogler, L. H. (1972). *Migrant in the city.* New York: Basic Books.

Rohde, E. S. (1922, 1971). *The Old English herbs.* New York: Dover.

Rose, P. I. (1981). *They and we: Racial and ethnic relations in the United States* (3rd ed.). New York: Random House.

Rosen, P. (1980). *The neglected dimension: Ethnicity in American life.* Notre Dame, London: University of Notre Dame Press.

Rosenbaum, B. Z. (1985). *How to avoid the evil eye.* New York: St. Martin's Press.

Ross, N. W. (1960). *The World of Zen.* New York: Vintage Books.

Rossbach, S. (1987). *Interior design with feng shui.* New York: Arkana.

Roter, D. L., & Hall, J. A. (1993). *Doctors talking with patients.* Westport, CT: Auburn House.

Rude, D. (Ed.). (1972). *Alienation: Minority groups.* New York: Wiley.

Russell, A. J. (1937). *Health in his wings.* London: Metheun.

Ryan, W. (1971). *Blaming the victim.* New York: Vintage Books.

S., E. M. (1927). *The house of wonder: A romance of psychic healing.* London: Rider.

Santillo, H. (1983). *Herbal combinations from authoritative sources.* Provo, UT: NuLife.

Santino, J. (1994). *All around the tear.* Chicago: University of Illinois Press.

Santoli, A. (1988). *New Americans.* New York: Ballantine.

Sargent, D. A. (1904). *Health, strength, and power.* New York: HM Caldwell.

Saunders, L. (1954). *Cultural difference and medical care: The case of the Spanish-speaking people of the Southwest.* New York: Russell Sage Foundation.

Saunders, R. (1927). *Healing through the spirit agency.* London: Hutchinson.

Schneider, M. (1987). *Self healing: My life and vision.* New York: Routledge & Kegan Paul.

Scholem, G. G. (1941). *Major trends in Jewish mysticism.* New York: Schocken Books.

School, B. F. (1924). *Library of health complete guide to prevention and cure of disease.* Philadelphia, PA: Historical.

Schrefer, S. (Ed.). (1994). *Quick reference to cultural assessment.* St. Louis, MO: Mosby.

Scott, W. R., & Volkart, E. H. (1966). *Medical care.* New York: Wiley.

Senior, C. (1961). *The Puerto Ricans, strangers—then neighbors.* Chicago: Quadrangle Books.

Serinus, J. (Ed.). (1986). *Psychoimmunity and the healing process.* Berkeley, CA: Celestial Arts.

Sexton, P. C. (1965). *Spanish Harlem.* New York: Harper & Row.

Shaw, W. (1975). *Aspects of Malaysian magic.* Kuala Lumpur, Malaysia: Naziabum. Nigara.

Sheinkin, D. (1986). *Path of the Kabbalah.* New York: Paragon House.

Shelton, F. (1965). *Pioneer comforts and kitchen remedies: Oldtime highland secrets from the Blue Ridge* and *Great Smoky Mountains*. High Point, NC: Hutcraft.

Shelton, F. (Ed.). (1969). *Pioneer superstitions*. High Point, NC: Hutcraft.

Shenkin, B. N. (1974). *Health care for migrant workers: Policies and politics*. Cambridge, MA: Ballinger.

Shepard, R. F., & Levi, V. G. (1982). *Live and be well*. New York: Ballantine Books.

Shih-Chen, L. (1973). *Chinese medicinal herbs*. Trans. F. P. Smith & G. A. Stuart. San Francisco: Georgetown Press.

Shor, I. (1986). *Culture wars: School and society in the conservative restoration 1969–1984*. Boston, MA: Routledge & Kegan Paul.

Shorter, E. (1987). *The health century*. New York: Doubleday.

Shostak, A. B., Van Til, J., & Van Til, S. B. (1973). *Privilege in America: An end to inequality?* Englewood Cliffs, NJ: Prentice Hall.

Silver, G. (1976). *A spy in the house of medicine*. Germantown, MD: Aspen Systems Corp.

Silverman, D. (1989). *Legends of Safed*. Jerusalem: Gefen.

Silverstein, M. E., Chang, I-L., & Macon, N., trans. (1975). *Acupuncture and moxibustion*. New York: Schocken Books.

Simmen, E. (Ed.). (1972). *Pain and promise: The Chicano today*. New York: New American Library.

Simmons, A. G. (n.d.). *A witch's brew*. Coventry, CT: Caprilands Herb Farm.

Skelton, R. (1985). *Talismanic magic*. York Beach, ME: Samuel Weiser.

Slater, P. (1970). *The pursuit of loneliness*. Boston: Beacon Press.

Smith, H. (1958). *The religions of man*. New York: Harper & Row.

Smith, L. (1963). *Killers of the dream*. Garden City, NY: Doubleday.

Smith, P. (1962). *The origins of modern culture, 1543–1687*. New York: Collier Books.

Sowell, T. (1981). *Ethnic America*. New York: Basic Books.

Sowell, T. (1996). *Migrations and cultures*. New York: Basic Books.

Spann, M. B. (1992). *Literature-based multicultural activities*. New York: Scholastic Professional Books.

Spector, R. E. (1983). "A Description of the Impact of Medicare on Health-Illness Beliefs and Practices of White Ethnic Senior Citizens in Central Texas." Ph.D. diss., University of Texas at Austin School of Nursing, 1983; Ann Arbor, MI: University Microfilms International.

Spector, R. E. (1998). *CulturalCare: Maternal infant issues*. Baltimore: Williams & Wilkins (video).

Spicer, E. (Ed.). (1977). *Ethnic medicine in the Southwest*. New York: Russell Sage Foundation.

Stack, C. B. (1974). *All our kin*. New York: Harper & Row.

Starr, P. (1982). *The social transformation of American medicine*. New York: Basic Books.

Steele, J. D. (1884). *Hygienic physiology*. New York: A. S. Barnes.

Steinberg, M. (1947). *Basic Judaism*. New York: Harcourt, Brace and World.

Steinberg, S. (2001) *The ethnic myth: Race, ethnicity, and class in America*. Boston, MA: Beacon Press.

Steiner, S. (1969). *La Raza: The Mexican Americans*. New York: Harper & Row.

Steinsaltz, A. (1980). *The thirteen petalled rose*. New York: Basic Books.

Stephan, W. G., & Feagin, J. R. (1980). *School desegregation past, present, future*. New York: Plenum.

Stevens, A. (1974). *Vitamins and remedies*. High Point, NC: Hutcraft.

Stewart, J. (Ed.). (1973). *Bridges not walls*. Reading, MA: Addison-Wesley.

Still, C. E., Jr. (1991). *Frontier doctor medical pioneer*. Kirksville, MO: Thomas Jefferson University Press.

Stoll, R. I. (1990). *Concepts in nursing: A Christian perspective*. Madison,

WI: Intervarsity Christian Fellowship.

Stone, E. (1962). *Medicine among the American Indians*. New York: Hafner.

Storlie, F. (1970). *Nursing and the social conscience*. New York: Appleton-Century-Crofts.

Storm, H. (1972). *Seven arrows*. New York: Ballantine Books.

Strauss, A., & Corbin, J. M. (1988). *Shaping a new health care system*. San Francisco: Jossey-Bass.

Styron, W. (1966). *The confessions of Nat Turner*. New York: Random House.

Swazey, J. P., & Reeds, K. (1978). *Today's medicine, tomorrow's science*. Washington, DC: U.S. Government Department of Health, Education, and Welfare.

Sweet, M. (1976). *Common edible plants of the west*. Happy Camp, CA: Naturegraph.

Szasz, T. S. (1961). *The myth of mental illness*. New York: Dell.

Takaki, R. (1993). *A different mirror: A history of multicultural America*. Boston, MA: Little, Brown.

Tallant, R. (1946). *Voodoo in New Orleans*. New York: Collier Books.

Tan, A. (1989). *The Joy Luck Club*. New York: Ivy Books.

Tan, A. (2001). *The bonesetter's daughter*. New York: Putnam & Sons.

Te Selle, S. (Ed.). (1973). *The rediscovery of ethnicity: Its implications for culture and politics in America*. New York: Harper & Row.

ten Boom, C. (1971). *The hiding place*. Washington Depot, CT: Chosen Books.

Thernstrom, S. (Ed.). (1980). *Harvard encyclopedia of American ethnic groups*. Cambridge: Harvard University Press.

Thomas, C. (1983). *They came to Pittsburgh*. Pittsburgh: Post-Gazette.

Thomas, P. (1958). *Down these mean streets*. New York: Signet Books.

Thomas, P. (1972). *Savior, Savior, hold my hand*. Garden City, NY: Doubleday.

Tierra, M. (1990). *The way of herbs*. New York: Pocket Books.

Titmuss, R. M. (1971). *The gift relationship*. New York: Vintage.

Tomasi, S. M. (Ed.). (1980). *National directory of research centers, repositories, and organizations of Italian culture in the United States*. Torino: Fondazione Giovanni Agnelli.

Tompkins, P., & Bird, C. (1973). *The secret life of plants*. New York: Avon.

Tooker, E. (Ed.). (1979). *Native American spirituality of the eastern woodlands*. New York: Paulist Press.

Torres, E. (1982). *Green medicine: Traditional Mexican-American herbal remedies*. Kingsville, TX: Nieves Press.

Torres-Gill, F. M. (1982). *Politics of aging among elder Hispanics*. Washington, DC: University Press of America.

Touchstone, S. J. (1983). *Herbal and folk medicine of Louisiana and adjacent states*. Princeton, LA: Folk-Life Books.

Trachtenberg, J. (1939). *Jewish magic and superstition*. New York: Behrman House.

Trachtenberg, J. (1983). *The devil and the Jews*. Philadelphia, PA: The Jewish Publication Society of America. (Original publication, New Haven, CT: Yale University Press, 1945.)

Trattner, W. I. (1974). *From poor law to welfare state: A history of social welfare in America*. New York: Free Press.

Trotter, R., II, & Chavira, J. A. (1981). *Curanderismo: Mexican American folk healing*. Athens, GA: University of Georgia Press.

Tucker, G. H. (1977). *Virginia supernatural tales*. Norfolk, VA: Donning.

Tula, M. T. (1994). *Hear my testimony.* Boston, MA: South End Press.

Twining, M. A., & Baird, K. E. (Eds.). (1991). *Sea Island Roots: African presence in the Carolinas and Georgia.* Trenton, NJ: Africa World Press.

Unger, S. (Ed.). (1977). *The destruction of American Indian families.* New York: Association on American Indian Affairs.

U.S. Commission on Civil Rights. (1976). *Fulfilling the letter and spirit of the law.* Washington, DC: Government Printing Office.

U. S. Commission on Civil Rights. (1970). *Mexican Americans and the administration of justice in the Southwest.* Washington, DC: Government Printing Office.

U.S. Department of Commerce, Bureau of the Census. (1980). *Ancestry of the population by State: 1980.* Washington, DC: Government Printing Office.

U. S. Department of Commerce, Bureau of the Census. (1982, September). *Population profile of the United States: 1981.* "Population Characteristics," ser. 20, no. 374.

U.S. Department of Health and Human Services. (1997). *Comprehensive health care program for American Indians and Alaska Natives.* Rockville, MD: Public Health Service, Indian Health Service.

U. S. Department of Health and Human Services. (1997). *Regional differences in Indian health.* Rockville, MD: Public Health Service, Indian Health Service.

U. S. Department of Health and Human Services. (1997). *Trends in Indian Health.* Rockville, MD: Public Health Service, Indian Health Service.

U. S. Department of Health and Human Services. (1993). *Health United States 1992 and healthy people 2000 review.* Washington, DC: United States Department of Health and Human Services, Public Health Service Centers for Disease Control and Prevention. DHHS Pub. No. (PHS) 93-1232.

U. S. Department of Health and Human Services. (1992). *Healthy people 2000 national health promotion and disease prevention objectives: Full report with commentary.* Boston: Jones and Bartlett.

U.S. Department of Health, Education, and Welfare. *Health in America: 1776–1976.* Washington, DC: DHEW pub. (HRA) 76-616, 1976.

U.S. Department of Justice, Immigration and Naturalization Service. (1979). *Immigration literature: Abstracts of demographic economic and policy studies.* Washington, DC: Government Printing Office.

Valentine, C. A. (1968). *Culture and poverty.* Chicago: University of Chicago Press.

Wade, M. (1946). *The French-Canadian outlook.* New York: Viking Press.

Wade, M. (1955). *The French-Canadians, 1876–1945.* New York: Macmillan.

Walker, A. (1994). *The temple of my familiar.* New York: Harcourt, Brace, Jovanovich.

Wall, S. (1994). *Shadowcatchers.* New York: HarperCollins.

Wall, S., & Arden, H. (1990). *Wisdomkeepers meetings with native American spiritual elders.* Hillsboro, OR: Beyond Words Publishing Co.

Wallace, R. B. (Ed.). *Public health and preventive medicine* (14th ed.). Stamford, CT: Appleton & Lange.

Wallnöfer, H., & von Rottauscher, A. (1972). *Chinese folk medicine.* Trans. M. Palmedo. New York: New American Library.

Warner, D. (1979). *The Health of Mexican Americans in South Texas.* Austin, TX: Lyndon Baines Johnson School of Public Affairs, University of Texas at Austin.

Warner, D., & Red, K. (1993). *Health care across the border*. Austin, TX: LBJ School.

Warren, N. (Ed.). (1980). *Studies in cross-cultural psychology*. New York: Academic Press.

Weible, W. (1983). *Medjugore: The message*. Orleans, MA: Paraclete Press.

Wei-kang, F. (1975). *The story of Chinese acupuncture and moxibustion*. Peking: Foreign Languages Press.

Weil, A. (1983). *Health and healing*. Boston, MA: Houghton Mifflin.

Weinbach, S. (1991). *Rabbenu Yisrael Abuchatzira: The story of his life and wonders*. Brooklyn, NY: ASABA-FUJIE publication.

Weinberg, R. D. (1967). *Eligibility for entry to the United States of America*. Dobbs Ferry, NY: Oceana.

Wiebe, R., & Johnson, Y. (1998). *Stolen life—The journey of a Cree woman*. Athens: Ohio University Press.

Weiss, G., & Weiss, S. (1985). *Growing and using the healing herbs*. New York: Wings Books.

Wheelwright, E. G. (1974). *Medicinal plants and their history*. New York: Dover.

Wilen, J., & Wilen, L. (1984). *Chicken soup and other folk remedies*. New York: Fawcett Columbine.

Williams, R. A. (Ed.). (1975). *Textbook of black-related diseases*. New York: McGraw-Hill.

Williams, S. J., & Torrens, P. R. (1990). *Introduction to health services* (3rd ed.). New York: Wiley.

Wilson, F. A., & Neuhauser, D. (1982). *Health services in the United States* (2nd ed.). Cambridge, MA: Ballinger.

Wilson, S. G. (1992). *The drummer's path: Moving the spirit with ritual and traditional drumming*. Rochester, VT: Destiny Books.

Winkler, G. (1981). *Dybbuk*. New York: Judaica Press.

Wolfson, E. (1993). *From the earth to the sky*. Boston, MA: Houghton Mifflin.

Wright, E. (1984). *The book of magical talismans*. Minneapolis, MN: Marlar Publishing, Co.

Wright, R. (1937). *Black boy*. New York: Harper & Brothers.

Wright, R. (1940). *Native son*. New York: Grosset & Dunlop.

Wright-Hybbard, E. (1977–1992). *A brief study course in homeopathy*. Philadelphia: Formur.

Yambura, B. S. (1960). *A change and a parting*. Ames: University of Iowa Press.

Young, J. H. (1967). *The medical messiahs*. Princeton, NJ: Princeton University Press.

Zambrana, R. E. (Ed.). (1982). *Work, family, and health: Latina women in transition*. New York: Fordham University.

Zborowski, M. (1969). *People in pain*. San Francisco: Jossey-Bass.

Zeitlin, S. J., Kotkin, A. J., & Baker, H. C. (1977). *A celebration of American family folklore: Tales and traditions from the Smithsonian collection*. New York: Pantheon Books.

Zolla, E. (1969). *The writer and the shaman*. New York: Harcourt Brace Jovanovich.

Zook, J. (1972). *Exploring the secrets of treating deaf-mutes*. Peking: Foreign Languages Press.

Zook, J. (1899). *Oneida, The people of the stone*. The Church's Mission to the Oneidas. Oneida Indian Reservation, WI.

Zook, J. (1972). *Your new life in the United States*. Washington, DC: Center for Applied Linguistics.

Zook, J., & Zook, J. (1978). *Hexology*. Paradise, PA: Zook.

Index

1 YEAR UPGRADE
BUYER PROTECTION PLAN

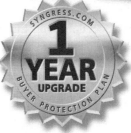

MANAGING
Cisco Network
Security Second Edition

Eric Knipp

Brian Browne

Woody Weaver

C. Tate Baumrucker

Larry Chaffin

Jamie Caesar

Vitaly Osipov

Edgar Danielyan Technical Editor

KEY	SERIAL NUMBER
001	42397FGT54
002	56468932HF
003	FT6Y78934N
004	2648K9244T
005	379KS4F772
006	V6762SD445
007	99468ZZ652
008	748B783B66
009	834BS4782Q
010	X7RF563WS9

PUBLISHED BY
Syngress Publishing, Inc.
800 Hingham Street
Rockland, MA 02370

Managing Cisco® Network Security, Second Edition

Printed in the United States of America

1 2 3 4 5 6 7 8 9 0

ISBN: 1-931836-56-6

Technical Editor: Edgar Danielyan   Cover Designer: Michael Kavish
Technical Reviewer: Sean Thurston   Page Layout and Art by: Shannon Tozier
Acquisitions Editor: Catherine B. Nolan   Copy Editor: Michael McGee
Developmental Editor: Jonathan Babcock   Indexer: Nara Wood

Distributed by Publishers Group West in the United States and Jaguar Book Group in Canada.

Acknowledgments

We would like to acknowledge the following people for their kindness and support in making this book possible.

Ralph Troupe, Rhonda St. John, Emlyn Rhodes, and the team at Callisma for their invaluable insight into the challenges of designing, deploying and supporting world-class enterprise networks.

Karen Cross, Lance Tilford, Meaghan Cunningham, Kim Wylie, Harry Kirchner, Kevin Votel, Kent Anderson, Frida Yara, Bill Getz, Jon Mayes, John Mesjak, Peg O'Donnell, Sandra Patterson, Betty Redmond, Roy Remer, Ron Shapiro, Patricia Kelly, Andrea Tetrick, Jennifer Pascal, Doug Reil, and David Dahl of Publishers Group West for sharing their incredible marketing experience and expertise.

Jacquie Shanahan, AnnHelen Lindeholm, David Burton, Febea Marinetti, and Rosie Moss of Elsevier Science for making certain that our vision remains worldwide in scope.

Annabel Dent and Paul Barry of Elsevier Science/Harcourt Australia for all their help.

David Buckland, Wendi Wong, Marie Chieng, Lucy Chong, Leslie Lim, Audrey Gan, and Joseph Chan of Transquest Publishers for the enthusiasm with which they receive our books.

Kwon Sung June at Acorn Publishing for his support.

Ethan Atkin at Cranbury International for his help in expanding the Syngress program.

Jackie Gross, Gayle Voycey, Alexia Penny, Anik Robitaille, Craig Siddall, Darlene Morrow, Iolanda Miller, Jane Mackay, and Marie Skelly at Jackie Gross & Associates for all their help and enthusiasm representing our product in Canada.

Lois Fraser, Connie McMenemy, Shannon Russell and the rest of the great folks at Jaguar Book Group for their help with distribution of Syngress books in Canada.

Thank you to our hard-working colleagues at New England Fulfillment & Distribution who manage to get all our books sent pretty much everywhere in the world. Thank you to Debbie "DJ" Ricardo, Sally Greene, Janet Honaker, and Peter Finch.

Contributors

F. William Lynch (SCSA, CCNA, LPI-I, MCSE, MCP, Linux+, A+) is co-author of *Hack Proofing Sun Solaris 8* (Syngress Publishing, ISBN: 1-928994-44-X), and *Hack Proofing Your Network, Second Edition* (Syngress Publishing, ISBN: 1-928994-70-9). He is an independent security and systems administration consultant and specializes in firewalls, virtual private networks, security auditing, documentation, and systems performance analysis. William has served as a consultant to multinational corporations and the federal government including the Centers for Disease Control and Prevention headquarters in Atlanta, GA as well as various airbases of the United States Air Force. He is also the Founder and Director of the MRTG-PME project, which uses the MRTG engine to track systems performance of various UNIX-like operating systems. William holds a bachelor's degree in Chemical Engineering from the University of Dayton in Dayton, OH and a master's of Business Administration from Regis University in Denver, CO.

Robert "Woody" Weaver (CISSP) is a Principal Architect and the Field Practice Leader for Security at Callisma. As an information systems security professional, Woody's responsibilities include field delivery and professional services product development. His background includes a decade as a tenured professor teaching mathematics and computer science, as the most senior network engineer for Williams Communications in the San Jose/San Francisco Bay area, providing client services for their network integration arm, and as Vice President of Technology for Fullspeed Network Services, a regional systems integrator. Woody received a bachelor's of Science from Caltech, and a Ph.D. from Ohio State. He currently works out of the Washington, DC metro area.

Larry Chaffin (CCNA, CCDA, CCNA-WAN, CCDP-WAN, CSS1, NNCDS, JNCIS) is a Consultant with Callisma. He currently provides strategic design and technical consulting to all Callisma clients. His specialties include Cisco WAN routers, Cisco PIX Firewall, Cisco VPN, ISP design and implementation, strategic network planning, network architecture and design, and network troubleshooting and optimization. He also provides Technical Training for Callisma in all technology areas that include Cisco, Juniper, Microsoft, and others. Larry's background includes positions as a Senior LAN/WAN Engineer at WCOM-UUNET, and he also is a freelance sports writer for *USA Today* and ESPN.

Eric Knipp (CCNP, CCDP, CCNA, CCDA, MCSE, MCP+I) is a Consultant with Callisma. He is currently engaged in a broadband optimization project for a major US backbone service provider. He specializes in IP telephony and convergence, Cisco routers, LAN switches, as well as Microsoft NT, and network design and implementation. He has also passed both the CCIE Routing and Switching written exam as well as the CCIE Communications and Services Optical qualification exam. Eric is currently preparing to take the CCIE lab later this year. Eric's background includes positions as a project manager for a major international law firm and as a project manager for NORTEL. He is co-author on the previously published *Cisco AVVID and IP Telephony Design and Implementation* (Syngress Publishing, ISBN: 1-928994-83-0), and the forthcoming book *Configuring IPv6 for Cisco IOS* (Syngress Publishing, ISBN: 1-928994-84-9).

Jamie Caesar (CCNP) is the Senior Network Engineer for INFO1 Inc., located in Norcross, GA. INFO1 is a national provider of electronic services to the credit industry and a market leader in electronic credit solutions. INFO1 provides secure WAN connectivity to customers for e-business services. Jamie contributes his time with enterprise connectivity architecture, security, deployment, and project management for all WAN services. His contributions enable INFO1 to provide mission-critical, 24/7 services to customers across all of North America. Jamie holds a bachelor's degree in Electrical Engineering from Georgia Tech. He resides outside Atlanta, GA with his wife, Julie.

Vitaly Osipov (CISSP, CCSA, CCSE) is a Security Specialist with a technical profile. He has spent the last five years consulting various companies in Eastern, Central, and Western Europe on information security issues. Last year Vitaly was busy with the development of managed security service for a data center in Dublin, Ireland. He is a regular contributor to various infosec-related mailing lists and recently co-authored *Check Point NG Certified Security Administrator Study Guide*. Vitaly has a degree in mathematics. Currently he lives in the British Isles.

C. Tate Baumrucker (CISSP, CCNP, Sun Enterprise Engineer, MCSE) is a Senior Consultant with Callisma. He is responsible for leading engineering teams in the design and implementation of complex and highly available systems infrastructures and networks. Tate is industry recognized as a subject matter expert in security and LAN/WAN support systems such as HTTP, SMTP, DNS, and DHCP. He has spent eight years providing technical consulting services in enterprise and service provider industries for companies including American Home Products, Blue Cross and Blue Shield of Alabama, Amtrak, Iridium, National Geographic, Geico, GTSI, Adelphia Communications, Digex, Cambrian Communications, and BroadBand Office.

Brian Browne (CISSP) is a Senior Consultant with Callisma. He provides senior-level strategic and technical security consulting to Callisma clients, has 12 years of experience in the field of information systems security, and is skilled in all phases of the security lifecycle. A former independent consultant, Brian has provided security consulting for multiple Fortune 500 clients, and has been published in *Business Communications Review*. His security experience includes network security, firewall architectures, virtual private networks (VPNs), intrusion detection systems, UNIX security, Windows NT security, and public key infrastructure (PKI). Brian resides in Willow Grove, PA with his wife, Lisa and daughter, Marisa.

Technical Reviewer

Sean Thurston (CCDP, CCNP, MCSE, MCP+I) is an employee of Western Wireless, a leading provider of communications services in the Western United States. His specialties include implementation of multi-vendor routing and switching equipment and XoIP (Everything over IP installations). Sean's background includes positions as a Technical Analyst for Sprint-Paranet and the Director of a brick-and-mortar advertising dot com. Sean is also a contributing author to *Building a Cisco Network for Windows 2000* (Syngress Publishing, ISBN: 1-928994-00-8) and *Cisco AVVID & IP Telephony Design and Implementation* (Syngress Publishing, ISBN: 1-928994-83-0). Sean lives in Renton, WA with his fiancée, Kerry. He is currently pursuing his CCIE.

Technical Editor

Edgar Danielyan (CCNP Security, CCDP, CSE, SCNA) is a self-employed consultant, author, and editor specializing in security, UNIX, and internetworking. He is the author of *Solaris 8 Security* available from New Riders, and has contributed his expertise as a Technical Editor of several books on security and networking including *Hack Proofing Linux* (Syngress Publishing, ISBN: 1-928994-34-2) and *Hack Proofing Your Web Applications* (Syngress Publishing, ISBN: 1-928994-31-8). Edgar is also a member of the ACM, IEEE, IEEE Computer Society, ISACA, SAGE, and the USENIX Association.

Contents

Chapter 2 What Are We Trying to Prevent?   61

Answers to Your Frequently Asked Questions

Q: Is a vulnerability assessment program expensive?

A: Not necessarily. The Cisco product is not terribly expensive, and there exist open source solutions which are free to use. The actual assessment program is probably less expensive than the remediation efforts: Maintaining all your hosts on an ongoing basis is a steep maintenance requirement, and one that not all enterprises have accepted. But ever since the summer of 2001, there has been clear evidence that you have to manage your hosts and keep their patch levels up-to-date just to stay in business.

NOTE

Make sure the COM port properties in the terminal emulation program match the following values:

- 9600 baud
- 8 data bits
- No parity
- 1 stop bit
- Hardware flow control

Chapter 4 Traffic Filtering in the Cisco Internetwork Operating System 163

Logging Commands

There are also eight different levels of messages, which will be listed from most severe (Emergency - Level 0) to least severe (Debugging - Level 7):

- Emergency – Level 0

- Alerts – Level 1

- Critical – Level 2

- Errors – Level 3

- Warning – Level 4

- Notification – Level 5

- Informational – Level 6

- Debugging – Level 7

Chapter 5 Network Address Translation/Port Address Translation   233

Configuration Commands

Before NAT can be implemented, the "inside" and "outside" networks must be defined. To define the "inside" and "outside" networks, use the *ip nat* command.

```
ip nat inside |
   outside
```

- **Inside** Indicates the interface is connected to the inside network (the network is subject to NAT translation).

- **Outside** Indicates the interface is connected to the outside network.

Chapter 6 Cryptography   **273**

Encryption Key Types

Cryptography uses two types of keys: *symmetric* and *asymmetric*. Symmetric keys have been around the longest; they utilize a single key for both the encryption and decryption of the ciphertext. This type of key is called a *secret key*, because you must keep it secret. Otherwise, anyone in possession of the key can decrypt messages that have been encrypted with it. The algorithms used in symmetric key encryption have, for the most part, been around for many years and are well known, so the only thing that is secret is the key being used. Indeed, all of the really useful algorithms in use today are completely open to the public.

Chapter 7 Cisco LocalDirector and DistributedDirector   313

LocalDirector Product Overview

The LocalDirector product is available in three different ranges:

- **LocalDirector 416**
  This is both the entry-level product as well as the medium-size product. It supports up to 90 Mbps throughput and 7,000 connections per second.

- **LocalDirector 430**
  This is the high-end product. It supports up to 400 Mbps throughput and 30,000 connections per second.

- **LocalDirector 417**
  Newer platform with different mounting features. It is even more productive than 430 series and has more memory—two Fast Ethernet and one Gigabit Ethernet interfaces.

Chapter 8 Virtual Private Networks and Remote Access   **335**

Overview of the Different VPN Technologies

- A *peer* VPN model is one in which the path determination at the network layer is done on a hop-by-hop basis.

- An *overlay* VPN model is one in which path determination at the network layer is done on a "cut-through" basis to another edge node (customer site).

- Link Layer VPNs are implemented at link layer (Layer 2) of the OSI Reference model.

Chapter 9 Cisco Authentication, Authorization, and Accounting Mechanisms   379

WARNING

The SRVTAB is the core of Kerberos security. Using TFTP to transfer this key is an IMPORTANT security risk! Be very careful about the networks in which this file crosses when transferred from the server to the router. To minimize the security risk, use a cross-over cable that is directly connected from a PC to the router's Ethernet interface. Configure both interfaces with IP addresses in the same subnet. By doing this, it is physically impossible for anyone to capture the packets as they are transferred from the Kerberos server to the router.

Chapter 10 Cisco Content Services Switch   455

FlowWall Security

FlowWall provides intelligent flow inspection technology that screens for all common DoS attacks, such as SYN floods, ping floods, smurfs, and abnormal or malicious connection attempts. It does this by discarding packets that have the following characteristics:

- Frame length is too short.

- Frame is fragmented.

- Source IP address = IP destination (LAND attack).

- Source address = Cisco address, or the source is a subnet broadcast.

- Source address is not a unicast address.

- Source IP address is a loop-back address.

- Destination IP address is a loop-back address.

- Destination address is not a valid unicast or multicast address.

**Searching the
Network for
Vulnerabilities**

There are three primary
steps in creating a session
to search your network for
vulnerabilities:

1. Identifying the network
   addresses to scan

2. Identifying
   vulnerabilities to scan
   by specifying the TCP
   and UDP ports (and
   any active probe
   settings)

3. Scheduling the session

**Frequently Asked
Questions**

Q: Which IDS platforms
are supported in
CSPM?

A: Only Cisco Secure IDS
sensors (former
NetRanger sensors) are
supported, either in
standalone
configuration or as
Catalyst 6000 blades.
Embedded IDS features
of Cisco PIX firewalls
and Cisco IOS routers
are not supported.

Distributed Denial of Service Attacks

Recently, distributed denial of service (DDoS) attacks have become more common. Typical tools used by attackers are Trinoo, TFN, TFN2K and Stacheldraht ("barbed wire" in German). How does a DDoS attack work? The attacker gains access to a Client PC. From there, the cracker can use tools to send commands to the nodes. These nodes then flood or send malformed packets to the victim. Coordinated traceroutes from several sources are used to probe the same target to construct a table of routes for the network. This information is then used as the basis for further attacks.

Network Security Management

To overcome security management issues, Cisco has developed several security management applications including these:

- PIX Device Manager

- CiscoWorks2000 Access Control Lists Manager

- Cisco Secure Policy Manager

- Cisco Secure Access Control Server

Chapter 14 Network Security Management   593

Chapter 15 Looking Ahead: Cisco Wireless Security

Understanding Security Fundamentals and Principles of Protection

Security protection starts with the preservation of the *confidentiality*, *integrity*, and *availability* (CIA) of data and computing resources. These three tenets of information security, often referred to as "The Big Three," are sometimes represented by the CIA triad.

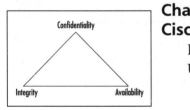

Foreword

Today's Security Environment

Information security has become an extremely important topic for everyone over the past few years. In today's environment the number of touch points between an organization's information assets and the outside world has drastically increased: millions of customers can interact via a Web site, thousands of employees and partners may connect using Virtual Private Network s (VPNs), and dozens of critical applications may be completely outsourced to application service providers (ASPs). The deployment of wireless LANs also means that users no longer even need a physical connection to the network to gain access.

In addition to an explosion of touch points, we are faced with an infinitively complex and rapidly changing web of networks, applications, systems, client software, and service providers. Under these circumstances, absolute security cannot be guaranteed since it's impossible to test the security implications of every configuration combination of hardware and software under every set of conditions.

A critical strategy for reducing security risk is to practice defense-in-depth. The essence of defense-in-depth is to create an architecture that incorporates multiple layers of security protection. Recognizing this requirement, Cisco Systems has placed a high priority on security and offers a wide range of stand-alone and integrated security products. *Managing Cisco Network Security, Second Edition* is important to anyone involved with Cisco networks, as it provides practical information on using a broad spectrum of Cisco's security products. Security is not just for "security geeks" anymore. It is an absolute requirement of all network engineers, system administrators, and other technical staff to understand how best to implement security.

About This Book

In addition to providing a general understanding of IP network security and the threat environment, this book offers detailed and practical information on how to use Cisco's suite of security products. Callisma's contributing authors are industry experts with real world implementation experience. Each chapter will guide you through a particular aspect of security, from the family of PIX firewalls, to the Cisco Secure Intrusion Detection System (IDS), to traffic filtering in IOS, to the Cisco Secure Policy Manager (CSPM). In reading this book, you will obtain a firm understanding of how to secure your Cisco network.

About Callisma

Callisma is setting a new standard for network consulting, helping today's enterprises and service providers design and deploy networks that deliver strategic business value. By providing its clients with a broad base of technical practices, a flexible, results-oriented engagement style, and the highest quality documentation and communication, Callisma delivers superior solutions—on time and on budget. Callisma practices include IP Telephony, Internetworking, Optical Networking, Operations Management, Project Management, and Security and Storage Networking. Callisma is headquartered in Silicon Valley, with offices located throughout the United States. For more information, visit the Callisma Web site at www.callisma.com or call 888-805-7075

—*Ralph Troupe*
President and CEO, Callisma

Introduction to IP Network Security

Introduction

This book is intended to help people implement IP network security in a Cisco environment. It will provide the language, architectural framework, technical insight, technical configuration, and practical advice to ensure best practice security implementation. Successfully digesting the material presented in this book will allow you to protect your environment and client services using a wide array of Cisco security technologies and equipment.

What Role Does Security Play in a Network?

This book is about IP network security. Though you probably already know something about networking, we'll go over some of the language to be sure we are all working from the same concepts. Let's begin by discussing what we are trying to accomplish with IP network security.

Goals

The goals of security usually boil down to three things, represented by the acronym CIA:

- **Confidentiality** Confidentiality protects sensitive information from unauthorized disclosure or intelligible interception. Information should only be seen by the intended parties in a conversation, not by eavesdroppers.

- **Integrity** Integrity ensures that information or software is complete, accurate, and authentic (in other words, it isn't altered without authorization). We want to ensure mechanisms are in place to protect against accidental or malicious changes, and may wish to produce documented trails of which communications have occurred.

- **Availability** Availability ensures that information and services are accessible and functional when needed and authorized. There is a related concept of trust. The formal definition of trust concerns the extent to which someone who relies on a system can have confidence that the system meets its specifications (that is, the system does what it claims to do and does not perform unwanted functions).

Different systems and businesses will place differing levels of importance on each of these three characteristics. For example, while Internet service providers (ISPs) may be concerned with confidentiality and integrity, they will be more concerned with protecting availability for their customers. The military, by contrast, places more emphasis on confidentiality, with its system of classifications of information, and the clearances for people who need to access it. Most businesses must be concerned with all three elements, but will be concerned primarily with the integrity of their data.

Confidentiality

Confidentiality protects sensitive information from unauthorized disclosure or intelligible interception. Cryptography and access control are used to protect confidentiality. The effort applied to protecting confidentiality depends on the sensitivity of the information and the likelihood of it being observed or intercepted.

Damage & Defense...

Cleartext Passwords

Passing passwords in cleartext that permits administrative access to systems is a severe security risk. Use access control mechanisms, and where possible, encryption controls (such as SSH) to communicate with infrastructure devices. Many Cisco devices will support SSH with a modern image.

Network encryption can be applied at any level in the protocol stack. Applications can provide end-to-end encryption, but each application must be adapted to provide this service. Encryption at the transport layer is used frequently today. Virtual private networks (VPNs) can be used to establish secure channels of communication between two sites or between an end user and a site. (VPNs are covered in more detail in Chapter 5.) Encryption can be used at the OSI data-link layer, but doesn't scale easily; every networking device in the communication pathway would have to participate in the encryption scheme. Data-link layer encryption is making a comeback in the area of wireless security, such as in IEEE 802.11. Physical security, meanwhile, is used to prevent unauthorized access to network ports or equipment rooms. One of the risks at the physical level is violation of access control through the attachment of promiscuous packet capture devices to the network, particularly with the widespread use of open source tools such as Ethereal (www.ethereal.com) and tcpdump (www.tcpdump.org) that permits nearly any host to become a packet decoder.

Integrity

Integrity ensures that information or software is complete, accurate, and authentic. We want to keep unauthorized people or processes from making any changes to the system, and keep authorized users from making changes that exceed their authority. These changes may be intentional or unintentional, and similar mechanisms can protect a system from both.

For network integrity, we need to ensure that the message received is the same message that was sent. The content of the message must be complete and unmodified, and that the link is between a valid source and destination nodes. Connection integrity can be provided by cryptography and routing control. Simple integrity assurance methods to detect incidental changes, like adding up all the bytes in a message and recording that as an element in the packet, are used in everyday IP flows. More robust approaches, such as taking the output from a hash function like message digest (version) 5 (MD5) or secure hash algorithim (SHA) and adding that to the message, as is used in IPSec, can detect attempted malicious changes to a communication.

For host integrity, cryptography can also come to the rescue. Using a secure hash can identify whether an unauthorized change has occurred. However, of fundamental importance are careful use of audit trails to determine what changed, when the change occurred, and who made the change. Sound security design includes a centralized log server, and policy and procedure around safe handling of audit data.

Integrity also extends to the software images for network devices that are transporting data. The images must be verified as authentic, and that they have not been modified or corrupted. Just as a transported IP packet has a checksum to verify it wasn't accidentally damaged in transit, Cisco provides a checksum for IOS images. When copying an image into flash memory, verify that the checksum of the bundled image matches the checksum listed in the README file that comes with the upgrade.

Availability

Availability ensures that information and services are accessible and functional when needed. Redundancy, fault tolerance, reliability, failover, backups, recovery, resilience, and load balancing are the network design concepts used to assure availability. If systems aren't available, then integrity and confidentiality won't matter. Build networks that provide high availability.

Your customers or end users will perceive availability as being the entire system—application, servers, network, and workstation. If they can't run their applications, then it is not available. To provide high availability, ensure that security processes are reliable and responsive. Modular systems and software, including security systems, need to be interoperable.

Denial of service (DoS) attacks are aimed at crippling the availability of networks and servers, and can create severe losses for organizations. In February, 2000, large Web sites such as Yahoo!, eBay, Amazon, CNN, ZDNet, E*Trade, Excite, and Buy.com were knocked offline or had their availability reduced to about 10 percent for many hours by distributed denial of service attacks (DDoS). The attacks were not particularly sophisticated—they were launched by a teenager—but were disastrously effective.

NOTE

Having a good inventory and documentation of your network is important for day-to-day operations, but in a disaster, you can't depend on having it available. Business Continuity/Disaster Recovery is an important aspect of security design. Store the configurations and software images of network devices *offsite* with your backups from servers, and keep them up to date. Include documentation about the architecture of your network. All of this documentation should be available in printed form because electronic versions may be unavailable or difficult to locate in an emergency. Such information will save valuable time in a crisis.

Cisco makes many products designed for high hardware availability. These devices are characterized by a long mean time between failure (MTBF) with redundant power supplies, and hot-swappable cards or modules. For example, devices that provide 99.999 percent availability would have about five minutes downtime per year.

Availability of individual devices can be enhanced by their configuration. Using features such as redundant uplinks with Hot Standby Router Protocol (HSRP), fast convergent Spanning Tree, or Fast EtherChannel provide a failover if one link should fail. Uninterruptible power supplies (UPSs) and backup generators are used to protect mission-critical equipment in the event of a power outage. These are not security features per se—and in some instances may work against security, such as using HSRP to force a router offline to allow the bypassing of access controls—but are a valid part of a security design.

Although not covered in this book, Cisco IOS includes reliability features such as:

- Hot Standby Router Protocol (HSRP)
- Simple Server Redundancy Protocol (SSRP)
- Deterministic Load Distribution (DLD)

Philosophy

The underlying philosophy behind security is different from what most network managers face. There are three common perspectives behind the design of networks:

- **User perspective** Get it out fast, and as inexpensively as possible. Make it work. If it breaks, fix it.

- **Operations management perspective** Get it out to meet all needs, and do it as reliably as possible. Document how it's working. Don't let it break, or at least recover from breaks transparently.

- **Security perspective** Get it out in a controlled fashion, meeting authorized needs. Allow only authorized services to work. If it breaks, make sure it fails in a fashion that doesn't allow unauthorized services.

The way to think of the user perspective is to imagine you are programming a computer: Write code to make it work, and move on. If the code is a little buggy, that's okay—it's less expensive, and you get most of what you need. The way to think of the operations management perspective is to see yourself programming Murphy's computer: Write code with the understanding that things will break at the worst possible time, and deal with it gracefully. You spend time developing useful error messages, and help the user understand what is happening inside the program. It costs more, but it's a better "quality" program. The way to think of the security perspective is to imagine yourself programming Satan's computer: Write code with the understanding that there is an actively malicious agent at the heart of the environment trying to break things; protect yourself and your clients. You spend time checking for buffer overflows or impossible inputs. It's more difficult of course, but hey, it's a dangerous world out there…

None of these perspectives is best; they all have advantages. Working from an operations management perspective is expensive; it means you usually have to buy two of everything, provide redundant routes, and spend time thinking about command and management issues. Working from a security perspective is inconvenient; in addition to the increased complexities, we often have to reduce features and try to streamline systems to provide the necessary controls. Maintaining all three perspectives simultaneously is the challenge that network managers face.

Cisco has documented its fundamental blueprints in the SAFE program (see www.cisco.com/warp/public/779/largeent/issues/security/safebprint.html for further information). A quick summary might state that security does not come from a single product but is based upon a triad of people, processes, and technology; and that security should not be in a single location but be handled by a distributed, defense-in-depth approach that's spread across the enterprise. Though security policy and its procedural issues are outside the scope of this book, be warned that some sidebars may creep into these pages from time to time. What we will do is show how the various pieces of security technology can be deployed across your environment to enhance your security posture.

What if I Don't Deploy Security?

Security costs significant money, and is rather inconvenient. These are rather good reasons not to deploy security, and for many enterprises that was the standard operating procedure. Unfortunately, that turned out to be a shortsighted decision. According to an Information Week / Price Waterhouse Cooper survey (the Security Benchmarking Service), losses due to security breaches cost over 1.39 *trillion* dollars last year. The Computer Security Institue (CSI)/FBI survey showed that the average annual loss per company exceeded *two million* dollars. One interesting study is Egghead Software: On the day a security breach was announced, their stock dropped 25 percent, and they never recovered. What is a fourth of your company's capitalization? If you can reduce or eliminate this number, that can fund a pretty significant security program.

An effective security program *can* make a difference. Computer Economics estimated the three most costly mobile code events were CodeRed and its variants at 2.62 billion dollars; SirCam at 1.15 billion dollars; and Nimda at 635 million dollars. The first and last could have been stopped by an effective vulnerability assessment program, such as a solid Cisco Secure Scanner deployment, while the SirCam could have been stopped by an effective antivirus filtering program at the perimeter of the network.

Some enterprises argue that they aren't a target, so they don't have to protect themselves. How wrong they are. Automated tools probe the Internet looking for vulnerable hosts. If you put an unpatched Microsoft Internet Information Server (IIS) on the Internet, (even via dialup or DSL) you have between 30 minutes and two hours, on average, before a Nimda probe will compromise your machine. Script kiddies and commercial crooks alike look for innocuous hosts, called *zombies*, that they can compromise and control to use in attacks on other systems. Even if you don't handle credit card information, if you care about your system being available for your own use, you have to take steps, and if you care about the "public health" of the Internet, you have to be diligent.

The Fundamentals of Networking

Information security deals primarily with the CIA of information. IP network security addresses these issues as information passes over IP networks. Consequently, to talk about security we first have to talk about IP networking.

A good place to start is the underlying information architecture on which networking is based. A good reference point is the Department of Defense (DoD) networking model; this was the original seed for the ideas on which the Internet was founded, and IP protocols tend to be based upon this model.

The four layers of the DoD model, moving up from low-level transport to high-level application are:

- **Network Access Layer** Describes how computers talk to other locally attached devices. Focuses on issues of frames, which is the fundamental data unit passed along a physical network interface. In network security, we look at media, hub, and switch issues for security.

- **Internetwork Layer** Describes how frames are encapsulated into packets, and packets into datagrams; and how the datagram is transported between local networks. In network security, we look at switches, routers, and firewalls, such as the Cisco PIX for security.

- **Host-to-Host Transport Layer** Describes how hosts can achieve a reliable information stream. In network security, we look at routers, firewalls, and application devices such as load balancers or content managers, in conjunction with detective controls such as an Intrusion Detection System (IDS—for example, the Cisco Secure IDS) for security.

- **Process Application Layer** Describes how end users and end applications interact with the transported data. In network security, we look at end applications, together with IDS and Vulnerability Assessment tools such as the Cisco Secure Scanner, as well as auxiliary applications such as authentication servers like Cisco Secure Access Control Server (ACS).

Security can be applied in each layer and at the interface between layers; for example:

- **Network Access Layer** Examples of network access security issues are physical media access address resolution protocols and broadcast issues (for example, Address Resolution Protocol (ARP) cache poisoning and Virtual LANs (VLANs)/Multiprotocol Label Swtiching (MPLS) design).

- **Internetwork Layer** Examples of internetwork layer issues are packet routing security and transport control issues (for instance, IP address spoofing, IP address-based Access Control Lists (ACLs), source routing, fragment handling, and ICMP message handling).

- **Host-to-Lost Layer** Examples of host-to-host transport layer issues are communication stream initialization, transport confidentiality and integrity, and communication stream closure (for example, three-way handshake spoofing, packet snooping, and session hijacking).

- **Process Application Layer** Examples would be the SMTP or HTTP protocols (such as unsolicited commercial e-mail eradication or mobile code stripping).

Where Does Security Fit in?

To protect your infrastructure, you must apply security in layers. This layered approach is also called defense in depth. The idea is that you create multiple systems, so that a failure in one of them does not leave you vulnerable, but is caught in the next layer. You should create appropriate barriers inside your system so intruders that gain access to one part of it, do not automatically acquire access to the rest of the system. Use firewalls to minimize the exposure of private servers from public networks. Firewalls are the first line of defense. Packet filtering on routers can supplement the protection of firewalls and provide internal access boundaries.

Access to hosts that contain confidential information needs to be carefully controlled. Inventory the hosts on your network, and use this list to categorize the protection they will need. Some hosts will be used to providing public access, such as the corporate Web site or online storefront. Others will contain confidential information that may be used only by a single department or workgroup.

Plan the type of access needed and determine the boundaries of access control for these resources.

A good way to develop a defense in depth is to look at each layer of the DoD model, and apply security accordingly.

Network Access Layer Security

Network access layer security is done locally. One form of security addresses point-to-point communication, such as over a leased line or Frame Relay permanent virtual circuit. Dedicated hardware devices attached to each end of the link do encryption and decryption. Military, governments, and banking are the most common users of this approach. Though it is not scalable to large internetworks, because the packets are not routable in their encrypted state, this method does have the advantage that an eavesdropper cannot determine the source or destination addresses in the packets. It can also be used for upper-layer protocols.

A second form of security addresses controlling access to the shared media of the local LAN. At its simplest, if you have two machines that shouldn't communicate without controls (for example, a machine that handles Top Secret data and a machine that handles Unclassified data), don't put them on the same LAN. The military is known for building completely separate and partitioned networks, and having people with two machines on their desk to prevent information from spilling from one network into the other. Even in networks with less stringent requirements, the modern style is to develop separate, out-of-band management networks for controlling infrastructure equipment.

Configuring & Implementing...

NSA Router Security Guides

The National Security Agency of the United States has developed guidance on deploying Cisco routers in a secure fashion. They provide strategic design elements and tactical configurations for Cisco equipment. As of this writing, the guides are available online at http://nsa2 .www.conxion.com/cisco/index.html.

In a modern enterprise, it's not always possible to completely isolate machines on separate networks. They may need to communicate directly, or we may not have the resources to deploy separate routers, switches, and communication channels for all the equipment. In that environment, the most reasonable solution is judicious use of VLANs and virtual wide area networks through MPLS. For example, suppose you want to manage your firewalls, routers, switches, IDS, and other security devices from a management station on your desktop. You could buy a separate T1 to connect to your remote sites, and run separate wires to management interfaces on all these devices. Since that isn't practical, you can use MPLS and VLAN tags, combined with physically isolating management interfaces on separate switched ports, to provide that virtually partitioned network.

NOTE

Don't carry this process to the extreme. In security, there is a concept known as the Trusted Computing Base (TCB), its formal definition being "The totality of protection mechanisms within a computer system, including hardware, firmware, and software, the combination of which is responsible for enforcing a security policy." (Orange book). The goal is to make the TCB as small as possible—and ensure the components of the TCB are security devices, carefully reviewed, and so on.

For critical placements, you want the TCB to be the firewall and its software, and nothing else. It's important to remember that a switch is not a security device. As the SAFE architecture notes, "Avoid using VLANs as the sole method of securing access between two subnets. The capability for human error, combined with understanding that VLANs and VLAN tagging protocols were not designed with security in mind, makes their use in sensitive environments inadvisable. When VLANs are needed in security deployments, be sure to pay close attention to the configurations and guidelines mentioned above."

So, don't interconnect the router outside your firewall with a device inside the firewall via VLANs—there is a risk that if the switch is compromised, the firewall will be bypassed and the security of the whole enterprise will be placed in jeopardy. Make reasonable tradeoffs in the way of convenience, elegant design, and security.

Internetwork Layer Security

The easiest place to enforce a technical control is at the Internetwork layer—since you can inspect and forbid information from passing between separate networks and machines. Controlling access to the network with firewalls, routers, switches, remote access servers, and authentication servers can reduce the traffic getting to critical hosts to just authorized users and services. Security considerations can have an effect on the physical design of the network. Networks can be segmented to provide separation of responsibility. Departments, such as finance, research, or engineering, can be restricted so only the people that need access to particular resources can enter a network. You need to know the specifications that will be used to purchase network equipment, software features or revision levels that need to be used, and any specialized devices used to provide encryption, quality of service, or access control. You need to determine the resources to protect, the origin of threats against them, and where your network security perimeters should be located. Install devices and configurations at the perimeter—the internetwork layer between networks—that meets your security requirements.

Jon Postel, one of the godfathers of the Internet, wrote: "be conservative in what you do, be liberal in what you accept from others." Unfortunately, this principle of robustness has lead to security problems, particularly at the application and internetwork layers. At the Internetwork layer, it is important to validate the information you receive before routing. Of special importance is preventing simple fraud: a particularly pernicious problem today is based upon the *smurf* attack. This is a variant of the real-world "pizza order" attack, where you call a dozen pizza delivery companies and have them all deliver a pizza to someone's home at the same time. In a smurf attack, one computer makes requests for service from a large number of sites on the behalf of another host. There are details in terms of minimization of the bandwidth consumed by the attacker and maximization of the tidal wave of responses that hits the victim host, but it's all based upon sending outgoing requests as if for another person. If the pizza company could use caller ID to not accept requests from places other than where the call originates, the "pizza order" attack would fail. Similarly, if end routers did not route packets that could not have originated locally, the smurf attack would never get off the ground. In a modern internetworking environment, be cautious in what you accept from others; if it doesn't make sense, log it and drop it.

Access Control Lists

Access Control Lists (ACLs) are an effective way to address the filtering problem mentioned earlier. ACLs are packet filters that can be implemented on routers and similar devices to control the source and destination IP addresses allowed to pass through the gateway. Standard access lists can filter on source address. Extended access lists can filter ICMP, IGMP, or IP protocols at the Network layer. ICMP can be filtered based on the specific message. IP filtering can include port numbers at the transport (TCP/UDP) layer to allow or disallow specific services between particular addresses. Access lists can also control other routed protocols such as AppleTalk or IPX, and they are your first and best way to eliminate inappropriate traffic.

Configuring & Implementing...

Martian Filtering

The router requirements of RFC 1812 talk about "martian filtering," and notes "A router SHOULD NOT forward any packet that has an invalid IP source address or a source address on network 0." Large chunks of IP space—not just the RFC 1918's of the 10, 172.16, and 192.168 networks, are invalid addresses and should be dropped. An effective way of achieving this is to null route the logon, like this:

```
ip route 1.0.0.0 255.0.0.0 null0

ip route 2.0.0.0 255.0.0.0 null0

ip route 5.0.0.0 255.0.0.0 null0

ip route 7.0.0.0 255.0.0.0 null0

ip route 10.0.0.0 255.0.0.0 null0

ip route 23.0.0.0 255.0.0.0 null0

ip route 27.0.0.0 255.0.0.0 null0

ip route 31.0.0.0 255.0.0.0 null0

ip route 36.0.0.0 255.0.0.0 null0

ip route 37.0.0.0 255.0.0.0 null0

ip route 39.0.0.0 255.0.0.0 null0

ip route 41.0.0.0 255.0.0.0 null0

ip route 42.0.0.0 255.0.0.0 null0
```

An extremely useful consensus document on secure router templates for the Internet is Rob Thomas' *Secure IOS Template*, available at www.cymru.com/~robt/Docs/Articles/secure-ios-template.html.

Host-to-host Layer Security

Host-to-host layer security can be applied to secure traffic for all applications or transport protocols in the above layers. Applications do not need to be modified since they communicate with the Transport layer above. Confidentiality and integrity are easily obtained through encryption and authentication protocols, and availability and other reliability issues are addressed through reliable transport protocols.

IPSec

The security architecture for IP (IPSec) is a suite of security services for traffic at the IP layer. It is an open standard, defined in RFC 2401 and several following RFCs. It has received widespread adoption, and clients are generally available for many hosts and network infrastructure devices. It is integrated into Cisco IOS, and available on most routers and firewalls. It is the single most common, least expensive, and most widely deployed technical security control at the host-to-host layer.

IPSec protocols can supply access control, authentication, data integrity, and confidentiality for each IP packet between two participating network nodes. IPSec can be used between two hosts (including clients), a gateway and a host, or two gateways. No modification of network hardware or software is required to route IPSec. Applications and upper-level protocols can thus be used unchanged.

IPSec adds two security protocols to IP, Authentication Header (AH) and Encapsulating Security Payload (ESP). AH provides connectionless integrity, data origin authentication, and anti-replay service for the IP packet. AH does not encrypt the data, but any modification of the data would be detected. ESP provides confidentiality through the encryption of the payload. Access control is provided through the use and management of keys to control participation in traffic flows.

IPSec was designed to be flexible so different security needs could be accommodated. The security services can be tailored to the particular needs of each connection by using AH or ESP separately for their individual functions, or combining the protocols to provide the full range of protection offered by IPSec. Multiple cryptographic algorithms are supported. The algorithms that must be present in any implementation of IPSec are listed next. The null algorithms provide no protection, but are used for consistent negotiation by the protocols. AH and ESP cannot both be null at the same time.

- Data Encryption Standard (DES) in Cipher Block Chaining (CBC) mode

- HMAC (Hash Message Authentication Codes) with MD5

- HMAC with SHA

- Null Authentication Algorithm

- Null Encryption Algorithm

A security association (SA) forms an agreement between two systems participating in an IPSec connection. A security association represents a simplex connection to provide a security service using a selected policy and keys, between two nodes. A Security Parameter Index (SPI), an IP destination address, and a protocol identifier are used to identify a particular SA. The SPI is an arbitrary, 32-bit value selected by the destination system that uniquely identifies a particular security association among several associations that may exist on a specific node. The protocol identifier can indicate either AH or ESP, but not both. Separate security associations are created for each protocol, and for each direction between systems. If two systems were using AH and ESP in both directions, then they would form four security associations.

Each protocol supports a transport mode and a tunnel mode of operation. The transport mode is between two hosts. These hosts are the endpoints for the cryptographic functions being used. Tunnel mode is an IP tunnel, and is used whenever either end of the security association is a security gateway. A security gateway is an intermediate system, such as a router or firewall, which implements IPSec protocols. A security association between a host and a security gateway must use tunnel mode. If the connection traffic is destined for the gateway itself, such as management traffic, then the gateway is treated as a host, because it is the endpoint of the communication.

In transport mode, the AH or ESP header is inserted after the IP header, but before any upper-layer protocol headers. As shown in Figure 1.1, AH authenticates the original IP header, but does not protect the fields that are modified in the course of routing IP packets. ESP only protects what comes after the ESP header. If the security policy between two nodes requires a combination of security services, the AH header appears first after the IP header, followed by the ESP header. This combination of security associations is called an *SA bundle*.

In tunnel mode, the original IP header and payload are encapsulated by the IPSec protocols. A new IP header that specifies the IPSec tunnel destination is prepended to the packet. The original IP header and its payload are protected by the AH or ESP headers. From Figure 1.2, you can see that, as in transport mode, AH offers some protection for the entire packet, but does not protect the fields that are modified in the course of routing IP packets between the IPSec tunnel endpoints. It does, however, completely protect the original IP header.

Figure 1.1 The IPSec Transport Mode in IPv4

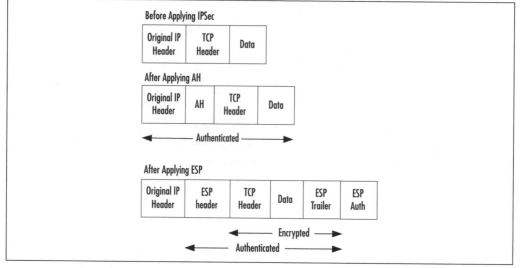

Figure 1.2 The IPSec Tunnel Mode in IPv4

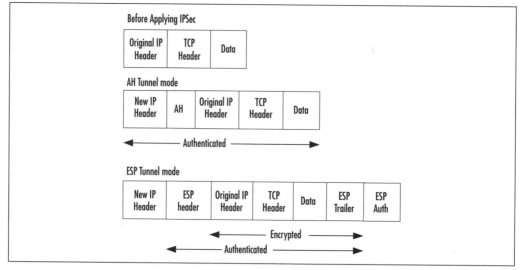

Key management is another major component of IPSec. Manual techniques are allowed in the IPSec standard, and might be acceptable for configuring one or two gateways, but typing in keys and data is not practical in most environments. The Internet Key Exchange (IKE) provides automated, bidirectional SA management, key generation, and key management. IKE negotiates in two phases. Phase 1 negotiates a secure, authenticated channel over which the two systems can communicate for further negotiations. They agree on the encryption algorithm, hash algorithm, authentication method, and Diffie-Hellman group to exchange keys and information. A single phase 1 association can be used for multiple phase 2 negotiations. Phase 2 negotiates the services that define the security associations used by IPSec. They agree on IPSec protocol, hash algorithm, and encryption algorithm. Multiple security associations will result from phase 2 negotiations. An SA is created for the inbound and outbound of each protocol used.

Process Application Layer Security

Any vendor's software is susceptible to harboring security vulnerabilities. Security can be seen as an arms race, with the bad guys exploiting vulnerabilities and the good guys patching them. Every day, Web sites that track security vulnerabilities, such as CERT, are reporting new vulnerability discoveries in operating systems, application software, server software, and even in security software or devices. Last year, CERT advertised an average of over six vulnerabilities a day. Figure 1.3 shows the increase in reported incidents over the years.

Figure 1.3 CERT Reporting Statistics

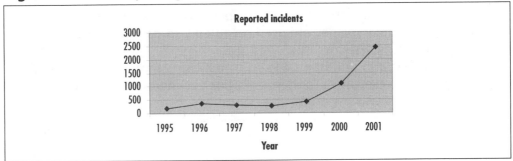

Patches are implemented for these known bugs, but new vulnerability discoveries continue. Sometimes patches fix one bug, only to introduce another. Even open source software that has been widely used for ten years is not immune to harboring serious vulnerabilities. In June 2000, CERT reported that MIT Kerberos had multiple buffer overflow vulnerabilities that could be used to gain root access, and in Feb of 2002, widespread vulnerabilities were announced in the fundamental ASN.1 encoding schema common to all SNMP agents, allowing the compromise of nearly all infrastructure devices across the Internet.

Many sites do not keep up when it comes to applying patches and so leave their systems with known vulnerabilities. It is important to keep all of your software up to date. Many of the most damaging attacks have occurred in end-user software such as electronic mail clients. Attacks can be directed at any software and can seriously affect your network.

The default configuration of hosts makes them easy to get up and running, but many default services are unnecessary. These unnecessary services increase the vulnerabilities of the system. On each host, all unnecessary services should be shut down. Misconfigured hosts also increase the risk of an unauthorized access. All default passwords and community names must be changed.

NOTE

The SANS (System Administration, Networking, and Security) Institute in conjunction with the National Infrastructure Protection Center (NIPC) has created a list of the top 20 Internet security threats as determined by a group of security experts. The list is maintained at www.sans.org/top20.htm. This guide is an excellent list of the most urgent and critical vulnerabilities to repair on your systems. Two of the problems listed earlier—unnecessary default services and default passwords—are on this list.

This effort was started because experience has shown that a small number of vulnerabilities are used repeatedly to gain unauthorized access to many systems.

SANS has also published a list of the most common mistakes made by end users, executives, and information technology personnel. It is available at www.sans.org/mistakes.htm.

The increased complexity of systems, the shortage of well-trained administrators, and a lack of resources all contribute to reducing the security of hosts and applications. We cannot depend on hosts to protect themselves from all threats. A useful approach is to use automated scanning devices, such as Cisco Secure Scanner (formerly NetSonar) to help identify the vulnerabilities from a network perspective, and work with the information owner to apply the necessary remediation.

All is not lost, however. Application layer security can provide end-to-end security from an application running on one host through the network to the application on another host. It does not care about the underlying transport mechanism. Complete coverage of security requirements, integrity, confidentiality and non-repudiation, can be provided at this layer. Applications have a fine granularity of control over the nature and content of the transactions. However, application layer security is not a general solution, because each application and client must be adapted to provide the security services. Several examples of application security extensions are described next.

PGP

Phil Zimmerman created Pretty Good Privacy (PGP) in 1991. It is widely used by individuals worldwide for privacy and the digital signing of e-mail messages. PGP provides end-to-end security from the sender to the receiver. It can also be used to encrypt files. PGP has traditionally used RSA public key cryptography to exchange keys, and IDEA to encrypt messages.

PGP uses a Web of trust or network trust model, where any users can vouch for the identity of other users. Getting the public keys of the intended person can be difficult to achieve in a secure manner. You can get a person's public key directly from that person, and then communicate the hash of the key in an out-of-band pathway. Keys are stored in files called key rings. Some Internet servers, in fact, have public key rings. They do not authenticate the keys—merely store them. You should not trust keys that have an unknown heritage.

S-HTTP

S-HTTP is not widely used, but it was designed to provide security for Web-based applications. Secure HTTP is a secure message-oriented communications protocol, and can transmit individual messages securely. It provides transaction confidentiality, authentication, and message integrity, and extends HTTP to include tags for encrypted and secure transactions. S-HTTP is implemented in some commercial Web servers and most browsers. As an S-HTTP server, it negotiates with the client for the type of encryption that will be used, several types of which exist.

S-HTTP does not require clients to have public key certificates because it can use symmetric keys to provide private transactions. The symmetric keys would be provided in advance using out of band communication.

Secure Sockets Layer and Transport Layer Security

Secure Sockets Layer (SSL) was designed by Netscape and is widely used on the Internet for Web transactions such as sending credit card data. It can be utilized for other protocols as well, such as Telnet, FTP, LDAP, IMAP, and SMTP, but these are not commonly used. Transport Layer Security (TLS), on the other hand, is an open, IETF-proposed standard based on SSL 3.0. RFCs 2246, 2712, 2817, and 2818 define TLS. The name is misleading, since TLS happens well above the transport layer. The two protocols are not interoperable, but TLS has the capability to drop down into SSL 3.0 mode for backwards compatibility, and both can provide security for a single TCP session.

SSL and TLS provide a connection between a client and a server, over which any amount of data can be sent securely. Server and browser generally must be SSL- or TLS-enabled to facilitate secure Web connections, while applications generally must be SSL- or TLS-enabled to allow their use of the secure connection. However, a recent trend is to use dedicated SSL accelerators as VPN terminators, passing the content on to an end server; the Cisco Content Services Switch Secure Content Accelerator 1100 is an example of this technique.

For the browser and server to communicate securely, each needs to have the shared session key. SSL/TLS use public key encryption to exchange session keys during communication initialization. When a browser is installed on a workstation, it generates a unique private/public key pair.

The Secure Shell Protocol

The Secure Shell protocol (SSH) is specified in a set of Internet draft documents. SSH provides secure remote login and other secure network services over an insecure network. It's being promoted free as a means for reducing cleartext passwords on networks. One excellent Windows client is PuTTY, available at www.chiark.greenend.org.uk/~sgtatham/putty. The IOS on a modern Cisco router supports SSH, but only SSH version 1. SSH version 2 is completely rewritten to use different security protocols and has added public key cryptography. Both versions provide confidentiality of passwords and other commands during sessions.

The SSH protocol provides channels for establishing secure, interactive shell sessions and tunneling other TCP applications. There are three major components to SSH:

- **Transport layer protocol** Provides authentication, confidentiality, and integrity for the server. It can also compress the data stream. The SSH transport runs on top of TCP. The transport protocol negotiates the key exchange method, public key, symmetric encryption, authentication, and hash algorithms.

- **User authentication protocol** Authenticates the user-level client to the server and runs on top of the SSH transport layer. It assumes that the transport layer provides integrity and confidentiality. The method of authentication is negotiated between the server and the client.

- **Connection protocol** Multiplexes an encrypted tunnel into several channels. It is run on top of SSH transport and authentication protocols. The two ends negotiate the channel, window size, and type of data. The connection protocol can tunnel X11 or any arbitrary TCP port traffic.

Figure 1.4 shows how various security controls can interact with network traffic, and shows several of the areas where controls can be placed—from directly encrypting signals as they are applied to the Network Access Layer (link encryption) all the way up to encrypting the contents of a mail message (PGP):

Figure 1.4 The Layers of Security Controls

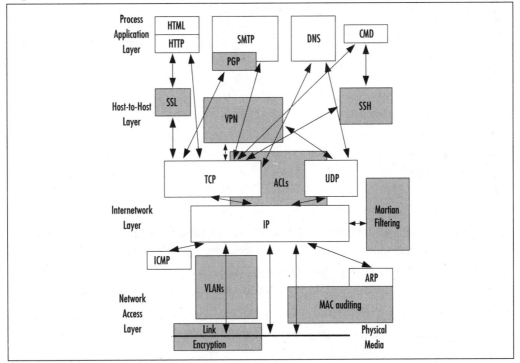

Authentication

Authentication can be used as a security control at any layer in the protocol stack, but is typically deployed at the application process layer. (Often, the application process layer then makes changes to controls at the internetworking layer, establishing sessions or opening ACLs to permit traffic.)

Authentication can be provided locally on each device on your network, but using an authentication server offers improved scalability, flexibility, and control. Firewalls, routers, and remote access servers enforce network access security. Configuring these devices to use one, centralized database of accounts is easier on the administrator and the users who may access the network through multiple pathways.

A Cisco Network Access Server (NAS), firewall, or router acts as the client and requests authentication from an authentication server. The access server or router will prompt the user for a username and password, and then verifies the password with the authentication server. TACACS+, RADIUS, and Kerberos are widely used authentication servers supported by Cisco. TACACS+ and RADIUS can also provide services for authorization, and accounting.

Terminal Access Controller Access System Plus

Terminal Access Controller Access System Plus (TACACS+) is an enhanced version of TACACS developed by Cisco. The enhancements include the separation of authentication, authorization, and accounting into three distinct functions. These services can be used independently or together. For example, Kerberos could be used for authentication, and TACACS+ used for authorization and accounting. Some of the characteristics of TACACS+ are:

- While older versions of TACACS and RADIUS use UDP for transport, TACACS+ uses TCP (port 49) for reliable and acknowledged transport.

- TACACS+ can encrypt the entire payload of the packet, so it protects the password, username, and other information sent between the Cisco access client and the server. The encryption can be turned off for troubleshooting. Communication from the workstation to the Cisco client providing access services is not encrypted.

- TACACS+ supports multiple protocols such as IP, AppleTalk Remote Access (ARA), Novell, Asynchronous Services Interface (NASI), X.25 PAD connection, and NetBIOS.

- You can use TACACS+ to provide greater control over router management in either nonprivileged or privileged mode, because you can authenticate individual users or groups rather than a shared password. Router commands can be specified explicitly on the TACACS+ server to allow specific commands.

Remote Dial-in User System

Remote Dial-in User System (RADIUS) is an open standard and available from many vendors. It was originally designed for ISPs to support dial-in clients, and provides the authorization and billing information for those needs. RADIUS can be a good choice in a heterogeneous network environment because of its widespread support, but some vendors have implemented proprietary attributes in RADIUS that hinder interoperability.

- RADIUS uses UDP, so it only offers best effort delivery at a lower overhead.

- For authentication, RADIUS encrypts only the password sent between the Cisco access client and RADIUS server. RADIUS does not provide encryption between the workstation and the Cisco access client.

- RADIUS does not support multiple protocols, and only works on IP networks.

- RADIUS does not provide the ability to control the commands that can be executed on a router: It provides authentication, but not authorization to Cisco devices.

Kerberos

Kerberos protocol can be used for network authentication and host authentication. It uses a *trusted third-party* approach, where users identify themselves to a central server, and the server then provides "tickets," that the user can present to gain access to servers; the end server trusts that the Kerberos server is granting authority correctly.

A Kerberos realm includes all users, hosts and network services that are registered with a Kerberos server. Kerberos uses symmetric key cryptography and stores a shared key for each user and each network resource that is participating in its realm. Host-based applications must be "kerberized," with modules adapted to use the Kerberos protocol. Kerberized versions of Telnet, ftp, mail, and several others exist, and APIs exist for updating code. Every user and network resource needs a Kerberos account. Kerberos stores all passwords encrypted with a single system key. If that system key is compromised, all passwords need to be recreated.

The process of authenticating using Kerberos involves three systems: a client, a network resource, and the Kerberos server. The Kerberos server is called the Key Distribution Center (KDC). The KDC has two functions: an Authentication

www.syngress.com

Service (AS) and a Ticket Granting Service (TGS). The basic process is a six-step sequence:

1. **Alice to KDC** Hi, I'm Alice. Could I have access to the AS?

2. **AS to Alice** Here is your "ticket-granting ticket." If you aren't Alice, it's useless. If you are Alice, decrypt this, and come back with the answer.

3. **Alice to TGS** Okay, I figured out your secret. Give me a "service-granting ticket" so I can talk to server Bob.

4. **TGS to Alice** You have it! It's encrypted using the same mechanism as before, and then encrypted with Bob's password. This ticket will be accepted by Bob for eight hours.

5. **Client to Bob** The KDC gave me this ticket, and it is encrypted using your password. Validate me.

6. **Bob to Alice** Hello, Alice! I've decrypted what you got from the KDC, I trust the KDC, and he trusts you, so your access is granted. It is worth noting that under Kerberos, passwords are never sent in the clear; there is a preshared secret between the client and the KDC, and the client uses that to unlock the "ticket-granting ticket." This allows the client to request tickets that can be provided to individual servers to obtain that service.

As an example, let's look at remote network access. The remote user establishes a PPP connection to the boundary device, and the device prompts the user for username and password. The device, acting as the client, requests a ticket-granting ticket from the Kerberos authentication server. If the user has an account, the authentication server generates a session key, and sends a ticket-granting ticket (TGT) to the client encrypted with the password stored on the AS for that account. The Cisco access server will attempt to decrypt the TGT with the password that the user entered. The TGT is a credential that specifies the user's verified identity, the Kerberos server identity, and the expiration time of the ticket. By default, tickets expire after eight hours. The TGT is encrypted with a key known only to the ticket-granting server and the authentication server. The TGT is presented back to the TGS with a request for access to the Cisco access server. Now the roles reverse, and the Cisco access server becomes the server. The Cisco access server accepts the service ticket, decrypts it to verify it is valid, and provides service. If successful, the user is authenticated to the access server, and the user's workstation becomes part of the protected network.

Note that at this point, the only authenticated "user" is the Cisco access server. Users, who want to access services that are part of the Kerberos realm on the network, must now re-authenticate against the Kerberos server and get authorization to access the services. The user first gets a ticket-granting ticket as previously described, which is used to request access to other services. The difference is that the client is now the user's workstation.

More details on AAA can be found in Chapter 9.

OSI Model

The DoD model is very helpful for thinking about security. Unfortunately, it's the Betamax of security models—internetworking professionals tend to prefer the OSI model; it adds more specific layers at the low and high ends, and more naturally maps to certain kinds of equipment. It is worth reviewing the OSI model to set up the language that will be used in the later chapters of the book, and to correspond to materials you will read elsewhere.

The OSI Reference Model consists of seven layers:

- The physical layer (Layer 1)

- The data-link layer (Layer 2)

- The network layer (Layer 3)

- The transport layer (Layer 4)

- The session layer (Layer 5)

- The presentation layer (Layer 6)

- The application layer (Layer 7).

This convention has been developed to provide an initial framework to simplify network design and to provide a systematic approach to troubleshooting. As our discussion progresses, the functionality of each layer and how these layers communicate will become increasingly clear. The OSI model was an extension of the more Internet focused DoD model, and provides additional structure, particularly at the higher layers.

A nice mnemonic for the OSI layers is the expression "All People Seem To Need Data Processing." The first initials correspond to "Application, Presentation, Session, Transport, Network, Data, Physical."

In our discussion of how each layer functions, we look at the parallels between human communication and that of computer systems, breaking down

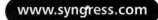

the communication process into its components to allow more granular comparisons. Imagine yourself as a student in a classroom listening to an instructor's lecture. This constitutes our example of human communication; we then address how computer communications correspond to that example. Keep in mind that when we talk about computer systems communicating, we are really referring to one device talking to another.

Layer 1: The Physical Layer

The *physical layer* is identified as the physical medium that facilitates communication. In our classroom example, air is considered the physical medium. It carries the sound waves produced by the instructor to the students. Both the air and the sound waves being transmitted are considered part of the physical layer. In the computer world, where traditional wired technology is implemented, copper is the primary mode of transmission. It carries a designated electrical pattern to the other computers in the local network. Again, the electrical waves are a component of the physical layer. This layer is also responsible for specifying the shape and intensity of the electrical wave.

Layer 2: The Data-link Layer

The *data-link layer,* in our human analogy, formats thoughts passed from the instructor's brain into a simplified, and hopefully more organized structure. The structures at this phase are blocks of verbal syllables. These syllables are the simplest elements of the message from the higher layers. In order to ensure that the instructor emits sound waves comprehensible to the audience, there is a "think before you speak" process, the human equivalent of error checking. This layer then hands these blocks of syllables, or *frames*, to the physical layer, which translates these messages into sounds that the students can understand. Lastly, sound waves are produced from the instructor and transmitted via air compression waves to the intended audience—the students in the class.

Another characteristic of communication at this layer, called *flow control*, is evidenced when a student has a question during a lecture. The instructor can either stop the lecture and address the question immediately or request that the student hold the question until the instructor is finished—that is, the instructor is managing the flow of the lecture. This function is important because it optimizes communication within the classroom. The instructor might think that the material needs to be presented in its entirety to maximize the level of understanding. On the other hand, the instructor could find that questions from the audience enhance the lecture. The flow of the class all depends on the instructor.

These same attributes are found in the computer world as well. Information from higher-level layers is formatted into frames, just as the instructor's concept from the instructor's mental processes is formatted into syllables the instructor speaks. In addition to formatting, the intended destination (the students) and source identifier (their instructor) are attached. The destination and source information are represented as addresses, formally referred to as *media access control* (MAC) addresses. The Ethernet MAC address is a 48-bit number known as the hardware address, which is mostly unique and that is "burned into" the device. Also included in the frame created by the data-link layer is the *cyclical redundancy checksum* (CRC). The CRC provides a metric allowing the receiving device a way of determining whether the data has been damaged in the transmission process or in transit. This parallels the "think before you speak" process, making sure that the instructor didn't mumble (valid transmission) and loud noises didn't drown out the lecture (not damaged during transit). Note that in our example, the destination address is a *broadcast address*, intended for multiple recipients. In the Ethernet world, this is achieved by using a special MAC—either the all 1s MAC as a general broadcast, or through the use of a specialized MAC and techniques such as group messaging controls to indicate the intended audience.

Damage & Defense...

Hardware Address Spoofing

Hardware MAC addresses are supposed to be unique, and some systems use them as unique security identifiers. The problem is that the transmitted address can be manipulated by software. Sometimes this is a good thing: if a network is designed with a particular fixed MAC address in mind, and a piece of hardware fails, then another device can "take over" that role—this is used for highly available systems or to comply with licensing constraints. It can also be used to indicate particular functions—for example, one popular "sticky honeypot" uses a forged MAC address for its virtual hosts. On the other hand, if a system trusts a MAC address to identify a host, and someone else interferes with that process—either by interrupting the hardware address resolution request or killing the victim host and spoofing its address—unintentional and inappropriate communications may occur.

The physical layer is actually divided into two sublayers: the logical link control (LLC) and the MAC. The LLC is the liaison between the protocols within the network layer and the media access control sublayer. The media access controls access the physical medium. An example of a protocol that works with MAC is the carrier sense multiple access/collision detect (CSMA/CD). This protocol performs a measure of flow control.

NOTE

Watch for unusual changes in the physical port locations of your hardware addresses. If devices "move around" mysteriously or large numbers of devices suddenly appear, you probably have a network problem or a security event.

Layer 3: The Network Layer

The primary function of the *network layer* is to determine the best-known path for information to reach its intended destination. In our classroom example, the information is intended for the local audience. The instructor knows that all the students in the class are there to hear the information in the lecture. The information is formatted, error-checked, and translated into a message via the data-link layer. Subsequently, the frame is transmitted into the physical medium. Because the students are local, no particular treatment is required; they are directly available to hear the message.

What if there is an emergency phone message for the instructor? The person taking the call knows the instructor and the location of the classroom and will deliver the information. The messenger knows the information in the message is important and needs to find the best—in this case, the fastest—way to the classroom. Perhaps the elevator is the fastest, but there are many students in the building, which could cause delay. The stairs seem to be the most reliable and the fastest route. These decisions are similar to the decisions the network layer makes in order to deliver traffic as effectively as possible.

The network layer deals with *packets*, which are eventually encapsulated into frames by the data-link layer. The packets contain information from the layer above the network layer. This is also where the logical IP addresses reside. They are considered logical because, unlike the MAC address that is permanently "burned" into the network interface card (NIC), IP addressing provides a method of grouping devices regardless of their physical location. This is an important aspect of network design.

Layer 4: The Transport Layer

The *transport layer* provides methods of flow control, ordering of received data, and acknowledgement of correctly received data. It relates to our classroom scenario in that it establishes the way that the instructor presents the lecture. For instance, the instructor might look to the audience for an indication of whether or not they understand the lecture. The instructor could invite questions, look for body language indicating agreement, or perhaps even count sleeping students. The instructor attempts to give each student a chance to be involved in the lecture emulating one-on-one attention. On the other hand, it is also possible that the instructor does not desire feedback and will lecture regardless of audience reactions. This type of presentation could be necessary when there is an excessive amount of information and inadequate time to present the material. These two approaches are both appropriate for certain situations and audiences. You will see this type of communication in the computer world as well.

The transport layer can be categorized into *connection-oriented* and *connectionless* protocols. An example of a connection-oriented protocol is TCP. The term *connection-oriented* refers to communications that establish an interaction between the two ends of the connection; they shake hands and agree upon some basic conventions, and then pass along service information about the ongoing communication. It implies a level of reliability and a guarantee of delivery of services, much like the first method of presentation in the classroom. The processes involved in the protocol function to provide a virtual one-on-one appearance. Connectionless protocols, like UDP, do not provide these measures of reliability. In a connectionless communication, information is simply dropped on the wire and a "best effort" delivery is assumed to get the information to its recipient. This method is analogous to the second method in our classroom example, in which the instructor continues to lecture whether the students hear and understand everything or not. Generally speaking, what is lost in reliability is gained in efficiency; connectionless protocols are generally chosen when high throughput is necessary and some information loss is acceptable.

Designing & Planning...

ISN Spoofing

As part of the connection establishment process, a TCP session identifies an initial sequence number (ISN) that is used to provide a marker into how much data has been transmitted and received. Because this is information negotiated as part of the session, some people assume that possession of the ISN means that you are rightfully one of the parties of the communication.

The problem is that ISNs are often predictable. Originally, ISNs were designed to be clock-driven—which provides uniqueness, but also a high degree of predictability. Later implementations simply used the next available number, so systems that were relatively quiet were easily predicted. A malicious user would use this predictability to forge a communication from a trusted host, bypassing local security measures. The most famous of these was Kevin Mitnick, who used this technique to steal research data, documented in Tsutomu Shimomura and John Markoff's book, *Takedown*.

NOTE

Don't assume that because a TCP session has been successfully established, the end IP addresses are valid. Enforce IP address antispoofing techniques whenever possible to prevent rogue packets from coming onto your network.

Layer 5: The Session Layer

The *session layer* establishes the parameters of any upcoming communication. The parameters include the language that will be used and the style of the lecture (whether or not questions are acceptable intermittently or need to be held until the end of the lecture)—those being parameters that need to be predetermined. Another issue to resolve is setting time limits: When the lecture will conclude, for example, which could be at an established time or simply whenever all the topics and questions have been addressed. These parameters are established to set the expectations for everyone involved, a critical aspect of effective communication.

These types of parameters are also established prior to the exchange of data among computer systems. First, protocols need to be agreed on. Some examples of session-layer protocols are Network File System (NFS), Structured Query Language (SQL), and X Windows. Protocols are important because if the devices are not using the same protocols, they are essentially speaking different languages. Next, they decide on the communication flow. There are three types: *single mode*, *half-duplex mode*, and *full-duplex mode*. Single-mode communication occurs when only one device at a time transmits information, and it transmits until all the information has been completely sent. Half-duplex mode occurs when the devices take turns transmitting. This is comparable to a conversation between two people using walkie-talkies in which only one person can talk at any given time. (If both people push the Talk button at the same time, neither person will hear anything.) Full-duplex mode occurs when the devices transmit and receive simultaneously. An example of full-duplex communication is when two people talk on a phone—both parties can talk at the same time.

Once all the preliminary details have been established, data exchange can proceed. After the exchange is complete, the devices systematically disengage the session.

The session layer can be either *connection-oriented* or *connectionless*. A connection-oriented session contains checkpoints or activity management. This system provides a way to efficiently retransmit any data that is lost or is erroneous on receipt. It is efficient because only the data that needs to be transmitted is sent, rather than the entire session. Connectionless sessions, as with IP and UDP, are a best-effort delivery. As with the two other examples, in a connectionless session, the layer above (the presentation layer) is responsible for providing reliability.

Layer 6: The Presentation Layer

The *presentation layer* establishes the way in which information is presented, typically for display or printing. Data encryption and character set conversion (such as ASCII to EBCDIC) are usually associated with this layer. The primary reason for someone to attend a class is that the presentation of information is designed to help that person learn. Students could, theoretically, pick up the literature and learn the material on their own; however, the value comes with the instructor's interpretation of the material. The instructor translates the information in such a way that students understand it. The presentation layer provides this functionality in computer systems.

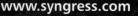

The presentation layer translates information in a way that the application layer understands. Likewise, this layer translates information from the application layer to the session layer. Some examples of presentation layer protocols are SSL, HTTP/ HTML (agent), FTP (server), AppleTalk Filing Protocol, Telnet, and so on.

Layer 7: The Application Layer

The *application layer* is where user space programs make requests of network services. In our metaphor, this represents the overall point or concept of the instructor's lecture—this is what use the student makes of the lecture. All the layers of communication we have talked about to this point are transparent to the student, for the most part. However, the overall effectiveness of the course could depend on the way the material is communicated and how the class is structured. For instance, if the instructor is difficult to understand, for whatever reason, the content of the material is meaningless to the students. The same is true if the situation were reversed: the instructor could be a sensational communicator, but if the material being covered is inappropriate for the desired goal of the class, the content is worthless.

A good example of an application layer protocol is the HTTP/HTML browser. The end look and feel of a Web page is highly dependent upon the application. Using Microsoft Internet Explorer may cause certain things to break that look normal under Netscape; using lynx provides a text-based view; other browsers are designed for the visually impaired, and read the text out loud or provide displays to Braille screens. The end-user experience is very different in each case—but if we looked at what is happening on the network, it's still the same HTTP GET requests.

Another good example is FTP. At the application layer, an FTP server provides a user interface. You can see the output from an FTP command line client next:

```
ftp> help
Commands may be abbreviated. Commands are:
!              delete         literal        prompt         send
?              debug          ls             put            status
append         dir            mdelete        pwd            trace
ascii          disconnect     mdir           quit           type
bell           get            mget           quote          user
binary         glob           mkdir          recv           verbose
bye            hash           mls            remotehelp
cd             help           mput           rename
close          lcd            open           rmdir
```

Some of these commands are completely local—for example, the command *help* produced the output shown in the code and no network traffic. However, several correspond to a network interface, as specified in various RFCs. These are listed in Table 1.1 that follows.

Table 1.1 FTP Session Layer Commands

Type of Command	Applicable Commands
Access Control Commands	USER, PASS, ACCT, CWD, CDUP, SMNT, REIN, QUIT
Transfer Parameter Commands	PORT, PASV, TYPE, STRU, MODE
FTP Service Commands	RETR, STOR, STOU, APPE, ALLO, REST, RNFR, RNTO, ABOR, DELE, RMD, MKD, PWD, LIST, NLST, SITE, SYST, STAT, HELP, NOOP

Take a look at this output:

```
ftp> ascii
200 Type set to A.
ftp> get icmpmask.c
200 PORT command successful.
150 Opening ASCII mode data connection for icmpmask.c (7565 bytes).
226 Transfer complete.
ftp: 7852 bytes received in 1.09Seconds 7.20Kbytes/sec.
```

It was produced by the following TCP stream:

```
C: TYPE A
S: 200 Type set to A.
C: PORT 165,247,113,42,9,142
S: 200 PORT command successful.
C: RETR icmpmask.c
S: 150 Opening ASCII mode data connection for icmpmask.c (7565 bytes).
S: 226 Transfer complete.
```

Thus FTP is both a Layer 6 (session) and Layer 7 (application) layer protocol.

Some protocols exist only at Layer 7. For example, online gaming, such as Doom, typically only has one standard client, so all requests are handled directly by the application.

How the OSI Model Works

Now that we've looked at the overview of the OSI model with metaphors to make things more natural, let's address some of the specifics of IP communication over Ethernet networks.

Transport Layer Protocols

The transport layer provides duplex, end-to-end data transport services between applications. Data sent from the application layer is divided into segments appropriate in size for the network technology being used. TCP and UDP are the protocols used at this layer.

TCP

TCP provides reliable service by being connection-oriented and including error detection and correction. The connected nature of TCP is used only for two end points to communicate with each other. The connection must be established before a data transfer can occur, and transfers are acknowledged throughout the process. Acknowledgements assure that data is being received properly. The acknowledgement process provides robustness in the face of network congestion or communication unreliability. TCP also determines when the transfer ends and closes the connection, thus freeing up resources on the systems. Checksums assure that the data has not been accidentally modified during transit. Figure 1.5, taken from RFC 793, shows the format of the TCP header.

Figure 1.5 The TCP Header

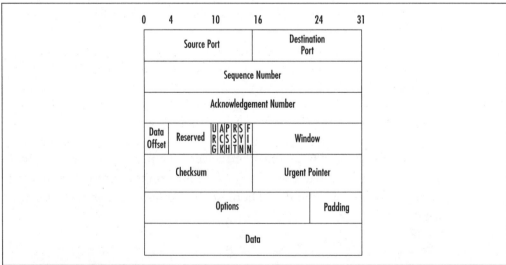

TCP ports are used to multiplex this protocol layer to the layer above with multiple applications on the same host. A source port and a destination port are associated with the sending and receiving applications, respectively. The ports from 0 to 1023 are Well Known Ports, and are assigned by Internet Assigned Numbers Authority (IANA). Ports from 1024 to 49151 are Registered Ports, while ports from 49152 through 65535 are Dynamic/Private Ports. The Well Known and Registered Port numbers are available at www.isi.edu/in-notes/iana/assignments/port-numbers.

Bits 10 through 15 at word offset 3 correspond to the TCP control bits, or flags. They provide information about the importance of the Sequence Number, Acknowledgement Number, and Urgent Pointer fields. They also provide information about how the packet should be treated by the receiving host. These are reflected in Table 1.2.

Table 1.2 TCP Control Bits

Control Bit	Description
URG	Urgent control bit indicates that Urgent Pointer is a valid offset to add to the Sequence Number. The sender of data can indicate to the receiver that there is urgent data pending.
ACK	Acknowledgement control bit indicates that the Acknowledgement Number contains the value of the next sequence number the sender of the segment is expecting to receive. ACK is always set for an established connection.
PSH	Push all data received to this point up to the receiving application. This function expedites the delivery of urgent data to the destination.
RST	Reset the connection. This function flushes all queued segments waiting for transmission or retransmission, and puts the receiver in listen mode.
SYN	Synchronize sequence numbers. The SYN control bit indicates that the Sequence Number contains the initial sequence number.
FIN	Sender has finished sending data. The FIN control bit is set by the application closing its connection.

The sequence numbers allow recovery by TCP from data that was lost, damaged, duplicated, or delivered out of order. Each host in the TCP connection selects an Initial Sequence Number (ISN), and these are synchronized during the establishment of the connection. The sequence number is incremented for each byte of data transmitted across the TCP connection, including the SYN and FIN flags. Sequence numbers are 32 bits and will wrap around to zero when they overflow. The ISN should be unpredictable for a given TCP connection. Some TCP implementations have exhibited vulnerabilities of predictable sequence numbers. Predicting the sequence number can allow an attacker to impersonate a host.

The acknowledgement number has a valid entry when the ACK flag is on. It contains the next sequence number that the receiver is expecting. Since every data segment sent over a TCP connection has a sequence number, it also has an acknowledgement number.

The ACK and RST play a role in determining whether a connection is established or being established. Cisco uses the established keyword in Access Control Lists (ACLs) to check whether the ACK or RST flags are set. If either flag is set, the packet meets the test as established. If neither the ACK nor the RST flags are set, then this packet is not part of an existing connection, but an attempt to establish a new connection to the device at the destination TCP address.

Damage & Defense...

Penetrating "Established" ACLs

One problem with using simple ACLs for a network firewall is that inbound at your perimeter router you have to allow "established" packets, as noted above. Unfortunately, this means a crafted packet that has an ACK bit set will pass through to an end host. This allows various sorts of network mapping to occur, and is a demonstration of why keeping state, either through stateful packet filters or application gateways, is needed to fully conceal protected networks.

HTTP, SMTP, FTP, Telnet, and rlogin are examples of applications that use TCP for transport. Applications that need reliability support from the transport layer use Remote Procedure Calls (RPC) over TCP. Applications that do not depend on the transport layer for reliability use RPC over UDP.

TCP Connections

Figure 1.6 shows the establishment of a TCP/IP connection. Establishing a TCP connection requires three segments, known as the "three-way handshake."

1. To initiate the connection, the source host sends a SYN segment (SYN flag is set), and an ISN in the sequence number field to the destination port and host address.

2. The destination host responds with a segment containing its initial sequence number, and both the SYN and ACK flags set. The acknowledgement number will be the source's sequence number, incremented by one.

3. The source host acknowledges the SYN from the destination host by replying with an ACK segment and an acknowledgement number that is the destination's sequence number incremented by one.

Figure 1.6 Establishing a TCP Connection

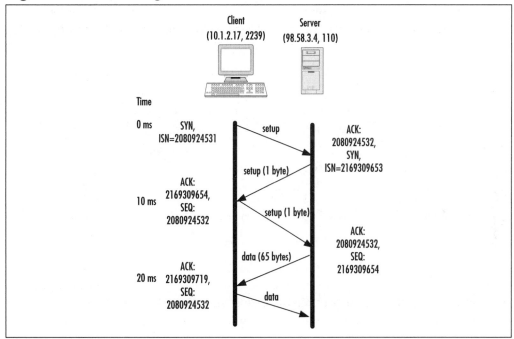

This sequence—SYN, SYN-ACK, ACK—characterizes the handshake.

This diagram represents the first few packets in a TCP session. The packets marked "setup" represent the establishment of the TCP session. The packets marked "data" represent the first few packets in the data stream. In this case, the session represents a typical Windows POP3 session between a host on a private network and a server on the Internet. The host establishes a local socket using its IP address (here, 10.1.2.17) and an ephemeral port, chosen for this session (here, 2239). The server, at IP address 98.58.3.4, is listening on port 110.

The client generates a packet with source IP 10.1.2.17, source port 2239, and destination address 98.58.3.4, destination port 110. The sequence number field is filled with an Initial Sequence Number chosen randomly—for this example, the ISN is 2080924531. Note that the ISNs are 32-bit unsigned integers, between zero and about four billion, and so, in general, are quite large. The acknowledgement number field is not used in the initial packet; by convention it is set to zero. The data offset field is set to a value that describes where in the TCP packet the data begins; in the sample diagram describing packets above, the offset would be 6 (since there is one 32-bit word consisting of options plus padding); other implementations will vary. The reserved field must be set to zero. With regards to the control fields, the SYN bit (offset 4, bit 14) is set to one; all other bits are set to zero. The window size is set to a value suitable for the client; 16K is typical. The checksum is computed based upon the TCP packet plus the source and destination address, the protocol, and the TCP length. Since the Urgent control bit is not set, the urgent pointer field is conventionally set to zero. The options field is set to implementation-specific values; communicating the maximum segment size is common. In this case, there will be no data (other than the fact of the SYN request) so the data field will be empty, and our packet is ready for transmission!

When the client receives the packet, it will make note of the request for communication. It will store in its TCP acceptance queue a request with sequence number 2080924531. It will also generate an ISN for its data; in this case, the randomly chosen number is 2169309653. Filling in the fields one at a time:

- Source port: 110 (its POP3 server)

- Destination port: 2239 (client request)

- Sequence number: 2169309653 (its ISN)

- Acknowledgement number: 2080924532 (client's ISN + 1)

- Data offset: 5 (depends on TCP implementation)

- Reserved: 0 (always)

- Control Bits: SYN, ACK (acknowledging the client data, requesting client synchronize)

- Window size: 17520 (depends upon server implementation)

- Checksum (computed based upon packet values)

- Urgent pointer: 0 (urgent control bit not set)

- Options, padding: Depends upon TCP implementation

- Data: Empty (no data yet)

When the client receives the SYN-ACK, the client needs to acknowledge the server request. Back comes a packet with only the ACK bit set, with sequence number set to its ISN + 1, and acknowledging client's ISN + 1.

Once a TCP connection between the two systems exists, data can be transferred. As data is sent, the sequence number is incremented to track the number of bytes. In the previous example, the first packet after establishment sends 65 bytes of data. Acknowledgement segments from the destination host increment the acknowledgement number as bytes of data are received; in this case, the client ACKs reception through 2169309719 = 2169309654 + 65 bytes.

The states that TCP goes through in establishing its connection allows firewalls to easily recognize new connections versus existing connections. Access lists on routers also use these flags in the TCP header to determine whether the connection is established.

A socket is the combination of IP address and TCP port. A local and remote socket pair (quadruplet) determines a connection between two hosts uniquely:

- The source IP address
- The source TCP port
- The destination IP address
- The destination TCP port

Firewalls can use this quadruplet to track the many connections on which they are making forwarding decisions at a very granular level. During the establishment of the connection, the firewall will learn the dynamic port assigned to the client for a particular connection. For the period of time that the connection exists, the dynamic port is allowed through the firewall. Once the connection is finished, the client port will be closed. By tracking the state of a particular connection in this way, security policy rules don't need to compensate for dynamic port assignments.

UDP

UDP is a simple, unreliable transport service. It is connectionless, so delivery is not assured. Look at the simple design of the UDP header in Figure 1.7, and you will understand the efficiency of this protocol. Since connections aren't set up and torn down, there is very little overhead. Lost, damaged, or out of order segments will not be retransmitted unless the application layer requests it. UDP is used for fast, simple messages sent from one host to another. Due to its simplicity, UDP packets are more easily spoofed than TCP packets. If reliable or ordered delivery of data is needed, applications should use TCP.

Figure 1.7 The UDP Header

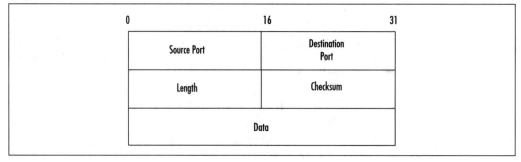

Simple Network Management Protocol (SNMP), Trivial File Transfer Protocol (TFTP), BOOTstrap Protocol (BOOTP), Network File System (NFS), and Dynamic Host Control Protocol (DHCP) are examples of applications that use UDP for transport. UDP is also used for multimedia applications. Unlike the connection-oriented TCP which can only connect between two hosts, UDP can broadcast or multicast to many systems at once. The small overhead of UDP eases the network load when running time-sensitive data such as audio or video.

The Internet Layer

The Internet layer is responsible for addressing, routing, error notification, and hop-by-hop fragmentation and reassembly. It manages the delivery of information from host to host. Fragmentation could occur at this layer because different network technologies have a different Maximum Transmission Unit (MTU). IP, ICMP, and ARP are protocols used at this layer.

IP

IP is an unreliable, routable packet delivery protocol. All upper layer protocols use IP to send and receive packets, which receives segments from the transport layer, fragments them into packets, and passes them to the network layer.

The IP address is a logical address assigned to each node on a TCP/IP network. IP addressing is designed to allow routing of packets across internetworks. Since IP addresses are easy to change or spoof, they should not be relied upon to provide identification in untrusted environments. As shown in Figure 1.8, the source and destination addresses are included in the IP header.

Figure 1.8 The IP Header

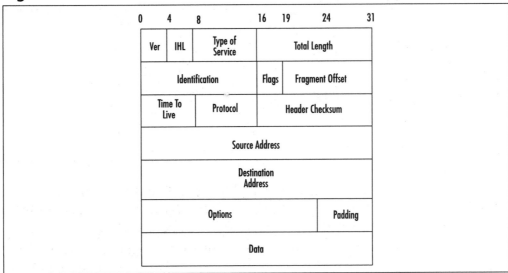

Let's take a look at each of these fields in Figure 1.8:

- *Ver* documents the IP version number. This template is for IP version 4, commonly deployed across the Internet.

- *IHL* is the Internet Header Length, in 32-bit words, and points to the beginning of the data segment. Note that the minimum valid IHL is 5, when there are no options.

- The *Type of Service* provides a suggestion for the desired quality of service. Across the Internet, no particular type of service can be guaranteed; generally, this field is set to zero.

- The *Total Length* specifies the length of the datagram. Based upon size, the largest datagram is 65535 bytes; this does (rarely) occur across some cores. Typically, the largest size one sees is 1500.

- The *Identification* field provides a unique identifier prepared by the sender to help in the reassembly of packets.

- There are three *Flags*. The first bit is reserved, and always set to zero. The second bit is the "Don't Fragment" bit, set if routers are not permitted to fragment the packet as it is passed along. The third bit is the "More Fragments" bit, set if additional fragments of this packet exist, or unset if this is the last fragment in the packet.

- The *Fragment Offset* field suggests where this packet exists in the datastream, measured in units of eight octets. The first fragment has offset zero.

- The *Time To Live* field indicates the maximum number of router hops the packet will survive before being discarded. The host generating the packet will set the value to some number—Windows often uses 128, some Unixes use 64—and as the packet is routed, the number is decremented.

- The *protocol* parameter indicates the upper level protocol that is using IP. The decimal value for TCP is 6 and UDP is 17. The list of assigned numbers for this field is available at www.isi.edu/in-notes/iana/assignments/protocol-numbers.

- The *checksum* is computed only on the header, so it does not check the integrity of the data payload.

- The *source address* and *destination address* fields are filled with the IP address of the respective devices; note an IP address is four octets, so this can be viewed as a 32-bit number.

- The *options* field resembles the TCP options field, and similarly allows for zero byte padding to bring options plus *padding* to a multiple of 32 bits.

Damage & Defense...

Penetrating with Sharp Fragments

Because not all links allow transmission of the same size of fragments, occasionally routers have to fragment datagrams (segment the data portion and place them into multiple packets) and end hosts have to reassemble the fragments into the original datagram. Packet reassembly can be a time-consuming task for detective systems, and so malicious users often artificially fragment their packets before delivery to evade firewalls and intrusion detection systems. One trick involved negative packet fragments, to create a packet with rewritten source and destination addresses!

Ensure that your defenses include packet reassembly before passing uncontrolled traffic onto your unsuspecting hosts.

ICMP

ICMP provides diagnostic functions and error reporting for IP. ICMP is protocol type 1. For example, ICMP can provide feedback to a sending host when a destination is unreachable or time is exceeded (TTL=0). A ping is an ICMP echo request message, and the response is an ICMP echo reply.

ARP

ARP is responsible for resolving the logical IP address into the hardware address for the network layer. (Note that an ARP packet is not an IP packet, and works below that layer.) If the destination IP address is on the same subnet as the source host, then IP will use ARP to determine the hardware address of the destination host. If the destination IP address is on a remote subnet, then ARP will be used to determine the hardware address of the default gateway. The ARP cache, a table of translations between IP address and hardware, stores its entries dynamically and flushes them after a short period of time.

SECURITY ALERT!

Some attacks have been based upon gratuitous or forged ARP replies and redirecting IP traffic to a system that sniffs for cleartext passwords or other information. One such attack tool is available at www.monkey.org/~dugsong/dsniff/. This attack disables the benefit of a switched Ethernet environment because ARP requests are broadcast to all local network ports. The spoofing machine can respond with its hardware address and become a man-in-the-middle. Research is being conducted on a new ARP protocol that would be resistant to these types of attacks. However, it is best to assume that switches do not provide access control, and avoid the use of cleartext passwords or other sensitive information.

The Network Layer

The network layer includes the network interface card and device driver. These provide the physical interface to the media of the network. The network layer controls the network hardware, encapsulates and transmits outgoing packets, and accepts and demultiplexes incoming packets. It accepts IP packets from the Internet layer above.

Composition of a Data Packet

In the IP world, the term *data packet* is generic. To be more formal, we often talk about a *protocol data unit* (PDU) that is wrapped into a frame—a representation of the data defined by physical characteristics. Collections of frames are integrated (or sometimes split) with the extraneous framing information removed into datagrams. Using the lecture metaphor again, the underlying thoughts are the PDUs, the physical manifestation of syllables the frames, and the words (an assembled collection of syllables) are the datagram.

Before considering the security of the packet, first we will look at the physical issues of the frame.

Ethernet

Ethernet refers broadly to a wide variety of data link implementations. Originally, this referred to the Dec, Intel, and Xerox implementation of Version 1 or Version 2 Ethernet. When IEEE developed the 802.3 standard, the term was applied to it as well, and characterizes Carrier Sense Multiple Access, Collision Detect (CSMA/CS) technology. Today, this protocol is used as a general reference to several different types of data link protocols, including the 802.3u or *Fast Ethernet* and the 802.3x or *Full Duplex*. It has evolved from transmission rates of 1/10/100 Mbps to 1 Gbps. Ethernet is even used as a model for 802.11, Carrier Sense Multiple Access, Collision Avoidance (CSMA/CA) within wireless networks.

Looking at the structure of an Ethernet frame is important to better understand the functions this layer provides. There are four common types of Ethernet frames found in networks today: Version II, 802.3 SNAP, 802.3 raw, and 802.3 LLC. Figure 1.9 examines the "Original Style," described on Cisco equipment as Ethernet frame type ARPA, which is probably the most common—it is the default in "pure-play IP" Windows NT and 2000 installations.

The Preamble consists of 62 bits of alternating 1s and 0s that allow the NIC to synchronize with the beginning of the frame. The Start Frame Delimiter is the bit pattern 10101011, and indicates the start of the frame. The Ethertype distinguishes between various types of frames, and its values can be found in RFC 1340. For example, IP packets have Ethertype 08 00 while ARP packets have Ethertype 08 03. The Frame Check Sequence (FCS) is a checksum computed by a Cyclic Redundancy Check polynomial (CRC) based upon the address fields, Ethertype, and data, and is designed to detect errors in transmission.

One interesting observation about the structure of Ethernet packets is that the destination MAC comes first in the frame, unlike in IP packet headers. The reason for this engineering is to allow bridges and switches earliest access to the destination so they can copy the packet to the correct port as quickly as possible.

Figure 1.9 An Ethernet Frame: Original Style (Digital, Intel, Xerox)

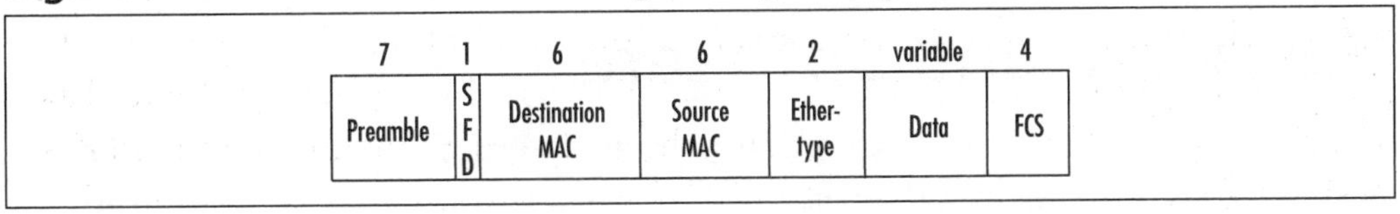

7	1	6	6	2	variable	4
Preamble	S F D	Destination MAC	Source MAC	Ether-type	Data	FCS

Figure 1.10 examines an 802.3 SNAP Ethernet frame, described on Cisco equipment as Ethernet frame type SNAP. This is an extension of the earlier LLC format, which had only a limited number of Ethertypes.

Figure 1.10 An Ethernet Frame: IEEE-Style SNAP

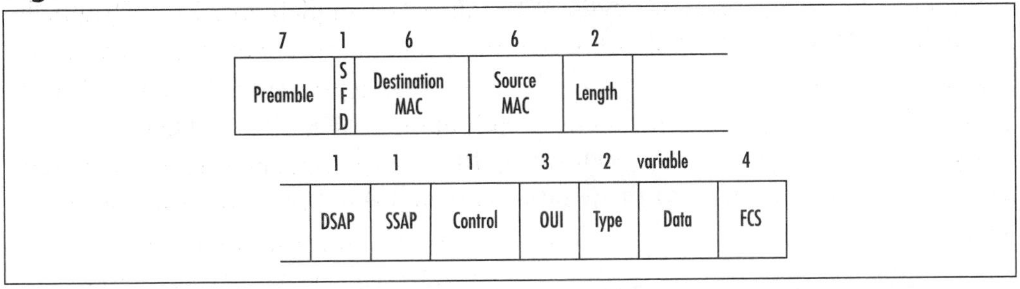

7	1	6	6	2	
Preamble	S F D	Destination MAC	Source MAC	Length	

1	1	1	3	2	variable	4
DSAP	SSAP	Control	OUI	Type	Data	FCS

The new fields here are the Destination and Source Service Access Points, which describe the upper protocol type for the frame; the Control field, generally unused but designed for administrative purposes; the Organizationally Unique Identifier (OUI), to distinguish protocols from different vendors—the OUI is the same value used in the MAC addresses—and finally a two-byte Type identifier to specify the actual protocol, and maintain compatibility with the earlier Ethernet II frame type.

Security in TCP/IP

The Internet provides no guarantee of privacy or integrity for data. Because of this, cryptography should be considered for private, valuable, or vulnerable data. This way, data is encrypted as it is transmitted, and decrypted as it is received. In fact, most layers in the ISO model can be used to provide data integrity and confidentiality. The application of security to each layer has its own particular advantages and disadvantages. The characteristics of security applied at a particular layer provide features that can be used as a decision point in determining the applicability of each technique to solve a particular problem.

Cisco IP Security Hardware and Software

Firewalls are typically placed at borders of security groups to create a security perimeter. Most frequently, they are used to protect an internal network from external access. Firewalls may also be used internally to control network access to specific departments or resources. The Cisco Secure PIX Firewall series of products are dedicated firewall appliances. All models offer VPN, IPSec, and firewall capabilities. The three models, 506, 515, and 520, provide performance levels ranging from small offices up to large enterprises and Internet service providers (ISP). Choose the appropriate model based on the throughput and number of interfaces needed for your application.

Information flow control policies can be enforced consistently across large enterprises and ISPs with the Cisco Secure Policy Manager (CSPM). It can centrally manage up to 500 Cisco Secure PIX firewalls. Organizations providing managed network security to many customers will also appreciate this centralized management feature.

The Cisco Secure PIX Firewall

The Cisco Secure PIX Firewall 506 has two integrated 10BaseT ports. The 515-R is limited to two 10/100 Ethernet interfaces. The 515-UR and the 520 provide up to six 10/100 Ethernet interfaces, while the 520 also gives the option of up to four 4/16 Mbps token ring or two dual-attached, multimode FDDI interfaces.

Common features shared by all models are as follows:

- **Embedded, Real-Time Operating System** The proprietary operating system was developed specifically for the PIX firewall. It provides high performance, and is generally immune to Unix security breaches. The code is a trade secret held by Cisco.

- **Stateful Inspection** Cisco calls it Adaptive Security Algorithm (ASA). ASA tracks the state of connections based upon source address, destination address, sequence numbers, ports numbers, and TCP flags. Forwarding decisions are based on applying the configured security policy to these parameters.

- **VPN Tunnels Using DES or 3DES** This feature provides confidentiality across untrusted networks. The addition of the PIX Private Link encryption card allows the PIX to create and/or terminate VPN tunnels between two PIX firewalls, between a PIX and any Cisco VPN enabled router, and between a PIX and the Cisco Secure VPN Client. The 506 supports up to four VPN peers. The 515 and 520, meanwhile, support up to 256 peers.

- **Java Applet Filter** Java applets can be blocked when delivered in HTTP content. More sophisticated filtering requires a third-party product.

NOTE

There are three basic types of firewalls available today, Packet Filters, Application Gateways, and Hybrids.

- **Packet Filters (PF)** look at various pieces of information and decide whether or not to forward the packet. A PF can be stateless or stateful. In a stateless environment, the PF looks at the protocol, address, or port information and other pieces of information in each packet and makes a forwarding decision for that packet based on static rules. Access Control Lists (ACLs) on routers are an example of stateless packet filters. Access control lists are useful for blocking source or destination addresses, solving the problems of spoofed source addresses, and can restrict the services accessible.

- **Stateful Inspection (SPF)** analyzes all the communication layers, extracts the relevant communication and application state information, and dynamically maintains the state of communications in tables. Forwarding decisions are based upon the configured security policy. Stateful inspection offers flexibility and increased applicability to enforcement of information flow control rules.

- **Application Gateways (AG)** use a specific application for each service that will be forwarded through the firewall. The AG takes requests on one interface, and terminates the service request; it then forwards a request, as appropriate, on to the device on another network. In particular, with a Web server protected by an AG, the Web server sees the IP stack of the AG, not the end client; this means that low-level packet attacks that might pass through a packet filtering firewall will be stopped by the AG. All other things being equal, an AG offers the best security, but you must have an application for each service that will be processed by the firewall.

Most modern firewalls are a hybrid of the three types. For example, the PIX uses primarily packet filtering for reasons of performance. However, some applications (the "fixup commands") invoke application gateways to sanitize particular services. This provides heightened capabilities, such as the Java content blocking ability mentioned earlier.

The 515 and 520 models offer additional features of interest to larger organizations:

- **Network Address Translation (NAT)** NAT conserves the IP address space by translating up to 64,000 internal hosts to a single external IP address. The PIX firewall uses port address translation (PAT) to multiplex each internal host with a different port number. PAT does not work with H.323 applications, multimedia applications, or caching nameservers.

- **Failover/Hot Standby Option** This feature improves availability of the network. It is not available on the 515-R. Cisco has created a Fail-Over Bundle (515-UR only) to add software and a second chassis to create a redundant firewall configuration.

- **Cut-through User Authentication** A cut-through proxy is used to authenticate users with a TACACS+ or RADIUS server. This feature improves performance for authentication, authorization, and accounting. When the username and password are correct, the PIX firewall lets further traffic between the specified authentication server and the connection interact directly.

- **URL Filtering** A NetPartners WebSENSE server is needed to utilize this feature. The PIX firewall permits or denies connections based on the outbound URL requests and the policy on the WebSENSE server.

Table 1.3 compares the performance of the PIX firewalls offered by Cisco.

Table 1.3 Cisco Secure PIX Firewall Performance Comparison

Model	Throughput	Simultaneous Sessions
506	10 Mbps	N/A
515-R	120 Mbps	50,000
515-UR	120 Mbps	125,000
520	370 Mbps	250,000

You will find configuration details on Cisco Secure PIX firewalls in Chapter 3. Additional information on related topics is found in Chapter 8, 9, and 5.

Cisco Secure Integrated Software

Cisco Secure Integrated Software (formerly called Cisco IOS Firewall Feature Set) is a bundle of security features that integrate with Cisco IOS software. It can add firewall, intrusion detection, Data Encryption Standard (DES) (56-bit) encryption, and secure administration capabilities to most of the following routers:

- 800
- UBR900 series
- 1600
- 1720
- 2500
- 2600
- 3600
- 7100
- 7200
- 7500
- RSM (Route Switch Module)

The 800, UBR904, 1600, and 2500 do not support authentication proxy or intrusion detection.

The authentication proxy can use TACACS+ or RADIUS protocols, which can be applied per-user on LAN or dial-up communication links.

The Cisco Secure Intrusion Detection System described next is a separate appliance and merely watches the network traffic. The Cisco Secure Integrated

Software is an integral part of Cisco IOS. This difference can affect performance because the Cisco Secure Integrated Software lies in the critical packet path.

Cisco Secure Integrated VPN Software

Cisco Secure Integrated VPN Software adds 3 DES (168-bit) encryption, and authentication through digital certificates, one-time password tokens, and pre-shared keys to the Cisco Secure Integrated Software features described earlier. The package is available for the following routers:

- 1720
- 2600
- 3600
- 7100

VPNs can be established over remote access, intranet, or extranets.

The Cisco Secure VPN Client

The Cisco Secure VPN Client enables secure connectivity for remote access VPNs. It can be used for applications such as e-commerce, mobile user, and telecommuting. It provides Microsoft Windows 95/98/2000 and NT users with a complete implementation of IPSec, including support for DES (56-bit) and 3DES (168-bit) encryption, and authentication through digital certificates, one-time password tokens, and preshared keys.

The security policy for end-users can be centrally managed, and protected as read-only for the client. This feature prevents users from bypassing the policy that has been put in place and ensures that policy is applied consistently among users.

More details about VPNs can be found in Chapter 8.

Cisco Secure Access Control Server

The Cisco Secure Access Control Server (ACS) provides authentication, authorization, and accounting (AAA) for users accessing network services. Cisco Secure ACS supports TACACS+ and RADIUS protocols, and the Windows NT version can also do pass-through authentication to the NT user accounts. The ACS can be used as a centralized server or a distributed system comprised of multiple ACS systems. It can also interface to other third-party RADIUS or TACACS+ systems in a distributed configuration. In a distributed environment, the ACS can act as a proxy and automatically forward an authentication request to another AAA server.

The accounting function can record each user session that was authenticated by the server. The accounting information can be used by ISPs to provide billing or usage reports for customers. It can also serve as data for security or forensic analysis.

More details about AAA can be found in Chapter 9.

Cisco Secure Scanner

Cisco Secure Scanner (formerly called NetSonar) is a vulnerability assessment tool for network hosts. This scanner software package is available to run on Windows NT, Solaris, and Solaris x86. It will map all devices connected to the scanned network. Vulnerability assessment can be performed on:

- Unix hosts
- Windows NT hosts
- Network TCP/IP hosts
- Mail servers
- Web servers
- FTP servers
- Routers
- Firewalls
- Switches

The scanner comes with a database of known security vulnerabilities. The database contains information about repairing any of the vulnerabilities it finds, and is updated periodically as new vulnerabilities are discovered. You can also create customized scanning rules tailored to your environment or security policies.

More details about Cisco Secure Scanner can be found in Chapter 11.

Cisco Secure Intrusion Detection System

An intrusion detection system (IDS) can help make you aware of the nature and frequency of attacks against your network and systems. From the information provided by the IDS, you can design an appropriate response to reduce the risks to your systems from these attacks.

Cisco Secure Intrusion Detection System (formerly called NetRanger) is a real-time, network intrusion detection system (NIDS) consisting of sensors and one or more managers. A system can be implemented with a single sensor at a strategic location, or multiple sensors placed at many well-chosen locations in the network. Sensors operate in promiscuous mode and passively analyze the network traffic that appears on its interface for unauthorized activity. The IDS sensor will report traffic matching attack signatures to the director. The sensor can also be configured to actively change ACLs on Cisco routers in response to attack signatures, a process called "shunning." The sensor is a hardware and software appliance that is available for five network technologies:

- Ethernet
- Fast Ethernet
- Token Ring
- Single attached FDDI
- Dual attached FDDI

The Cisco Secure Policy Manager (CSPM) is the management station. It receives the alerts from sensors locally or remotely located. You can have one central director—which can be configured to send alarms to a pager or e-mail address—or you can have multiple directors receiving alerts from any of your network sensors.

A recent addition to the IDS product line is the host-based IDS (HIDS), an OEM of Entercept technologies. The host-based approach allows for detection of malicious activity at the target itself—and the HIDS can be configured to prevent malicious activity. These sensors are also controlled by a centralized console mechanism.

More details about intrusion detection can be found in Chapter 13.

Cisco Secure Policy Manager

The Cisco Secure Policy Manager (formerly called Cisco Security Manager) is a comprehensive security management system for Cisco Secure products. You can define, distribute, enforce, and audit security policies for multiple security devices from a central location. Cisco Secure Policy Manager supports IPSec VPN, user authentication, and in a future version will support intrusion detection and vulnerability scanning technologies. Its use on routers requires that Cisco Secure Integrated Software be installed.

Policy Manager centralizes the management of security policies, the monitoring of status, and reporting of policy events. It can help to ensure a consistent application of policies across hundreds of devices, and will save you time by automating portions of the policy creation and distribution.

More details about Cisco Secure Policy Manager can be found in Chapter 12.

Cisco Secure Consulting Services

Cisco Secure Consulting Services are targeted to large corporate and government customers, and though consulting services are beyond the scope of this book, they do round out the Cisco Secure product line for those of you who need expert assistance. It offers two types of professional services:

- **Security Posture Assessments** This service provides comprehensive security analysis of large, complex networks. Cisco will test your network security from the perspective of external attackers, disgruntled employees, or contractors. They will then make recommendations on needed security measures to improve your network security.

- **Incident Control and Recovery** This service is an emergency response to a hostile network incident. Cisco can provide short-notice assistance to restore control and availability of your network.

Summary

Security plays a key role in a network. The fundamental goals of network security usually boil down to three issues, coded by CIA: Confidentiality, Integrity, and Availability of data and services. Confidentiality is usually achieved through access control and encryption. Integrity, meanwhile, is attained by cryptographic means and careful use of audit trails. Lastly, availability is accomplished by using high-quality Cisco equipment configured to carefully provide redundancy, as well as designing services that can survive or rapidly recover from attack.

Security is one of three common perspectives in designing networks. These perspectives are: the user perspective, where the goal is to get a fast, cheap solution; the ops management perspective, where the goal is to get a complete and reliable solution; and the security perspective, where the goal is to get a controlled, authorized solution. All perspectives are valid, and a good network architect will balance all three.

An excellent source of security design is the Cisco SAFE program, available at www.cisco.com/warp/public/779/largeent/issues/security/safebprint.html.

You don't *have* to deploy security. However, this means your site is assuming some significant risks—corporate losses per company per year averaged over two million dollars, according to CSI/FBI statistics. Simple programs can eliminate the most expensive risks, but remember, every enterprise is a target.

One of the most effective ways of thinking about network security is the DoD model. This breaks the net into four layers: Network Access, Internetwork, Host-to-host Transport, and Process Application. Security techniques can be applied at each of these layers to improve the security posture of your network.

At the Network Access Layer, you can control accesses to shared media, and provide link encryptors where appropriate. It's best to partition where possible, virtually using VLAN or MPLS technologies.

At the Internetwork Layer, controls can be enforced over the packets routed between layers. The old adage "be conservative in what you do, be liberal in what you accept from others" needs to be updated: Be cautious in what you accept from others, and if it doesn't make sense, log it and drop it.

At the Host-to-host Layer, transport protocols such as IPSec are widely used and quite effective. IPSec is a flexible protocol that is part of a best practices mechanism for transport across uncontrolled networks. It has two modes: transport mode, useful when both endpoints of the IPSec tunnel are capable of using the data, and tunnel mode, useful as a passive encapsulated, encrypted path across the uncontrolled network.

At the process application layer, the key message is that it is an arms race, and constant vigilance is required. Last year, an average of six vulnerabilities a day were reported. To keep on top of the situation, information owners must consistently update their software with vendor patches, and information security officers should apply vulnerability scanners on a regular basis to identify problems before they are exploited.

Some approaches to providing application security include Pretty Good Privacy (PGP), a standalone encryption package that can be integrated into mail transport and file storage. Secure Sockets Layer (SSL) can provide on-the-fly transport encryption to an application. Secure Shell (SSH), meanwhile, can provide confidentiality and session integrity for a command channel.

Some controls can be applied through all layers. Authentication protocols, for instance, can help with identity management using common authentication protocols such as TACACS+, RADIUS, and Kerberos. TACACS+ is a proprietary protocol that is especially useful in controlling access to Cisco infrastructure equipment. RADIUS is effective in a heterogeneous environment, as it is widely supported. Kerberos, on the other hand, is a sophisticated and trusted third-party solution that does not require passwords be sent in the clear, and has vendor neutral support.

While the DoD model is perhaps best for thinking about security issues, the OSI model is more commonly adopted by internetworkers, and is useful for discussing what occurs with security equipment. The seven layers are: Physical Layer, Data-link Layer, Network Layer, Transport Layer, Session Layer, Presentation Layer, Application Layer. The following is a brief description of each: Physical Layer—handles physical characteristics of signal transport; Data-link Layer—handles encoding and decoding of data from bits into transmitted frames, and address access to the physical layer; Network Layer—handles transport of datagrams across local networks to remote networks; Transport Layer—addresses flow control, ordering of received data, and acknowledgement of data; Session Layer—establishes the parameters of any upcoming communication; Presentation Layer—establishes the way information is presented, typically for display or printing; Application Layer—where user space programs make requests of network services.

Some specific aspects of the OSI model that are important: key layer 4 protocols are TCP and UDP.

TCP provides a reliable, connection-oriented service with data sequencing, congestion control, error detection, and retransmission. TCP communicates on "ports," distinguished by a number between 0 and 65535. It achieves sequencing, congestion control, error detection, and retransmission by sequence numbers and corresponding acknowledgements. Individual flags provide additional information to the receiving host about the nature of the packet. TCP sessions are initialized through three packets, SYN, SYN-ACK, and ACK—known as the "three-way handshake." A TCP session is uniquely identified by the local and remote socket pair.

UDP provides a connectionless but low overhead transport protocol. Some typical applications are SNMP, TFTP, DHCP, and many multimedia applications.

A key Layer 3 protocol is the IP protocol. TCP and UDP packets are encapsulated in IP packets. Other examples of IP packet types are ICMP and ARP.

Firewalls are typically placed at borders of security groups to create a security perimeter, and to offer firewall services such as VPN termination. Information flow control policies can be enforced consistently across large enterprises with a centralized security management platform such as the Cisco Secure Policy Manager. The Cisco Secure Integrated Software (formerly Cisco IOS Firewall Feature Set) allows integration of security controls across the enterprise by building it into the infrastructure. Several models also incorporate native VPNs, which interoperate with the Cisco Secure VPN client. The Cisco Secure ACS allows for centralized authentication of these structures.

Other tools, such as the Cisco Secure Scanner and Cisco Secure IDS, allow for detective analysis of an enterprise environment. Both the Cisco Secure IDS and HIDS allow for detective and preventative controls, unlike most IDSs on the market.

Solutions Fast Track

What Role Does Security Play in a Network?

☑ The fundamental goals for a security information processing network generally boil down to the acronym CIA: Confidentiality, Integrity, and Availability.

☑ Networks are typically designed from a user perspective—get it out fast and cheap—or from an operations management perspective—get it out reliably, and recover from faults gracefully. Add to this a third perspective: the security perspective—get it out in a controlled fashion, and fail safely.

☑ You don't have to deploy security. You can assume the risks yourself, just remember that they are high—average annual costs are around two million dollars per company for security breaches, and in some instances, said security events have destroyed the company.

The Fundamentals of Networking

☑ The DoD network model was the source for the design of the Internet.

☑ It is based upon four layers: the Network Access Layer, Internetwork Layer, Host-to-host Layer, and Process Application Layer.

☑ Security controls typically are applied within a layer.

Where Does Security Fit in?

☑ Applying security at multiple layers—defense in depth—means that a failure in one control doesn't invalidate your security policy. Look back to Figure 1.4 to see the various places security controls can be deployed.

☑ Unlike most security controls that are specific to a single layer, authentication applies at all layers.

☑ While most security types are like the DoD model, most networking types resemble the OSI model. It is based upon seven layers: Physical and Data-Link, corresponding to the Network Access Layer; Network corresponding to the Internetwork Layer; Transport, Session, and Presentation corresponding to the Host-to-Host Layer; and Application corresponding to the Process Application Layer.

☑ Application designers don't want to reinvent the wheel, so instead they generally depend upon two well-defined Transport Layer protocols: TCP and UDP. TCP is used for reliable, connection-oriented traffic; while UDP is employed for efficient, connectionless traffic.

☑ Two additional protocols to be aware of are the ICMP protocol, which provides control messages for IP, and ARP, which provides name services between physical media addresses and IP addresses.

Cisco IP Security Hardware and Software

☑ Cisco's primary appliance for providing information flow control policy enforcement is the PIX firewall. This is an IOS-like, high-performance firewall based upon stateful packet filtering combined with application gateways for specified protocols.

☑ Because Cisco has a wide variety of infrastructure products, Cisco has integrated security features into those devices to provide comprehensive protection for the whole enterprise. Cisco Secure Integrated Software and Integrated VPN Software are IOS features that permit protective and detective controls in the existing router and switch hardware; the VPN client allows termination of IPSec tunnels on end-user equipment.

☑ Authentication is provided by the Cisco Secure ACS, a combination RADIUS and TACACS+ server that runs on Unix or Windows platforms.

☑ The Cisco Secure Scanner (formerly NetSonar) provides vulnerability assessment services to identify problems on hosts before they can be exploited.

☑ The Cisco Secure IDS, both host- and network-based, provides ongoing reporting of intrusions and inappropriate traffic as it occurs.

☑ The Cisco Secure Policy Manager is the management console that provides control features for the security equipment at the site.

Frequently Asked Questions

The following Frequently Asked Questions, answered by the authors of this book, are designed to both measure your understanding of the concepts presented in this chapter and to assist you with real-life implementation of these concepts. To have your questions about this chapter answered by the author, browse to **www.syngress.com/solutions** and click on the **"Ask the Author"** form.

Q: I've deployed a firewall/IDS/VPN. Am I safe now?

A: No. Security is a process, not a product. It takes careful design, integrated personnel support, and multiple technologies. For example, the recent Nimda event would blow through most firewalls protecting corporate Web servers—the exploit was a conventional Web request, and firewalls are designed to allow Web requests into Web servers. Firewalls help with many things, but in this case, you would have needed a vulnerability assessment tool, like the Cisco Secure Scanner, combined with a remediation program, to dodge this particular bullet.

Q: I've deployed a firewall/IDS/VPN. Why should I put ACLs on my routers? Isn't that overkill?

A: Deploying multiple technologies is known as "defense in depth." The idea is that if one defense slips—due to human errors and omissions, or weaknesses in technology—another defense can cover the gap. It's also important to realize that sometimes the router is outside the firewall, and needs protection too, so it doesn't hurt to provide some protections for the firewall as well. Many systems, all working together, make the likelihood of a security incident less likely.

Q: My Web servers are on a service network, protected by a third interface off the PIX. I need to get them to talk to an SQL back-end, which lives within my corporate network. The Web guy wants to put another NIC in the Web server and use that to communicate into my corporate network because he says the PIX is too slow. He says he'll turn off packet routing on the Web server. Should I do that?

A: Some network engineers do use that architecture. It's probably not the best approach, however. The problem is that now the Web server is part of your trusted computing base – if the "Web guy" forgets to turn off packet routing, or for some reason the Web server is compromised, a direct path from the outside will open into the heart of your network. The PIX is a high-performance device. It can generally be quite effective at routing traffic back to the back-end server. An even better approach, however, is to put the SQL servers on their own service network, and enforce traffic to the SQL servers that way. Now, even if the Web server is compromised, the attack is contained. If for some reason something evil breaks out in your user community, the SQL servers are still protected.

Q: I'm designing a high-speed Web farm. Should I put in a PIX?

A: Some network architects use that design. However, consider this: in that environment, the PIX would limit access to Web services, and provide you with an audit trail of the transactions. You can achieve the same facilities with access lists on your routers and host logs on the servers. A careful Web farm design will incorporate load balancers, redundant routers and switches, VPN terminators for management, and IDS for detective controls. Assuming there are ACLs on the perimeter, firewalls are optional.

Q: Which firewall/IDS/VPN should I buy?

A: Your choice of product depends upon many factors, including cost, performance, support, the long-term viability of the company, the feature set, and so on. Cisco has an advantage in several of these arenas, and, of course, if you have a Cisco network already, a reduced number of vendors and the ability to integrate security features into your infrastructure can be very helpful. The best approach, however, is to identify what issues are important to you, and then review how equipment and support compares between vendors on these issues, ranking them accordingly. Be a smart consumer of security, and remember to design security natively and ubiquitously across your network!

## Chapter 2

What Are We Trying to Prevent?

Solutions in this chapter:

- **What Threats Face Your Network?**
- **Malicious Mobile Code**
- **Denial of Service**
- **Detecting Breaches**
- **Preventing Attacks**

- ☑ **Summary**
- ☑ **Solutions Fast Track**
- ☑ **Frequently Asked Questions**

Introduction

An attentive network administrator is always looking for the right strategy for information services security. You need to understand the risks you are facing, and assign resources to reduce and manage those risks. To do this correctly, one needs a *quantitative* security risk assessment. You write down all the potential adverse events, estimate the loss from such events, and calculate the probability of such events occurring. Multiplying the latter and then adding up the results gives a value known as the "Annual Loss Expectation" or "Expected Annual Costs."

For information security, this is a difficult problem on several levels. Writing down every potential adverse event is a complex and time-consuming task. Estimating the loss from such events is no trivial feat either. For risks like fire or earthquake, we at least have data culled over a long period of time. Risks due to information security events, on the other hand, are highly variable, and change over time as new tools emerge and new malicious code is distributed. Insurance companies are busy developing data for new information security insurance, but that data remains regrettably limited.

On the upside, undertakings of this sort produce hard numbers—the kind a CEO can appreciate. It's a type of exercise that can be helpful when considering strategies or identifying where security resources should be deployed. Even a simple first-pass approach—identify the crucial assets, think about what can go wrong for those assets, figure out some likely scenarios and assign likelihood—can help with the decision-making process. Quantitative risk analysis is a path that many enterprises do follow, particularly in high-risk environments such as financial institutions, or highly-regulated environments such as health care.

Given the drawbacks, an alternative *qualitative* security business risk assessment is often more cost effective. The idea here is that probability data and cost impacts are not required, but instead, a rough estimate is employed—for instance, evaluating threats, vulnerabilities, and controls. This allows you to take a look at what risks you are facing (threats), the potential impacts of those threats (vulnerabilities), and potential ways to minimize both the threats and the vulnerabilities (controls). Controls that correspond to events of high probability and high impact are generally worth exploring first, while controls that correspond to events of low probability and low impact are worth examining later. A vulnerability approach is generally followed (rather than an asset protection approach) because the vulnerabilities usually are a smaller set of things to consider, and more directly relate to the controls that will be proposed.

When conducting security environmental vulnerability assessments in a qualitative environment, one associates a Risk Mitigation Factor with each device.

This factor is based upon two elements: The potential impact of the security violation on functional operations (severity of the hazard) and the probability that the violation will occur. The severity of the risk is classified in one of four categories: Critical, Severe, Moderate, and Low. The probability ranking is also categorized in one of four different classifications: Frequent, Probable, Occasional, and Possible. Table 2.1 lists the different levels of risk severity, while Table 2.2 shows the different levels of risk probability.

Table 2.1 Risk Severity

Level of Severity	Description
Critical	Business impact is considered Critical when exploitation of the vulnerability would result in a total system compromise, which may include complete loss of management control and/or use of the compromised system to launch attacks or intrusions against other companies. In addition to direct costs, there may be significant indirect financial loss, due in part to litigation or damaged reputation. An example of vulnerabilities of this nature would be installation of remote control software that would permit a remote intruder full access to the machine.
Severe	The business impact is considered Severe when exploitation of the vulnerability would result in a partial system compromise, potentially losing control over a delivered service or prompting unauthorized distribution of sensitive information. The primary impact of this sort of vulnerability is the direct cost associated with loss of service or information. An example of vulnerabilities of this nature would be a weakness in Web server configuration that allowed for Web page defacement.
Moderate	Impact is considered Moderate when exploitation of the vulnerability would result in degraded performance and loss of system integrity. Primary impact of this sort of vulnerability is the indirect cost associated with event normalization. An example of vulnerabilities of this nature would be a server subject to a Denial of Service attack.
Low	Business impact is considered Low when exploitation of the vulnerability results in degraded performance without loss of integrity, or which prompts an inability to control integrity in a functioning host. The primary impact of this sort of vulnerability is the indirect cost associated with higher maintenance. An example of vulnerabilities of this nature would be user-controlled desktops.

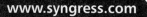

Table 2.2 Risk Probability

Level of Probability	Description
Frequent	The probability is considered Frequent when the event is likely to happen often. This might occur if the vulnerability has been widely publicized, automated tools are available, and/or if a worm using the exploit is available.
Probable	The probability is considered Probable when the event is likely to happen several times during the life cycle of the host system. This might occur because the vulnerability is well known, but "user friendly" exploit tools are not available, and thus require a higher level of skill to compromise the system.
Occasional	The probability is considered Occasional when the event is likely to occur sometime during the host system's life cycle. This would occur when the vulnerability is not well known, or when specific circumstances would be required for a breach (such as a maintenance window when certain protections are not in place).
Possible	The probability is considered Possible when it is unlikely but possible to occur in the system's lifecycle. A classification may be such when the vulnerability is of a theoretical nature and no exploit code is known, or specific circumstances of low probability are required, or when the vulnerability is of a theoretical nature and no way to exploit the vulnerability is currently known.

More information about identifying vulnerabilities is given in Chapter 11, where the Cisco Secure Scanner is discussed.

What Threats Face Your Network?

A threat to your network might come from actual intent to do harm to it, or from a malicious source a user may inadvertently activate. Both arise as a result of violations to a security policy.

Policy is driven by goals. Back in the summer of 1986, Hal Tipton, Richard W. Owen, Jr., and Ross Leo coined the term CIA—Confidentiality, Integrity, and Assurance—as a compact and succinct description of the things that matter in a secure information delivery/processing system. (The fact that it provides a nice chuckle at the expense of the U.S. Central Intelligence Agency only helps to make it more memorable.) Looking at harm from the perspective of a breakdown in CIA is a good way to approach potential problems.

Loss of Confidentiality

Loss of confidentiality is often the most serious form of harm. For example, when a merchant has customer credit card numbers compromised, he can expect a serious loss of customer confidence. The owner of the credit card loses, due to potential charges on their account, and the hassle of getting them cleared. The credit card company loses, due to absorbing the risk of fraud. In December of 2000, Egghead lost control of its 3.7 million customer database. Some clients lost access to their cards during the Christmas season, while the card's issuing companies were forced to cancel and reissue cards. Other credit card companies absorbed the risk of the fraud – and the estimate was that millions of dollars were lost. The biggest loser was Egghead itself: It saw its stock drop twenty-five percent overnight, and shortly thereafter ceased to be a viable company. Loss of confidentiality is usually due to human actions, but at least one worm (SirCam) will actively e-mail out potentially sensitive documents from an infected host.

Loss of Integrity

Loss of integrity is one of the most insidious forms of harm. Perhaps the earliest widespread example was the XM_COMPAT virus, which spread through macro code in Excel during the fall of 1998, making subtle changes to the spreadsheet data it infected. Since the computations of spreadsheets can affect device controls, including medical equipment, this was a potentially life-threatening virus and not easily detected by simple inspection (modern antivirus software easily controls this sort of problem, as long as the signatures are current.)

Another form of loss of integrity arises when authentication systems are poorly designed or are ineffective. If a VPN's server logs are not readily available, you won't be able to tell who is crawling through your system. If passwords are poorly chosen, mail may be compromised, and if something bad does happen, you may lose the ability to associate actions with individuals. Both of these events add to the cost of dealing with network problems.

Loss of Availability

Loss of availability is the most high-profile of the visible forms of harm. This category has its own classification—a denial of service (DoS) attack. More on this type of attack will be described later. Unfortunately, this sort of harm is generally the easiest to execute.

Sources of Threats

Donn Parker, in his book *Fighting Computer Crime, a New Framework for the Protection of Information*, recommends breaking down potential attackers by SKRAM, which stands for skills, knowledge, resources, authority, and motives. For example, one type of person that presents a serious threat to any network is the "script kiddie"—someone who downloads tools written by others, perhaps does some trivial modifications, and then launches those scripts without a deep understanding of their mechanisms or impact. These people are low in skill and authority and usually have limited knowledge of the target. However, they are high in resources, and often operate with a motive more related to chaos than financial gain. Another common threat is the disgruntled system administrator. These people most likely have a high level of skill and possess a deep knowledge of the target with enough authority to do some serious harm. Yet another threat to consider is mobile code, such as viruses, worms, Trojan horses, and the like. These have varying degrees of skill (worms are typically badly coded, and bugs are common) and generally have no particular knowledge of the target. They do have amazing resources, however, based upon the sheer number of machines they can infect and mobilize to help in their malicious work.

In these examples, the primary motive is to sow chaos. Other harm is possible, of course. We are starting to see a rise in computer-based crime: individuals or syndicates that utilize sophisticated programming techniques to commit extortion against information owners. For example, in the fall of 1999 the FBI arrested two members of the "Phonemasters," an international group that penetrated many of the computers at well-known corporations such as MCI, Sprint, AT&T, and Equifax. They stole Sprint calling card numbers that ended up in the hands of organized crime groups in Italy. Even if your network does not have such juicy targets, it can still be used as an attack platform against other systems, as the companies listed here were.

Perhaps an even more curious motive was documented in Clifford Stoll's book, *The Cuckoo's Egg*. There, Soviet foreign intelligence agents tapped into the resources of West German crackers to penetrate United States military and paramilitary organizations. It should not be a surprise that foreign agents might use such methods to acquire private sector intellectual property as well.

A final threat worth describing is automated crime. Over the past half-century, we've used computing technology to automate our business processes. These days, the direct deposit of payroll checks, the ordering of supplies, and other routine business transactions often occur without human intervention. With the proper

SKRAM, payroll checks can be sent to inappropriate accounts, supplies might arrive at inappropriate locations, and other breakdowns in business transactions will occur with the speed and scale of electronic activity. This means new kinds of responses to these threats are required.

Malicious Mobile Code

Malicious code, or malware, is software that does you harm. Malicious mobile code deals with viruses, worms, Trojan horses, and similar problems of rogue code that might compromise your security policy. Because the code is mobile, using your network to cause harm, it's your responsibility to bring it to heel. Due to its ability to infect many computers simultaneously and automatically, the vast resources available to this threat mean you must deal with it seriously in your defense strategies.

Trojan Horses

The term Trojan horse is a reference to a stratagem used in the siege of Troy, as told in the Iliad. The attacking Greeks found the city's walls impenetrable. They built a wooden horse and presented it to the citizens of Troy as a peace offering, concealing a force of one hundred Greek warriors inside. Even though one of the Trojan High Priests, Laocoön, warned against "Greeks bearing gifts," and the King's own daughter, Cassandra, warned of disaster, the horse was brought into the city. Later that night, the warriors concealed within crept out and opened the gates of the city, letting the Greeks in to sack and loot Troy.

In information technology, a Trojan horse is a computer program that appears to have a useful function, but in truth has a hidden and potentially malicious function that evades security mechanisms, sometimes by exploiting legitimate authorizations of the system entity that invoked the program in the first place. IT departments frequently warn their users against accepting files and e-mails from the Internet—yet warnings even from senior executives fail to be heeded. Trojan horses continue to be the most expensive vector for malicious code.

Viruses

A biological virus is a piece of DNA or RNA code that attaches itself to the surface of a healthy cell. The code then injects itself into the cell's functions, causing the cell to produce the viral fragments. In a similar vein, a computer virus is a piece of code that searches out other programs and inserts itself into them; these other programs then become Trojan horses that proceed to infect their neighbors. The chief difference between a computer virus and a Trojan horse is that the virus is not a complete program in and of itself, but requires resources of the victim program to replicate itself. In theory, computer viruses should be more widespread than Trojan horses, since they can reproduce via a wide variety of programs, while Trojans do so via a single program. In practice, computer environments are so highly homogeneous, with similar operating systems and applications, and the human part of the equation is so ready to execute unknown programs, that Trojan horses constitute more serious risks to the enterprise.

Worms

The term worm appears to have originated by John Brunner in his book "Shockwave Rider," a novel written in 1975 which anticipated many of the information tracking and privacy issues of the modern Internet. In the modern parlance, a worm is a computer program that can run independently, can propagate a complete working version of itself onto other hosts on a network, and may consume computer resources destructively. Common vectors today are open (or accessible) network shares and vulnerabilities in network services. As an example, the high profile (and still quite common) Nimda worm used both techniques to spread itself from machine to machine.

Worms can be classified into several subtypes.

- **Intelligent, Data-driven** These use databases provided by the infected host (for example, Outlook mail addresses) to pass code to the victim host. These have the advantage of drawing upon information that the author of the worm code didn't possess, and so can act in unanticipated ways. The may avoid some controls—for example, if you get a piece of mail from someone you know, you are more likely to execute Trojan code. They can be detected through unusual behavior, however. For example, it would be considered unusual for a user to suddenly send e-mails out to the first 50 names in his address book, leading a system administrator to suspect a compromised host.

- **Intelligent, Activity-driven** These sense activity from the infected host (for example, Web page clients, network file shares) to pass code to the victim host. These can be even more subtle; the hidden Trojan transaction is masked by an existing client transaction, so they would bypass controls to detect anomalous activity.

- **Unintelligent** These use search techniques to identify additional targets. They can be identified by a process in which they contact machines that aren't running vulnerable services, or in which they attempt to contact nonexistent IP addresses. This is the most general infective technique, and currently the most destructive.

Designing & Planning…

Tracking and Taming Unintelligent Worms

It is helpful to track attempts to contact a host on unused ports or unused IP addresses, which can indicate either a misconfiguration or a potentially malicious activity. Most worms don't use IP spoofing techniques, so it can be a good way to identify an infected host.

In addition, one can apply inverse TCP quality of service techniques to reduce the infection rate of hosts. Programs such as Tom Liston's LaBrea (at www.hackbusters.com) or the use of Cisco's Network-Based Application Recognition (NBAR) will allow system administrators time to get to the source of infection before it spreads farther.

A worm can be countered at several locations. The most traditional approach is to arrest the worm at the perimeter, through antivirus software on firewalls, mail servers, Web caches, and the like. Layered security through desktop antivirus software is also a common practice; the problem is ensuring that the antivirus software remains current. Perhaps the most cost-effective approach is to engage the end user, and ensure they communicate effectively with the security personnel.

The biggest threat of a worm lies in its automated capability to replicate. With a human attacker, replication works in terms of human reaction times. People have to receive and execute the malicious program. With a worm, the replication works in terms of computer reaction times. In November of 1988, Robert Tappan Morris released the "Great Worm," a coding experiment that was designed to seek out and contact Unix hosts, and then use those hosts to repeat that process. Unfortunately, some coding errors caused multiple copies of the worm to spawn, clogging process tables; like today's Nimda, the worm was everywhere, and sites took the unprecedented step of disconnecting themselves to address event normalization needs. For the first (and hopefully only) time in the history of the Internet, it was down, though not for a long time.

One traditional defense is the use of antivirus signatures at the perimeter. It is important to keep your antivirus software frequently updated, so that when a problem tries to penetrate your perimeter, it is recognized and blocked. When a "day zero" virus is announced, antivirus researchers update their signatures (which typically takes about a day) and the signatures are pushed out to the enforcement points. This keeps your window of exposure small, and hopefully provides a managed risk. However, an interesting paper by Nicholas Weaver at www.cs.berkeley .edu/~nweaver/warhol.html describes Warhol worms, sometimes called Flash worms, which by initially targeting highly connected hosts have the potential to infect every vulnerable machine across the Internet in about 15 minutes. Traditional antivirus approaches can not be successful in this sort of environment.

Current Malicious Code Threats

Commercial antivirus companies provide data on the most frequent malicious code they see from their clients. This information is relevant to the risk probability computation mentioned previously. As of this writing, the most common threats include the following:

1. A JavaScript Trojan horse that alters a browser's home page.

2. A Visual Basic Trojan horse that alters a browser's home page.

3. An e-mail Trojan horse and network shares worm.

4. An e-mail Trojan horse that executes upon viewing in certain mail viewers.

5. The Nimda Trojan horse/worm.

6. An e-mail Visual Basic script Trojan horse.

What should you draw from this list? None of these threats are new; all are based upon virus engines from the previous year. All of these have Trojan components. It should be clear that user education (not just warnings provided by Laocoön) is an important part of your malicious code defense strategy. None of these are viruses—instead, it should be taken as a statement about the efficiency of modern antivirus software rather than the potential vulnerability of the threat model.

Current Malicious Code Impacts

The threat associated with malicious mobile code is very high. Code executed via a Trojan runs with the privileges of the person who launched the code; this means, at the very least, user files are at risk. The second point of the CIA triad is integrity, and it's a crucial breakdown in information integrity. In a modern operating system, protections are in place so that an ordinary user does not have the ability to seriously harm the underlying system—but it turns out that operating system permissions are often frangible. Fred Cohen, one of the early virus researchers, noted in his PhD thesis how Unix viruses can break through the protective mechanisms of Unix operating system permissions. This is a reflection of rule number one of Microsoft's *Ten Immutable Laws of Security*, available at: www.microsoft.com/technet/columns/security/essays/10imlaws.asp

"If a bad guy can persuade you to run his program on your computer, it's not your computer anymore." Theory aside, we do see that the impact is critical. If you place a machine on the Internet, you will be probed on port 80 by a Nimda-infected machine. Nimda installs a "back door," a service that provides remote access to the machine. Take the IP address of the machine that probed you, and you can turn around and exploit that back door, and then use that machine to launch attacks across the Internet.

In 1988, the Great Worm required sites to disconnect themselves from the Internet. In the fall of 1999, Melissa spread like wildfire through e-mail systems globally. In the 11 years since the earlier event, networks had become much more robust, but e-mail was still a weak spot. Again, many enterprises had to shut mail systems down to clear queues and apply protective techniques. In the summer of 2001, Nimda proved an even more dangerous opponent: once infected, Nimda aggressively attempted to contact and infect additional vulnerable servers. The aggression produced ARP storms that brought down cable systems; the traffic overloaded enterprise LANs which prevented any other traffic. Try to imagine the traffic utilization associated with network backups running on every machine across the core of the network during the middle of the day. One representative case is a developer of Web-based customer relationship software, who had about a sixth of their six thousand machines running vulnerable Web servers. They were unable to talk to their clients for four days, during which "all hands on deck" emergency action with staff and outside consultants was carried out. The business impact of four days of downtime, along with the PR impact of a customer relationship management (CRM) developer being unable to talk to customers, is incalculable.

Denial of Service

A network-based denial of service (DoS) attack is a direct attack on system availability. There are two types of denial of service attacks: triggers and floods. The trigger class uses a vulnerability inherent in the operating system or application to make a system or component unavailable. A flood generally uses normal system functions but generates so much traffic that the target is overwhelmed. The target can be a client, service, or system. A target client would be a specific application, such as a Web browser or instant messaging client, which is made unavailable as a result of the attack. A target service would be when the attack prevents normal functioning of a particular service, such as Web browsing or file shares, without harming the underlying operating system. A target system would be when the underlying operating system itself is damaged and the entire host is made unavailable.

A nice example of a trigger attack on a client is a JavaScript bomb: very simply, the requested Web page invokes a new browser window inside a JavaScript loop, as in the following example:

```
<script language="JavaScript">
while(true) window.open("http://www.someone.com");
</script>
```

The effect of this code is to open an endless series of browser windows, exhausting the resources available to the browser. An interesting variant uses a lengthy list of pornographic sites as the URL to be opened, thus not only making the browser unusable but also getting the user in trouble with the local administration when URL filtering software is enabled.

A good example of a trigger attack on a service was seen by many AVVID clients as an incidental consequence of the IIS server attacks, such as CodeRed and Nimda. The Call Manager server is based upon IIS, and as Cisco observed in its security notice www.cisco.com/warp/public/707/cisco-code-red-worm-pub.shtml:

> the management of a Cisco CallManager product is disabled or severely limited until the defaced Web page is removed and the original management Web page is restored. Cisco CSS 11000 Content Services Switch, Cisco IP/VC 3510 H.323 Videoconference Multipoint Control Units, Cisco Aironet Wireless Bridge/Access Point, Cisco IP phone models 7960, 7940, and 7910, and Cisco 600 series DSL routers are vulnerable to a repeatable denial of service until the software is upgraded, or workarounds are applied.

An example of a trigger attack on a target system from a couple of years ago is the "Land" attack. If you craft a SYN packet with a source IP and port equal to the destination IP and port, the operating system may try to synchronize with itself—a Windows 95 PC will freeze and require a reboot, and an NT Workstation will be unusable for about a minute before it recovers.

Flood attacks are less subtle. They attempt to overwhelm by sheer volume of traffic. An example of a flood attack on a client would be to send an overly large mail attachment when an end user is on a dial-up system; if they can't control the browser to delete the rogue file without downloading it, it would deny mail services until the download is completed.

An example of a flood attack on a service would be the "Host Announcement Frame" vulnerability for Microsoft Common Internet File System (CIFS) documented in Microsoft Security Bulletin MS00-036. In essence, what happens is that if someone sends a large number of announcements for hosts, then those announcements need to be processed by a machine that is doing essential tasks, thereby degrading its performance. That host then replicates that information among its peers, again consuming large amounts of network bandwidth. Any other hosts that try to use that service need to process the large tables, degrading their performance. This is a common theme: The best floods have a natural multiplier effect that allows the user to exert a force on the network, while the effect is tenfold more severe.

The most common flood attacks are based upon simple volume-of-traffic tricks. The attacker generates packets, sometimes bouncing them off other hosts to conceal his tracks, and perhaps uses a multiplier trick to make his traffic more effective. The receiver must then deal with this heavy wave of traffic. Two attacks deserve special recognition: the Smurf attack and the SYN flood attack.

The Smurf Attack

The smurf attack uses an unfortunate default behavior of routers to swamp a victim host. Recall that ICMP is used to provide control messages over IP. One control message is an *echo request*, that asks a host to provide an *echo reply*, responding with the body of the message. Here lies the start of the problem: Suppose our evil host wants to take out a target host. He finds a well-connected intermediary, and forges an echo request to the intermediary host apparently from the target host. The intermediary responds, and the target receives a flood of traffic from the intermediary, potentially overwhelming the target. One additional trick makes this more deadly: the original echo request can be targeted not just at a single host, but at a broadcast request—and under a default configuration, *all* hosts on that network will reply. This allows a host to multiply itself by the number of hosts on that network: with a 200-fold multiplication, a single host on a 256K DSL line can saturate a 10Mb Ethernet feed.

The recommended guidance is to prevent broadcast addresses from being expanded, at least from packets on the Internet. On your Cisco routers, for each interface, apply the following configuration:

```
no ip directed-broadcast
```

This will prevent broadcast packets from being converted. Blocking ICMP doesn't help: A variant, *fraggle*, uses UDP packets in a similar fashion to flood hosts. An even more vicious approach, described in CERT advisory CA-1996-01, uses forged packets to activate the *chargen* port, ideally connecting to the *echo* port on the target. The two hosts are then locked in a fatal embrace of a packet stream until one or both of the machines are reset.

The SYN Flood Attack

The SYN flood attack consumes a limited resource on the victim server—the ability to establish TCP sessions—to prevent service. The idea is again fairly simple: Recall that a TCP session begins with a three-packet handshake. The idea is to spoof a new, incoming connection. The SYN packet prompts a response SYN-ACK from the server. The old approach, still followed by the Microsoft IP stack, is to maintain a small list of pending responses so that the server can remember which packets have already been received.

The vulnerability is to thus send a large number of SYN requests without receiving any response. The usual technique is to forge the return address on the request; since the end host doesn't exist, the server is never going to receive a response from its SYN-ACK, thus limiting the resource. In a surprisingly short time, this can prevent a host from accepting connections.

A PIX firewall can provide protection against this sort of attack. In a typical environment, one would specify the target IP with a *static* statement and use ACLs to pass traffic inside. For example, suppose the IP address 63.122.40.140 is a Web server off a DMZ interface of a PIX. The configuration would look something like:

```
static (dmz,outside) 63.122.40.140 63.122.40.140 netmask 255.255.255.255
     10000 500
access-list acl_out permit tcp any host 63.122.40.140 eq www
access-group acl_out in interface outside
```

The key line here is the first one; this allows the IP address 63.122.40.140 to allow traffic through the PIX. (The traffic is limited to Web traffic in the following line.) The last two values provide the protection. The first is the *max_cons* parameter; this is the maximum number of simultaneous connections through the PIX to the Web server. This allows a maximum of 10,000 simultaneous sessions. The second is the *em_limit*, and is the maximum number of uncompleted handshakes that will be passed to the inner host. If the number exceeds this limit, the PIX's TCP Intercept feature takes over. For each SYN received, the PIX captures the request, and responds for the server. It then waits for the handshake, and if the connection was false, doesn't bother the protected server. If the handshake is completed, it opens a connection with the inner host, establishes the handshake in a proxy fashion, and then forwards the packet appropriately.

If you don't have a PIX, another approach is to use an operating system that is not subject to this kind of attack. An approach known as *syn-cookies* uses a specialized ISN to record the state of the handshake. This means that the server does not need to remember any of the SYN packets it has received, therefore there is no resource for the attacker to consume. This is similar to the approach the PIX uses internally in its TCP Intercept feature.

Damage & Defense...

Don't Be a Participant in a Spoofed DoS Attack!

If a flood of traffic hits the victim, there is little they can do—the packets have already overwhelmed their link. To help lessen the damage, everyone should be a good corporate citizen, and prevent inappropriate packets from leaving their network.

The best current practice is to prevent packet spoofing. This is documented in RFC 2267. The idea is to ensure that packets that leave your network are stamped with a return address appropriate for your network. Don't let forged traffic onto the Internet!

Distributed Denial of Service (DDoS) Attacks

As described earlier, a fair amount of technical complexity is required to make these denial of service attacks work. A fair amount of labor is necessary to multiply an individual attacker's bandwidth enough that it swamps the end user. From this, network managers are becoming more and more careful, and denial of service attacks are becoming less and less successful.

Unfortunately, a simpler approach for the bad guys exists. A large number of hosts on the Internet are owned by individuals who do not exert proper care over their systems. They allow their hosts to become compromised, and permit remote-controlled software to be installed. After which, malicious agents can use these systems against others, providing remote computing power to help them facilitate brute force cracking attacks, or enough raw network bandwidth to be used against a host.

In underground parlance, a compromised host is known as a *zombie*, while the surreptitious controller is known as the *zombie master*.

The most famous example of a zombie attack was the spring 2000 attack on Yahoo!, eBay, Amazon, and others. Apparently, a ping flood tool known as *imp* was employed in the attack; the strategy was to launch a combined attack from hundreds of zombies, many located at the University of California in Santa Barbara. The attack hit like sledgehammer, flooding the target sites with hundreds of megabytes per second of traffic, and effectively bringing them to a standstill.

The only way to remedy such attacks is to find each of the zombies and release them from the control of the zombie master—a slow and tedious task. The only way to protect against this kind of traffic is to detect the compromise, and address remediation before the zombie can be put to use. This can be difficult, but, conveniently, it does provide an introduction to the next section.

Detecting Breaches

In any network exposed to an uncontrolled environment like the Internet, there will always be risk of a systems compromise—and over time, that risk approaches a level of certainty. Every system administrator should be prepared to detect breaches, and take appropriate action.

What is the appropriate action? That depends. In some environments, you clean it up and forget about it. It's usually helpful to document the attack, if possible, and report it to the originating ISP: This helps put pressure on the originator, and may reduce further attacks. In some cases, a detailed analysis of the event is prepared, to ensure the proposed remediation will be effective. In still others, detailed forensics with an eye to civil or criminal prosecution is required. This section delves into the detection and documentation of network attacks, as well as the strategies for addressing results.

Initial Detection

The bad way to find out a breach has occurred is to discover that your Web site isn't accessible, your Human Resources database has been zeroed out, or your President's private correspondence is duplicated in everyone's e-mail in-basket. Unfortunately, finding out that site service confidentiality, integrity, or availability has been compromised is not an uncommon way to detect the problem.

A better approach is through the use of file system integrity or network traffic anomaly tools. The former detects changes in the static configuration of a system, while the latter detects changes in network behavior. This sort of preparation allows for a more rapid and effective response to a breach.

File System Integrity Software

The idea behind file system integrity software is to take a snapshot of the configuration and file contents of a device, and then see what changes over time. A fundamental principle of security is that of secure change management: If a system starts in a known secure state, and the only changes to the system occur securely, then the system will always be in a secure state. So, take those snapshots, and periodically compare them against what actually exists on the device. If a change has occurred, and it doesn't match the expected changes as documented under the secure change control process, then you have a problem—either the change control didn't provide accurate documentation, or your systems have been breached.

The first software to perform this task was developed as an academic project by Gene Kim (a student) and Gene Spafford (professor) at Purdue University. The idea is fairly straightforward: develop a size, timestamp, and checksum for every file on the system. If a change occurs, you would like one of these three values to change. Crafting the change so that size and timestamp aren't altered isn't that difficult. However, the third element is what makes the bad guy's job hard: Using a cryptographically strong function to compute the checksum will ensure a change in the file will cause a change in the checksum. The original description of the idea is available at www.cerias.purdue.edu/homes/spaf/tech-reps/gkim. Tripwire still exists in an open source form as well as a commercial product; in addition, there are many other products such as AIDE, or fcheck. There are important details, such as ensuring the signature information is properly protected, that the signatures are computed correctly, that the tool is executed frequently enough to detect changes in near real time, that the results are available to security management in a useful format (and so on)—all of which should be specific to the product.

An alternative approach has recently become popular, based upon something called *host-based intrusion detection*. It boils down to that secure change concept: If we have a piece of software running that detects all inappropriate changes, we are safe. There is a Cisco product, manufactured by Entercept, which not only provides that detective capability, but also has the potential to prevent unauthorized changes from occurring. This change detection approach can provide real-time alerting of a security breach.

Network Traffic Anomaly Tools

A network traffic anomaly tool views traffic or reacts to traffic on the wire, and attempts to determine if something peculiar, abnormal, or otherwise inappropriate is occurring. Several approaches are valid: conventional network intrusion detection, log analysis, and honeypot approaches.

The most commonly deployed tool is a network intrusion detection system (IDS). Again, there is a Cisco product for intrusion detection, the Cisco Secure IDS, which is discussed in more detail in Chapter 13.

Log analysis depends on configuring systems to record traffic that doesn't match normal parameters, and then using scripted tools to analyze the resulting logs. For example, placing a "log" clause on an extended access list will send information about matching traffic via syslog to a central log server. A text-based search of those records can identify unusual traffic.

A honeypot, meanwhile, is a system (or systems) designed to decoy, detect, and trap an attacker on your network. Because these systems are not in use as production servers, simple use is an indication of inappropriate traffic. The systems are thus designed with more alarms than a conventional server, and often contain attractive elements that encourage an attacker to spend time on the system, increasing the likelihood of detection and tracking. An easily deployed tool is Tom Liston's "LaBrea" project, which is a "sticky honeypot" that reacts to TCP connection attempts on unused IP addresses.

Are Forensics Important?

The previous steps for initial detection involved a planning phase. You deployed integrity tools or a detective control, and hoped you found out about the breach before the users did. But perhaps the first inkling of the problem was when you found your Web site defaced. What do you do next?

Before you can answer that, you have to decide if preservation of forensic evidence is a goal. That means collecting data regarding the nature of the attack so you can prove to an independent third party your conclusions about how the attack occurred. Common reasons for preservation of forensic evidence are:

- To determine just how the breach occurred to improve your defenses.

- To document the event for an internal "lessons learned" document.

- To document the event for management to provide a root cause analysis.

- To prepare for a civil or criminal action (including a personnel action).

These require a careful handling of evidence, and correspondingly, a more expensive and time-consuming response to the security event. You should get guidance from management about the most appropriate response; if they want to follow up with legal action and you've already formatted the hard drive containing the breach, you're pretty much out of luck.

Some techniques apply to all levels of forensics. Probably the most important one involves careful documentation. Write everything down! Having good notes available will not only allow for the preparation of any reports required, but also help you review the steps you've followed, and assist in the analysis of the system.

It is worth observing that if you are preparing for legal action, it is important to not merely document what occurred but to preserve evidence. When preparing notes, start with a bound book in which you write your notes, subsequently signing and dating each page as you complete it. When working with hard drives, do not work on the original equipment! Prepare two copies of the disk. Remove the original, tag it, and place it into secure storage. Give one copy back to the information owner so they can get on with business, and retain one scratch copy for your own analysis.

What Are the Key Steps after a Breach Is Detected?

After detecting a breach, several steps should be followed. Precise details will vary depending upon site security policy, the nature of the event, and other constraints, but most should adhere to the following steps:

1. **Identification and Classification** This step requires determining whether or not a breach has actually occurred, and analyzing the circumstances of the breach. If a Web site is defaced, this is clearly a smoking gun. If one of the host integrity or networking intrusion detection tools dispatches an alarm, it may not be as obvious that the event

has occurred. The security analyst needs to review the tool's alarm, and determine if this is inappropriate traffic, or just an artifact of the tool.

2. **Containment**   As soon as an event is detected, the next step is usually containment, in order to limit potential damage from the event. You generally want to limit the scope and magnitude of the breach, to keep the cost of event normalization as small as possible.

3. **Eradication**   Eradication involves eliminating the cause of the breach. The most complete approach involves finding the human or humans responsible and hauling them into court to prevent them from further action. It is difficult to do this in a timely fashion, unfortunately. For the threats of malware, removing the software or using antivirus software is usually the best approach. For network-based threats, reconfiguring the perimeter as well as applying controls internally is usually effective. Other eradication techniques may depend upon the exact nature of the incident.

4. **Recovery**   Recovery is the process of returning status to normal after the event. If it was a simple Web defacement, it may be as easy as restoring the data from a recent backup. In a more complex incident, it may require complete rebuilds of the affected servers. Recovery also means restoring faith in your system, something which may require new procedures or updated software be put in place to ensure the original problem doesn't reoccur.

5. **Follow-up**   This final step involves analysis and the production of whatever ongoing reports are required for the future. This is a critical step! There is no better time to improve the security posture of your site than just after an incident. You generally have the attention of the principals involved, and your own attention is closely focused on the security of your environment. It is helpful to estimate the cost involved in the incident, both for future planning issues and to update law enforcement personnel for their own statistics.

Preventing Attacks

You've now seen several of the threats your network faces, and what to do when a breach occurs. While you can never eliminate the need to plan for security breaches, there are several things you can do to prevent certain types of attacks and reduce the likelihood of others.

The easiest step is to reduce vulnerabilities, places where the threat can take hold. There is an old joke in security: Protecting against network threats is often like being with a group of hikers in the woods who suddenly come across a bear. To be safe, you don't have to run faster than the bear—you just have to run faster than your fellow hikers. In a network environment, this means you don't have to be "completely" bulletproof—you just have to offer less vulnerability than the next guy. As a result, worms and other threats that flourish on the Internet will often pass you by for other targets.

The next easiest step is to "keep it simple," and provide a security architecture that is easy to diagnose, and offers enough visibility into your network that you can detect inappropriate activity early in the process. Good use of access controls to partition your network will help with simple, controlled designs.

Another step (generally the most cost-effective but not the easiest to implement) is to develop a culture of security within your company. Get your fellow employees working for you, and you'll have both fewer opportunities for security events and more eyes watching the store.

Perhaps the most important step, and one often overlooked, is clear documentation and explicit policy. Documentation on your intended security policy allows you to plan your security architecture, and helps you recover after an incident. It helps you better understand how you are achieving your goals, and thus allows you to catch errors before the bad guys find them for you!

Reducing Vulnerabilities

The security of a system is never greater than the security of its weakest element. Thus before getting clever about additional security controls, the first step should be to conduct an assessment and clean up any identified vulnerabilities.

This generally is an ongoing process. If you are running a particular service and have applied all known vendor patches, you can consider yourself free of known vulnerabilities to that service, which should provide some peace of mind. Six months later, a bug in the code may have been identified, and a new patch may have been released, which should prompt new activity on your part. Your security should be reviewed periodically over time to determine any new issues.

The easiest way to do this is through an automated tool such as the Cisco Secure Scanner, also known as NetSonar. This is a subscription-based software, where, just as antivirus signatures are maintained over time, Cisco manages the vendor alerts and patch information for you, so all you have to do is keep the scanner current and run it periodically. Automated vulnerability assessment is an easy way to identify problems inherent in the system.

Of course, the scanner doesn't fix problems, it merely identifies them. You must also institute a tracking program, so that when problems are identified, they are remedied. This is not always easy—often security personnel are separate from the people who actually own the assets. You may need cooperation from senior management to encourage other employees throughout the company to patch or otherwise address their system's vulnerabilities. Running the scanner on a regular basis and providing management level reports documenting when a vulnerability was first identified, and when notification to the asset owner occurred is important. It should be combined with an assessment of the risk this poses to the company, and generally prompt executive management to ensure the vulnerability is addressed.

Besides patching necessary systems to the current vendor recommended levels, another important strategy is that of "least privilege." The common concept is that a security architecture should be designed so that each system entity is granted the minimum system resources and authorizations that the entity needs to do its work. For system design, this means you should encourage removal of all unnecessary services on servers. The idea behind this is twofold. First, with fewer services is place, you can spend more time focusing on the security of the services you do provide. Second, fewer services means fewer things to go wrong, thus limiting the number and impact of systemic vulnerabilities.

Providing a Simple Security Network Architecture

We saw at the beginning of this chapter that an important part of risk management is "what if" planning, trying to understand what can go wrong in a system. If you have a complex environment, there may be too many variables, meaning too many things that can go wrong, preventing you from providing effective analysis. By reducing complexity, you can bring the number of "what ifs" down to a manageable level.

An example of this that nearly everyone follows is the use of firewalls on the perimeter to protect user and host servers. Since we removed all vulnerabilities in the previous step, this really isn't required, right? Wrong. Things still might go wrong. We might miss a vulnerability. Because of this, most people deploy perimeter controls to limit the exposure of their internal machines to the Internet. We would certainly still like to remove vulnerabilities wherever possible, but now we can provide some realistic planning about what might go wrong. The environment has been simplified to the "inside," the "outside," and the traffic that flows between those networks.

This idea can be extended. In the 80s and early 90s, most network designs had the approach we just described: a hostile network (the Internet), a friendly network (the inside), and a DMZ marked by a pair of routers that severely limited traffic between the two zones. Traffic that passed first had to be inspected by an armed guard—a bastion host—before it was allowed transit.

In the late 90s, the style was to introduce a centralized firewall and a services network. The idea would be that if a site wanted to provide public services, they would be isolated to their own network. The public services might access private databases through a three-tier architecture—external client on the Internet, talking to front-end Web server, talking to back-end database. Communication from the Web server back to the database would still be controlled by a firewall, so that in the event the Web server was compromised, this wouldn't provide unfettered access to the database. It also meant you could plan what protections were required, since you had a pretty good idea of the information flow patterns between the hosts because your information flow control policy could be enforced at that central firewall.

The cost of another interface off a firewall has decreased rapidly, and performance through firewalls has increased significantly. The modern style is to provide as many security zones as are required by functional properties or level of trust, and to separate each from the other with an access control device such as a firewall. Firewalls no longer are limited to external perimeters, but multiple, internal firewalls can protect the corporate "crown jewels" from the rest of the network. Also, part of the modern style is to support a partitioned administrative network to manage the infrastructure. Ideally, you would like this to be completely out of band, but in practice, a combination of VLAN and MPLS technologies are used to provide some traffic isolation.

A sample network is shown in Figure 2.1. The scenario is that of an enterprise that has an "operations network," a backbone that directly relates to the operation of the business. For example, a bioinformatics company might need a dedicated network that has a distributed storage network designed to support their internal databases; a circuit design company might need a compute server network; or a manufacturing company might need a fabrication control network. Developers are provided with a test network so they can develop new applications or experiment with existing ones without being required to change control procedures for the production network. In the diagram that follows, the operations network is drawn as distributed, so it can hook up with operations networks at other sites via internal point-to-point links. The scenario also assumes a business-to-business relationship, where the company hosts key servers on their site (the "crown jewel" DMZ) for client services and data. Typical user services are provided, so that individuals can do their local work as well as provide developers access to the test network, and managers access to the admin network.

Figure 2.1 A Sample "Simple" Network Design

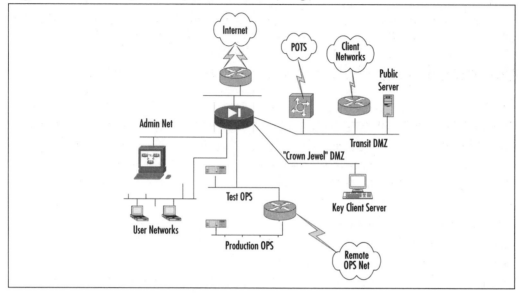

This probably doesn't look that simple. But the simplicity is not in the configuration of the hardware—after all, no firewalls provide a *really* simple network diagram. What it does provide is simplicity in information flow. The outside world (including dial-in or VPN users, clients, and the public) only talks to devices on the transit DMZ. No one talks to the production OPS network except the administration network, and no one talks to the "crown jewel DMZ" except system administrators from the admin network, who are possibly pulling content from the test network. The allowed communication is very controlled, with a limited number of patterns, and it is this simplicity that makes for a secure network.

What if something goes wrong? You have compartmentalization. Suppose a user accidentally executes a Trojan and contaminates his desktop. He would have full access to the other user machines, which could be a problem. Unfortunately, you can't put firewalls everywhere, and if he is an administrator, he might have limited access to the administrator network. Nevertheless, it definitely slows the spread, and if, for example, strong authentication is required to access the administration network, you are protected against all worms and viruses that don't have specific knowledge of your environment. Suppose a developer makes an error of omission on a test machine and it explodes, spewing packets everywhere? No problem, the test network is isolated from the production network (and the rest of the environment). But what if everything goes *really* sour? You can simply power down that central firewall, and provide complete isolation, while still preserving the physical integrity of the production operations net.

Yes, this provides more gear to manage. But in the long run, it offers a simpler security architectural model, and that translates to reduced risk.

Developing a Culture of Security

There is a wonderful apocryphal story of a new security officer who was unhappy that the written security policy of requiring badges for access through the building was not being universally enforced. The rules stated everyone should be badged, and technical controls would control access to certain rooms. However, once inside the perimeter, people would generally flow freely, making it next to impossible to determine if a visitor got away from his escort and was viewing unauthorized materials.

He had an interesting solution. Being new to the company, and not well known, the fellow stopped wearing his badge. Occasionally, someone would stop him and ask for identification. When that did occur, he would produce his identification—and a $20 bill. He would explain who he was, and present the money as a prize for complying with the company guideline on verifying identification. The story got around. He stopped the practice, but compliance remained high: It was a simple object lesson underlining the fact that the company cared about security, that it cared about people wandering the corridors unbadged; and reminded the community that it was their job to help with the enforcement of security.

You may not have $20 bills to hand out, but the concept of engaging the community, and providing a reminder that security matters and that it's a part of everyone's job is an essential element of any security program. It can be relatively inexpensive. Security is a very hot topic at the moment, and makes the front pages of the newspaper all the time. Start a brown bag lunch program, where a talk is provided on current security events, either nationally or within the company, and discuss how the company's policies and procedures might impact those events.

Getting the community on your side has many significant effects. There is the first order effect described previously: People will keep their eyes open, and if you gain their trust and let it be known you are receptive to alerts, you will have a highly effective security event alarming system. It is not at all uncommon for a breach to be detected because a user noticed someone he'd never seen before accessing a service; if that information gets back to you, and you can classify the event, it's a more effective approach than any network or host-based IDS.

A second order effect is even more profound: People start working with the system to get their job done, instead of working around it. Your employees are probably very clever when it comes to getting what they want. Security is generally inconvenient, so employees often try to bypass security to get their jobs done, and that can lead to headaches and vulnerabilities. Get them to work with you, having patience if it takes a little longer to bring a service up or a little more work to gain access to a system, and the vulnerabilities won't occur. A similar effect occurs when you publish policy on acceptable use, and then start providing feedback through technical controls like firewall filtering or an IDS deployment. Provide guidance, and demonstrate that the company takes this seriously, and people start complying with acceptable use guidelines, which will reduce overall maintenance costs dramatically.

Developing a Security Policy

Developing a security policy is the single most important step in security risk management. Security policy is the glue that binds the various efforts together. It provides the statement of goals and intent that the security infrastructure is designed to enforce. In many respects, it is better to have a policy and no firewall rather than firewall and no policy. With policy, you can know what it is you need to do, and take the necessary steps to ensure your goals are achieved. Without policy, any control you deploy will be hit or miss, and there is no guarantee you will achieve your purpose. Because the fundamental issues of security come from control of the details, your overall security is probably weakened.

All sites have some policy, of course. If nothing is written down, then the policy exists in the consensual cultural expectation. People probably have some expectations: That their PC will turn on in the morning, that they can access their e-mail without it being distributed to competitors, that the file they were working on yesterday will still be there and contain the same information when they closed the application. Sometimes policy can be inferred: For example, many sites adopt an "arbitrary network traffic can go out; only a specified set of traffic—mail to the mail server, Web clients to the public Web server can go in as a default information flow-control policy. Most people understand and accept the principle of least permission, and these are probably in the informal policy.

Documentation is important, however. People need guidance on how to handle the information, services, and equipment around them. Is it acceptable to load games on the office PC? Allowing uncontrolled applications runs the risk of a potential loss of system integrity. Many sites discourage such behavior, but then allow it on field worker laptops as an acceptable compromise when it comes to security, utility, and morale. Is it acceptable to receive personal e-mail on your corporate account? Allowing such things runs the risk of increased network utilization, and the transport of Trojans into the corporate network, but at the same time encourages increased literacy and raises morale. Policy needs to be written down so consensual policy can be made clear to all members of the community. Likewise, managers ideally need to make trade-offs to ensure due protection of corporate assets while optimizing worker efficiency.

Policy does not need to be overly complex. Indeed, it's best to make policy short. A policy framework can establish the overall guidelines—to borrow a Judeo-Christian metaphor: The Ten Commandments of security might be better than the security Bible. Most people only need those Ten Commandments. Where necessary, there can be a security Bible, which provides more detailed guidance, and provides documentation on security control configuration or security architecture strategies, but policy, at its best, should be holistically integrated into the people, processes, and technology that provides secure business information flow.

Summary

A professional network administrator or security officer makes plans for their security architecture. Effective planning requires an assessment of the risks. Two types of risk assessment are: quantitative, where hard numbers are developed to identify annual loss expectations and return on security investment; and qualitative, where relative values rank the importance of various threats, vulnerabilities, and controls for planning purposes. Because of the difficulty of the former, the latter is usually followed.

Threats are the actors or programs that may do harm to your network. Harm usually flows from a breakdown in CIA—confidentiality, integrity, and assurance. Loss of confidentiality is often the most serious type of harm: losing control over proprietary or third-party data hurts everyone involved, and can lead to the demise of the company. Loss of integrity is perhaps the most insidious harm: often the most difficult to detect, it means you can't trust your own data. Loss of availability is the most visible kind of harm: not everyone understands how bad things are if a credit card number is lost or a spreadsheet is altered, but if you can't get to your e-mail, it has a personal impact.

Sources of threats come from many categories. A good way to classify threats is via Skills, Knowledge, Resources, Authority, and Motive, which is also known as SKRAM. Examples of threat models are "script kiddies," disgruntled system administrators, dedicated cyber-criminals, foreign intelligences, and even automated programs that attack without human intervention.

A particular example of the latter is malicious mobile code. This is a special case of malicious code, or malware, that can spread across network boundaries to harm your assets. Malicious mobile code is usually broken into one of three types: Trojan horses, viruses, and worms. A Trojan horse is a piece of code that appears to do one thing, but actually has an unsuspected and inappropriate secondary function. A computer virus is a piece of code that is less than a program, but can attach itself to a program to turn it into a Trojan horse. A worm is a complete working program that can propel itself across a network, producing copies and potentially using computer resources destructively. Trojan horses and worms have been responsible for some dramatic losses over the past years, from the Great Worm that caused the Internet to crash in 1988, to Melissa that shut down many e-mail systems in 1999, to modern plagues like Nimda which appear to have permanently polluted port 80 across the Internet.

The threat associated with malicious mobile code is very high. Rule number one of Microsoft's *Ten Immutable Laws of Security* states: If a bad guy can persuade you to run his program on your computer, it's not your computer anymore." This is the integrity that malicious code violates.

Currently, while Trojan horses can be tamed by effective user training, worms must be defended through network means. They can be classified by intelligent worms that are either data-driven (using intelligence inherited from the host configuration) or state-driven (using activity provided by the host). Unintelligent worms simply reproduce through search strategies. Currently, the most widespread technique is the unintelligent worm.

Denial of service attacks, or DoS, are harm caused through loss of availability. Network denial of service attacks are based either on triggers, where a specific circumstance causes the end server to fail, or on floods, where the bulk nature of the communication causes the end server to fail. The target of the DoS can be a client application, a host service, or the entire system. Trigger attacks can have unexpected effects—for example, the Nimda worm caused trigger attacks on some Cisco infrastructure products, prompting instability and failure. Floods can affect a client (for example, an excessively large mail attachment causing a DoS on client mail downloads), a service (for instance, the CIFS Host Announcement Frame vulnerability that can cause Windows Domain Controllers to function poorly), or on a system and infrastructure (such as a smurf attack, which consumes all bandwidth heading toward a site). Floods are particularly difficult to address, as they often have no effective defense.

Of growing concern is the Distributed Denial of Service, or DDoS, attack. The chief problem is that a large number of unsophisticated users have placed their computers on the Internet, allowing unscrupulous attackers to take over their machine. These large numbers of machines can be used to harm networks or systems of networks in very simple ways—by launching DoS floods—and in such a fashion that the end site can not protect itself from the attack.

Any network exposed to an uncontrolled environment will eventually experience a systems compromise. System administrators should prepare to detect and address the breach of security. The first phase should be preparation, so that you find out about the compromise before the end user. Two common techniques are the use of file system integrity software and network traffic anomaly tools. File system integrity software takes a snapshot of the file system, in an efficient manner, and then periodically compares that snapshot against the current status to see what has changed. Network traffic anomaly tools scan traffic and attempt to identify evidence of a breach. System integrity software includes a new approach to host-based intrusion detection, detecting changes as they occur and potentially preventing those changes. Traffic anomaly tools include network intrusion detection systems, log analysis, and honeypots. The Cisco product, Cisco Secure Intrusion Detection System, is an example of a network IDS tool.

If you believe a breach has occurred, then you probably want to do more than just reformat the hard drives and start over. It is usually a good idea to produce a document analyzing the event, and you may also be asked to provide forensic evidence in support of legal action. The first thing to remember if forensics is required (or in most any event handling) is to take detailed and copious notes. The second is that if legal action is anticipated, preserve the evidence. This means carefully handling your notes to ensure they have not been tampered with. Physical evidence, meanwhile, should have the chain of custody preserved: original materials (not copies) should be kept in your possession and not tampered with until they can be placed into a secure storage facility.

After a breach has been detected, there are five steps you should take:

1. **Identification and Classification** Determine the extent and type of the breach.

2. **Containment** Prevent the breach from getting farther into your network.

3. **Eradication** Stop the source of the breach.

4. **Recovery** Return to a known good state.

5. **Follow-up** Use this as an opportunity to understand what went wrong and improve your security.

There are several things you can do to prevent some classes of attacks and reduce the likelihood of others. The easiest step is to reduce the number of vulnerabilities present on your network. This is an ongoing process, due to the continually changing status of software. Ongoing automated vulnerability assessment is an effective tool. The Cisco Secure Scanner (NetSonar) is an effective tool, in conjunction with a vulnerability remediation tracking program, so you can ensure that problems are fixed over time.

The next easiest step is to provide a simple security network architecture, meaning an environment with as few interactions as possible. This is an extension of the security principle of least privilege. Reduce complexity in the number of possible interactions between devices, and you improve control over the network. Provide compartmentalization, so that if something goes wrong, the problem is limited in scope, and controls are put in place to protect critical portions of your network.

A third step is to develop a culture of security. Get users on your side and you will have fewer incidents and more support. The final recommended step is to ensure that policy is developed, kept current, and disseminated to the users to ensure that security people, policy, and technologies at a site are kept consistent and work together.

Solutions Fast Track

What Threats Face Your Network?

☑ The sources of harm are related to the goals of information security: loss of confidentiality, loss of integrity, and loss of availability. Loss of confidentiality is serious and has destroyed companies. Loss of integrity is insidious, and makes your data untrustworthy. Loss of availability has a high visibility among the user community.

☑ There are a wide variety of sources that threats can come from. A good way to classify them is Skills, Knowledge, Resources, Authority, and Motives.

☑ Several kinds of threats include:

- **Script kiddies** Low skills but high resources, with a motive for chaos.

- **Disgruntled system administrators** Large knowledge base due to a position of high authority; motive is revenge.

- **Worms** Similar to script kiddies, but on a potentially wider scale.

- **Organized crime rings** High skills, motive is financial gain.

- **Automated crime** High skills, knowledge; motive is financial gain.

Malicious Mobile Code

☑ Malicious mobile code is usually classified as one of three types: Trojan horse, virus, or worm.

☑ A Trojan horse is a program that seems to do one thing, while performing another unexpected action. Users are notorious for not listening to the advice of system administrators to be on the lookout for Trojan horses.

☑ A virus is a fragment of a computer code that inserts itself into a normal program, turning it into a Trojan horse. At one time, viruses were the most frequent vector for malicious code; today worms and Trojan horses are much more common.

☑ A worm is a complete program that self-replicates over network resources. There is a risk that worms may reproduce so fast that conventional defenses may prove inadequate.

☑ Malicious code is a real and present danger. The fundamental problem is that uncontrolled code is running on your computer. As Microsoft puts it, "If a bad guy can persuade you to run his program on your computer, it's not your computer anymore."

☑ Worms can be classified into intelligent and unintelligent types. Slightly different defensive techniques are used to tame these different classes of worms.

Denial of Service

☑ Denial of service (DoS) attacks are direct attacks on system availability. They fall into two basic types: triggers, which require only a limited amount of traffic to cause a target to fail, and floods, in which the sheer amount of communication prompts failure.

☑ Targets of DoS include client, service, and host(s). An example of a client DoS would be a Web browser open loop, causing the browser to open windows indefinitely until resources were exhausted. An example of a service DoS would be Nimda's attack on Cisco's CallManager product, in which management was unavailable until the system was patched. An example of a host flood would be the massive ICMP floods perpetrated on commercial servers during February of 2001.

☑ Two DoS attacks of particular importance are the smurf attack and the TCP SYN flood attack. You can help protect yourself and others against smurf by removing directed broadcasts from all interfaces. You can protect others and be a good Internet citizen by enforcing antispoofing criteria, as recommended in RFC 2267.

☑ An extension of DoS is the distributed DoS. This occurs when an unscrupulous attacker compromises many individual hosts, called zombies, and then uses those zombies to attack a central target. This is a particularly destructive attack, since all of the zombies have to be addressed before the situation is returned to normal.

Detecting Breaches

☑ Every system will experience breaches. It is a good idea to be prepared and deploy detection software before the breach occurs so you can find it before your users do.

☑ Two types of controls exist: host-based, such as file system integrity; and network-based, such as IDS, log analysis, and honeypots. Cisco has an effective host-based product, manufactured by Entercept, as well as an effective network-based product, the Cisco Secure Intrusion Detection System (IDS).

☑ After detection, an important consideration is forensics. In all cases, take careful notes. If you are going to collect evidence for legal action, be sure to preserve the chain of evidence.

☑ The next steps vary slightly from site to site, but are generally: identification and classification, to determine the nature of the event; containment, to limit the damage; eradication, to eliminate the cause; recovery, to provide event normalization; and follow-up, to find lessons in the event.

Preventing Attacks

☑ The four recommended steps to prevent attacks are: reduce vulnerabilities, provide a simple security network architecture, develop a culture of security, and develop security policy.

☑ Reducing vulnerabilities can be achieved by automated vulnerability programs. The Cisco Secure Scanner (NetSonar) is an effective tool in identifying vulnerabilities. This should be combined with a security event management program to ensure that vulnerabilities are tracked and resolved over time.

☑ A simple network architecture provides heightened control over the network. This reduces the number of vulnerabilities by reducing the complexity of system interactions, and allows for compartmentalization of the site.

☑ A culture of security can enhance your environment in many ways. Getting people on your side will allow them to help support the security environment through shared effort. In addition, people working with the system instead of working around it will mean fewer security exceptions. People will start complying with acceptable use guidelines, which reduces overall maintenance costs dramatically.

☑ All sites have a policy—even if not written down, sites have a way of doing business. Documenting the policy allows for improved planning, clear communications of intent, and thoughtful management guidance to preserve corporate assets and make efficient decisions about corporate culture and worker efficiency.

Frequently Asked Questions

The following Frequently Asked Questions, answered by the authors of this book, are designed to both measure your understanding of the concepts presented in this chapter and to assist you with real-life implementation of these concepts. To have your questions about this chapter answered by the author, browse to **www.syngress.com/solutions** and click on the **"Ask the Author"** form.

Q: I've got antivirus software. Am I safe from malicious code?

A: Not completely. It certainly helps, since many pieces of code circulate over time, and the antivirus software will detect it. You do have to ensure your antivirus software is current, with current signatures, and that it is integrated with your mail client so it prevents the launch of a Trojan horse before clicking it. However, antivirus software won't protect you from flaws in your software—you need to patch your code to current vendor recommended standards. Even then, there is a window of vulnerability in which you might be affected.

Q: Does "virus" mean all of these things, worms and Trojan horses included?

A: The language is flexible, and antivirus software makers provide protection against the three types of malware, so it is natural that their name is associated with all three. However, the mechanisms for infection are different, and the best ways to protect against the codes are different. Because of this, security professionals tend to use the more specific names where possible.

Q: How can I protect against denial of service floods?

A: You can't, completely. If the packet is already crossing your WAN link and saturating it, then blocking it at your perimeter router won't help. Your best protection is a good relationship with your upstream, so they can block it at their routers, and leave your link free for traffic. They can apply specific blocks, or rate limiting techniques to ensure your traffic will continue to flow. Multihoming is also often a good idea, since sometimes you can control the inbound flow of traffic through BGP announcements or the like, and it gives you another tool in combating the flood.

Q: Is a vulnerability assessment program expensive?

A: Not necessarily. The Cisco product is not terribly expensive, and there exist open source solutions which are free to use. The actual assessment program is probably less expensive than the remediation efforts: maintaining all your hosts on an ongoing basis is a steep maintenance requirement, and one that not all enterprises have accepted. But ever since the summer of 2001, there has been clear evidence that you have to manage your hosts and keep their patch levels up-to-date just to stay in business.

Q: Should I use an IDS?

A: Only by sitting down with your security policy can you identify the necessary controls. However, it is worth noting that according to CSI/FBI statistics, about two thirds of all sites have IDSs in place, with another 10 percent due to be installed this year. Market statistics show that IDS products are among the top sellers, and external mandates such as HIPAA and Presidential Decision Directive 63 should provide even more drivers. Another observation is that IDSs are not yet well integrated into the enterprise: only limited traffic is exposed to IDSs, and IDS event management is generally not well operationalized. However, market forces and the effectiveness of an IDS as a tool will lead to improved devices in the near future.

## Chapter 3

Cisco PIX Firewall

Solutions in this chapter:

- Overview of the Security Features
- Initial Configuration
- The Command-Line Interface
- Configuring NAT and PAT
- Security Policy Configuration
- PIX Configuration Examples
- Securing and Maintaining the PIX

☑ Summary

☑ Solutions Fast Track

☑ Frequently Asked Questions

Introduction

A firewall can be described as a security mechanism located on a network that protects resources from other networks and individuals. It controls access to a network and enforces a security policy that can be tailored to suit the needs of a company.

There is some confusion on what the difference is between a Cisco PIX firewall and a router. Both devices are capable of filtering traffic with access control lists, and both devices are capable of providing Network Address Translation. PIX go above and beyond simply filtering packets, based on source/destination IP addresses, as well as source/destination TCP/UDP port numbers. PIX are a dedicated hardware device built to provide security. Although a router can also provide some of the functions of a PIX by implementing access control lists, it also has to deal with routing packets from one network to another. Depending on what model of router is being used, access lists tend to burden the CPU, especially if there are numerous access lists that must be referenced for every packet that travels through the router. This can impact the performance of the router, causing other problems such as network convergence time. A router is also unable to provide security features such as URL, ActiveX, and Java filtering, Flood Defender, Flood Guard, and IP Frag Guard, DNS Guard, Mail Guard, Failover, and FTP and URL logging.

Cisco Systems offer a number of security solutions for networks. Included in those solutions are the Cisco Secure PIX Firewall series. The PIX firewall is a dedicated hardware-based firewall that utilizes a version of the Cisco IOS for configuration and operation. This chapter will introduce and discuss security features, Network Address Translation (NAT), Network Address Port Translation (NAPT, referred to as PAT on the PIX firewall IOS), developing a security policy for your network, applying the security policy on the PIX and finally, maintaining your PIX and securing it from unauthorized individuals.

The PIX Firewall series offers several models to meet the needs of networks today. These range from the Enterprise class Secure PIX 535 Firewall to the newly introduced Small Office/Home Office (SOHO) class Secure PIX 501 Firewall model. A specification and description chart is shown in Table 3.1 that follows.

- **Cisco PIX 535 Firewall** Intended for large enterprise and service provider environments. It will provide over 1 Gbps of firewall throughput with the ability to handle up to 500,000 simultaneous connections. Some PIX 535 models include stateful high-availability capabilities, as well as integrated hardware acceleration for VPNs. This provides up to 95 Mbps of 3DES VPN and support for 2,000 IPSec tunnels. The Cisco PIX 535 provides a modular chassis with support for up to ten 10/100 Fast Ethernet interfaces or nine Gigabit Ethernet interfaces.

- **Cisco PIX 525 Firewall** Intended for large enterprise and service provider environments. It will provide over 360 Mbps of firewall throughput with the ability to handle as many as 280,000 simultaneous sessions. Some PIX 525 models include stateful high-availability capabilities, as well as integrated hardware acceleration for VPN. This will provide up to 70 Mbps of 3DES VPN and support for 2,000 IPSec tunnels. The PIX 525 provides a modular chassis with support for up to eight 10/100 Fast Ethernet interfaces or three Gigabit Ethernet interfaces.

- **Cisco PIX 515E Firewall** Intended for small-to-medium business and enterprise environments. It will provide up to 188 Mbps of firewall throughput with the ability to handle as many as 125,000 simultaneous sessions. Many PIX 515E models include stateful high-availability capabilities, as well as integrated support for 2,000 IPSec tunnels. The PIX 515E provides a modular chassis with support for up to six 10/100 Fast Ethernet interfaces.

- **Cisco PIX 506E Firewall** Intended for remote office/branch office environments. These PIX will provide up to 20 Mbps of firewall throughput and 16 Mbps of 3DES VPN throughput. The PIX 506E uses a compact, desktop chassis and provides two auto-sensing 10Base-T interfaces.

- **Cisco PIX 501 Firewall** Intended for small office and enterprise teleworker environments. These PIX will provide up to 10 Mbps of firewall throughput and 3 Mbps of 3DES VPN throughput. The PIX 501 delivers great security in a compact security appliance. It includes an integrated four-port Fast Ethernet (10/100) switch and one 10Base-T interface.

Table 3.1 Specifications for Cisco PIX Firewalls

Description	PIX 501	PIX 506	PIX 515	PIX 525	PIX 535
Processor	133MHz	200MHz	200MHz	350MHz	1GHz
RAM	16MB	32MB	32MB or 64MB	128MB or 256MB	512MB or 1GB

Continued

Table 3.1 Continued

Description	PIX 501	PIX 506	PIX 515	PIX 525	PIX 535
Flash Memory	8MB	8MB	16MB	16MB	16MB
PCI Slots	None	None	2	3	9
Fixed Interfaces	One 10BaseT Ethernet, four-port 10/100 switch	Two 10BaseT Ethernet	Two 10/100 Fast Ethernet	Two 10/100 Fast Ethernet	None
Max Interfaces	One 10BaseT Ethernet, four-port 10/100 switch	Two 10BaseT Ethernet	Six 10/100 Fast Ethernet or Gigabit Ethernet	Eight 10/100 Fast Ethernet or Gigabit Ethernet	Ten 10/100 Fast Ethernet
VPN Accelerator Card	No	No	Yes	Yes	Yes
Failover Support	No	No	Yes; UNRE-STRICTED only	Yes; UNRE-STRICTED only	Yes; UNRE-STRICTED only
Rack Mountable	No	No	Yes	Yes	Yes
Size	Desktop	Desktop	One RU	Two RU	Three RU

Overview of the Security Features

With the enormous growth of the Internet, companies are beginning to depend on having an online presence on the Internet. With that presence, there will be security risks that allow outside individuals to gain access to critical information and resources.

Companies are now faced with the task of implementing security measures to protect their data and resources. The resources to protect can be much diversified, such as Web servers, mail Servers, FTP servers, databases, or any type of networked devices. Figure 3.1 displays a typical company network with access to the Internet via a leased line without a firewall in place.

Figure 3.1 A Typical LAN with no Firewall

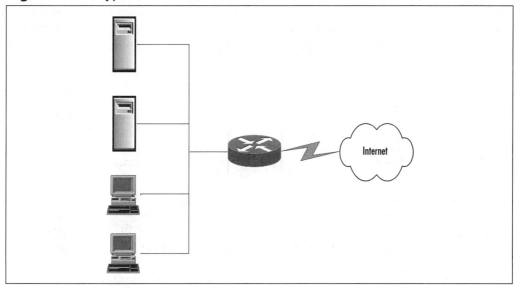

As you can see in Figure 3.1, company XYZ has a direct connection to the Internet. They are also using a class C public IP address space for their network, therefore making it publicly available to anyone who wishes to access it. Without any security measures, individuals are able to access each of the devices on the network with a public IP. Private information can be compromised, while malicious strikes such as denial of service (DoS) attacks may be launched against the company. If a firewall was placed between company XYZ's network and the Internet, security measures could be taken to filter and block unwanted traffic. Without access control at the network perimeter, a company's security relies on the proper configuration and security of each individual host and server. This can be an administrative nightmare if hundreds of devices need to be configured for this purpose.

Routers have the ability to filter traffic based on source address, destination address, and TCP/UDP ports. Using this ability as well as a firewall can provide a more complete security solution for a network.

Another example of how a PIX firewall can secure a network is in a company's intranet. Figure 3.2 illustrates a network in which departments are separated by two different subnets. What is stopping an individual in the Human Resources network from accessing resources on the Finance network? A firewall can be put in place between the two subnets to secure the Finance network from any unauthorized access, or restrict access to certain hosts.

Figure 3.2 A LAN Segmented by a Department with no Firewall

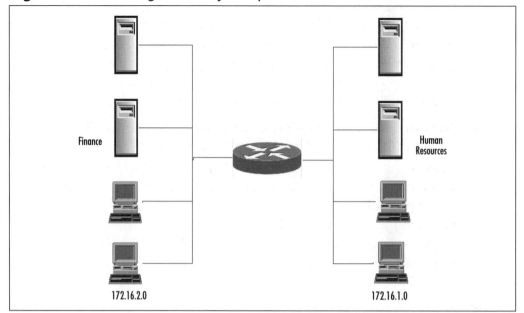

Since the PIX are designed as a security appliance, it provides a wealth of features to secure a network. These features include:

- **Packet filtering** A method for limiting inbound information from the Internet. Packet filters employ access control lists (ACL) similar to those used in routers to accept or deny access based on packet source address, destination address, and TCP/UDP sources and destination ports.

- **Proxy Server** A device that examines higher layers of the Open System Interconnection (OSI) model. This will act as an intermediary between the source and destination by creating a separate connection to each. Optionally, authentication can be achieved by requiring users to authenticate with a secure system by means of a proxy such as a Cisco IOS Firewall Authentication Proxy Server. Some of the drawbacks for this method of security are that it provides authentication at the cost of performance, and a proxy only supports a limited number of protocols.

- **Stateful Filtering** A secure method of analyzing packets and placing extensive information about that packet in a table. Each time a TCP connection is established from an inside host accessing an outside host through the PIX firewall, the information about the connection is automatically logged in a stateful session flow table. The table contains the source and destination addresses, port numbers, TCP sequencing information, and additional flags for each TCP connection associated with that particular host. Inbound packets are compared against the session flows in the table and are permitted through the PIX only if an appropriate connection exists to validate their passage. Without stateful filtering, access lists would have to be configured to allow traffic originating from the inside network to return from the outside network.

- **Network Address Translation and Network Address Port Translation** Another feature of the PIX. Usage of NAT is often mistaken as a security measure. Translating private IP addresses into global IP addresses was implemented to assist in the problem of rapidly depleting public IP addresses. Even though private IP addresses are used for an inside network, an ISP is still directly connected. It is not unheard of that a sloppy routing configuration on behalf of the ISP will leak a route to your network to other clients. NAT will hide your network, but it should not be relied upon as a security measure.

- **IPSec** Provides VPN (Virtual Private Network) access via digital certificates or preshared keys.

- **Flood Defender, Flood Guard, and IP Frag Guard** Features used to protect a network from TCP SYN flood attacks, controlling the AAA service's tolerance for unanswered login attempts, and IP fragmentation attacks.

- **DNS Guard** Identifies an outbound DNS resolve request, and only allows a single DNS response.

- **FTP and URL Logging** Allows you to view inbound and outbound FTP commands entered by users, as well as the URLs they use to access other sites.

- **Mail Guard** Provides safe access for SMTP (Simple Mail Transfer Protocol) connections from the outside to an inside e-mail server.

- **ActiveX Blocking** Blocks HTML *object* commands and comments them out of the HTML Web page.

- **Java Filtering** Allows an administrator to prevent Java applets from being downloaded by a host on the inside network.

- **URL Filtering**   When used with NetPartners WebSENSE product, PIX checks outgoing URL requests with policy defined on the WebSENSE server, which runs on either Windows NT/2000 or Unix.

- **AAA**   Provides authentication, authorization, and accounting with the aid of an AAA server such as a RADIUS or TACACS+ server.

Differences between PIX OS Version 4.x and Version 5.x

The following describes new features available in the recent release of the PIX OS:

- Cisco IOS Access Lists

- IPSec

- Stateful Failover

- Voice over IP (VoIP) Support

Cisco IOS access lists can now be specified in support of the IPSec feature. In addition, access lists can now be used to specify the type of traffic permitted through the PIX in conjunction with the *access-group* command. PIX OS 4.x used *conduit* and *outbound* statements to limit the type of traffic permitted through the interface. For example, the following command set can be rewritten using *access-list* and *access-group* statements.

```
pixfirewall(config)#write terminal
static (inside,outside) 207.139.221.10 192.168.0.10 netmask
    >255.255.255.255
```

Creates a static translation for private 192.168.0.10 to globally unique IP 207.139.221.10.

```
conduit permit tcp any host 207.139.221.10 eq www
```

Specifies that only HTTP traffic will be permitted to reach host 207.139.221.10.

```
outbound 10 permit any any 80 tcp
outbound 10 permit any any 23 tcp
outbound 10 deny any any any tcp
outbound 10 deny any any any udp
```

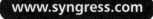

Specifies that HTTP and Telnet traffic will be permitted from a higher-level security interface to a lower-level security interface (inside, outside), followed by an explicit *deny all* statement.

```
apply (inside) 10 outgoing_src
```

Applies outbound list 10 to an inside interface. This configuration can be rewritten using *access-list* and *access-group* commands available in 5.x PIX OS.

```
pixfirewall(config)#write terminal
static (inside,outside) 207.139.221.10 192.168.0.10 netmask
   >255.255.255.255
```

This creates a static translation for private 192.168.0.10 to a globally unique IP 207.139.221.10.

```
access-list acl_out permit tcp any any eq www
access-list acl_out permit tcp any any eq telnet
access-list acl_out deny tcp any any
access-list acl_out deny udp any any
```

This specifies that HTTP and Telnet traffic will be permitted, followed by an explicit *deny all* statement:

```
access-list acl_in permit tcp any host 207.139.221.10 eq www
access-list acl_in permit tcp any host 207.139.221.10 eq ftp
```

This specifies that HTTP and FTP traffic will be permitted from any source to host 207.139.221.10.

```
access-group acl_out in interface inside
```

This applies access list *acl_out* to the inside interface.

```
access-group acl_in in interface outside
```

This applies access list acl_in to the outside interface.

The purpose of using the *access-list* and *access-group* commands instead of the *outbound* and *conduit* statements is to provide a common operating environment across various platforms. If an individual is able to implement access lists on a router, then implementing access lists on PIX should be no different.

The IPSec feature is based on the Cisco IOS IPSec implementation and provides functionality with those IPSec-compliant devices. IPSec offers a mechanism for secure data transmission by providing confidentiality, integrity, and authenticity of data across a public IP network. Refer to Chapter 8 for more information on IPSec.

The Stateful Failover feature provides a mechanism for hardware and software redundancy by allowing two identical PIX units to serve the same functionality in case one fails in an unattended environment. One PIX is considered an active unit while the other is in standby mode. In the event the active unit fails, the standby unit will become active, therefore providing redundancy.

PIX provides support for VoIP in its H.323 RAS feature—however, Cisco CallManager is not supported. For more information on VoIP, please refer to Cisco's Web site (www.cisco.com).

Other new commands introduced in the PIX 5.x OS are as follows:

- **ca** Provides access to the IPSec certification authority feature.

- **Clear flashfs** Clears Flash memory. Use before downgrading to any version 4.x release.

- **Crypto-map** Provides IPSec cryptography mapping.

- **Debug crypto ca** Debugs Certification Authority (CA) processing.

- **Debug crypto ipsec** Debugs IPSec processing.

- **Debug crypto isakmp** Debugs ISAKMP processing.

- **Domain-name** Changes the domain name.

- **Failover link** Enables Stateful Failover support.

- **ipsec** Shortened form of the *crypto ipsec* command.

- **Isakmp** Lets you create an IKE security association.

- **Sysopt connection permit-ipsec** Specifies that the PIX implicitly permit IPSec traffic and bypass the checking of the *conduit* or *access-group* commands associated with IPSec connections.

Differences between PIX OS Version 6.0 and Version 5.x

The newest version of Cisco PIX OS is Version 6.0. This version delivers the latest PIX capabilities and security improvements as well as some new features. The following is a list of new features for 6.0:

- PIX Device Manager

- VPN Client v3.x

- CPU Utilization Statistics

- Dynamic Shunning with the Cisco Intrusion Detection System

- Port Address Translations

- Skinny Protocol Support

- Session Initiation Protocol

- Stateful Sharing of HTTP (port 80) Sessions

- Ethernet Interfaces

Each of these new features are discussed in greater detail in the following sections.

Cisco PIX Device Manager

The Cisco PIX Device Manager is a Web browser-based configuration tool that enables you to set up, configure, and monitor your PIX firewall graphically over the Web browser—all without requiring any real knowledge of the command-line interface of the PIX firewall.

VPN Client v3.x

The Cisco VPN Client enables customers to establish secure end-to-end encrypted tunnels. The client can be preconfigured for deployment, and initial logins require very little user help. VPN access policies and configurations are downloaded from the PIX and pushed to the client when a connection is established, allowing simple setup and manageability.

CPU Utilization Statistics

The ability to monitor the CPU load on the PIX firewall has been added to version 6.0. The *show* command and PIX Device Manager can monitor and obtain five-second to five-minute CPU utilization statistics.

Dynamic Shunning with Cisco Intrusion Detection System

This feature allows PIX, when combined with a Cisco Intrusion Detection System Sensor, to dynamically respond to an attacking host by preventing new connections and disallowing packets from any existing connection. A Cisco

Intrusion Detection System device instructs the PIX firewall to shun sources of traffic when those sources of traffic are determined to be malicious by rule. The *shun* command applies a "blocking function" to the interface receiving the attack for a defined period of time by the user. Packets containing the IP source address of the attacking host are dropped and logged until the blocking function is removed by the Cisco Intrusion Detection System. No traffic from that IP source address will be allowed to traverse to the PIX firewall; also, any remaining connections time out. The *shun* command is applied whether or not a connection with the specified host IP address is currently active.

Port Address Translations

The PIX firewall now provides static Port Address Translation capability, enabling you to send multiple inbound TCP or UDP services to different internal hosts through a single global IP address. The global IP address can be a unique address or a shared outbound Port Address Translation.

Skinny Protocol Support

Cisco Secure PIX Firewall application handling has been enhanced to support the Skinny Client Control Protocol used by Cisco IP phones for VoIP call signaling. This capability dynamically opens pinholes for media sessions and Network Address Translation embedded IP addresses. Skinny Client Control Protocol supports IP telephony and can reside in an H.323 environment. An application layer ensures that all Skinny Client Control Protocol signaling and media packets can traverse the PIX firewall and interoperate with H.323 terminals.

Session Initiation Protocol

Session Initiation Protocol as defined by the Internet Engineering Task Force enables call handling sessions, particularly two-party audio conferences. Session Initiation Protocol works with Session Description Protocol, which defines the calls prior to call handling. Using Session Initiation Protocol, the PIX firewall can support VoIP and any proxy server using VoIP.

Stateful Sharing of HTTP (port 80) Sessions

The PIX firewall supports high-availability with the deployment of a redundant hot standby unit. This failover option maintains concurrent connections through automatic stateful synchronization. This ensures that even in the event of a system failure, sessions are maintained, and the transition is completely transparent to network users. PIX Firewall version 6.0 adds the ability to maintain HTTP (port 80) sessions.

Ethernet Interfaces

The PIX Firewall series supports single or four-port 10/100 Fast Ethernet, as well as Gigabit Ethernet network interface cards. The PIX 6.0 on PIX Firewall 535 with an unrestricted license may support up to ten Ethernet interfaces. Restricted licenses can support up to eight interfaces.

Initial Configuration

The initial configuration of the Secure PIX Firewall greatly resembles that of a router. A console cable kit consisting of a rollover cable and DB9/DB25 serial adapter is needed to configure the device out of the box. It is recommended that the initial configuration not take place on a live network until the initial setup has been completed and tested. Initial configuration should take place in a test bed environment, which is isolated from any production network. If initial configuration takes place on a production network and an incorrect IP address that is already in use on the network is assigned to an interface on the PIX, IP address conflicts will occur. It is generally a bad idea to set up a firewall or other security device on a non-isolated network. The default configuration is often not secure and can be compromised between the setup stage and security policy stage. Installing the PIX consists of removing the unit from the packaging, installing any optional hardware, such as an additional NIC, mounting the PIX in a rack (optional), and connecting all the necessary cables such as power and network cables. Once the hardware portion of the PIX setup has been completed, the software portion of the setup can begin.

Before configuring the software, be sure to have a design plan already in place. Items such as IP addresses, security policies, and placement of the PIX should already be mapped out. With a proper design strategy, the basic configuration will only have to be done once to make the PIX functional.

Installing the PIX Software

In this section, we will discuss the initial software configuration of the PIX to allow traffic to pass through it. Other features such as configuring NAT, PAT, and security policies will be covered later in this chapter.

When the PIX is first powered on, the software configuration stored in Flash memory permits the PIX to start up, but will not allow any traffic to pass through it until configured to do so. Newer versions of the PIX OS may be available from Cisco depending on what version shipped with the PIX, so it may be a good idea to complete the basic configuration to establish connectivity and then upgrade the version of the PIX OS.

Connecting to the PIX—Basic Configuration

In order to upgrade the IOS or begin allowing traffic to pass through the PIX, some basic configuration is needed to make the PIX operational.

1. Connect the serial port of your PC to the console port on the PIX firewall with the serial cable supplied with the PIX.

2. Using a Terminal Emulation program such as HyperTerminal, connect to the COM port on the PC.

NOTE

Make sure the COM port properties in the terminal emulation program match the following values:
- 9600 baud
- 8 data bits
- No parity
- 1 stop bit
- Hardware flow control

3. Turn on the PIX.

4. Once the PIX has finished booting up, the following prompt will appear:

   `pixfirewall>`

5. Type **enable** and press the **Enter** key. The following prompt appears:

   `Password:`

6. Press the **Enter** key again and you will now be in privileged mode, which is represented by the following prompt:

   `pixfirewall#`

7. Set an enable password by going into configuration mode. A strong, non-guessable password should be chosen. The example uses *<password>* to designate where your password should be typed:

```
pixfirewall#configure terminal
pixfirewall(config)#enable password <password>
```

8. Permit Telnet access to the console from the inside network:

```
pixfirewall(config)#telnet 0.0.0.0 0.0.0.0 inside
```

9. Set the Telnet console password. This password should be different from the enable password chosen in step 7.

```
pixfirewall(config)#passwd  <password>
```

10. Save your changes to your non-volatile RAM (NVRAM) with the *write* command:

```
pixfirewall(config)#write memory
```

NOTE

The configuration used in the following examples is based on IOS version 5.1(1).

Identify Each Interface

On new installations with only two interfaces, PIX will provide names for each interface, by default. These can be viewed with the *show nameif* command. The *show nameif* command output will resemble the following:

```
pixfirewall# show nameif
nameif ethernet0 outside security0
nameif ethernet1 inside security100
```

If additional NICs are going to be used, you must assign a unique name and security value to each additional interface.

The default behavior of the PIX includes blocking traffic originating from the *outside* interface destined for the *inside* interface. Traffic originating from the *inside* interface destined to the *outside* interface will be permitted until access lists are implemented to restrict traffic. The inside interface will be assigned a security value of 100 and the outside interface will be assigned a value of 0. These values are important when creating security policies in which traffic will flow from a lower security interface to a higher security level interface. If additional interfaces are added to the PIX, it is important to properly plan which interfaces will be used for what purposes. For example, in a situation where three interfaces are used to separate an inside network, outside network, and DMZ (Demilitarized Zone; discussed later in this chapter), assign the DMZ interface a security value between the inside and outside interfaces such as 50. This configuration will reflect the purpose of the DMZ, which is a network separated from the inside and outside networks, yet security can still be controlled with the PIX.

In order to assign a name to an interface, use:

Nameif hardware_id name security_level

- **Hardware_id** Either ethernet*n* for Ethernet, or token*x* for Token Ring interfaces where *n* and *x* are the interface numbers.
- **Name** The name to be assigned to the interface.
- **Security_level** A value such as security40 or security60. You can use any security value between 1 and 99.

```
pixfirewall#configure terminal
pixfirewall(config)#nameif ethernet2 dmz1 security40
pixfirewall(config)#show nameif
pixfirewall(config)#nameif ethernet0 outside security0
pixfirewall(config)#nameif ethernet1 inside security100
pixfirewall(config)#nameif ethernet2 dmz1 security40
```

NOTE

Be sure to use a naming convention that will easily describe the function of each interface. The dmz1 interface represents a "demilitarized zone" which is intended to be an area between the inside and outside networks. This is a common implementation for companies that host Web servers, mail servers, and other resources.

By default, each interface is in a shutdown state and must be made active. Use the *interface* command to activate the interfaces.

Interface hardware_id hardware_speed [**shutdown**]

- **Hardware_id** Either ethernet*n* for Ethernet, or token*x* for Token Ring interfaces where *n* and *x* are the interface numbers.

- **Hardware_speed** Either 4 Mpbs or 16 Mpbs for Token Ring, depending on the line speed of the Token Ring card. If the interface is Ethernet, use auto.

- **Auto** Activates auto-negotiation for the Ethernet 10/100 interface.

- **Shutdown** Disables the interface. When the PIX are configured for the first time, all interfaces will be shut down, by default.

The following examples will enable the *ethernet0* interface into auto-negotiation mode, and the Token Ring interface *token0* into 16 Mbps mode.

```
pixfirewall(config)#interface ethernet0 auto
pixfirewall(config)#interface token0 16mpbs
```

Installing the IOS over TFTP

The following steps will guide you through upgrading the PIX IOS.

1. Download the latest version of the IOS from Cisco's Web site (www.cisco.com).

2. Download and install the TFTP Server application which can also be found on Cisco's Web site. The TFTP server is an application installed on a host computer to provide a TFTP service. This service is used by the PIX firewall to download or upload software images and configuration parameters.

NOTE

You need to download the TFTP server software if you are using a Windows NT/2000 machine as a server. A Unix server has a TFTP server, by default.

3. Make sure the TFTP software is running on a server. Also confirm that the server is on the same subnet as one of the interfaces.

4. Once the connection to the PIX console port has been established, power on the PIX.

5. Immediately send a BREAK character by pressing the **Esc** key. The monitor prompt will appear.

6. Use the *address* command to specify an IP address on the interface in the same network where the TFTP resides.

7. Use the *server* command to specify the IP address of the TFTP server.

8. Use the *file* command to specify the name of the file to download from the TFTP server.

9. If the TFTP server resides on a different subnet then that of the PIX interface, use the *gateway* command to specify the IP address of the default gateway in order to reach the TFTP server.

10. In order to test connectivity, use the *ping* command to ping the TFTP server.

11. Finally, use the *TFTP* command to start the TFTP download of the IOS.

For example, assuming that the TFTP server has been configured with the IP address 172.16.0.39, and that a new software image file *pix512.bin* is stored on that server. We can download this new image on the PIX as follows:

```
monitor>
monitor>address 172.16.0.1
monitor>server 172.16.0.39
monitor>file pix512.bin
monitor>ping 172.16.0.39
Sending 5, 100-byte 0x5b8d ICMP Echoes to 172.16.0.39, timeout is 4
    seconds:
!!!!!
Success rate is 100 percent (5/5)
monitor>tftp
tftp pix512.bin@172.16.0.39
Received 626688 bytes

PIX admin loader (3.0) #0: Mon July 10 10:43:02 PDT 2000
Flash=AT29C040A @ 0x300
Flash version 4.9.9.1, Install version 5.1.2

Installing to flash
```

The following is a list of commands available while in monitor mode:

- **Address** Sets the IP address.

- **File** Specifies the boot file name.

- **Gateway** Sets the IP gateway IP address.

- **Help** Lists help messages.

- **Interface** Specifies the type of interface (Ethernet, Token Ring).

- **Ping** Tests connectivity by issuing echo-requests to specified IP addresses.

- **Help** Lists available commands and syntax.

- **Reload** Halts and reloads system.

- **Server** Specifies the server by IP address in which the TFTP application is running.

- **Tftp** Initiates the TFTP download.

- **Trace** Toggles packet tracing.

The Command-Line Interface

The command-line interface (CLI) used on the PIX is very similar to that used on routers. Three modes exist to perform configuration and troubleshooting steps. These three modes are:

- Unprivileged mode

- Privileged mode

- Configuration mode

When you first initiate a console or Telnet session to the PIX, you will be in user mode. Virtually no commands will be available in user mode. Only the *enable, pager,* and *quit* commands are permitted. Once in privileged mode, commands such as *show, debug,* and *reload* are available. From privileged mode, configuration tasks may take place by entering the *configure* command, followed by where the PIX will accept configuration commands from. For example, when you first connect to the PIX, either through a Telnet or console session, you will be in user mode (the user mode password must be entered when accessing the PIX by Telnet). User mode is represented by the following prompt:

```
Pixfirewall>
```

In order to access privileged mode, you must type **enable** at the prompt. After providing the required authentication, you will enter privileged mode. Privileged mode is represented by the following prompt:

```
Pixfurewall>enable
Password:  ********
Pixfirewall#
```

If the system did not request a password after typing **enable**, it means no enable password has been configured as described in the *Basic Configuration* section. It is very important that an enable password be configured.

Finally, in order to perform configuration tasks, you must be in configuration mode. This mode is represented by the following prompt:

```
Pixfurewall#configure terminal
Pixfirewall(config)#
```

Table 3.2 lists some of the shortcut key combinations available on the PIX CLI.

Table 3.2 Key Combination Shortcuts

Command	Result
TAB	Completes a command entry
Ctrl+A	Takes cursor to beginning of the line
Ctrl+E	Takes cursor to end of the line
Ctrl+R	Redisplays a line (useful if command gets interrupted by console output)
Arrow up or Ctrl+P	Displays previous line
Arrow up or Ctrl+n	Displays next line
Help or ?	Displays help

IP Configuration

Once the interfaces on the PIX have been named and assigned a security value (additional interfaces only), the IP must be configured on the interfaces in order to allow traffic to pass through the PIX.

IP Addresses

Once the interfaces have been named and are activated, an IP address needs to be assigned to them. To assign an IP address to an interface, use the command:

`ip address` interface-name netmask

To further explain:

- **Interface-name** The name assigned to the interface using the *nameif* command.

- **Netmask** The network mask assigned to the interface.

```
pixfirewall(config)#interface ethernet0 auto
pixfirewall(config)#interface ethernet1 auto
pixfirewall(config)#ip address inside 172.16.0.1 255.255.255.0
pixfirewall(config)#ip address outside 207.139.221.1 255.255.255.0
pixfirewall(config)#show interface ethernet1
interface ethernet1 "inside" is up, line protocol is up
   Hardware is i82559 ethernet, address is 0050.54ff.2aa9
   IP address 172.16.0.1, subnet mask 255.255.255.0
   MTU 1500 bytes, BW 100000 Kbit full duplex
          147022319 packets input, 3391299957 bytes, 0 no buffer
          Received 12580140 broadcasts, 0 runts, 0 giants
          0 input errors, 0 CRC, 0 frame, 0 overrun, 0 ignored, 0
abort
          166995559 packets output, 1686643683 bytes, 0 underruns
          0 output errors, 0 collisions, 0 interface resets
          0 babbles, 0 late collisions, 0 deferred
          0 lost carrier, 0 no carrier
```

Once the interfaces have been configured, test them to make sure they have been configured properly. A simple connectivity test is to ping another interface on your network or test lab environment. To do this:

`Ping` interface ip_address

In this case, the following is true:

- **Interface** The interface in which you want the ping to originate from (similar to an extended ping on a router).

- **Ip_address** The target IP address to ping.

```
pixfirewall#ping inside 172.16.0.2
            172.16.0.2 response received — 0ms
            172.16.0.2 response received — 0ms
            172.16.0.2 response received — 0ms
```

If no response is received, confirm that the network cables are connected to the interfaces and the interfaces have been configured correctly.

```
pixfirewall#ping inside 172.16.0.4
        172.16.0.4 NO response received — 940ms
        172.16.0.4 NO response received — 900ms
        172.16.0.4 NO response received — 920ms
```

Default Route

Now that all the interfaces have been configured, a default gateway must be assigned. A typical implementation will have a PIX firewall positioned between the ISP and company's networks (Figure 3.3).

Figure 3.3 Default Route

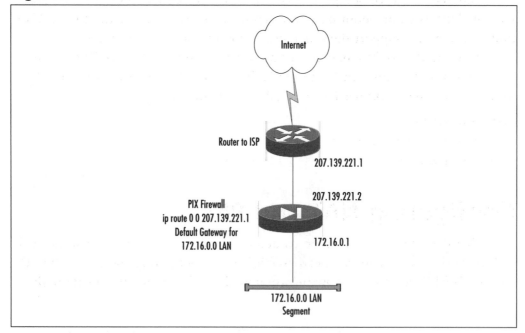

A default gateway must be assigned to the outside interface to allow traffic to reach the ISP. To do this, use the command:

```
route interface_name ip_address netmask gateway_ip [metric]
```

To further explain:

- **Interface_name** The internal or external network interface name.

- **Ip_address** ID of the internal or external IP address. Use **0.0.0.0** to specify a default route. The **0.0.0.0** can be abbreviated as **0**.

- **Netmask** Specifies a network mask to apply to *ip_address*. Use **0.0.0.0** to specify a default route. The **0.0.0.0** can be abbreviated as **0**.

- **Gateway_ip** The IP address of the gateway router (the next hop address for this route).

- **Metric** Specifies the number of hops to *gateway_ip*.

    ```
    pixfirewall>enable
    pixfirewall#configure terminal
    pixfirewall(config)#route outside 0 0 207.139.221.1
    ```

If different networks are present on the inside or outside interface, the PIX will need information about how to reach those networks. Since the PIX is not a router, it does not support the different routing protocols a router does. Currently, the PIX only supports RIP as its routing protocol. Since PIX it is not a router, it is not recommended to use RIP. Instead, add static routes to the PIX to make other networks reachable. To add a static route:

```
pixfirewall>enable
pixfirewall#configure terminal
pixfirewall(config)#route inside 192.168.1.0 255.255.255.0 172.16.0.2 1
```

Configuring NAT and PAT

Now that the interfaces have been named and security values have been assigned, and network connectivity has been established by configuring and testing the IP settings, NAT and PAT can now be configured to allow traffic to pass through.

Permit Traffic Through

When an outbound packet arrives at a higher security level interface (inside), the PIX checks the validity of the packet based on the Adaptive Security Algorithm (ASA), and then whether or not a previous packet has come from that host. If no packet has originated from that host, then the packet is for a new connection, and PIX will create a translation in its table for the connection.

The information that PIX stores in the translation table includes the inside IP address and a globally unique IP address assigned by the Network Address Translation, or Network Address Port Translation. The PIX then changes the packet's source IP address to the global address, modifies the checksum and other fields as required, and forwards the packet to the lower security interface (outside, or DMZ).

When an inbound packet arrives at a lower security level interface (outside, or DMZ), it must first pass the PIX Adaptive Security criteria. If the packet passes the security tests (static and Access Control Lists), the PIX removes the destination IP address, and the internal IP address is inserted in its place. The packet is then forwarded to the higher security level interface (inside). Figure 3.4 illustrates the NAT process on the PIX.

Figure 3.4 NAT Example

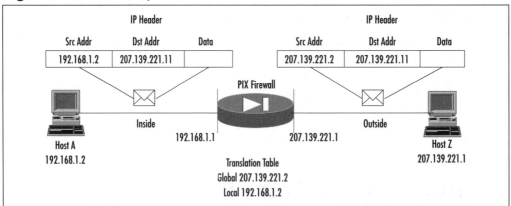

In the example, Host A initiates a session with Host Z. Since Host A is not on the same subnet as host Z, the packet must be routed. When the packet arrives at the inside interface of the PIX, it examines the Source address. NAT has been enabled on the PIX and a global pool of IP addresses has been allocated for translations. The PIX then modifies the IP header and alters the source address of the IP header to an IP address from the global pool of IP addresses. Once the translation occurs, the packet is then routed to Host Z. When Host Z replies to Host A, the PIX examines the packet that arrives on the outside interface. Since there is an active translation for Host A, the PIX knows that packets destined for IP address 207.139.221.2 must be translated back to 192.168.1.2. Once the PIX alters the IP header, it then routes the packet back to Host A. This process occurs until no more traffic needs to be translated between the two devices and the translation times out.

In order to allow traffic to flow from a higher-level security interface to a lower-level security interface (inside, outside), you must use the *nat* and *global* commands. In order to permit traffic from a lower-level security interface to flow through a higher-level security interface, you must use the *access-list* and *access-group* command.

NAT or Network Address Translation is a feature that dynamically maps IP addresses originating from the higher-level security interface into IP addresses on the same subnet as the lower-level security interface. For more information on NAT and PAT, refer to Chapter 5.

To enable NAT on an interface, use the command:

```
nat [(interface_name)] nat_id local_ip [netmask [max_conns [em_limit]]]
[norandomseq]
```

To further explain:

- **Interface_name** The internal network interface name.

- **Nat_id** Used in the *global* command statement. All *nat* commands with the same *nat_id* are in the same *nat* group.

- **Local_ip** The internal network IP address to be translated. You can use **0.0.0.0** to allow all hosts to start an outbound connection originating from the inside interface. The **0.0.0.0** IP can be abbreviated as **0**.

- **Netmask** The network mask for *local_ip*. You can also use the **0.0.0.0** to allow all outbound connections originating from the inside interface.

- **Max_cons** The maximum TCP connections limit. The default is 0, which will allow unlimited connections.

- **Em_limit** The embryonic connection limit. The default is also 0, which will allow unlimited connections.

■ **Norandomseq** Specifies not to randomize TCP packet sequence numbers. Because this is one of the security features of PIX, it is not recommended this option be used.

```
pixfirewall(config)#nat (inside) 1 0.0.0.0 0.0.0.0
pixfirewall(config)#nat (inside) 2 172.16.0.0 255.255.0.0
```

The first *nat_ id* will translate all traffic from the inside interface, whereas the second *nat_id* will translate only traffic originating from the 172.16.0.0 subnet.

NOTE

When PAT is used, the PIX will keep track of each translation by adding a unique source port number to the source IP address for each translation. This feature is valuable when only limited IP address space is available from the service provider. To display the active translations, use the command *show xlate* from the enable prompt.

Once the traffic to be translated has been specified on the inside interface, it is now time to specify the IP address pool that the inside traffic will be translated to. To do this, the *global* command will be used.

```
global [(interface_name)] nat_id global_ip[-global_ip] [netmask global_mask]
```

In this case:

■ **Interface_name** The external network interface where these global addresses will be used.

■ **Nat_id** The number shared with the *nat* command that will group the *nat* and *global* statements together.

■ **Global_ip** One or more global IP addresses that the PIX will translate the inside interface traffic to. If the external network interface is connected to the Internet, each global IP must be registered with the Network Information Center (NIC). You can specify either a single IP address or a range of addresses by separating the addresses with a dash (-). You can create a Network Address Port Translation (PAT) by specifying a single IP address in the *global* statement.

■ **Global_mask** The network mask for the *global_ip* statement.

```
pixfirewall(config)#global (outside) 1 207.139.221.1-207.139.221.254 netmask
    >255.255.255.0
Global 207.139.221.1-207.139.221.254 will be Network Address Translated
pixfirewall(config)#global (outside) 1 207.139.221.1 255.255.255.255
Global 207.139.221.128 will be Port Address Translated
```

WARNING

If PAT is used, the IP address must be different from the IP address assigned to any of the interfaces on the PIX.

In the first statement, inside IP addresses will be translated to an IP address in the range of 207.139.221.1 to 207.139.221.254. In the second statement, the inside IP address will be port address translated in a single IP address, 207.139.221.128.

NOTE

When NAT is used, the PIX have a specified range of global IP addresses to perform translations with. Once the last available global IP is used, no other traffic from the inside interface will be permitted through until one of the translations times out. It is a good idea to use both a NAT statement followed by a PAT statement. This way, when all IP addresses are used in NAT, the PAT will then be used until a NAT address has timed out. However, keep in mind that not all protocols work with PAT.

Security Policy Configuration

Security policy configuration is probably one of the most important factors in establishing a secure network. The following sections present security strategies and best practice policies that you can implement to ensure the best possible security.

Designing & Planning…

The Importance of Security Policies

A security policy is the most important aspect in network security. As a manager, you must take many things into careful consideration when planning your policy. Tasks such as identifying the resources to protect, balancing security risks with cost/productivity, and the ability to log items are very important. Creating regular reports on usage will assist in identifying possible weaknesses in your security policy. If weaknesses have been overlooked, they can then be quickly remedied. PIX allows you to utilize a feature called a syslog. With the addition of third-party software such as Open Systems Private I, detailed analysis on the contents of a syslog can be achieved. The ability to generate reports on the types of traffic being permitted or denied by the PIX is crucial to a security policy. If you suspect your network is being attacked, the ability to look at logs over certain time periods is invaluable in proving your suspicions.

As a manager, proactive measures are always better then reactive measures. Instead of generating reports and looking for weaknesses after the fact, it may be beneficial to create a strict policy and then remove elements of that policy as necessary. For example, if a company has set up a Web server on the inside network and has used PIX to translate that inside address to a globally unique address on the outside, the server has now become fully exposed. To reduce the risk of the server being compromised, access lists can be used to limit the type of TCP/UDP traffic that will be permitted to reach the server through the PIX. By only allowing HTTP traffic to reach the Web server from the outside network and explicitly denying all other traffic, the risk of it being comprised has been greatly reduced. If the server becomes an FTP server as well as a Web server, the security policy can be modified to permit FTP as well as HTTP traffic to the server from the outside interface by adding another access list which permits FTP traffic. A security policy can take many forms depending on the needs of an organization, and careful planning is a necessity prior to implementing the PIX firewall.

Security Strategies

In order for the PIX to protect a network, managers and administrators must figure out what type of security strategy to employ. Do we deny everything that is not explicitly permitted, or do we allow everything and deny only certain things? The security policy is the most important element when designing a secure network. Without a policy, the necessary devices and configurations cannot be implemented properly. The security policy should aim for a balance between security and cost/productivity. It is impossible for a network to be totally secure, but the security policy should reflect the biggest potential security risks the company is willing to take. For example, by allowing users the ability to browse Web sites to perform research on the Internet, a company opens itself up to numerous security risks that can be exploited. Weigh this against restricting access to browsing Web sites in a company which relies heavily on that information to function. If the security policy is designed and implemented properly, these risks will be minimal. Once a security policy has been established, a firewall can then be used as a tool to implement that security policy. It will not function properly at protecting your network if the security policy is not carefully defined beforehand.

Designing & Planning...

The Cost of Security

One thing to remember when working on your security policy is how much will it cost? This can be the biggest factor in deciding which policy you choose for your company. Here are some questions to ask yourself when pondering the numbers of your future policy:

- Does the cost of protection outweigh the value of what you are trying to protect?
- Could the cost of a one-time security breach and restore of data be more than the cost of a new policy?
- What is the average amount of data you will lose on an annual basis due to security breaches?
- Does a new policy outweigh the cost of all breaches put together?

Deny Everything that Is Not Explicitly Permitted

One of the most common strategies used for security policies, is to permit only certain IP traffic, and deny the rest. For example, Company XYZ wishes to permit HTTP, FTP, and Telnet traffic for users. Managers and administrators agreed that as a company policy only these three types of traffic are to be permitted. All other traffic, such as Real Audio, ICQ, and MSN Messenger, will be blocked. Using Access Control Lists (ACLs) similar to those employed on routers, the PIX will allow an administrator to specify which type of IP traffic to permit or deny based on the destination address/network, source address/network, TCP port number, and UDP port number. This implementation makes configuring the security policy for the administrator very simple. The administrator only has to worry about entering statements to permit HTTP, FTP, and Telnet traffic, and then at the end of the ACL he/she will add an explicit *deny all* statement.

Allow Everything that Is Not Explicitly Denied

On a network where many different types of IP traffic will be permitted, it may be easier for an administrator to use a different approach for a security policy. This strategy is to allow all types of traffic and deny specific IP traffic. For example, if Company XYZ is not concerned as to what types of traffic the users are going to access, but managers and administrators have agreed that since they only have a T1 connection to their Internet service provider that services one thousand users, they do not wish their users to use RealPlayer because it is bandwidth intensive. In order to implement this strategy, only one ACL needs to be implemented on the PIX. This ACL will deny the TCP/UDP port that RealAudio uses while allowing everything else.

> **WARNING**
>
> This is not a recommended strategy. Be sure to carefully plan in advance what types of traffic will be permitted through the firewall. This example was shown as an alternative to the "Deny Everything that Is Not Explicitly Permitted" strategy, and in some network scenarios may be useful. By using this type of implementation in a situation where the ISP charges by the byte may cause quite a shock when the first bill from the ISP arrives. This is also less secure than the deny all, permit some approach.

Identify the Resources to Protect

In the context of a security policy, a resource can be defined as any network device susceptible to attack which can cost a company financially or otherwise. Examples of resources are Web servers, mail servers, database servers, and servers which contain sensitive information such as employee records. If any of these servers are attacked, functionality can be affected which then costs a company money.

It is important to carefully evaluate the assets a company wishes to protect. Are some resources more important that others, therefore requiring higher security? Is a mail server more important to the operation of the company than a print server?

Areas of weakness must also be identified prior to implementing the security policy. If a company uses an ISP for Internet access, a pool of modems for dial-in access, and remote users tunneling into the LAN via the Internet through VPN, each of these points of entry must be looked at as a potential source of security issues. Once weaknesses have been identified, a security policy can be shaped to protect a company's LAN from those various weaknesses. For example, using the previous scenario of an ISP, dial-in access, and remote VPN access, placement of the PIX will be critical to the overall security of the LAN. If the PIX are placed between the LAN and the ISP, how does this protect the LAN from unauthorized dial-in users? By adding an additional NIC to the PIX, a DMZ (covered later) can be used to isolate the dial-in and VPN users from the rest of the LAN. An example of protecting a resource is in a situation where a public Web site is hosted internally by the company. The Web server is definitely considered an asset and must be protected. Because of this, some decisions will need to be made as to how the PIX will secure the Web server. Since only one Web site is hosted by the company, and it uses a private IP address space, a static translation in which the Web server is assigned an internal IP address is then translated by the PIX firewall with a global IP address allowing outside users to gain access to it.

Depending on the security policy, having servers on an internal network which are then translated to global IP addresses may be too risky. An alternative is to implement a demilitarized zone in which the public resources will reside.

Demilitarized Zone

A DMZ (demilitarized zone) is a zone that is logically and physically separated from both the inside network and outside networks. A DMZ can be created by installing additional NICs to the PIX. By creating a DMZ, it allows administrators to remove devices that need to be accessed publicly from the inside and outside zones, and place them into their own zone. By implementing this type of configuration, it helps an administrator establish boundaries on the various zones of their network.

NOTE

Remember that only the PIX 515 and 520 models allow additional interfaces to be added. The PIX 501 is a SOHO class firewall and currently does not support additional interfaces.

Figure 3.5 illustrates how a DMZ is used to secure public resources.

Figure 3.5 Securing Public Resources with a DMZ

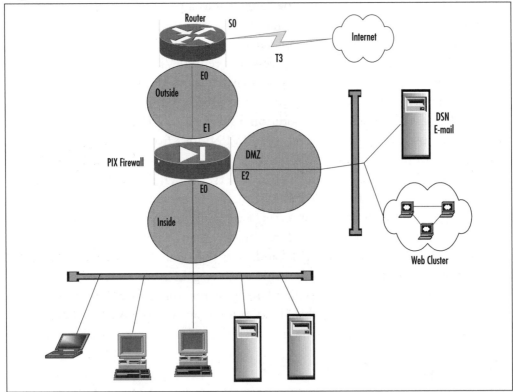

In this scenario, a DMZ has been used to separate the public servers from the inside and outside zones. This will allow administrators to control the flow of traffic destined for the DMZ zone. Since all traffic must pass through the outside interface in order to reach the DMZ, ACLs can be applied to the outside interface specifying the type of traffic permitted to reach the DMZ. For example, since the public servers are Web, e-mail, and DNS servers, HTTP, DNS, and SMTP traffic will be permitted to reach the DMZ. Everything else will be denied.

It is very difficult to secure a server. The Operating System (OS) and software applications can contain bugs and security flaws and need to be continuously updated. As soon as you install a server that offers a public service, there is always a risk the server can be compromised. Creating a new perimeter (DMZ) where the public servers are located, allows more control over the traffic permitted into the internal network. For example, once a DMZ has been set up and the public servers have been removed from the inside network, a rule can be created that denies all traffic destined for the inside network, therefore increasing security.

No matter what type of network a company has, careful planning is needed well in advance to implement a successful security policy. Planning in advance helps avoid making unnecessary changes in the way the PIX operates while in production. If a company continuously alters how resources are to be protected, availability of those resources will fluctuate. In a situation where a company relies heavily on that availability, careless planning may cost the company money.

Identify the Security Services to Implement

Depending on how your security policy is designed will reflect on how you design and implement your network. Various factors such as resources to protect, user authentication, traffic filtering, and confidentiality all come into play when designing the security policy.

Authentication and Authorization

Authentication is a mechanism which verifies a user is who they say they are, authorization is a mechanism which will determine what services a user can employ to access a host. An administrator must design a security policy which specifies the resources that need to be protected, what type of user will be able to access those resources, and which services a user will be able to employ to access those resources. Once a security policy has been outlined, an authentication server such as a RADIUS or TACACS+ server must be put in place in order to implement the security policy.

Once authentication and authorization have been enabled on the PIX, it will provide credential prompts on inbound and outbound connections for FTP, Telnet, and HTTP access. The actual decision about what users are permitted or denied use of, and the services used will be done by the authentication and authorization server. For more information on AAA, please refer to Chapter 6.

Access Control

In a network of any size, various administrators have control over different areas of the network. How does one administrator know where their responsibility stops and another administrator's responsibility begins? It is important to lay out the perimeters either inside a network, or surrounding a network. For example, if a network is connected to the Internet via a T1 leased line, does the administrator maintain the network on the other side of the T1? Probably not. This is where the ISP takes over. Perimeters must be established in order to help design a security policy. By defining perimeters, an administrator can secure resources under their control, which will also aid in the decision of where traffic should be filtered. ACLs are used to permit or deny traffic based on various criteria. These ACLs are used to assist in securing various resources by filtering the traffic that will get to them.

Confidentiality

Confidentiality is achieved by encrypting the information that travels along the network. If an individual used a network monitoring tool, there is a good chance they would be able to look at the data in the packets. An example of this is PAP. When using PPP (Point-to-Point Protocol) with PAP (Password Authentication Protocol), information is sent in clear text during the authentication phase. If a network monitor is used to capture these packets, the password used to authenticate the two parties would be readily available. To remedy this problem CHAP (Challenge Handshake Authentication Protocol) encrypts the negotiation phase. IPSec was developed to provide confidentiality, access control, authentication and integrity for data traversing a network. IPSec is a suite of protocols to assist in the encryption of data across a network. Commonly found in VPN tunnels, IPSec uses various encryption algorithms, keys, and certificates to validate information passed throughout a network. For more information on IPSec, refer to Chapter 5.

URL, ActiveX, and Java Filtering

ACLs are limited to certain criteria; destination address, source address, and ports are all taken into consideration for ACLs. ActiveX blocking occurs by the PIX commenting out HTML *<object>* commands on Web pages. As a technology, ActiveX creates many potential problems for clients—prompting workstations to fail, introducing network security problems, or causing servers to fail.

Java filtering is accomplished by denying applets downloaded to a client once they access a URL.

URLs themselves can also be filtered. Typically a company will introduce an AUP (Acceptable Usage Policy) that dictates usage of the Internet for their employees. This can be somewhat enforced by the PIX as well as third-party applications. The PIX can redirect URL requests to a server running a third-party application. This application will decide whether to permit or deny access to that URL and then pass responses back to the PIX.

> **NOTE**
>
> URL filtering can be accomplished with addition of a server running WebSENSE (www.websense.com). The configuration on the PIX will allow URLs to be forwarded to the WebSENSE server, which will then permit or deny the destination URL.

Implementing the Network Security Policy

Once a security policy has been created, it is now time to implement that security policy on the PIX. In order to completely implement a policy, other devices (such as AAA server and IPSec) will need to be used. This section will cover the commands to enable these features on the PIX, but the actual configuration on other devices will be discussed in later chapters.

Authentication Configuration in PIX

In order to configure Authentication on the PIX, it must first be enabled. To enable AAA authentication, use the *aaa-server* and *aaa* commands.

`aaa-server` *group_tag if_name* `host` *server_ip key* `timeout` *seconds*

In this case:

- **Group_tag** An alphanumeric string which is the name of the server group. Use the *group_tag* in the *aaa* command to associate *aaa authentication* and *aaa accounting* command statements to an AAA server.

- **If_name** The interface name on which the server resides.

- **Host** *server_ip* The IP address of the TACACS_ or RADIUS server.

- **Key** A case-sensitive, alphanumeric keyword of up to 127 characters. The key must be the same one used on the TACACS+ server.

- **Timeout** *seconds* A retransmit timer that specifies the duration in which the PIX can retry access four times to the AAA server before choosing the next AAA server.

- **Protocol** *auth_protocol* The type of AAA server, either tacacs+ or radius.

```
aaa authentication include | exclude authen_service inbound | outbound |
     if_name local_ip local_mask foreign_ip foreign_mask group_tag
```

In this case:

- **Accounting** Enables or disables accounting services with an authentication server.

- **Include** Creates a new rule with the specified service to include.

- **Exclude** Creates an exception to a previously stated rule by excluding the specified service from authentication, authorization, or accounting to the specified host.

- **Acctg_service** The account service. Accounting is provided for all services, or you can limit it to one or more services. Possible values are *any*, *ftp*, *http*, *telnet*, or *protocol port*.

- **Authentication** Enables or disables user authentication, prompts user for username and password, and verifies information with the authentication server.

- **Authen_service** The application with which a user accesses a network. Use *an*, *ftp*, *http*, or *telnet*.

- **Authorization** Enables or disables TACACS+ user authorization for services (PIX does not support RADIUS authorization).

- **Author_service** The services which require authorization. Use *any*, *ftp*, *http*, *telnet*, or *protocol port*.

- **Inbound** Authenticates or authorizes inbound connections.

- **Outbound** Authenticates or authorizes outbound connections.

- **If_name** The interface name from which users require authentication. Use *if_name* in combination with the *local_ip* address and the *foreign_ip* address to determine where access is sought and from whom.

- **Local_ip** The IP address of the host or network of hosts that you want to be authenticated or authorized. Set this to **0** for all hosts.

- **Local_mask** The network mask of *local_ip*. If IP is 0, use **0**. Use **255.255.255.255** for a host.

- **Foreign_ip** The IP address of the hosts you want to access the *local_ip* address. Use **0** for all hosts and **255.255.255.255** for a single host.

- **Foreign_mask** The network mask of *foreign_ip*. Always specify a specific mask value. Use **0** if the IP address is 0, use **255.255.255.255** for a single host

- **Group_tag** The group tag set with the *aaa-server* command.

```
pixfirewall>enable
pixfirewall#configure terminal
pixfirewall(config)#aaa-server AuthOutbound protocol tacacs+
pixfirewall(config)#aaa-server tacacs+ (inside) host 172.16.0.10
cisco  >timeout 20
pixfirewall(config)#aaa authentication include any outbound 0 0 0 0
>AuthOutbound
pixfirewall(config)#aaa authorization include any outbound 0 0 0 0
```

The first *aaa-server* statement specifies TACACS+ as the authentication protocol to use, and the second *aaa-server* statement specifies the server that is performing the authentication. The last two statements indicate that all traffic outbound will need to be authenticated and authorized.

Access Control Configuration in PIX

Access control can be achieved through the use of ACLs. Similar to those used on routers, ACLs can limit the traffic able to traverse the PIX based on several criteria, including source address, destination address, source TCP/UDP ports, and destination TCP/UDP ports.

In order to implement ACLs on PIX, the *access-list* and *access-group* commands are used:

```
access-list acl_name deny | permit protocol src_addr src_mask operator
    port dest_addr dest_mask operator port
```

- **Acl_name** The name of an access list.

- **Deny** Does not allow a packet to traverse the PIX. By default, PIX denies all inbound packets unless explicitly permitted.

- **Permit** Allows a packet to traverse the PIX.

- **Protocol** The name or number of an IP protocol. It can be one of the keywords, *icmp, ip, tcp,* or *udp.*

- **Src_addr** The address of the network or host from which the packet originated. To specify all networks or hosts, use the keyword *any*, which is equivalent to a source network and mask of 0.0.0.0 0.0.0.0. Use the *host* keyword to specify a single host.

- **Src_mask** The netmask bits to be applied to the *src_addr* if the source address is for a network mask. Do not apply if the source address is a host.

- **Dst_addr** The IP address of the network or host to which the packet is being sent. Like the *src_addr*, the keyword *any* can be applied for a destination and a netmask of 0.0.0.0 0.0.0.0, as well as the *host* abbreviation for a single host.

- **Dst_mask** The netmask bits to be applied to the *dst_addr* if the destination address is for a network mask. Do not apply if the destination address is a host.

- **Operator** A comparison that lets you specify a port or port range. Use without the operator and port to indicate all ports. Use *eq* and *port* to permit or deny access to just that single port. Use *it* to permit or deny access to all ports less than the port specified. Use *gt* and a *port permit*, to deny access to all ports greater than the port you specify. Use *neq* and a *port permit*, or deny access to every port except the ports you specify. Finally, use *range* and *port range* to permit or deny access to only those ports named in the range.

- **Port** Service or services you permit to be used while accessing *src_addr* or *dest_addr*. Specify services by port number or use the literal name.

- **Icmp_type** Permits or denies access to ICMP message types.

  `access-group` *acl_name* `in interface` *interface-name*

- **Acl_name** Name associated with an access list.

- **In interface** Filters inbound packets at the given interface.

- **Interface_name** Name of the network interface.

```
pixfirewall>enable
pixfirewall#configure terminal
pixfirewall(config)#access-list acl_out permit tcp any any eq http
pixfirewall(config)#access-list acl_out permit tcp any any eq ftp
pixfirewall(config)#access-list acl_out permit tcp any any eq ftp-data
pixfirewall(config)#access-list acl_out permit tcp any any eq telnet
pixfirewall(config)#access-list acl_out permit tcp any any eq smtp
pixfirewall(config)#access-list acl_out deny tcp any any
pixfirewall(config)#access-list acl_out deny udp any any
pixfirewall(config)#access-group acl_out in interface inside
```

The *access-list* statements for ACL *acl_out* will permit http, ftp, ftp-data, telnet, and smtp traffic. The last two statements of the *access-list* will explicitly deny all traffic.

The *access-group* statement will apply ACL *acl_out* to the inside interface.

Securing Resources

An example of securing resources would arise if Company XYZ has numerous consultants that need access to a resource on the internal LAN. Previously, the consultants have been using a RAS connection to dial in but have complained several times that the link is too slow for their work. To remedy this, administrators have decided to permit terminal access to the server via the Internet. The internal server is a Windows NT 4.0 Terminal Server and the consultants have been provided with the Terminal Server client. For security reasons, administrators have also requested the IP and subnet from which the consultants are going to be connecting.

This configuration example will explain the commands necessary to protect a server with a private IP address that is translated to a global IP address.

In order to create a translation for an internal IP address to a public IP address, use the *static* command.

```
static (internal_if_name, external_if_name) global_ip local_ip netmask
    network_mask max_conns em_limit norandomseq
```

To further explain:

- **Internal_if_name** The internal network interface name. The higher security level interface you are accessing.

- **External_if_name** The external network interface name. The lower security level interface you are accessing.

- **Global_ip** A global IP address. This address cannot be a Port Address Translation IP address.

- **Local_ip** The local IP address from the inside network.

- **Netmask** Specifies the network mask.

- **Network_mask** Pertains to both *global_ip* and *local_ip*. For host addresses, always use 255.255.255.255. For networks, use the appropriate class mask or subnet mask.

- **Max_cons** The maximum number of connections permitted through the static at the same time.

- **Em_limit** The embryonic connection limit. An embryonic connection is one that has started but not yet completed. Set this limit to prevent attack by a flood of embryonic connections.

- **Norandomseq** Specifies not to randomize the TCP/IP packet's sequence number. Only use this option if another inline firewall is also randomizing sequence numbers. Employing this feature opens a security hole in the PIX.

Once a translation for an internal IP to an external IP has been made, you must specify the type of traffic that will be permitted to access it. To do this, use the *access-list* command.

```
access-list acl_name deny | permit protocol src_addr src_mask operator
    port dest_addr dest_mask operator port
```

- **Acl_name** The name of an access list.

- **Deny** Does not allow a packet to traverse the PIX. By default, PIX denies all inbound packets unless explicitly permitted.

- **Permit** Allows a packet to traverse the PIX.

- **Protocol** The name or number of an IP protocol. It can be one of the keywords, *icmp, ip, tcp,* or *udp.*

- **Src_addr** The address of the network or host from which the packet originated. To specify all networks or hosts, use the keyword *any*, which is equivalent to a source network and mask of 0.0.0.0 0.0.0.0. Use the *host* keyword to specify a single host.

- **Src_mask** The netmask bits to be applied to the *src_addr* if the source address is for a network mask. Do not apply if the source address is a host.

- **Dst_addr** The IP address of the network or host to which the packet is being sent. Like the *src_addr*, the keyword *any* can be applied for a destination and netmask of 0.0.0.0 0.0.0.0, as well as the *host* abbreviation for a single host.

- **Dst_mask** The netmask bits to be applied to the *dst_addr* if the destination address is for a network mask. Do not apply if the destination address is a host.

- **Operator** A comparison that lets you specify a port or port range. Use without the operator and port to indicate all ports. Use *eq* and port to permit or deny access to just that single port. Use *it* to permit or deny access to all ports less than the port specified. Use *gt* and a port permit or deny access to all ports greater than the port you specify. Use *neq* and a port to permit or deny access to every port except the ports you specify. Finally, use *range* and port range to permit or deny access to only those ports named in the range.

- **Port** A service or services you permit to be used while accessing *src_addr* or *dest_addr*. Specify services by port number or use the literal name.

- **Icmp_type** Permits or denies access to ICMP message types.

```
pixfirewall>enable
pixfirewall#configure terminal
pixfirewall(config)#static (inside,outside) 207.139.221.10 172.16.0.32  >
    netmask 255.255.255.255
pixfirewall(config)#access-list acl_consult permit tcp 198.142.65.0 >
    255.255.255.0 host 207.139.221.10 eq 3389
pixfirewall(config)#access-list acl_consult permit tcp 64.182.95.0 >
    255.255.255.0 host 307.139.221.10 eq 3389
pixfirewall(config)#access-group acl_consult in interface outside
```

The first *static* statement will provide a translation for the inside server with an IP address of 172.16.0.32 to a global IP address of 207.139.221.10.

The *access-list* statements specify that the ACL *acl_consult* will only permit Microsoft Terminal Server client traffic originating from 198.142.65.0 and 64.182.95.0.

NOTE

TCP port 3389 is the corresponding port for Microsoft Terminal Server client. For a listing of valid TCP and UDP port numbers, refer to: www.isi.edu/in-notes/iana/assignments/port-numbers.

Finally, the *access-group* statement will apply the *acl_consult* Access Control List to the outside interface.

It is also important to note that implementing a security policy does not revolve around configuration of the PIX. In the previous example, PIX will not assist as a security measure if the information passed from terminal server to terminal server client is not encrypted. If information is passed as cleartext, a network monitoring tool could be used to capture packets which could then be analyzed by other individuals. Once a consultant has connected to the terminal server, how is the authentication handled? What permissions does that account have? Have various Windows NT security flaws been addressed with the latest service packs?

Confidentiality Configuration in PIX

This configuration example will explain the commands necessary to enable IPSec on the PIX. For more detailed information on IPSec refer to Chapter 5.

URL, ActiveX, and Java Filtering

To implement URL, ActiveX, and Java filtering, use the *filter* command:

```
filter activex port local_ip mask foreign_ip mask
```

In this case:

- **Activex** Blocks outbound ActiveX tags from outbound packets.

- **Port** Filters Activex only at the point which Web traffic is received on the PIX firewall.

- **Local_ip** The IP address of the highest security level interface from which access is sought. You can set this address to **0** to specify all hosts.

- **Mask** The network mask of *local_ip*. You can use **0** to specify all hosts.

- **Foreign_ip** The IP address of the lowest security level interface to which access is sought. You can use **0** to specify all hosts.

- **Foreign_mask** The network mask of *foreign_ip*. Always specify a mask value. You can use **0** to specify all hosts.

`filter java` port[-port] *local_ip mask foreign_ip mask*

To further explain:

- **Java** Blocks Java applets returning to the PIX firewall as a result of an outbound connection.

- **Port[-port]** Filters Java only on one or more ports on which Java applets may be received.

- **Local_ip** The IP address of the highest security level interface from which access is sought. You can set this address to **0** to specify all hosts.

- **Mask** The network mask of *local_ip*. You can use **0** to specify all hosts.

- **Foreign_ip** The IP address of the lowest security level interface to which access is sought. You can use **0** to specify all hosts.

- **Foreign_mask** The network mask of *foreign_ip*. Always specify a mask value. You can use **0** to specify all hosts.

`filter url http|except` *local_ip local_mask foreign_ip foreign_mask* [**allow**]

Here we see:

- **url** Filters URLs from data moving through the PIX firewall.

- **http** Filters URL only Filter HTTP URLs.

- **except** Filters URL only and creates an exception to a previous *filter* condition.

- **Local_ip** The IP address of the highest security level interface from which access is sought. You can set this address to **0** to specify all hosts.

- **Mask** The network mask of *local_ip*. You can use **0** to specify all hosts.

- **Foreign_ip** The IP address of the lowest security level interface to which access is sought. You can use **0** to specify all hosts.

- **Foreign_mask** The network mask of *foreign_ip*. Always specify a mask value. You can use **0** to specify all hosts.

- **Allow** Filters URLs only when the server is unavailable; lets outbound connections pass through the PIX firewall without filtering. If you omit this option and if the WebSENSE server goes offline, PIX firewall stops outbound port 80 traffic until the WebSENSE server is back online.

Once filtering has been enabled on the PIX, to successfully filter URLs, you must designate a WebSENSE server with the *url-server* command.

url-server (*if_name*) **host** *ip_address* **timeout** *seconds*

To further explain:

- **If_name** The network interface where the authentication server resides. Default is inside.

- **Host *ip_address*** The server that runs the WebSENSE URL filtering application.

- **Timeout *seconds*** The maximum idle time permitted before PIX switches to the next server you specify. Default is 5 seconds.

```
pixfirewall>enable
pixfirewall#configure terminal
pixfirewall(config)#filter url http 0 0 0 0
pixfirewall(config)#filter activex 80 0 0 0 0
pixfirewall(config)#filter java 80 0 0 0 0
pixfirewall(config)#url-server (inside) host 172.16.0.38 timeout 5
```

The *filter url* statement specifies that all http traffic passing through the PIX will be filtered. In addition, the *url-server* statement will specify which server is running WebSENSE to provide the actual filtering.

The *filter activex* and *filter java* statements specify that all http traffic will be filtered for ActiveX controls and Java applets.

PIX Configuration Examples

The following examples illustrate how a PIX firewall can be used in various real-world scenarios as well as the configuration needed on the PIX.

Protecting a Private Network

Due to security reasons, Company XYZ management has decided to restrict access to the Finance servers. Management has assigned the task of securing the Finance network from unauthorized access. Only individuals who are in the Finance departments network will have access to any of the Finance resources, any traffic originating from the Finance LAN will be permitted to any destination and all other departments will not be permitted to access the Finance LAN. Figure 3.6 illustrates how the LAN will be set up.

Figure 3.6 Secure Department to Department

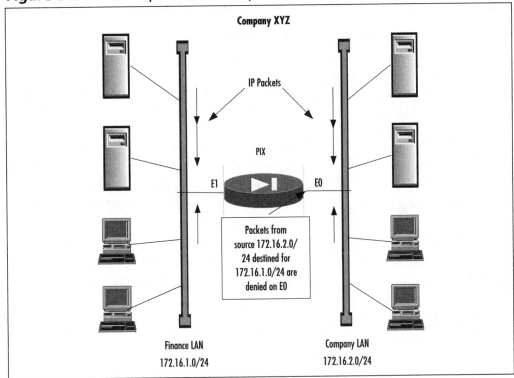

To begin, execute the following:

```
pixfirewall(config)#write terminal
nameif ethernet0 public security0
nameif ethernet1 finance security100
```

This assigns names and security values to each of the interfaces.

```
interface ethernet0 inside auto
interface ethernet1 outside auto
```

This sets each Ethernet interface to 10/100 auto negotiation.

```
ip address public 172.16.2.1 255.255.255.0
ip address finance 172.16.1.1 255.255.255.0
```

This assigns unique RFC 1918 IP addresses to each of the interfaces.

```
access-list deny tcp any 172.16.1.0 255.255.255.0
>eq any
```

```
access-list deny udp any 172.16.1.0 255.255.255.0
>eq any
```

This specifies that TCP and UDP traffic from any source will be denied if the destination is the network 172.16.1.0/24. By applying this access list inbound on the public interface (E0), traffic originating from the 172.16.2.0/24 subnet will be denied access to the Finance LAN.

This applies access-list acl_out to the public interface.

```
telnet 172.16.1.0 255.255.255.0 public
telnet 172.16.2.0 255.255.255.0 finance
```

This specifies that only clients from the 172.16.1.0/25 and 172.16.2.0/24 subnets will be able to Telnet to the PIX.

NOTE

This configuration, where two departments are separated for security reasons, can easily be achieved by using a router with Access Control Lists. The PIX is a very versatile device and can also be used to protect internal networks as shown in this example.

Protecting a Network Connected to the Internet

Company XYZ management has decided that in order to keep up with the rapidly evolving world of technology, Internet access is a necessity. Managers and administrators have decided that a T1 leased line will be sufficient for their users to access the Internet and an ISP has already been chosen. Since the LAN uses an IP address scheme employing the private 172.16.0.0 network, Network Address Translation, or Network Address Port Translation will be needed in order to translate internal IP addresses to global IP addresses. The ISP has also provided the company with eight public addresses which consist of 207.139.221.1 to 207.139.221.8. A Cisco Secure PIX 515 Firewall has been chosen to provide security for Company XYZ.

Management and administrators have established a security policy in which users will only be permitted to access HTTP, FTP, Telnet, e-mail, DNS, and News. Web site filtering will be performed by a third-party application called WebSENSE Web filtering software (www.websense.com). ActiveX controls will also be filtered due to the security problems associated with them. The ability to Telnet to the inside interface will be restricted to the administrator's workstation. Figure 3.7 shows how the network will be set up.

Figure 3.7 Two Interfaces

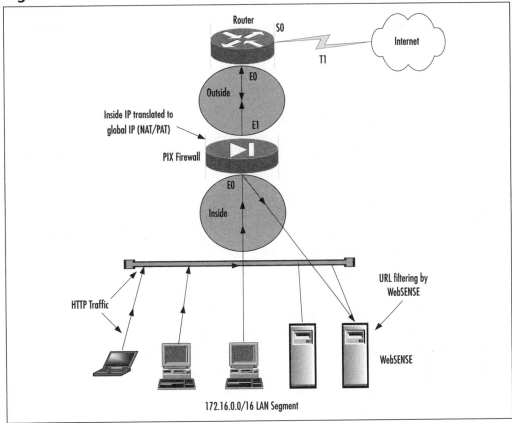

To begin, execute the following:

```
pixfirewall(config)#write terminal
interface ethernet0 inside auto
interface ethernet1 outside auto
```

This sets each Ethernet interface to 10/100 auto-negotiation ip address inside 172.16.0.1 255.255.0.0.

```
ip address outside 207.139.221.2 255.255.255.248
```

This assigns unique IP addresses to each of the interfaces.

```
route outside 0.0.0.0 0.0.0.0 207.139.221.1
```

This adds a static route for the outside interface.

```
nat (inside) 1 0.0.0.0 0.0.0.0
```

This allows any address on the inside interface to be NATed.

```
global (inside) 1 207.139.221.3
```

This sets up a global pool using the unique IP address 207.139.221.3 for NAPT.

```
filter url http 0 0 0 0
```

This filters any HTTP URL requests to any destination address.

```
filter activex 0 0 0 0
```

This filters any ActiveX controls in the HTML pages to any destination address.

```
url-server (inside) host 172.16.0.10 timeout 5
```

This specifies the server in which WebSENSE is running for URL filtering.

```
access-list acl_out permit tcp any any eq http
access-list acl_out permit tcp any any eq ftp
access-list acl_out permit tcp any any eq ftp-data
access-list acl_out permit tcp any any eq smtp
access-list acl_out permit tcp any any eq telnet
access-list acl_out permit tcp any any eq nntp
access-list acl_out permit tcp any any eq domain
access-list acl_out permit udp any any eq domain
access-list acl_out deny tcp any any
access-list acl_out deny udp any any
```

This specifies types of traffic that will be permitted through the PIX (inside, outside) with an explicit *deny all* statement to block any other traffic.

```
access-group acl_out in interface inside
```

Applies access-list acl_out to the inside interface.

```
telnet 172.16.0.50 255.255.255.255. inside
```

Only permits host 172.16.0.50 for Telnet sessions on the inside interface.

Protecting Server Access Using Authentication

The Finance department in Company XYZ is concerned about users in other departments accessing their Finance Web server. To alleviate this concern, IT has decided to limit access to the Finance server using the PIX firewall. A new server has been provided which will serve as the AAA server running Cisco Secure ACS. Figure 3.8 illustrates this scenario.

Figure 3.8 Protecting a Server Using AAA

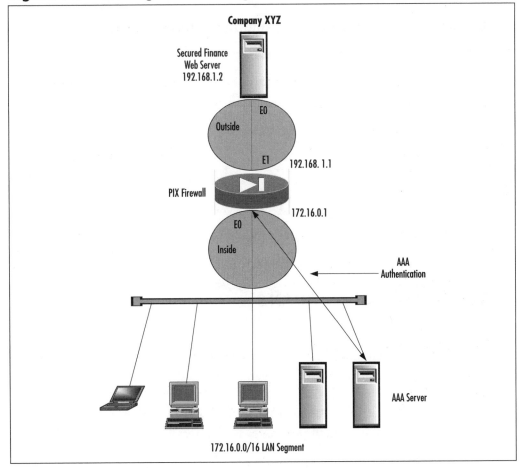

To begin, execute the following:

```
pixfirewall(config)#write terminal
interface ethernet0 inside auto
interface ethernet1 outside auto
```

This sets each Ethernet interface to 10/100 auto negotiation.

```
ip address outside 192.168.1.1 255.255.255.0
ip address inside 172.16.0.1 255.255.255.0
```

This assigns unique IP addresses to each of the interfaces.

```
nat (inside) 1 0 0
```

This allows any address on the inside interface to be NATed.

```
global (outside) 1 192.168.10-192.168.20 netmask >255.255.255.0
```

Sets up a global pool using address 192.168.10-192.168.20 for NAT.

```
global (outside) 1 192.168.10.21 netmask >255.255.255.255
```

Sets up a global pool using 192.168.10.21 for PAT. This is used when addresses from the NAT pool have been exhausted.

```
aaa-server AuthOutbound protocol tacacs+
```

Specifies TACACS+ for AAA protocol.

```
aaa-server AuthOutbound (inside) host 172.16.0.10 >cisco timeout 20
```

Specifies host 172.16.0.10 as the AAA server.

```
aaa authentication include any outbound host >192.168.1.2 0 0
```

Authorizes any traffic with a destination address of 192.168.1.2.

Protecting Public Servers Connected to the Internet

Company XYZ management has discussed the possibility of hosting their public servers internally. Currently the Web servers are hosted elsewhere by another company in which connectivity, security, and maintenance is provided by them. The security policy dictates that the risks of having public servers on the internal network are unacceptable. A new perimeter (DMZ) will need to be defined to secure the public servers.

Three Web servers, one e-mail server, and one DNS server will be placed in the DMZ.

A class C subnet has been assigned to the company by their ISP. To allow the company to utilize as many of the class C public addresses, PAT will be used instead of NAT.

Management would like to restrict the amount of traffic that traverses the PIX from their local LAN to the Internet. Administrators have decided that the only traffic permitted from the LAN will be HTTP, FTP, Telnet and DNS requests to their DNS server. Figure 3.9 illustrates how the LAN will be set up.

Figure 3.9 Three Interfaces without NAT

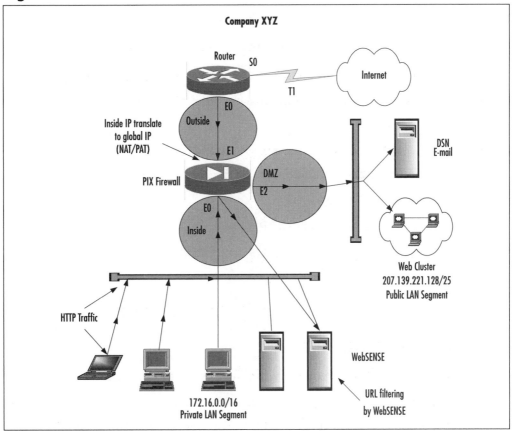

To begin, execute the following:

```
pixfirewall(config)#write terminal
nameif ethernet2 dmz security 50
```

Names and assigns security values to an ethernet2 interface.

```
interface ethernet0 inside auto
interface ethernet1 outside auto
interface ethernet2 dmz1 auto
```

Sets each Ethernet interface to 10/100 auto negotiation.

```
ip address inside 172.16.0.1 255.255.0.0
ip address outside 207.139.221.2 255.255.255.128
ip address dmz 207.139.221.129 255.255.255.128
```

Assigns unique IP addresses to each interface.

```
route (outside) 0.0.0.0 0.0.0.0 207.139.221.1
```

Sets static routes for the outside interface.

```
nat (inside) 1 0.0.0.0 0.0.0.0
```

Enables NAT for all traffic originating from the inside interface.

```
Nat (dmz) 0 0.0.0.0 0.0.0.0
```

Disables the NAT feature on the DMZ interface. Since hosts on the DMZ interface will be using global IP addresses, NAT translations are not necessary.

```
global (inside) 1 207.139.221.3
```

Sets up a global pool using global IP address 207.139.221.3 for NAPT.

```
static (dmz,outside) 207.139.221.129 207.139.221.129 >netmask 255.255.255.128
```

Creates a static translation for:

```
static (dmz,outside) 207.139.221.130 207.139.221.130 >netmask 255.255.255.128
static (dmz,outside) 207.139.221.131 207.139.221.131 >netmask 255.255.255.128
filter url http 0 0 0 0
```

Filters any HTTP URL requests with any destination address.

```
filter activex 0 0 0 0
```

Filters any ActiveX controls in HTML pages to any destination address.

```
url-server (inside) host 172.16.0.10 timeout 5
```

Specifies the server in which WebSENSE is running for URL filtering.

```
access-list acl_out permit tcp any any eq http
access-list acl_out permit tcp any any eq ftp
access-list acl_out permit tcp any any eq ftp-data
access-list acl_out permit tcp any any eq smtp
access-list acl_out permit tcp any any eq telnet
access-list acl_out permit tcp any any eq domain
```

```
access-list acl_out permit udp any any eq domain
access-list acl_out deny tcp any any
access-list acl_out deny udp any any
```

Specifies types of traffic that will be permitted through the PIX (inside, outside) with an explicit *deny all* statement to block any other traffic.

```
access-list dmz_in permit tcp any 207.139.221.128
>255.255.255.128 eq http
access-list dmz_in permit tcp any 207.139.221.128
>255.255.255.128 eq domain
access-list dmz_in permit udp any 207.139.221.128
>255.255.255.128 eq domain
access-list dmz_in permit tcp any 207.139.221.128
>255.255.255.128 eq smtp
access-list dmz_in permit tcp any 207.139.221.128
>255.255.255.128 eq pop3
```

Specifies types of traffic that will be permitted through the PIX (outside, dmz). All traffic not explicitly permitted will be denied.

```
access-group acl_out in interface inside
```

Applies *access-list acl_out* to the inside interface.

```
access-group dmz_in in interface outside
```

Applies *access-list acl_in* to the DMZ interface.

```
telnet 172.16.0.0 255.255.0.0 inside
```

Permits Telnet access on the inside interface from any host on the 172.16.0.0/16 network.

Figure 3.10 illustrates an example of a DMZ which uses private IP addresses, therefore requiring NAT.

To continue with the configuration:

```
pixfirewall(config)#write terminal
nameif ethernet2 dmz security 50
```

Names and assigns security values to an ethernet2 interface.

```
interface ethernet0 inside auto
interface ethernet1 outside auto
interface ethernet2 dmz1 auto
```

Figure 3.10 Three Interfaces with NAT

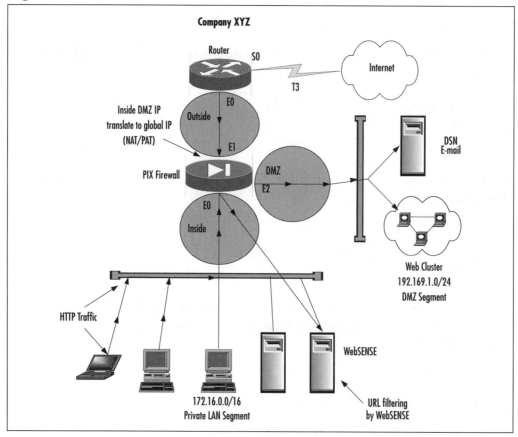

Sets each Ethernet interface to 10/100 auto negotiation.

```
ip address inside 172.16.0.1 255.255.0.0
ip address outside 207.139.221.2 255.255.255.0
ip address dmz 192.168.1.1 255.255.255.0
```

Assigns unique IP addresses to each interface.

```
route 0.0.0.0 0.0.0.0 207.139.221.1
```

Sets the static route for the outside interface.

```
nat (inside) 1 172.16.0.0 255.255.0.0
```

Enables NAT for all traffic originating from the inside interface.

```
nat (dmz) 1 0.0.0.0 0.0.0.0
```

Enables NAT for all traffic originating from the DMZ interface.

```
global (inside) 1 207.139.221.3
```

Sets up a global pool using the global IP address 207.139.221.3 for PAT.

```
global (dmz) 1 192.168.1.10-192.168.1.30
```

Sets up a global pool using IP addresses 192.168.1.10 thru 192.168.1.30 for DMZ.

```
static (dmz,outside) 207.139.221.129 192.168.1.2 >netmask 255.255.255.0
```

Creates a static translation for DMZ host 192.168.1.2 to global unique IP 207.139.221.129.

```
static (dmz,outside) 207.139.221.130 192.168.1.3 >netmask 255.255.255.0
```

Creates a static translation for DMZ host 192.168.1.3 to global unique IP 207.139.221.130.

```
static (dmz,outside) 207.139.221.131 192.168.1.4 >netmask 255.255.255.0
```

Creates a static translation for DMZ host 192.168.1.4 to global unique IP 207.139.221.131.

```
filter url http 0 0 0 0
```

Filters any HTTP URL requests with any destination address.

```
filter activex 0 0 0 0
```

Filters any ActiveX controls in HTML pages to any destination address.

```
url-server (inside) host 172.16.0.10 timeout 5
```

Specifies the server in which WebSENSE is running for URL filtering.

```
access-list acl_out permit tcp any any eq http
access-list acl_out permit tcp any any eq ftp
access-list acl_out permit tcp any any eq ftp-data
access-list acl_out permit tcp any any eq smtp
access-list acl_out permit tcp any any eq telnet
access-list acl_out permit tcp any any eq domain
access-list acl_out permit udp any any eq domain
access-list acl_out deny tcp any any
access-list acl_out deny udp any any
```

Specifies types of traffic that will be permitted through the PIX (inside, outside) with an explicit *deny all* statement to block any other traffic.

```
access-list dmz_in permit tcp any 207.139.221.129
>255.255.255.255 eq http
access-list dmz_in permit tcp any 207.139.221.130
>255.255.255.255 eq domain
access-list dmz_in permit udp any 207.139.221.130
>255.255.255.128 eq domain
access-list dmz_in permit tcp any 207.139.221.131
>255.255.255.131 eq smtp
```

Specifies types of traffic that will be permitted through the PIX (outside, dmz). All traffic not explicitly permitted will be denied.

```
access-group acl_out in interface inside
```

Applies *access-list acl_out* to the inside interface.

```
access-group dmz_in in interface outside
```

Applies *access-list acl_dmz* to the outside interface.

```
telnet 172.16.0.0 255.255.0.0 inside
```

Securing and Maintaining the PIX

Part of creating a security policy is not only protecting the network resources but also protecting the PIX itself. PIX provides several mechanisms to assist an administrator in limiting access to the PIX and reporting various items such as security violations.

System Journaling

As with most Cisco products, the system message logging feature can save messages in a buffer or redirect the messages to other devices such as a system logging server to be analyzed or archived. This feature allows administrators to reference these logs in case of security violations.

System journaling is an often overlooked security mechanism. Logging is essential to the security of the network. It can be used to detect security violations, and help determine the type of attack. If logging is done in real time, it can be used to detect an ongoing intrusion (more on this is covered in Chapter 13).

PIX also has the added feature that if for some reason or another, the syslog server is no longer available, the PIX will stop all traffic.

UNIX servers, by default, provide a syslog server. On Windows NT/2000 servers, a syslog server must be downloaded. Cisco provides a syslog server on their Web site (www.cisco.com).

By default, system log messages are sent to the console and Telnet sessions. In order to redirect logging messages to a syslog server use the *logging* command. Some of the variables used with the *logging* command are as follows:

- **On** Starts sending syslog messages to all output locations. Stop all logging with the *no logging on* command.

- **Buffered** Sends syslog messages to an internal buffer which can be viewed with the *show logging* command. To clear the buffer, use the *clear logging* command.

- **Console** Specifies that syslog messages appear on the console. You can limit which type of messages appear by using the *level* option.

- **Host** Specifies a syslog server that will receive the messages sent from the PIX. You may use multiple *logging host* commands to specify multiple syslog servers.

- **In_if_name** Interface in which the syslog server resides.

- **Ip_address** The IP address of syslog server.

- **Protocol** Protocol in which the syslog message is sent—either tcp or udp. PIX will only send TCP messages to the PIX syslog server unless otherwise specified. You cannot send both protocols to the same syslog server. Use multiple syslog servers in order to log both UDP and TCP traffic.

- **Level** Specifies the syslog message level as a number or string. See Table 3.2 for the different syslog levels.

- **Port** Port in which the PIX sends either UDP or TCP syslog messages. Default for UDP is port 514 and port 1470 for TCP.

- **Timestamp** Specifies that the syslog messages sent to the syslog server should have a time stamp value on each message.

Table 3.3 lists the different SNMP trap levels.

Table 3.3 SNMP Trap Levels

Level	Type	Description
0	Emergencies	System unusable messages
1	Alerts	Take immediate action
2	Critical	Critical condition
3	Errors	Error messages
4	Warnings	Warning message
5	Notifications	Normal but significant condition
6	Informational	Information message
7	Debugging	Debug messages, log FTP commands, and WWW URLs

An example of sending warnings to a syslog server is:

```
pixfirewall>enable
pixfirewall#configure terminal
pixfirewall(config)#logging trap 4
pixfurewall(config)#logging host inside 172.16.0.38 tcp
```

NOTE

Syslog is *not* a secure protocol. The syslog server should be secured and network access to the syslog server should be restricted.

Securing the PIX

Since the PIX is a security device, limiting access to the PIX to only those who need it is extremely important. What would happen if individuals where able to freely Telnet to the PIX from the inside network? Limiting access to the PIX can be achieved by using the *telnet* command. Telnet is an insecure protocol. Everything that is typed on a telnet session, including passwords, is sent in cleartext. Individuals using a network monitoring tool can then capture the packets and discover the password to log in and enable a password if issued. If remote management of the PIX is necessary, the network communication should be secured.

It is also a good idea to limit the idle-time of a Telnet session and log any connections to the PIX through Telnet. When possible, use a RADIUS, Kerberos or TACACS+ server to authenticate connections on the console or vty (telnet) ports.

```
telnet ip_address netmask interface_name
```

- **Ip_address** An IP address of a host or network that can access the PIX Telnet console. If an interface name is not specified, the address is assumed to be on the internal interface. PIX automatically verifies the IP address against the IP addresses specified by the *ip address* commands to ensure that the address you specify is on an internal interface.

- **Netmask** Bit mask of *ip_address*. To limit access to a single IP address, use 255.255.255.255 for the subnet mask.

- **Interface_name** The name of the interface to apply the security to.

- **Timeout** The number of minutes that a Telnet session can be idle before being disconnected by the PIX. Default is 5 minutes.

NOTE

When permitting Telnet access to an interface, be as specific as possible. If an administrative terminal uses a static IP address, only permit that IP address for Telnet access.

The following is an example of limiting Telnet access to the PIX to one host on the inside network.

```
pixfirewall>enable
pixfirewall#configure terminal
pixfirewall(config)#telnet 172.16.0.50 255.255.255.255 inside
pixfurewall(config)#telnet timeout 5
```

If features are not used on the PIX, they should then be disabled. If SNMP is not used, deactivate it. If it is used, change the default communities and limit access to the management station only.

Finally, a security measure that is often forgotten is to keep the PIX is a secure area. By locking it away in a server room or wiring closet, only authorized individuals will be able to physically reach the PIX. How would your security policy be enforced in an individual was able to walk up to the PIX and pull out the power cable?

Take the extra time to secure the PIX according to the security policy. The PIX is typically the device that enforces the majority of a company's security policy. If the PIX itself is not secured, and an unauthorized individual gains access to it, the security of the network will be compromised.

Summary

The Cisco PIX Firewall is a very versatile security device. From the PIX 501 SOHO model to the Enterprise class PIX 535 model, the PIX can fulfill the security needs of any size network.

In this chapter, we covered numerous topics including the design of a security policy and then implementing that security policy on the PIX. It is extremely important to thoroughly design a policy before implementing it. By identifying the resources to protect, the services you wish to allow (HTTP, FTP, and so on), and requiring users to be authenticated in order to access a resource ahead of time will permit an organization to implement a security policy in a quick and efficient manner. By creating a security policy on the fly, your resources can be compromised and data can be corrupted. Instead of being reactive to attacks and other security holes, creating a detailed security policy beforehand is a proactive, and superior, way of protecting your network.

Remember the key security features of the PIX, such as URL filtering, ActiveX and Java filtering, Access Control Lists, DMZs, AAA authentication and authorization, DNS Guard, IP Frag Guard, Mail Guard, Flood Defender, Flood Guard, IPSec, Stateful filtering, securing access to the PIX, and syslog. These features will aid you in creating and implementing your security policy. NAT and NAPT should not be relied on as a security measure. Using a syslog server will allow you to archive all of the traffic that passes through your firewall. By using syslog, you will always have a record of anyone attempting to attack your firewall from the inside or outside.

Solutions Fast Track

Overview of the Security Features

- ☑ PIX firewalls provide security technology ranging from stateful inspection to IPSec and L2TP/PPTP-based VPN. Also provides content filtering capability.

- ☑ Working with Cisco Intrusion Detection System can help secure the network environment.

- ☑ The PIX firewalls also contain the adaptive security algorithm. This maintains the secure perimeters between the networks controlled by the firewall.

Initial Configuration

☑ Easy setup with the use of Cisco PIX Device Manager.

☑ The same command-line interface spans all PIX firewalls.

☑ The PIX 501 is a basic Plug-and-Play for your SOHO network.

The Command-Line Interface

☑ The command-line interface (CLI) used on the PIX is very similar to that used on routers.

☑ Three modes exist in order to perform configuration and troubleshooting steps. These modes are unprivileged, privileged, and configuration mode.

Configuring NAT and PAT

☑ The information that PIX stores in the translation table includes the inside IP address and a globally unique IP address assigned by the Network Address Translation (NAT) or Network Address Port Translation (PAT).

☑ In order to allow traffic to flow from a higher level security interface to a lower level security interface (inside, outside), you must use the *nat* and *global* commands.

☑ NAT is a feature that dynamically maps IP addresses originating from the higher security level interface into IP addresses on the same subnet as the lower level security interface.

Security Policy Configuration

☑ The security policy is the most important element when designing a secure network.

☑ Remember, the PIX will deny everything that is not explicitly permitted.

☑ Planning in advance will help avoid making unnecessary changes in the way the PIX operates while in production.

☑ Once authentication and authorization have been enabled on the PIX, it will provide credential prompts on inbound and outbound connections for FTP, Telnet, and HTTP access.

☑ Perimeters must be established in order to help with designing a security policy.

☑ Java filtering is accomplished by denying applets downloaded to a client once they access a URL.

☑ In order to create a translation for an internal IP address to a public IP address, use the *static* command.

☑ Access control can be achieved through the use of Access Control Lists (ACLs).

PIX Configuration Examples

☑ **pixfirewall(config)#write terminal** shows configuration.

☑ **global (outside) 1 192.168.10.21 netmask 255.255.255.255** sets up a global pool using 192.168.10.21 for NAPT. This is used when addresses from the NAT pool have been exhausted.

☑ **access-list deny udp any 172.16.1.0 255.255.255.0 eq any** specifies that TCP and UDP traffic from any source will be denied if the destination is the network 172.16.1.0/24.

Securing and Maintaining the PIX

☑ Limit the access of the PIX to only those people who really need it. This will help the security of the network.

☑ Remember to give your PIX a unique name for the Interface Name.

☑ Be sure to put your Routers, Hubs, and PIXs in a secure location that is locked. This will stop any threats that are physical in nature, and will help secure your network.

Frequently Asked Questions

The following Frequently Asked Questions, answered by the authors of this book, are designed to both measure your understanding of the concepts presented in this chapter and to assist you with real-life implementation of these concepts. To have your questions about this chapter answered by the author, browse to **www.syngress.com/solutions** and click on the **"Ask the Author"** form.

Q: I have two inside networks. I would only like one of them to be able to access the Internet (outside network). How would I accomplish this?

A: Instead of using the NAT (inside) *1 0 0* statement which specifies all inside traffic, use the NAT (inside) 1 *xxx.xxx.xxx.xx yyy.yyy.yyy.yyy* statement where *x* is the source network you wish to translate, and *y* is the source network subnet mask.

Q: I am setting up my outbound Access Control Lists to specify which traffic I will permit users to use. How do I know which TCP or UDP port a particular application uses?

A: Usually the application vendor will have the TCP or UDP port(s) listed in the documentation, or available on their Web site. For a comprehensive list of Well Known Ports, Registered Ports, and Dynamic/Private ports, visit: www.isi.edu/in-notes/iana/assignments/port-numbers.

Q: My organization uses Microsoft Exchange server for our mail. How would I allow our Exchange server to receive external mail if the server is located on the inside network and a PIX firewall is in place?

A: Since the server is physically located on the inside network, a static translation will need to be created to assign the Exchange server a global IP address. Once the translation has been created, use ACLs to limit the type of traffic able to reach the server. In SMTP, for example, the Exchange server's internal IP address is 172.16.0.16, and the globally assigned IP address will be 207.139.221.40:

```
pixfirewall(config)#static (inside,outside) 207.139.221.40 172.16.0.16
    >netmask 255.255.255.255
pixfirewall(config)#access-list acl_mailin permit tcp any host
    207.139.221.40 eq smtp
pixfirewall(config)#access-group acl_mailin in interface outside
```

Q: If you were going to buy one new PIX for your office, but wanted to make sure you could expand or upgrade it sometime down the road. Which model would you chose?

A: PIX model 515 since the 501 and 506 are not upgradeable.

Q: While trying to connect to the PIX through the COM port, my connections keeps timing out. What are some settings to review on your terminal setup?

A: 9600 baud, 8 data bits, No parity, 1 stop bit, and Hardware flow control

Q: If I was looking to put a new server on my network but did not want to add it to the hidden network behind my PIX, where would be a good place to add it?

A: Adding it to the DMZ off of the PIX will put the new server on a different part of your network.

Q: Searching for a network interface that someone else has added to the network can be a problem. If you do not know the name of the interface you are looking for and would like to see a list of interface names on your PIX, what command would you use?

A: Type **show nameif** at the command prompt.

Q: What is the most important thing to remember when trying to sell your security plan to management?

A: Does the cost of the plan outweigh the cost of the data or network being protected?

## Chapter 4

Traffic Filtering in the Cisco Internetwork Operating System

Solutions in this chapter:

- Access Lists
- Lock-and-key Access Lists
- Reflexive Access Lists
- Context-based Access Control
- Configuring Port to Application Mapping

- ☑ Summary
- ☑ Solutions Fast Track
- ☑ Frequently Asked Questions

Introduction

As the use of technology continues to grow in business, the volume of data that companies need to exchange is increasing to match that growth. To facilitate the exchange of this data, a connection must be established between the networks of these companies. Without some form of security, each network will have complete access to the other with no way of controlling what data someone will be able to see.

One of the easiest ways to protect your network from unauthorized access is to filter the traffic at the point where it enters your network. By catching all traffic before it can be forwarded into your network, you can minimize the chance someone will be able to sidestep your security measures and find an alternate path to the data they are trying to access.

In many cases, the device used to connect two or more networks together is a router. To allow traffic filtering at the connection point to other networks, we need some method of filtering traffic on the router itself. This chapter will cover the different traffic filtering mechanisms available in a Cisco router.

In the simplest case, traffic filtering can consist of a list that permits or denies traffic based on the source or destination IP address. But very often, basic traffic filtering is not sufficient to provide adequate security in a network. Today, modern security products provide more control over the network traffic entering and exiting the network. To achieve that, the traffic must be inspected and the state of the connection must be kept. These advanced features require the router or firewall to understand the internal workings of the protocol it is trying to secure.

Access Lists

A very important step to security is the capability to control the flow of data within a network. A way to accomplish this is to utilize one of the many features of the Cisco Internetwork Operating System (IOS) known as an access list, or Access Control List (ACL). The function of an access list depends on the context in which it is used. For instance, access lists can:

- Control access to networks attached to a router or define a particular type of traffic allowed to pass to and from a network.

- Limit the contents of routing updates advertised by various routing protocols,

- Secure the router itself by limiting access to services such as SNMP and Telnet.

- Define "interesting traffic" for Dial on Demand routing. Interesting traffic defines which packets allow the dial connection to occur.

- Define queuing features by determining what packets are given priority over others.

An access list is comprised of a sequential series of filters defined globally on the router. Think of each filter as a statement you enter into the router. Each of these filters performs a comparison or match and permits or denies a packet across an interface. The decision to permit or deny is determined by the information contained inside the packets. This process is commonly referred to as *packet filtering*. The criteria that must be met for action to be taken can be based on only a source address or a source and destination address, a protocol type, a specific port or service type, or other type of information. This information is typically contained within the Layer 3 and Layer 4 headers.

Once an access list is defined, it will need to be applied on the interface where access control is required. It was previously stated that we define access lists globally on the router. The key here is to remember that after defining the access list, it must be applied on the interface or your access list will have no effect. Also remember that traffic moves both in and out of the interface of the router. So, access lists can be applied either in the inbound or in the outbound direction on a specific interface. One method commonly used to avoid confusion here is to assume you are inside the router. Simply ask yourself if you want to apply the access list statements as traffic comes in (inbound) or as traffic moves out (outbound). You can have one access list, per protocol, per interface, per direction. So, for example, it is possible to have one access list for outbound IP traffic and one access list for inbound IP traffic applied to the same interface. See Figure 4.1 for an illustration of this concept.

Figure 4.1 Inbound and Outbound Traffic on an Interface

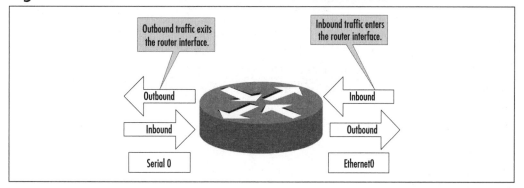

Access List Operation

When a packet enters a router, the destination address in the packet is compared to the routing table, and the exit interface for the packet is determined. When using access lists, before the packet can enter or exit the router there is a "stack" of filters applied to the interface in which the packet must pass through. The stack we are referring to here would be the commands you entered on your router with the *access-list* global configuration command. Think of each line of your access list as a filter. The following example represents a user-defined access list with three filters. A complete description on the access list syntax is given in a later section.

```
access-list 1 permit 192.168.10.15
access-list 1 permit 192.168.10.16
access-list 1 deny 192.168.10.17
```

Assuming this list is applied in the outbound direction, the packet exiting the router will be tested against each condition until a match occurs. If no match occurs on the first line, the packet moves to the second line and the matching process happens again. When a match is established, a permit or deny action, which is specified on each filter statements, will be executed. What happens if the packet ends up at the end of the stack, or last line of our access list, and a match has never occurred? There is an implicit *deny all* command at the end of every access list. So any packet that passes through an access list with no match is automatically dropped. You will not see this line on any access list you build, just think of it as a default line that exists at the end of your access list. In Figure 4.2, we can see the direction of a packet as it flows through the access list.

In some cases, you may want to enter the last line of the access list as a *permit any* statement, as shown next:

```
access-list 1 deny 192.168.10.15
access-list 1 deny 192.168.10.16
access-list 1 permit any
```

With this line in place all packets that don't match the first two lines will be permitted by the third line and will never reach the implicit *deny all*.

Figure 4.2 Flowchart of Packets Matching an Access List

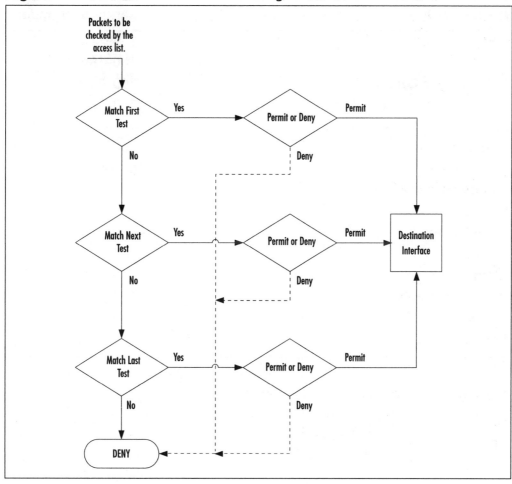

Types of Access Lists

There are several types of access lists available on Cisco routers, which can be used to filter just about any protocol that can run on the router. Access lists are usually referred to by a number, which uniquely identifies a particular list as well as specifying what type of access list it is. For example, when creating a standard IP access list, you must use any number between 1 and 99. If you use the number 100 for an access list, it will have to be an extended IP access list, which uses a different format. Table 4.1 shows the various number ranges of access lists, and what type of traffic they are meant to filter.

Table 4.1 Access List Numbers

Access List Type	Range of Numbers
Standard IP	1–99
Extended IP	100–199
Ethernet Type Code	200–299
DECnet and Extended DECnet	300–399
XNS	400–499
Extended XNS	500–599
AppleTalk	600–699
48-bit Ethernet Address	700–799
Standard IPX	800–899
Extended IPX	900–900
IPX SAP	1000–1099
Extended 48-bit Ethernet Address	1100–1199
NLSP route summary	1200–1299
Standard IP (IOS 12.1 number ranges were extended)	1300–1999
Extended IP (IOS 12.1 number ranges were extended)	2000–2699

Access lists may also be identified by name instead of a number. Named access lists are beneficial to the administrator when dealing with a large number of access lists for ease of identification and also if more than 99 standard or extended access lists are needed. Another advantage of a named access list over a numbered access list is in modifying the access list. With numbered access lists, the entire access list and all its statements are considered one entity. To delete or change a statement, you will have to delete the entire numbered access list and reenter the statements you want to keep. Named access lists allow you to delete one statement within the access list, although you are still limited to only adding new entries at the bottom of the list.

Although a Cisco router is designed to operate with multiple protocols, this chapter will only cover access lists as they relate to the IP protocol. We will discuss, in detail, the two basic types of IP access lists, standard and extended. In addition, we will cover more advanced filtering techniques that employ the use of access lists, such as lock-and-key access lists, reflexive access lists, and Context-based Access Control (CBAC).

Standard IP Access Lists

The standard IP access list is the most basic IP access list that can be created because it only looks at the source address and ignores all other information in the IP header. This allows you to easily permit or deny access to your entire network for a list of addresses and/or subnets.

As with all access lists, you must define the list in the global configuration mode of the router. In the following example any field represented by {} is mandatory for the access list. Any field represented by [] is optional. The syntax of the standard IP access list is:

```
access-list list-number {permit | deny} source-address [wildcard-mask][log]
```

Table 4.2 breaks down each section of this command and describes its function.

Table 4.2 Standard IP Access List Configuration

Command	Description
access-list list number	Defines the number of the access list. The standard access list numbers range from 1–99.
Permit	If conditions are met, traffic will be allowed.
Deny	If conditions are met, traffic will be denied.
source-address	Identifies the host or network from which the packet is being sent. The source can be specified by an IP address or by using the keyword *any*.
Wildcard-mask	By default, this field will be 0.0.0.0. This defines the number of wildcard bits assigned to the source address. The default value (0.0.0.0) specifies a single IP address. Wildcard masks will be explained further in the following section.
Log	This keyword results in the logging of packets that match the *permit* or *deny* statement.

Notice that a hyphen is required between the words *access* and *list*. Next is the list number. Since we are referencing a standard IP access list, the numbers would range from 1 to 99. The access list number actually serves a dual purpose here. Typically, you will find several access lists on one router, therefore the router must have a way to distinguish one access list from another. The number performs this purpose along with tying the lines of an access list together. The number also tells the router the type of access list it is.

The keywords *permit* or *deny* indicate the action to be performed if a match occurs. For example the keyword *permit* would allow the packet to be forwarded by the interface. The keyword *deny* will drop the packet if a match is found. If a packet is dropped, an ICMP error message of destination unreachable will be sent back to the source.

Source Address and Wildcard Mask

When using a standard IP access list, the source address must always be specified. The source address can refer to the address of a host, a group of hosts, or an entire subnet. The scope of the source address is specified by the wildcard mask.

The wildcard mask is typically one of the most misunderstood topics when dealing with access lists. When using the wildcard mask, think of the reverse manner in which a subnet mask works. The job of a subnet mask is to specify how many bits of an IP address refer to the subnet portion. Remember, a binary 1 in the subnet mask indicates the corresponding bit is part of the subnet range and a binary 0 in the subnet mask indicates the corresponding bit is part of the host portion. For example, take the following IP address and subnet mask:

```
Source address   - 10101100.00010000.10000010.01000110  =  172.16.130.77
Subnet Mask      - 11111111.11111111.11111111.00000000  =  255.255.255.0
Subnet           - 10101100.00010000.10000010.00000000  =  172.16.130.0
```

In the first three octets of the subnet mask, we have set all the bits to one (decimal 255 = 11111111 in binary). This tells us that all of the bits in the first three octets are now part of the subnet field, while the last eight bits are used for the host addresses.

Now, let's move from the subnet mask to the wildcard mask. When using a wildcard mask a zero is used for each bit that should be matched and a one is used when the bit position doesn't need to be matched. The easiest way to create a wildcard mask is to first decide what subnet mask applies to the traffic you want to filter, and then use it to create the wildcard mask. To get a wildcard mask for a subnet mask, all you need to do is change all the 1s to 0s, and the 0s to 1s. You will see this in the following example. Assume that we want to deny the IP entire subnet 172.16.130.0 with a mask of 255.255.255.0.

```
Source address   - 10101100.00010000.10000010.00000000 = 172.16.130.0
Subnet Mask      - 11111111.11111111.11111111.00000000 = 255.255.255.0
Wildcard Mask    - 00000000.00000000.00000000.11111111 = 0.0.0.255
```

So, the following access list line will deny any traffic that has a source address in the range 172.16.130.0 – 172.16.130.255, because the wildcard mask tells us that the first three octets (24 bits) must match, but the last octet (8 bits) can be anything.

```
Router(config)#access-list 5 deny 172.16.130.0 0.0.0.255
```

As a more complicated example, let's say we want to only deny the IP address range of 172.16.130.32 through 172.16.130.63. The mask associated with this range is 255.255.255.224, so we would write this in binary and derive the wild-card mask as shown next.

```
Source address  - 10101100.00010000.10000010.00100000 = 172.16.130.32
Subnet Mask     - 11111111.11111111.11111111.11100000 = 255.255.255.224
Wildcard Mask   - 00000000.00000000.00000000.00011111 = 0.0.0.31
```

So, to create an access list that allowed all traffic except those packets that come from the range 172.16.130.32 to 172.16.130.63, we would type the following:

```
Router(config)#access-list 8 deny 172.16.130.32 0.0.0.31
Router(config)#access-list 8 permit 0.0.0.0 255.255.255.255
```

Keywords *any* and *host*

In an effort to make access lists a little easier to deal with, the keywords *any* and *host* were created. For example, if you want to create a statement that allowed all traffic through, you would have to create the following command:

```
Router(config)#access-list 14 permit 0.0.0.0 255.255.255.255
```

In the previous section, we learned that a 1 bit in the wildcard mask means you don't match that bit in the source address. So, a wildcard mask of all 1s (255.255.255.255) means you do not match any of the bits in the source address, and it will permit all traffic. To save yourself from having to type all those 0s and 255s, you can use the *any* keyword, as seen in the command that follows.

```
Router(config)#access-list 14 permit any
```

Another example is when you only want to match one specific address. To do this, you would have to type in the command:

```
Router(config)#access-list 15 permit 172.16.134.23 0.0.0.0
```

Because the wildcard mask is all 0s, you are telling the router you want to match every single bit of the source address. So, you would permit

172.16.134.23, but it would deny any other address (due to the implicit *deny* statement at the end). Another way of typing this command is:

```
Router(config)#access-list 15 permit host 172.16.134.23
```

Using the *any* and *host* keywords in the *access-list* command makes them easier to read and saves you from having to type out the whole wildcard mask when you are matching on all of the bits, or on none of the bits.

Keyword Log

When including the keyword *log* in an *access-list* statement, a match of that statement will be logged. That is, any packet that matches the access list will cause a message to be sent to the console, memory, or to a syslog server.

Configuring & Implementing...

Logging Commands

You can control how your router handles log messages with the *logging* commands in global configuration mode. To see what logging features are configure on your router, use the *show logging* command as shown next:

```
Router#show logging
Syslog logging: enabled (0 messages dropped, 0 flushes, 0 overruns)
    Console logging: level debugging, 2966 messages logged
    Monitor logging: level debugging, 2695 messages logged
    Buffer logging: level informational, 54 messages logged
    Trap logging: level informational, 59 message lines logged
```

The preceding output shows us three different items: the destination of the log messages, the severity of messages logged to that destination, and the number of messages that have been logged.

As seen previously, there are four different destinations that the router can send logging messages. *Console logging* refers to the messages sent to the screen while connected to the console port. When you are connected to the router via Telnet, you cannot see console messages, but you can type **terminal monitor**, and you will be able to see any messages that are sent to *Monitor Logging*. The router also has in internal

Continued

buffer that can be used to store messages, which are collected by the *Buffer Logging* settings. When you use the *show logging* command, the buffered messages will be shown immediately after the preceding output. Finally, if you would like to keep a history of all messages generated, you can configure a syslog server and choose which messages are sent to it with the *Trap Logging* destination.

There are also eight different levels of messages, which will be listed from most severe (Emergency Level 0) to least severe (Debugging Level 7):

- **Emergency** Level 0
- **Alerts** Level 1
- **Critical** Level 2
- **Errors** Level 3
- **Warning** Level 4
- **Notification** Level 5
- **Informational** Level 6
- **Debugging** Level 7

The level set in the previous *show logging* output shows the least severe message type that will be logged. The router will also log all severity levels above what is shown. For example, Level 0 through Level 6 messages will be logged to the buffer in the preceding example. All messages generated by adding the *log* keyword to an access list are classified as Level 6, or informational messages.

This feature is available with standard access lists since IOS 11.3. Previously, this capability was only available in extended IP access lists. When using the *log* keyword, the first packet that matches the access list causes a logging message immediately. Following matching packets are gathered over a five-minute interval before they are displayed or logged. Let's look at how this would work in the following example:

```
Router(config)#access-list 17 deny 172.16.130.88 log
Router(config)#access-list 17 deny 172.16.130.89 log
Router(config)#access-list 17 deny 172.16.130.90 log
Router(config)#access-list 17 permit any
```

Suppose the interface receives 10 packets from host 172.16.130.88, 15 packets from host 172.16.130.89, and 20 packets from host 172.16.130.90 over a five-minute period. The first log would look as follows:

```
list 17 deny 172.16.130.88 1 packet
list 17 deny 172.16.130.89 1 packet
list 17 deny 172.16.130.90 1 packet
```

After five minutes, the log would display as follows:

```
list 17 deny 172.16.130.88 9 packets
list 17 deny 172.16.130.89 14 packets
list 17 deny 172.16.130.90 19 packets
```

When using the keyword *log,* we are provided with an observant capability. Here you are able to analyze not only who has tried to access your network but you are also able to tell the number of attempts. The log message will indicate the number of packets, whether the packet was permitted or denied, the source address, and the access list number. There will be a message generated for the first packet that matches the test and then at five-minute intervals you will receive a message stating the number of packets matched during the previous five minutes.

Applying an Access List

Now that we've learned how to structure the access list, we will learn how to apply it to an interface. In this section, we will assume we have a router with two interfaces: Serial0 and Ethernet0. The network we want to protect is on the Ethernet 0 interface and we want to filter traffic as it enters the router on the Serial0 interface. The only network we want to be able to pass through our router is the 192.168.10.0 255.255.255.0 network, while all other traffic is denied. In addition, the host 192.168.10.5 should also be denied access to our network, even though it is a part of the 192.168.10.0 subnet.

The first step is to create our access list. In this example, we've decided to use access list number 25. We create the list by typing:

```
Router(config)#access-list 25 deny host 192.168.10.5
Router(config)#access-list 25 permit 192.168.10.0 0.0.0.255
```

Our first statement in our access list is to deny the host 192.168.10.5. The next statement is to allow the entire Class C subnet 192.168.10.0. The implicit *deny* statement at the end of the access list will prevent any other traffic from being permitted through the list.

NOTE

Remember that access lists are processed in sequential order. If our first statement were to permit the 192.168.10.0 network, then 192.168.10.5 would be able to access our network, even though we want to deny it. This would happen because 192.168.10.5 would match the *permit* statement and would not process any farther. To remedy this situation, we must deny the specific IP first, and then allow the rest of the network.

Next, we must specify the interface where we plan to apply the access list. Since all traffic from outside our network must come to us over the Serial0 link, we want to apply this access list to that interface. To enter interface configuration mode, we would type:

```
Router(config)#interface serial 0
```

The next step is to apply the access list to the interface and define the direction of the access list. This is accomplished by using the *ip access-group* command. Table 4.3 describes the *ip access-group* command.

```
ip access-group {list number} {in|out}
```

Table 4.3 The *ip access-group* Command

Command	Description
ip	Defines the protocol used.
access-group	Applies the access list to the interface.
List number	Identifies the access list you wish to apply.
**in	out**	Keyword in or out defines the direction in which the access list will be applied. This indicates whether packets are examined as they leave the interface (outside), or as they enter the router (inside).

To complete our example, we would use the following command to apply the access list. This command will apply the access list we just created to filter traffic that comes towards us into the serial interface. Before it is routed to the Ethernet interface, it must pass through the access list or else it will be dropped.

```
Router(config-if)#ip access-group 25 in
```

Extended IP Access Lists

Although there are times when we only need to filter traffic based on the source address, more often than not we will need to match traffic with a higher level of detail. An option for more precise traffic-filtering control would be an extended IP access list. Here, both the source and destination address are checked. In addition, you also have the ability to specify the protocol and optional TCP or UDP port number to filter more precisely. In the following example, any field represented by {} is mandatory for the access list, while any field represented by [] is optional. The format of an extended IP access list is:

```
access-list access-list-number {permit | deny} protocol source
    source-wildcard [operator source-port] destination destination-wildcard
    [operator destination-port] [precedence precedence-number] [tos tos]
    [established] [log | log-input]
```

Bold items represent keywords that are part of the access list syntax. Table 4.4 lists the configuration for a standard IP access list.

Table 4.4 Extended IP Access List Configuration

Command	Description
Access-list list number	Defines the number of the access list. The extended access list numbers range from 100–199.
Permit	If conditions are met, traffic will be allowed.
deny	If conditions are met, traffic will be denied.
Protocol	Defines the Internet protocol for filtering. Available options here are keywords such as *TCP* or *UDP*, or the number of the protocol as seen in the IP header.
source-address	Identifies the host or network from which the packet is being sent. The source can be specified by an IP address or by using the keyword *any*.
source wildcard-mask	This defines the number of wildcard bits assigned to the source address. The source wildcard-mask can be specified by an IP address or by using the keyword *any*.

Continued

Table 4.4 Continued

Command	Description
Operator source-port	Defines the name or number of a *source* TCP or UDP port. A list of operators is shown next.
Destination-address	Identifies the host or network to which the packet is being sent. The destination can be specified by an IP address or by using the keyword *any*.
Destination wildcard-mask	This defines the number of wildcard bits assigned to the destination address. The destination wildcard-mask can be specified by an IP address or by using the keyword *any*.
Operator destination-port	Defines the name or number of a *destination* TCP or UDP port. A list of operators is shown next.
precedence precedence-number	Used for filtering by the precedence level name or number (0 thru 7).
tos tos-number	Used for filtering by the Type of Service level specified by a name or number (0 thru 15).
established	Allows established TCP sessions through the list.
log | log-input	Log the event when a packet matches the access list statement. Log-input shows the same information as the *log* keyword, except it also adds the interface name the packet was received on.

In the following access list, we get very specific about what host we want to access a particular network or host on a network. In the first three lines, we are permitting or allowing packets from individual hosts on subnet 172.16.130.0 to any host on network 10.0.0.0. In line 4, we are denying packets with the source address that belongs to subnet 172.16.130.0 to the destination of host 192.168.10.118. Line 5 tells us that we are permitting all IP packets with no concern of a source or destination address. The implicit *deny all* at the end of the list will never be matched against a packet because the previous *permit* statement will match all packets. In Figure 4.3, we would apply this access list on the serial 0 interface in the outbound direction as follows:

```
Router(config)# interface serial 0
Router(config-if)# ip access-group 141 out
```

Figure 4.3 An Example Network

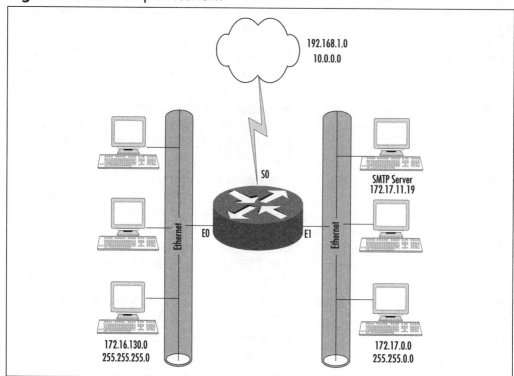

An example of an extended access list is as follows:

```
access-list 141 permit icmp host 172.16.130.88 10.0.0.0 0.255.255.255
access-list 141 permit tcp host 172.16.130.89 eq 734 10.0.0.0 0.
    255.255.255 range 10000 10010
access-list 141 permit udp host 172.16.130.90 10.0.0.0 0.255.255.255
    eq tftp
access-list 141 deny ip 172.16.130.0 0.0.0.255 host 192.168.10.118
access-list 141 permit ip any any
```

Table 4.5 describes the extended access list commands.

Table 4.5 A Description of *Access List* Commands

Command	Description
access-list 141 permit icmp host 172.16.130.88 10.0.0.0 0.255.255.255	Allows host 172.16.130.88 to send ICMP messages to any host on network 10.0.0.0.
access-list 141 permit tcp host 172.16.130.89 eq 734 10.0.0.0 0.255.255.255 range 10000 10010	Allows host 172.16.130.89 to initiate TCP sessions from port 734 to any port between 10000 and 10010 on any host on network 10.0.0.0.
access-list 141 permit udp host 172.16.130.90 10.0.0.0 0.255.255.255 eq tftp	Allows host 172.16.130.90 to send files via TFTP (UDP port 69) to any host on net-work 10.0.0.0.
access-list 141 deny ip 172.16.130.0 0.0.0.255 host 192.168.10.118	Denies any host on network 172.16.130.0 to host 192.168.10.118. Since we configured some *permit* statements from hosts within these previous two subnets, this entry will deny everything between these two networks that isn't explicitly permitted in the earlier listing.
access-list 141 permit ip any any	Allows all hosts from any network to any network, if it has not matched one of the preceding lists. Take a good look at the order of these commands to get a feel for the importance of the list order. Remember this is processed in a top-down manner, as shown in Figure 4.2.

Just as in our standard access list, the extended access list will require a hyphen between the words *access* and *list*. Next is the list number. Since we are referencing an extended IP access list, the numbers would range from 100 to 199.

The access list number serves the same dual purpose here as we looked at earlier with the standard access list. The router must have a way to distinguish between access lists. The number performs this purpose along with tying the lines of an access list together and designates which access list the filter is part of. The number also tells the router the type of access list.

Designing & Planning…

Placement of Access Lists

Often you have a few options about how to apply your access lists and still achieve the same affect on the traffic flowing through the router. In the case of the previous example, access list 141 was applied outbound on the serial 0 interface. Because access list 141 was designed to only filter traffic originating from the 172.16.130.0 network, and not traffic from 172.17.0.0, this list could have been applied in the inbound direction on Ethernet 0. Both approaches will have the same affect on the traffic flowing through the router.

There is a minor difference between these two approaches, though. When the ACL is applied outbound on the Serial0 interface, the traffic enters the Ethernet0 interface and is processed against the routing table. The packet is then passed to the outbound interface, where it is checked against any outbound ACLs. If the outbound interface is Serial 0, it checks packets against access list 141 and will permit or deny the traffic based on the rules defined in that list.

When the ACL is applied inbound on the Ethernet0 interface, the traffic is permitted or denied before it is processed against the routing table. On a router under heavy traffic loads, this could make a considerable difference in the delay that is introduced because the router does not have to process packets that will be dropped by the outbound interface.

Although inbound filtering has the advantage with respect to route processing, that does not necessarily make it the better way to apply access lists. Under different circumstances, you may want to prevent access to an external subnet from both Ethernet interfaces. In this case, it may be easier to apply the access lists in the outbound direction of Serial0 because packets from both Ethernet interfaces will have to pass through Serial0 to get to the external subnet. In other words, you are applying the access list to the bottleneck in traffic. Otherwise, you will

Continued

have to keep two separate access lists, one specific for Ethernet0 and the other specific for Ethernet1. If the router is under light traffic loads, it may be easier to maintain a single access list.

There is disagreement among network and security professionals about which approach is better, but neither approach should be considered better than the other in all cases. It is up to you to decide which is best for your situation.

Keywords *permit* or *deny*

A keyword *permit* or *deny* specifies to the router the action to be performed. For example, the keyword *permit* would allow the packet to exit or enter the interface, depending on whether you specify the filtering to be performed in or out. Again, this option provides the same function as in our standard access list. The last line of our extended access list example could have read as follows:

```
access-list 141 permit ip any any
```

Protocol

You have the option of filtering several different protocols using the extended access list. The protocol field in the IP header is an 8-bit number that defines what protocol is used inside the IP packet. TCP and UDP are only two of the possible protocols that can be filtered on, although they are most common. Other protocols, such as ICMP and EIGRP, have their own protocol numbers because they are not encapsulated inside TCP or UDP. If we use a question mark when defining an access list, we can see the protocol numbers that have been defined by name inside the router.

```
Router(config)#access-list 191 permit ?
  <0-255>  An IP protocol number
  ahp      Authentication Header Protocol
  eigrp    Cisco's EIGRP routing protocol
  esp      Encapsulation Security Payload
  gre      Cisco's GRE tunneling
  icmp     Internet Control Message Protocol
  igmp     Internet Gateway Message Protocol
  igrp     Cisco's IGRP routing protocol
  ip       Any Internet Protocol
```

```
ipinip    IP in IP tunneling
nos       KA9Q NOS compatible IP over IP tunneling
ospf      OSPF routing protocol
pcp       Payload Compression Protocol
pim       Protocol Independent Multicast
tcp       Transmission Control Protocol
udp       User Datagram Protocol
```

Protocols not on the preceding list may also be filtered with extended access lists, but they must be referenced by their protocol number. A full list of assigned IP protocol numbers can be found at www.iana.org/assignments/protocol-numbers.

It is important to remember that the IP keyword in the protocol field matches all protocol numbers. You must use a systematic approach here when designing your access list. For example, if your first line in the access list permits IP for a specific address, and the second line denies UDP for the same address, the second statement would have no effect. The first line would permit IP, including all the above layers. An option here may be to reverse the order of the statements. With the statements reversed, UDP would be denied from that address and all other protocols would be permitted.

Source Address and Wildcard-mask

The source address and source wildcard-mask perform the same function here as in a standard IP access list. So, in the preceding example we could have used the wildcard mask instead of the *host* and *any* keywords. The access list would then look as follows:

```
access-list 141 permit ip 172.16.130.88 0.0.0.0 10.0.0.0 0.255.255.255
access-list 141 permit ip 172.16.130.89 0.0.0.0 10.0.0.0 0.255.255.255
access-list 141 permit ip 172.16.130.90 0.0.0.0 10.0.0.0 0.255.255.255
access-list 141 permit ip 172.16.130.0 0.0.0.255 192.168.10.118 0.0.0.0
access-list 141 permit ip 0.0.0.0 255.255.255.255 0.0.0.0 255.255.255.255
```

In the first three lines, we are permitting or allowing packets from individual hosts on subnet 172.16.130.0 to any host on network 10.0.0.0. In line 4, we are permitting packets with the source address that belongs to subnet 172.16.130.0 to the destination of host 192.168.10.118. Line 5 tells us that we are permitting all packets regardless of the source or destination address. Remember that standard IP access lists have a default mask of 0.0.0.0. This does not apply to extended access lists so we must specify one.

Destination Address and Wildcard-mask

The destination address and wildcard-mask have the same effect and structure as the source address and wildcard-mask. So, here the keywords *host* and *any* are also available. You can utilize these keywords to specify any destination address as well as a specific destination without using the wildcard mask. Remember that extended access lists try a match on both source and destination. A common mistake here is trying to build an extended access list with the idea of only filtering the source address, and forgetting to specify the destination address.

Source and Destination Port Number

Many times, we don't want to deny all access to a particular server. When you put a Web server out on the Internet, you want everyone to be able to access it on port 80 (WWW), but you don't want to allow access to any other ports, because it gives hackers the opportunity to exploit other services you may not be aware of (although you should know of them in the first place). Restricting access to this level of detail is another benefit of extended ACLs. We have the option of specifying a source and destination port number in the access list. Let's look at a simple example:

```
Router(config)# interface Serial 0
Router(config-if)# ip access-group 111 in

Router(config)#access-list 111 permit tcp any host 172.17.11.19 eq 25
Router(config)#access-list 111 permit tcp any host 172.17.11.19 eq 23
```

These commands are explained in Table 4.6.

Table 4.6 Router Commands

Router Commands	Description
access-list 111 permit tcp any host 172.17.11.19 eq 25	Permits SMTP from anywhere to host 172.17.11.19.
access-list 111 permit tcp any host 172.17.11.19 eq 23	Permits Telnet from anywhere to host 172.17.11.19.
interface Serial 0	Enters interface submode.
ip access-group 111 in	Applies access list inbound on interface.

In line 1, we are permitting TCP packets from any source to the destination of host 172.22.11.19 if the destination port is 25 (SMTP). In line 2, we are permitting TCP packets from any source to the destination of host 172.22.11.19 if the destination port is 23 (Telnet). The implicit *deny* statement at the end of this access list will prevent all other traffic from making it into our network.

Let's take a look at filtering with TCP and UDP. When using TCP, for example, the access list will examine the source and destination port numbers inside the TCP segment header. So, when using an extended access list, you have the capability to filter to and from a network address and also to and from a particular port number. You have several options when deciding which operator to use, such as:

- **eq** equal to

- **neq** not equal to

- **gt** greater than

- **lt** less than

- **range** specifies an inclusive range or ports (Here, two port numbers are specified.)

Established

One of the options available for use with an extended access list is the established option. This option is only available with the TCP protocol. The idea here is to prevent someone outside your network from initiating a connection to a host on the inside, but still letting traffic through if it is a response to something that originated from inside your network. To demonstrate this, let's take a look at the following access list, which will apply later to Figure 4.4.

```
Router(config)# interface Serial 0
Router(config-if)# ip access-group 110 in


access-list 110 permit tcp any host 172.17.11.19 eq 25
access-list 110 permit tcp 12.0.0.0 0.255.255.255 172.22.114.0 0.0.0.255 eq
23
```

We created this access list so the server 172.17.11.19 can receive mail messages on the SMTP port, and to allow the 12.0.0.0 255.0.0.0 network Telnet access to the 172.22.114.0 255.255.255.0 network. What you may not realize is that while this access list will protect our network from access except on the specified servers and ports, it will also prevent anyone on our network from surfing the Web. It is important to realize that if you are permitting a very specific list of traffic, and denying everything else, responses to traffic initiated inside your network will be blocked. Let's go over the steps when the host 172.17.10.10 tries to visit a Web page at 10.15.25.35, which is somewhere on the Internet. (If you need a refresher on the TCP handshake process, you can look at Figure 4.5 later in this section.)

1. Host 172.17.10.10 initiates a TCP from a random port above 1024 (let's assume 10000) and tries to connect to port 80 (WWW) on server 10.15.25.35.

2. Host 10.15.25.35 will receive a TCP packet with the SYN flag set, destined for port 80 and sourced from 172.17.10.10:10000.

3. Host 10.15.25.35 will send a TCP packet with the SYN and ACK flag set to acknowledge the TCP session. The TCP segment will be sourced from port 80 and sent to port 10000 on 172.17.10.10.

4. The SYN/ACK TCP packet will enter the router through Serial0, which has access list 110 applied in the inbound direction

5. The packet will not match either the first or second lines in the access list, so it will match the implicit *deny all* and the packet will be dropped. This will prevent all hosts inside your network from communicating on the Internet.

In this case, we want to allow all workstations access to the Internet, but obviously, we cannot create individual lines in an access list to permit traffic back from every Web server on the entire Internet. To solve this problem, the established keyword was added to the extended access list. If the established keyword is used on a line of the access list, it will only allow a packet through if it matches the line of the list, and has either the ACK or RST bit set in the TCP header. Let's look at another access list to demonstrate this.

Figure 4.4 shows an example of our network with the access list applied inbound on interface Serial0 (S0). The first line of the access list permits TCP packets from any source to the network 172.17.0.0 with the TCP flag ACK or RST bit set. This will allow traffic back into our network if it is a response to something that was originated inside. The second line tells the router to permit TCP packets from any source if the destination is 172.17.11.19 and the destination port is 25 (SMTP). Line 3 is allowing a TCP segment with a source address from network 12.0.0.0 to port 23 (Telnet), to any address on subnet 172.22.114.0. What will happen to all other packets? Once again the implicit *deny all* will drop any other packets.

Figure 4.4 The Access List Applied to Serial 0 Inbound

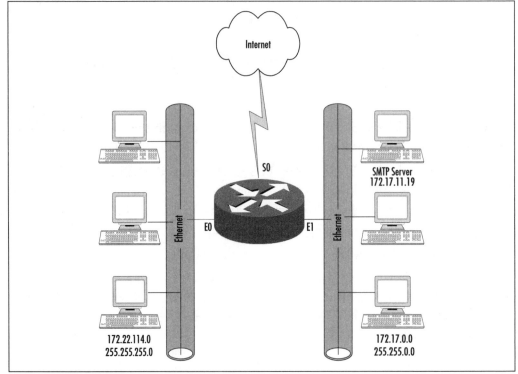

```
Router(config)# interface Serial 0
Router(config-if)# ip access-group 111 in

access-list 111 permit tcp any host 172.17.0.0 0.0.255.255 established
access-list 111 permit tcp any host 172.17.11.19 eq 25
access-list 111 permit tcp 12.0.0.0 0.255.255.255 172.22.114.0 0.0.0.255 eq
23
```

In the TCP segment there are 6 flag bits, two of which are the ACK and RST. If one of these two bits is set, then a match on the established keyword will occur. The SYN bit indicates that a connection is being established. A packet with a SYN bit without an ACK bit is the very first packet sent to establish a connection, and will be denied by a line with the established keyword due to the lack of an ACK flag. Figure 4.5 shows the TCP setup handshake.

Figure 4.5 A TCP Session Being Established

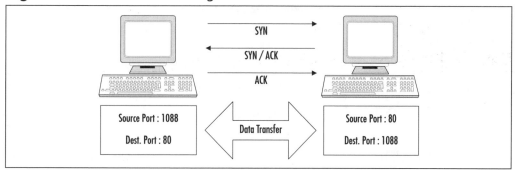

Another issue to consider here is that you, as the administrator, may not be certain what protocols the host may be using. However, we do know ports are chosen by workstations randomly between the port ranges of 1024 and 65535. Keeping that in mind, we could modify the first line of the access list as follows:

```
access-list 111 permit tcp any host 172.17.0.0 0.0.255.255 gt 1023
established
```

This would insure that no packets are accepted inbound to our network unless the destination port is higher that 1023. The hacker could spoof the ACK or RST bit in the packet but the destination port would still have to be higher that 1023. Typically, our servers running services such as DNS run below port 1024. However, it is not a good idea to let through all ports over 1023. You become vulnerable to network scans and denial of service attacks (RST).

SECURITY ALERT

The established keyword is not a secure way of protecting your network, because a hacker can easily forge a packet with the RST or ACK flag set and it will be allowed through the access list. To solve this problem, use either reflexive access lists or CBAC, which are covered later in this chapter.

Now, let's look at what happens when we decide to allow restricted TFTP access to host 172.17.11.19, unrestricted DNS access to host 172.17.11.20, and unrestricted SNMP access to the entire network. TFTP, DNS, and SNMP are UDP-based protocols. We have added to our extended access list again in the following example:

```
access-list 111 permit tcp any host 172.17.0.0 0.0.255.255 established
access-list 111 permit tcp any host 172.17.11.19 eq 25
access-list 111 permit tcp 12.0.0.0 0.255.255.255 172.22.114.0 0.0.0.255 eq
  23
access-list 111 permit udp 192.168.10.0 0.0.0.255 host 172.17.11.19 eq 69
access-list 111 permit udp any host 172.17.11.20 eq 53
access-list 111 permit udp any any eq 161
```

You will notice there is no keyword established on the lines for UDP packets. Remember that UDP is a connectionless protocol, therefore no connections will be established between hosts. A UDP packet is sent without any acknowledgement; the sending host just assumes the packet arrived at the destination. Since we have not changed the first three lines of our access list, we will begin by discussing line 4. Line 4 is allowing UDP datagrams from subnet 192.168.10.0 to port 69 (TFTP) on host 172.17.11.19. Line 5 is allowing UDP datagrams from any source to host 172.17.11.20 with a destination port of 53 (DNS). Line 6 allows all SNMP (port 161) to and from any destination. Remember, any packets not matching the list will be dropped by the implicit *deny all*. Figure 4.6 shows the addition of a DNS server in our network. Here, we would apply the access list inbound on interface serial 0. Also, be aware that the 172.22.114.0 network would still be unable to surf the Web with the current ACL applied.

Figure 4.6 Example Network with a DNS Server Added

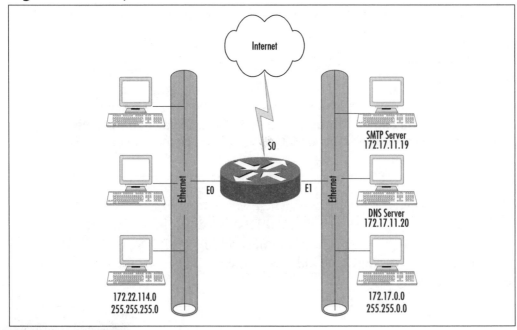

Log and Log-input

When we were discussing standard access lists we covered the *log* keyword, and what sort of information this presents us. This keyword is also available for extended access lists. Just as extended access lists allow us to filter on much more information than a standard access list, the *log* keyword gives us much more information when used with an extended access list, than a standard access list. When used with an extended ACL, we will be told the protocol, destination IP, source port and destination port, in addition to the other information returned from a standard ACL.

In some cases, for example when assigning an outbound ACL to an interface, we may not be able to tell where a packet has originated, especially in large networks. Of course, we will be given the source address, but to figure out where the packet originated, we would have to look at the routing table to see which interface the packet should have arrived on. To make this process a little easier, Cisco added the *log-input* keyword for the ACL. This will give us the interface name on which the packet arrived, in addition to all the information gathered from the *log* keyword.

The *log-input* command can also be useful in discovering if a source address has been spoofed. If your router logs are showing a packet entering on a different interface from where the route table says the network is supposed to be, you may be dealing with a packet that has a spoofed source address.

Named Access Lists

Each access list type has a range of acceptable numbers that can be used. For example, there are 99 standard (1 thru 99) and 100 extended (100 thru 199) access lists available in the Cisco IOS. This seems to be more than enough—however, maybe you need to create more that 100 extended IP access lists on your enterprise router. Named access lists provide an alternative to allow this. Also, named access lists provide a description that is typically more manageable than a large group of numbers.

Named access lists are just as the title implies, an access list that is referenced by name instead of a number. They also allow you to delete a specific entry in your access list. When using numbered access lists, this is not an option. When using a numbered access list, you must recreate the entire access list to remove an unwanted entry. When adding to an access list, both the named and numbered will place the new line at the bottom of the access list.

When creating a named access list, it must begin with a standard alphabetic character. Names are case sensitive so the access list SYDNEY and Sydney will be looked at as two unique names or two different access lists. Named access lists use the same syntax as numbered access lists, but the creation is slightly different. Notice that you must use the keyword *ip* before the main access list statement. You also enter a new configuration mode specifically for the named access lists. In this mode, you start with the *permit* or *deny* keyword, so you do not have to type **access-list** at the beginning of every line. Just type **exit** when you are finished to exit the named ACL configuration mode. Named access lists are applied with the *ip access-group* command just like numbered ACLs.

```
Router(config)#ip access-list extended filter_tx
Router(config-ext-nacl)#permit tcp any 172.17.0.0 0.0.255.255 established
Router(config-ext-nacl)#permit tcp any host 172.17.11.19 eq smtp
Router(config-ext-nacl)#permit tcp 12.0.0.0 0.255.255.255 172.22.114.0
    0.0.0.255 eq 23
Router(config-ext-nacl)#permit udp 192.168.10.0 0.0.0.255 host
    172.17.11.19 eq 69
Router(config-ext-nacl)#permit udp any host 172.17.11.20 eq 53
Router(config-ext-nacl)#permit udp any any eq 161
Router(config-ext-nacl)#exit
Router(config)#
```

Editing Access Lists

When applying access lists, there are several factors to consider. One of the most important things to remember is that access lists are evaluated from the top down. So packets will always be tested starting with the top line of the access list. Careful consideration should be taken regarding the order of your access list statements. The most frequent match should always be at the beginning of the access list.

Another thing to consider is the placement of the access list. When looking at your network, a standard access list should be placed closest to the destination of where you are trying to block the packets. Remember that a standard IP access list filters on the source IP address. If the IP address is blocked, then the entire protocol suite (IP) would typically be denied. So, if you denied an IP address close to the source, the user would basically be denied access anywhere on the network.

NOTE

Packets generated by the router are not affected by an outbound access list. So, to filter routing table updates or any traffic generated by the router, you should consider inbound access lists.

When using a named access list, we can delete a specific entry—however, with a numbered access list, we do not have this option. We have learned that when you need to add an entry into the access list in a specific position (such as the fifth line) the entire access list must be deleted and then re-created with new entries. This applies to both numbered and named access lists. So if this tells me I have just created a 35-line access list and need to make a change, is the only option I have to simply start over? Not really. There are several ways to avoid re-creating your entire access list. One option to explore here may be the use of the TFTP protocol. When utilizing TFTP we have the ability to copy our configuration to a server as a text file. Remember, when you copy from anywhere to the running configuration, a merge will occur. So, if your intention is to change line 14, make your changes to the configuration file while on the TFTP server, then when you copy the file to the running configuration, the merge will replace line 14 with your new changes. Once on the server, we can use a text editor to modify then reload the configuration to our router. Another option may be to have a template of an access list on your TFTP server. Having the template will help to ensure you enter the command correctly. Remember, the commands you use here will be the exact commands you would enter at the command line of the router. When copying this file to your running configuration, it will merge the new access list with your current configuration. If the syntax is incorrect, the operation will fail. The following is an example of how a session would look when loading an access list from a TFTP server. We will merge the access list with the running configuration.

```
Router# copy tftp running-config
Address or name of remote host []? 172.16.1.1
Source filename []? accesslist.txt
Destination filename [running-config]?
Accessing TFTP://172.16.1.1/accesslist.txt… OK - 1684/3072 bytes]
Loading accesslist.txt from 172.16.1.1 (via Ethernet 0): !!
    [OK - 1388/3072 bytes]
1388 bytes copied in 3 secs (462 bytes/sec)
```

If you do not have access to a TFTP server, another option for editing access lists is to just use the cut and paste feature of your terminal program. You can copy the current access list out of the *show running-config* output, and paste it into a text editor like Notepad. Once in Notepad, you can make the needed changes and paste the list back into the router.

WARNING

Be aware that if you want to paste the ACL back into the router with the same name or number, you must delete the old ACL first. If you do not, then the two access lists will combine and contain lines from both the new and old list. It is best to use a slightly different name or number for the revised ACL and then go back and change the *ip access-group* command to avoid any unexpected complications. This also avoids the small amount of time that you would be unsecured while you delete your old ACL and paste in the new one.

Problems with Access Lists

As you've seen so far, access lists are very useful in controlling what type of traffic is allowed to flow through the router. Unfortunately, in most situations, basic access lists cannot be relied upon to properly secure a network. Many times a basic access list is not flexible enough to provide a good solution for the problem. For example, using the access lists we've discussed thus far, we don't have any way of creating temporary entries in a list. Some other issues you may encounter with access lists are their limited capability to test information above the IP layer. Extended access lists have the capability to check on Layer 4, but not in the detailed sense.

Another problem to consider is that the access list will examine each packet individually and does not have the capability of detecting if a packet is part of an upper layer conversation. The keyword *established* can be used to match TCP packets that are part of an established TCP session, but you need to be cautious when using it. Remember that *established* only checks the TCP header for the presence of an RST or ACK flag, and does not perform any checks to verify that a packet is truly part of an established conversation. Although this filtering technique is suitable in many cases, it does not protect against forged TCP packets (commonly used to probe networks), nor does it offer any facility to filter UDP sessions. Reflexive access list and CBAC, introduced later in this chapter, offer better control and more facilities to do session filtering.

To help solve some of these problems, Cisco has added some advanced features to the IOS software. We will go through some of these features and discuss the problems they were designed to handle, as well as when it is best to use them.

Lock-and-key Access Lists

Lock-and-key is a traffic filtering security feature that can automatically create an opening in an access list on the router to allow incoming traffic from an authenticated source. These access lists are also referred to as dynamic access lists. When using the basic access lists discussed earlier in this chapter, the list will never change unless an administrator makes a change. With lock-and-key access lists, you can add dynamic entries that are only active after the user has been authenticated with the router. After the authentication process, the dynamic entry will disappear after the configured timeout value, or after the maximum lifetime of the temporary entry has been reached. Once the entry is terminated, the interface is configured back to its original state.

Let's say, for example, that a user in Figure 4.7 is working at a branch office and needs to log in to the corporate office. The user will attempt to log in from a PC that is connected to a router (typically via LAN). A Telnet session will be opened to the router to provide authentication. The router at the corporate site (which is configured for lock-and-key) receives the Telnet packet and opens a Telnet session. Next, the router will prompt for a password and then perform authentication by using a test that is configured by the administrator, such as a name and password. The authentication process can be done locally by the router using a local username/password configuration, or through an external AAA server such as TACACS+ or RADIUS. When the user successfully authenticates, the Telnet session closes and a temporary entry is created in the dynamic access list. This dynamic access list will typically permit traffic from the user's source IP address to some predetermined destination. This dynamic access list will be deleted when a timeout is reached, or can be cleared by the administrator. A timeout can be configured as an idle-timeout or maximum-timeout period expires.

A user may not have a static IP address in a situation where a DHCP is in use in a LAN environment or when a user is connected through a dialup to an Internet Service Provider (ISP). In both cases, users may typically get a different IP address. Lock-and-key access lists can be used to implement a higher level of security without creating large holes in your network. The format of a lock-and-key

ACL is identical to an extended access list, except for two extra fields, as seen in Table 4.7.

```
access-list access-list-number [dynamic dynamic-name[timeout minutes]]
    {deny | permit} protocol source source-wildcard destination
    destination-wildcard[precedence precedence] [tos tos] [established]
    [log | log-input]
```

Figure 4.7 Using Lock and Key

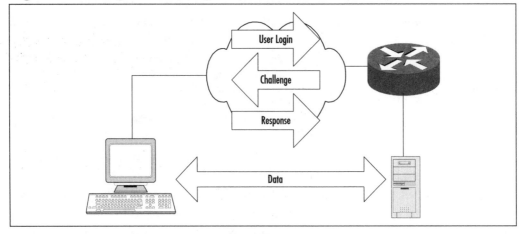

Table 4.7 Lock-and-Key Access List Configuration

Command	Description
access-list list number	Defines the number of the access list. The usable access list numbers range from 100–199.
dynamic dynamic-name	Designates this particular entry as part of a dynamic ACL. The *dynamic-name* field is a name assigned to the dynamic entries. If multiple entries need to be triggered at the same time, they all should have the same *dynamic-name*.
Timeout minutes	The *timeout* is optional and designates the absolute timeout for dynamic entries. No matter if the session is being used or not, the entry will be removed from the ACL after this timeout expires.
permit	If conditions are met, traffic will be allowed.
deny	If conditions are met, traffic will be denied.
Protocol	Defines the protocol for filtering, as discussed in the section about extended access lists.

Continued

Table 4.7 Continued

Command	Description
source-address	Identifies the host or network from which the packet is being sent. The source can be specified by an IP address or by using the keyword *any*.
source-wildcard	This defines the number of wildcard bits assigned to the source address. The source wildcard-mask can be specified by an IP address or by using the keyword *any*.
destination-address	Identifies the host or network to which the packet is being sent. The destination can be specified by an IP address or by using the keyword *any*.
destination-wildcard	This defines the number of wildcard bits assigned to the destination address. The destination wild-card-mask can be specified by an IP address or by using the keyword *any*.
precedence precedence-number	Used for filtering by the precedence level name or number.
tos	Defines filtering by service level, specified by a name or number (01-5).
established	When using TCP filtering, will occur if RST or ACK bits are set.
*log	log-input*	This keyword results in the logging of packets that match the *permit* or *deny* statement.

NOTE

Lock-and-key will only install one dynamic access list in any given access list. Although the router will allow you to specify multiple dynamic entries with different *dynamic-name* fields, these will not have any effect. You will see all the entries when viewing the list with *show ip access-list*, but if a user authenticates, it will only activate the first dynamic list. If you wish to use multiple lines when a user authenticates, make sure each entry has the same *dynamic-name* field.

Previously, when defining standard and extended access lists, we had two steps: Build the access list and apply it to an interface. Those steps are still required for lock-and-key access lists, but a few extra steps must be taken. Any entry in the ACL not marked as dynamic will filter just like a basic extended ACL. The dynamic entries will not be used until the authentication process takes place. To activate the dynamic entries, the user must Telnet into the router. With no additional configuration, the user will be at the standard user mode prompt. To open the temporary entries defined in the list, the user must type the *access-enable* command at the prompt. The format of the command is as follows:

```
access-enable [host] [timeout minutes]
```

We will look at each component of this command in Table 4.8.

Table 4.8 The Lock-and-key Access List Configuration

Command	Description
access-enable	Tells the router to activate the temporary entries in a lock-and-key ACL.
host	This keyword specifies that only the authenticating host should be allowed through the dynamic ACL, instead of activating the entire statement.
timeout minutes	This timeout value is an idle-timeout, unlike the one specified in the *access-list* command. If no traffic matches the dynamic entry in the number of minutes specified, the temporary entry will be removed from the list.

SECURITY ALERT

If your dynamic entries are configured to allow anyone to authenticate, you must make sure that the *host* keyword is used with the *access-enable* command. If not, you will open up your network to everyone. To avoid relying on the users to employ the command properly, configure the router with the *autocommand* feature. This will be discussed later in this section.

Under normal circumstances, you will be trusting the user to enter the correct command to allow himself access through the network. This can be a very dangerous thing to do because the user could accidentally open more access than you would wish.

Let's assume we have a router connected to the Internet. Our serial interface, which is connected to our ISP, has the address 10.10.100.2 assigned. The server that we are trying to protect is using the IP address 10.150.200.25. Let's also assume that we have users connecting to the Internet via dial-up accounts, and they could have IP addresses from almost any network connected to the Internet. In this case, we may decide to create a dynamic access entry such as:

```
Router(config)#access-list 120 dynamic remoteuser timeout 60 permit tcp
    any host 10.150.200.25 eq ftp
Router(config)#access-list 120 permit tcp any host 10.10.100.2 eq telnet

Router(config)#int s0
Router(config-if)#ip access-group 120 in
```

Next, we will verify the configuration.

```
Router#show ip access-list 120
Extended IP access list 120
    Dynamic remoteuser permit tcp any host 10.150.200.25 eq ftp
    permit tcp any host 10.10.100.2 eq telnet
```

In the preceding output, we see that only Telnet access to 10.10.100.2 is currently allowed. The preceding *dynamic* command will allow anyone who can authenticate with the router to FTP to the host 10.150.200.25. If the user types the command *access-enable host*, then they will allow their specific address through the access list. We can see this in the following output (assume that the user is assigned the address 192.168.100.43):

```
Router#show ip access-list 120
Extended IP access list 120
    Dynamic remote permit tcp any host 10.150.200.25 eq ftp
      permit tcp host 192.168.100.43 host 10.150.200.25 eq ftp
    permit tcp any host 10.10.100.2 eq telnet
```

Now we can see that a user has been authenticated and a specific IP is being allowed FTP access to the server. Now, let's assume that a second user wants to access the server. This user logs in correctly, but only types *access-enable* at the prompt, and does not include the *host* keyword. Let's look at the output from this command:

```
Router#show ip access-list 120
Extended IP access list 120
```

```
Dynamic remote permit tcp any host 10.150.200.25 eq ftp
   permit tcp host 192.168.100.43 host 10.150.200.25 eq ftp
   permit tcp any host 10.150.200.25 eq ftp
 permit tcp any host 10.10.100.2 eq telnet
```

Now we see that our second user has just opened up the FTP server to anyone on the Internet. Obviously, this just defeated the purpose of us setting up a lock-and-key access list to begin with. To solve this problem, we will rely on the *autocommand* feature of the Cisco IOS that will allow us to make a user automatically run a command upon login.

By default, the router has five Virtual Terminal (VTY) ports available for Telnet sessions, which are numbered 0 thru 5. When a user connects to a router, the connection will reserve a VTY port for the duration of that session. So five different Telnet sessions can be established on the router simultaneously. If you specify multiple VTY ports, they must all be configured identically because the software hunts for available VTY ports on a round-robin basis. If you do not want to configure all your VTY ports for lock-and-key access, you can specify access on a per-user basis.

First, we will cover the VTY configuration to allow users lock-and-key access:

```
Router(config)#line vty 0 4
Router(config-line)#login
Router(config-line)#password OpenUp
Router(config-line)#autocommand access-enable host timeout 10
```

Using the previous configuration, as soon as someone enters the appropriate password into the Telnet session, the command *access-enable host timeout 10* will be executed and the Telnet session will be disconnected. This will ensure that the appropriate command is used every time someone authenticates with the router. Unfortunately, this also means you will be unable to use the VTY ports for administrative purposes, so this solution isn't usually very appealing. A better way to configure the router for lock-and-key is as follows:

```
Router(config)#username susan password OpenUp
Router(config)#username susan autocommand access-enable host timeout 10
Router(config)#username admin password supersecret

Router(config)#line vty 0 4
Router(config)#login local
```

The previous commands create two users: *susan* and *admin*. If someone logs into the router as Susan, then the command *access-enable host timeout 10* will be executed and the session disconnected. If, on the other hand, someone logs in with the admin user, then they will have regular access to the router for configuration purposes.

Designing & Planning…

Security Risks Using Lock-and-key ACLs

One thing to consider is an attacker using IP spoofing. IP spoofing is where a hacker changes the source IP address of the packets that are sent to an IP address believed trusted by the network. When packets arrive at your router it is nearly impossible to determine if the packets are from a real host. Lock-and-key access lists play a big role in assisting here, due to the fact that the opening is only temporary. This lowers the chance of the hacker determining the trusted source IP address. It doesn't lower the chance of determining the source IP, but it does reduce the window of opportunity to exploit the temporary opening.

One drawback to consider is when a client is behind NAT or NAPT (PAT in Cisco nomenclature). If this user is allowed to authenticate using lock-and-key to access a remote site, the dynamic access list on the router will use the external or public address of the PAT device. That address is potentially used by a number of users and they will automatically be allowed access without any authentication. This is a serious security consideration.

You must also be extremely careful when configuring the dynamic statements in the access list. If you do not specify a timeout, then the dynamic opening will stay open until the router is reset. In addition, you want to take precautions to prevent a user from accidentally making a giant hole in your router security as discussed in this section.

Reflexive Access Lists

The reflexive access list alleviates some of the limitations of the basic and extended access list. Reflexive access lists allow IP packets to be filtered based on upper-layer session information as in extended access lists—however, the reflexive access list can do session filtering by creating dynamic openings for IP traffic that are part of the allowed session. By so doing, reflexive access lists provide a way to maintain information about existing connections. You have the option to permit

IP traffic for sessions originating from within your network, but to deny IP traffic for sessions originating outside your network. This sounds the same as an extended access list. Reflexive access lists are referred to as a separate type of access list, however it is important to note that a reflexive access list is a feature added to an extended access list and can only be defined using extended named IP access lists.

One instance where a reflexive access list could be used is when an IP upper-layer session (such as TCP or UDP) is initiated from inside the network, with an outgoing packet traveling to the external network. In this case, a new, temporary entry will be created to allow the return traffic back into the network. The ingoing traffic will only be permitted if it is part of the session and all other traffic will be denied. This happens because a temporary access list will be created inside the reflexive access list when an outbound TCP packet is forwarded outside of your network. This temporary access list will permit ingoing traffic corresponding to the outbound connection.

Reflexive access lists are similar to other access lists in several ways. As with other access lists, reflexive access lists contain entries that define criteria for permitting IP packets. These entries are evaluated in a top-down process in form until a match occurs. Reflexive access lists have significant differences—for example, they contain only temporary entries. The idea here is to create a reflexive access list that is embedded within the extended access list that is protecting an interface. As stated earlier, temporary entries are created within the reflexive ACL automatically when a new IP session begins and matches a reflexive permit entry (for example, with an outbound packet); the entries are removed when the session ends. Reflexive access lists are not applied directly to an interface. They are placed within an extended named IP access list that is applied to the interface. Reflexive access lists do not have the implicit *deny all* at the end of the list. Remember, they are nested in another access list, so once the reflexive ACL has been processed, the router will continue with the rest of the extended ACL.

The idea of a reflexive access list is to basically create a mirror image of the reflected entry. For example, in Figure 4.8, host0 on network 172.22.114.0 initiates a Telnet session to host1 on network 172.17.0.0. Telnet uses the TCP protocol, therefore host0 will pick a random source port number—let's use port 1028. Also, here we will have a source IP address, destination IP address, and destination TCP port number. Since we are using Telnet, the destination port number will be 23. So far, we have the following information:

Figure 4.8 Example Network Using Reflexive ACLs

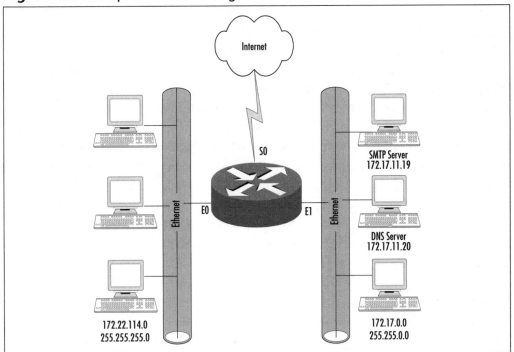

```
Source TCP port-1028
Destination TCP port-23
Source IP address-172.22.114.1
Destination IP address-172.17.0.1
```

In our configuration, we will have a *reflexive access-list* statement that will trigger a reflected access list entry. This will allow inbound return traffic and would look as follows:

```
Source TCP port-23
Destination TCP port-1028
Source IP address-172.17.0.1
Destination IP address-172.22.114.1
```

The following shows our information as a reflected access list entry:

```
permit tcp host 172.17.0.1 eq 23 host 172.22.114.1 eq 1028
```

In the preceding example of a reflected entry, the source and destination address have been swapped, along with the source and destination port numbers giving the "mirror image."

Building Reflexive Access Lists

When building a reflexive access list, we must first design an extended named access list. Remember from earlier that you must use an extended named access list when defining your reflexive access list and there is no implicit *deny all* at the end. Here, we enter a *permit* statement to allow all protocols in which you want a reflected entry created. So, what must we do to indicate a reflexive opening? You need to use the keyword *reflect* in each of your *permit* statements. This tells us that a reflexive opening will occur. The following example shows the format of a reflexive access list.

```
permit protocol source source-wildcard destination destination-wildcard
    reflect name [timeout seconds]
```

Table 4.9 describes reflexive access lists.

Table 4.9 Reflexive Access Lists

Command	Description
Permit	This entry will always use the keyword *permit*.
Protocol	Any TCP/IP protocol supported by an extended named IP access list.
Source	Identifies the host or network from which the packet is being sent. The source can be specified by an IP address or by using the keyword *any* or *host*.
Destination	Identifies the host or network to which the packet is being sent. The destination can be specified by an IP address or by using the keyword *any* or *host*.
Reflect	Allows the *permit* statement to create a temporary opening.
Name	This is the name of the reflexive access list. A name must be specified so the router can add the reflected entries into this list. This list will also be referenced within the ACL that filters traffic coming into the network.
Timeout	Timeout is optional and has a default value of 300 seconds.

The format here is very comprehensible:

- This entry will always use the keyword *permit*. The keywords *permit* and *reflect* work hand in hand. To allow the *permit* statement to create a temporary opening, you must use the *reflect* statement.

- The protocol field can depict any UDP, TCP, IP, and ICMP protocols supported by an extended named IP access list.

- The source field represents the source IP address. Keywords such as *any* and *host* are applicable here.

- The destination field represents the destination IP address. Keywords such as *any* and *host* are applicable here.

- You must include the name of the access list. Remember, a reflexive entry can only be used with an extended IP named access list.

- The timeout field is optional. If no value is specified, a default of 300 seconds will be used. The timeout is necessary when using connection-less protocols such as UDP. UDP offers nothing in the header to determine when the entry should be deleted. When using TCP, the timeout is not used. Instead, the reflexive access list is deleted after receiving a packet with the RST flag set—or when the TCP session closes (both ends have sent FIN packets), the reflexive access list is deleted within five seconds of detecting the bits.

To nest our reflexive access list within an access list, we use the *evaluate* command. By default, an access list does not evaluate. This command is used as an entry in the access list and points to the reflexive access list to be evaluated, therefore traffic entering your network will be evaluated against the reflexive access list.

NOTE

Reflexive access lists are *not* defined like extended access lists. They are created within an extended access list, although you will be able to see the reflexive ACL with the *show ip access-lists* command.

Given the information about the preceding Telnet session, we will be creating three access lists: *Outbound-List*, *Inbound-List*, and *Reflected-List*. The *Outbound-List ACL* will look at the outbound traffic and decide what should be reflected. *Inbound-List ACL* is the access list that will deny all inbound traffic to the network except for the traffic we will be evaluating. *Reflected-List ACL* is the reflexive access list.

```
Router(config)#ip access-list extended Outbound-List
Router(config-ext-nacl)#permit tcp any any reflect Reflected-List
```

```
Router(config-ext-nacl)#exit
Router(config)#ip access-list extended Inbound-List
Router(config-ext-nacl)#evaluate Reflected-List
Router(config-ext-nacl)#exit
```

Now we have created two extended access lists, and one reflexive access list. As traffic leaves our network, it will match the traffic in the *Outbound-List ACL*. The *reflect* statement will add the mirror image entry to the *Reflected-List ACL*. When return traffic is checked against the *Inbound-List ACL*, which runs the *evaluate* command on *Reflected-List ACL*, it will be allowed back to the original host. If the *evaluate* statement was not in place within *Inbound-List ACL*, then no traffic will be allowed back into the network.

Please note that while I have stated that there is not an *implicit deny* at the end of a reflexive access list, there is an *implicit deny* at the end of the *Inbound-List ACL*. If the *implicit deny* was at the end of *Reflected-List ACL*, then the router would never check any other statements that might be in *Inbound-List ACL* after the *evaluate* command.

You can use the keyword *timeout* to specify a timeout period for individual entries. If the timeout field is not used, a default value of 300 seconds is applied. Remember, this will not apply when using TCP. Also keep in mind that when using TCP, the access list will close immediately after receiving the RST bit or within five seconds after both ends have closed the TCP session. The timeout can be set on a line-by-line basis in the extended ACL configuration, or you can set a global timeout with the following command:

```
ip reflexive-list timeout seconds
```

Even though reflexive access lists give more control in our networks, they do have a major shortcoming. Reflexive access lists are only capable of handling single channel applications such as Telnet, which uses a single static port that stays the same throughout the conversation. Reflexive access lists do not offer the ability to support applications that change port numbers in a session. So how do we handle FTP? Normal mode FTP is a multichannel operation that uses one channel for control and the second channel for data transmission and is not supported by reflexive access lists because the server chooses the data port, not the client. If using the passive mode FTP, we can generally have a more favorable result. With passive mode, the server does not perform an active open to the client. Instead, the client uses the command channel to exchange port information. The client then performs an open to the server on an agreed port. So, both of the sessions we just discussed are outbound from the client, and the reflexive access list would create an additional entry. Here we would have success! FTP is not the only protocol that might be a potential problem here. Many other protocols with similar behavior, such as RPC, SQL★Net, Streamworks, and multimedia such as H.323 (Netmeeting, Proshare) will have problems.

Applying Reflexive Access Lists

The first step in applying a reflexive access list is to decide which interface the ACLs should be applied on. While referring to Figure 4.8, we need to determine which interface the ACLs, which we created previously, should be applied to. Because we want to be able to reflect sessions if they go out ethernet1 or serial0, we need to apply both ACLs to the ethernet0 interface as shown here:

```
Router(config)#interface ethernet0
Router(config-if)#ip access-group Outbound-List in
Router(config-if)#ip access-group Inbound-List out
```

Don't be confused by the names and directions in the *access-group* commands. Remember that access lists are applied with respect to the interface. So, any traffic that is heading outbound *from our network* will be considered inbound *to the ethernet0 interface*. The same logic applies to traffic flowing in the opposite direction.

In the preceding example, we must apply both ACLs to the ethernet0 interface, so we can use the reflexive operation regardless of which interface the traffic exits (serial0 or ethernet1). The previous configuration will allow any traffic that originates from the 172.22.114.0 network to the other interfaces, but only packets that are sent in response to that traffic will be allowed back onto the ethernet0 segment.

Normally, when a packet is tested against entries in an access list, the entries are tested in sequential order, and when a match occurs, no more entries are tested. When using a reflexive access list nested in an extended access list, the extended access list entries are tested sequentially up to the *evaluate* command. Then the reflexive access list entries are tested sequentially, and finally the remaining entries in the extended access list are tested sequentially. After a packet matches *any* of these entries, no more entries will be tested.

Context-based Access Control

As discussed earlier, the reflexive access list can only handle single channel applications. This could prove to be detrimental in your enterprise network. Now we will discus how CBAC overcomes some of these issues. Provided in Cisco Secure

Integrated Software, Context-based Access Control (CBAC) includes an extensive set of security features. The idea of CBAC is to inspect outgoing sessions and create temporary openings to enable the return traffic. Sound familiar? We just described a reflexive access list. The difference here is that CBAC can examine and securely handle various types of application-layer information. This is called stateful inspection, because it continually monitors the state of each connection to decide how it should be handled. For example, when the traffic you specify leaves the internal network through an interface, an opening is created that allows returning traffic based on the traffic being part of a data session that was initiated from an internal network. These openings are created when specified traffic exits your internal network through the router and allows returning traffic that would normally be blocked similar to a reflexive access list. The openings also allow additional data channels to enter your internal network back through the router if it is part of the same session as the originating traffic.

With other types of access lists, such as reflexive or extended access lists, traffic filtering is limited to filtering packets at the network layer or transport layer. CBAC examines the network layer and transport layer along with application-layer protocol information to learn about the state of the TCP or UDP session. Some protocols create multiple channels as a result of negotiations used in the control channel, and it is not possible to filter those protocols using only the information available in the IP and transport layers. By examining the information at the application layer, CBAC provides support for some of these protocols. As previously stated, CBAC inspects outgoing sessions and creates temporary openings to enable the return traffic just as a reflexive access list does. However, unlike reflexive access lists CBAC has the ability to make decisions based on the behavior of the application up to and including Layer 7. When using CBAC, the packets are examined when leaving or entering an interface on the router and the information will be placed in a packet state information table. The information may be an IP address and port numbers from Layer 4. This state table is used by CBAC to create a temporary opening in the access list for return traffic. This shows us another difference between CBAC and reflexive access lists. We had to specifically configure an access list to evaluate the reflexive ACL. With CBAC, the router will automatically determine which access lists would block the return traffic and will add the temporary entry as the very first line in the ACL. CBAC also inspects application-layer information to ensure that the traffic being allowed back through the router is applicable. Recall the issue we had with FTP earlier. Reflexive access list could only support passive mode where all communications are initiated from the client. Now we can use normal mode where multiple channels are used. CBAC would observe the outgoing session, then permit the data connection that will be established from the server to the client by creating an opening in the inbound access list. The following is a listing of the protocols where CBAC performs the equivalent function:

- Single-channel TCP
- Single-channel UDP
- CU-SeeME
- FTP
- H.323
- Java applets transported via HTTP
- Microsoft NetShow
- UNIX "r" commands
- RealAudio
- RPC
- SMTP
- SQL*Net
- StreamWorks
- TFTP
- VDOLive

Just as with everything, there are a few limitations when using CBAC.

- Any packets with the router as the source address or destination address will not be inspected. Only TCP and UDP packets are inspected. So traffic originating or in destination for the router itself cannot be controlled with CBAC.
- CBAC cannot inspect IPSec traffic. If the traffic needs to be inspected, the router must be configured as the IPSec tunnel endpoint.

UDP and ICMP traffic is stateless, so CBAC is unable to track state information for these types of sessions. UDP replies are allowed through temporary openings that timeout after a specified period of time, but ICMP traffic must be permitted or denied by extended ACL commands and will not be tracked by CBAC.

The Context-based Access Control Process

The following section describes a sample process of the events that occur when we configure CBAC on a router. We will assume that the router only has two interfaces: One that connects to the internal network we want to protect, and another connecting to the external network. Assume that *outbound* traffic is traveling from the internal to external network, and *inbound* traffic is flowing from the external to the internal network.

- The outgoing packet reaches the router and is evaluated against the outbound access list. If the access list allows the traffic, then it will be inspected by CBAC. Otherwise, it will be dropped and a CBAC inspection will never occur.

- During CBAC inspection, information is recorded, including the source and destination IP address and port numbers. The information is recorded in a state table entry created for the new connection.

- A temporary access list entry is created based on the previous state information. This access list entry is placed at the beginning of the extended access list that is configured to filter inbound traffic.

- This temporary opening is designed to permit inbound packets that are part of the same connection as the outbound packet that was inspected previously. The outbound packet now leaves the interface.

- The return packet is tested against the inbound access list and permitted because of the temporary entry created by CBAC. Here CBAC will modify the state table and inbound access list, if necessary.

- All inbound and outbound traffic in the future will be tested; therefore, the state table access list will be modified as required.

- When the connection is closed, the state table entry is deleted along with the temporary access list.

Configuring Context-based Access Control

There are several steps to follow here. We must specify which protocols you want inspected. We must also specify an interface and direction where the inspection originates. CBAC will only inspect the protocols we specify. As mentioned earlier, we must configure an outbound access list so that CBAC will know what traffic to inspect. This list can be either a standard or extended ACL, but the inbound ACL must be extended. This is because CBAC must have the facility to allow traffic back in based on Layer 4 header information. These steps are:

1. **Choose the interface** Here the decision is to configure CBAC on an internal or external interface, such as Ethernet0 or Serial0. The internal interface is where the client sessions originate. The external interface is where the client sessions exit the router. In the network shown in Figure 4.9, we will be inspecting traffic inbound to the Ethernet interface, and the return ACL will be applied inbound to the Serial interface.

Figure 4.9 Configuring Context-based Access Control

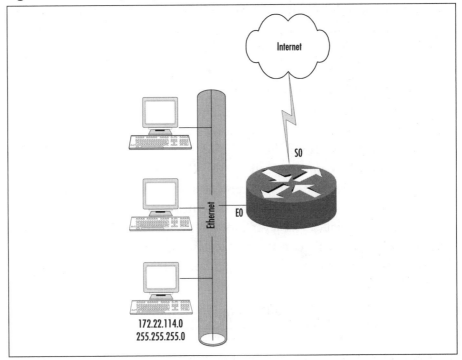

2. **Configure Access Lists** Next, we need to create the access lists for the CBAC configuration. One access list should define all traffic that will be allowed outbound to the Internet. This could be a very specific list, or just a single *permit any* command. The second list that must be created is the inbound list, which controls which traffic should be allowed through regardless of CBAC inspection. For example, you may want to allow certain types of ICMP in, or a connection to a Web server that needs to be initiated from the Internet.

3. **Configuring Global Timeouts and Thresholds** CBAC uses time-outs and thresholds to determine the duration of an inactive session before it is deleted. This helps prevent certain denial of service (DoS) attacks by monitoring the number and frequency of half-open connections. With TCP, a half-open session is one that has not completed the three-way handshake, or if using UDP, a session which the firewall has not detected returning traffic. CBAC counts both TCP and UDP when determining the number of half-open sessions. Half-open sessions are only monitored for connections configured for inspection by CBAC. These timeouts and thresholds apply globally to all sessions. You can use the default timeout and threshold values, or you can change to values more suitable to your security requirements. You should make any changes to the timeout and threshold values before you continue configuring CBAC. Table 4.10 lists available CBAC commands used to configure timeouts and thresholds.

4. **Inspection Rules** After configuring global timeouts and thresholds, you must define an inspection rule. This specifies which application-layer protocols will be tested by CBAC at an interface. Typically, you define only one inspection rule. One exception might be if you want to enable CBAC in two directions. In this case, you should define two rules, one in each direction. The inspection rule should specify each desired application-layer protocol, as well as TCP or UDP, if desired. The inspection rule consists of a series of statements, each listing a protocol and specifying the same inspection rule name.

Table 4.10 Available Timeout Commands and Thresholds

Command	Description	Default Values
ip inspect tcp synwait-time *seconds*	Length of time of wait for TCP session to be established	30 seconds
ip inspect tcp finwait time *seconds*	Length of time TCP is managed after FIN exchange	5 seconds
ip inspect tcp idle-time *seconds*	TCP idle timeout	3600 seconds
ip inspect udp idle-time *seconds*	UDP idle timeout	30 seconds

Continued

Table 4.10 Continued

Command	Description	Default Values
ip inspect dns-timeout *seconds*	DNS lookup idle timer	5 seconds
ip inspect max-incomplete high *number*	Max number of half-open connections before CBAC begins closing connections	500 sessions
ip inspect max-incomplete low *number*	Max number of half-open connections causing CBAC to stop closing connections	400 sessions
ip inspect one-minute high *number*	Rate of half-open sessions per minute before CBAC begins closing connections	500 sessions
ip inspect one-minute low *number*	Rate of half-open sessions per minute causing CBAC to stop deleting connections	400 sessions
ip inspect tcp max-incomplete host *number* block-time *seconds*	Number of existing half-open sessions with the same destination address before CBAC begins closing sessions	50 sessions

Inspection Rules

The following is the format for defining inspection rules:

```
ip inspect name inspection-name protocol [alert {on|off} [audit-trail
     {on|off}][timeout seconds]
```

The keyword *alert* allows CBAC to send messages to a syslog server when a violation occurs in a monitored application. Each application will have an individual alert that the router will send to the server for illegal conditions. The keyword *audit trail* permits the tracking of connections used for a protected application. Here, the router logs information about each connection, including ports used, number of bytes transferred, and source and destination IP address. A key issue here is if a large amount of traffic is being monitored, the logging produced will be significant!

www.syngress.com

Applying the Inspection Rule

Now that we have defined the inspection rule, the final step is to apply it to an interface. You will apply the inspection rule the same way you apply access lists on the interface. You must also specify inbound (for traffic entering the interface) or outbound (for traffic exiting the interface). The command is as follows:

```
ip inspect inspection-name {in | out}
```

The following is an example of Java blocking. A list of permitted IP addresses must be created using a standard IP access list. The following is an example:

```
access-list list-number {permit | deny} source-address [wildcard-mask]
    [log]
```

```
ip inspect name inspection-name http [java-list access-list] [alert
    {on | off}] [audit-trail {on | off}] [timeout seconds}
```

By default, an undefined access list in the java-list definition will deny all Java applets. CBAC can only block Java applets and not ActiveX.

There are several commands that are useful in gathering information about CBAC. The *show ip inspect config* command will be discussed first. This command allows all specific portions of a configuration. The following is an example:

```
Router# show ip inspect config
Session alert is enabled
One-minute (sampling period) thresholds are [400:500] connections
max-incomplete sessions thresholds are [400:500]
max- incomplete tcp connections per host is 50.
Block-time 0 minute.
tcp synwait-time is 30 sec - tcp finwait - time is 5 sec
tcp idle - time is 3600 sec - udp idle - time is 30 sec
dns - timeout is 5 seconds
```

The *show ip inspect interfaces* command shows the interfaces where CBAC inspection is configured. Here's an example:

```
Router# sh ip inspect interfaces
Interface FastEthernet 3/0
Inbound inspection rule is Protector
tcp alert is on audit-trail is off timeout 3600
udp alert is on audit-trail is CBAC off timeout 30
```

```
fragment Maximum 50 In Use 0 alert is on audit-trail is off timeout 1
Inbound access list is 114
Outbound access list is not set
```

Refer to the "Protecting Public Servers Connected to the Internet" section for the required configuration for CBAC.

Configuring Port to Application Mapping

A limitation of CBAC is the fact that only services running on standard ports can be controlled. For example, traffic going to a Web server running on a port other than the standard HTTP port (80) cannot be inspected and protected using CBAC. Port to Application Mapping (PAM) can be used to override this limitation. PAM gives you the capability to customize TCP or UDP port numbers for network services or applications. Upon startup, PAM will build a table of ports associated with their default application, known as a PAM table or database. Kept in this table are all of the services supported by CBAC. Here is where the link with CBAC comes into play. The information built into the PAM table will give CBAC the ability to function on a non-standard port. If you are running applications on non-standard ports, PAM and CBAC have the ability to work together to identify the ports associated with their applications. Without the use of PAM, CBAC is limited to well-known ports and their applications.

PAM comes standard with the Cisco Secure Integrated Software Feature Set. Network services or applications that use non-standard ports will require you to place entries in the PAM table manually. You can also specify a range of ports used by an application by establishing a separate entry in the PAM table for each port number in the range. All manual entries are saved with the default mapping information when you save the router configuration, so upon startup, the mapping will be in the PAM table. If you use an application that requires a non-standard port, you will need to enter this manually in the PAM table (for example, if you use the Telnet application with port 8000 instead of port 23).

Configuring PAM

When configuring PAM, the following format is used:

ip port-map application_name **port** port-number

The following is a mapping for well-known port 23 (Telnet) to port 8000, and may look as follows:

```
ip port-map telnet port 8000
```

Now let's take this example a step farther and define a range of non–standard ports for use with telnet. An example may look as follows:

```
ip port-map telnet port 8001
ip port-map telnet port 8002
ip port-map telnet port 8003
ip port-map telnet port 8004
```

We also have the option of mapping an application to a port for a specific host or subnet. Mapping an application to a host would look as follows:

```
access-list 1 permit host 172.16.144.1
ip port-map telnet port 8000 list 1
```

When mapping to a specific subnet, the list may look like this:

```
access-list 1 permit 172.16.144.0 0.0.0.255
ip port-map telnet port 8000 list 1
```

Protecting a Private Network

In this section, we will apply some of the concepts we discussed in this chapter to different situations. Please keep in mind that these solutions are meant to demonstrate the application of some of the different security techniques available in a Cisco router, and may not present the most secure or appropriate solution possible. Currently, CBAC is the most secure means of protecting your network, but the licensing cost for the firewall feature set (CBAC) may cause you to decide to use some other feature when deploying security on your network. You will have to weigh your options and decide which solution works best for your network.

In this first example, we are assuming a simple connection between two companies over a point-to-point T1 connecting to the Serial0 interface on your router. As far as this exercise is concerned, we either do not have an Internet connection, or we are using a separate device to secure the Internet connection, which we need not worry about here. We are focusing on securing the connection between our company, Company A, and the remote company, Company B.

Although the risk of being hacked is considerably less from a single company as compared with an Internet connection, we still need to apply some sort of security to prevent access to unauthorized services. Figure 4.10 shows a basic layout of this connection. I purposefully did not show anything beyond the router of Company B because in most cases you will not know the topology of the other company's network. You will know the next hop router you are connecting to, but nothing beyond that point. The following is a summary of requirements that need to be properly secured:

1. All hosts belonging to Company A need to be able to access 10.150.200.5 on TCP port 1000.

2. Host 172.20.100.130 needs access to 10.150.150.56 on TCP port 1299.

3. Company B server 10.150.100.5 needs to have access to 172.20.100.155 on TCP ports 13000 thru 13010.

4. Company B server 10.150.100.6 needs to have access to 172.20.100.156 on TCP port 12050.

Figure 4.10 Connection to a Private Network

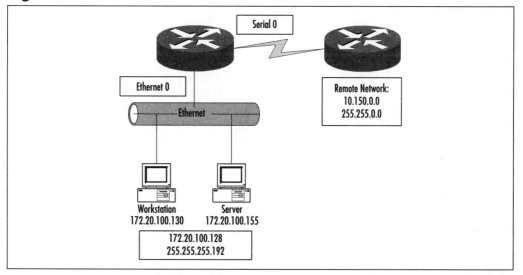

Fortunately, we have a fairly strict set of requirements defining the access between these two companies. This means that we can lock down the access lists to prevent unauthorized access to certain servers. For example, we know that only one server needs access to our 172.20.100.155 server, so we do not need to define the entire 10.150.0.0 subnet access to our servers.

We could filter traffic down to this specific list only using extended access lists, but we will use reflexive access lists to allow us to add a little extra security to the network. That way we do not have to define statements for return traffic that would be always open; we can just allow the reflexive list to handle that part. The reflexive list will prevent someone from having full access to our subnet if they source the packets from 10.150.200.5:1000. This is because if we were going to allow the return traffic through by hand, we would have to create an access list entry that permitted the one server on port 1000 to access our entire subnet on any port. The reflexive list will only allow traffic through if it is response traffic coming from, and going to, a very specific port, and the session was originated from our network.

Since we only have two interfaces on this router, we will apply the ACL that filters outgoing (from our network) traffic on Ethernet0 in the inbound direction. This will allow us to drop traffic we do not wish to pass before it reaches the route engine within the router. This will save CPU cycles. Also, we will apply the ACL that filters incoming traffic in the inbound direction on Serial0 for the same reasons as before.

The following is the configuration we will need to create to protect our network.

```
interface Ethernet0
ip address 172.20.100.129 255.255.255.192
ip access-group ToCompanyB in


interface Serial0
ip address 172.16.0.1 255.255.255.252
ip access-group FromCompanyB in


ip access-list extended ToCompanyB
   evaluate EstSessionB
   permit tcp 172.20.100.128 0.0.0.63 host 10.150.200.5 eq 1000 refelct
      EstSession
   permit tcp host 172.20.100.130 host 10.150.150.56 eq 1299 reflect
      EstSession
   deny ip any any log


ip access-list extended FromCompanyB
   evaluate EstSessionA
   permit tcp host 10.150.100.5 host 172.20.100.155 range 13000 13010
      reflect EstSessionB
```

```
   permit tcp host 10.150.100.6 host 172.20.100.156 eq 12050 reflect
      EstSessionB
deny ip any any log
```

Notice that we are reflecting in both directions. We could have easily allowed any access out of our network, but since we had a small and strict list of communications that should be allowed, we are securing both networks. We may not have a responsibility to protect Company B's network, but by doing so, we are decreasing the liability that our company is exposed to should one of our employees try to hack into a server at Company B.

Also be aware that we manually entered the *deny ip any any* statement so that we could use the *log* keyword with it. This will allow us to see any traffic that is denied by our access list and see if someone is attempting to find a way around it.

Protecting a Network Connected to the Internet

This next example will cover how to put basic protection in place when you have connected your network to the Internet. Due to the security risks associated with attaching your network to the Internet, we will use the Firewall IOS (CBAC) to secure our network. Another reason we would rather use CBAC is to cause less problems with applications that are in use on the network. For example, people may need to download files from an FTP server, or use RealAudio to stream a newscast. CBAC can handle these applications, while reflexive access lists cannot.

The following is the configuration we will use to protect our network, which is shown in Figure 4.11:

```
ip inspect name CompanyA-FW tcp
ip inpsect name CompanyA-FW udp
ip inspect name CompanyA-FW ftp
ip inspect name CompanyA-FW http
ip inspect name CompanyA-FW realaudio

interface ethernet 0
  ip address 10.150.130.0 255.255.255.0
  ip access-group Outbound in
  ip inspect CompanyA-FW in

interface serial 0
```

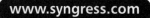

```
    ip address 192.168.5.1 255.255.255.252
    ip access-group Inbound in

ip access-list extended Outbound
    permit ip 10.150.130.0 0.0.0.255 any
    deny ip any any log

ip access-list extended Inbound
    permit icmp any 10.150.130.0 0.0.0.255 echo-reply
    permit icmp any 10.150.130.0 0.0.0.255 traceroute
    permit icmp any 10.150.130.0 0.0.0.255 time-exceeded
    permit icmp any 10.150.130.0 0.0.0.255 unreachable
    deny ip any any log
```

Figure 4.11 A Network Attached to the Internet

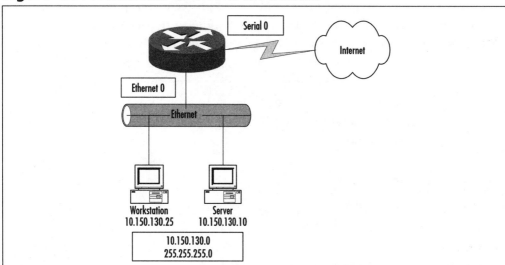

The previous configuration will allow all IP traffic outbound to the Internet. If we are worried about someone running a VPN connection from our network, we could allow protocols such as TCP, UDP, and ICMP but deny all other IP traffic. In this case, we do not care where our users go. One protective step we did take was to only allow traffic that is sourced from our subnet to be allowed through the router. We have done this to prevent someone on our network from launching an attack with spoofed source addresses. The only address spoofing that could make it through the router is if a host spoofed their address to an address used by another host on our network.

The CBAC portion of this will keep a state for all traffic that flows out to the Internet and allow the responses back in. As you can see, we specifically told CBAC to inspect FTP, HTTP, and RealAudio traffic because we think our users may be running applications that use those protocols. The other protocols CBAC can handle, such as SQLNet, are not expected to originate from our users toward the Internet. If we find that we need to use one of these protocols in the future, we can quickly and easily add another command to the inspect list.

We have also allowed specific types of ICMP traffic back through the router for troubleshooting purposes. While we don't want someone on the Internet to be able to ping our hosts, we do want to receive replies to the pings and tracer-outes that we send into the Internet. In addition to only allowing our users' replies to their pings, they can also see when a TTL has expired on their packets, indicating a routing loop, as well as unreachable messages if there are other routing or access problems somewhere on the Internet.

Protecting Server Access Using Lock-and-key

As a continuation of our last example, we need to allow two of our users access to a particular server from outside our network. This access will not be constant, so we do not want to make a permanent entry into our access lists. The best way to perform this with the tools we have available will be to use a lock-and-key access list. We are working in the same network shown in Figure 4.11, and the configuration from the previous example is applied, so we will need to modify our configuration to allow this access through.

Our two employees need to access the 10.150.130.10 server on port 110 (POP3) from their home computers. This will allow them to pull their e-mail from the server across the Internet, while prohibiting access to the mail server from everywhere else. We will be setting a very short idle timeout on the dynamic entry (one minute) because the user will only need to authenticate and then download his e-mail once during that session. If an e-mail has a large file attach-ment, the temporary entry will stay in place while the download occurs, but will be deleted after no traffic passes through for one minute. Since our users only need access from their home machines, we won't need to configure the dynamic ACLs to allow users to authenticate from everywhere (using the *any* keyword), and we can further reduce our risks by tightening down the dynamic lists. Their ISPs use DHCP, so they won't have the same IP every time they connect, but we do know which subnets our two users will be connecting from: 172.20.128.0 255.255.252.0, and 172.21.64.0 255.255.255.254.0.

After making the changes to our configuration, it should look like this:

```
username bill password needmyemail
username bill autocommand access-enable host timeout 1
username susan password letmein
username susan autocommand access-enable host timeout 1
username admin password supersecret


ip inspect name CompanyA-FW tcp
ip inpsect name CompanyA-FW udp
ip inspect name CompanyA-FW ftp
ip inspect name CompanyA-FW http
ip inspect name CompanyA-FW realaudio
!
interface Ethernet 0
 ip address 10.150.130.0 255.255.255.0
 ip access-group Outbound in
 ip inspect CompanyA-FW in
!
interface Serial 0
 ip address 192.168.5.1 255.255.255.252
 ip access-group Inbound in
!
ip access-list extended Outbound
  permit ip 10.150.130.0 0.0.0.255 any
  deny ip any any log
!
ip access-list extended Inbound
  permit icmp any 10.150.130.0 0.0.0.255 echo-reply
  permit icmp any 10.150.130.0 0.0.0.255 traceroute
  permit icmp any 10.150.130.0 0.0.0.255 time-exceeded
  permit icmp any 10.150.130.0 0.0.0.255 unreachable
  permit tcp 172.20.128.0 0.0.3.255 host 192.168.5.1 eq telnet
  permit tcp 172.21.64.0 0.0.1.255 host 192.168.5.1 eq telnet
  dynamic POPAccess permit tcp 172.20.128.0 0.0.3.255 host 10.150.130.1
```

```
      eq 110
   dynamic POPAccess permit tcp 172.21.64.0 0.0.1.255 host 10.150.130.1
      eq 110
   deny ip any any log
!
line vty 0 4
login local
exec-timeout 15 0
```

Protecting Public Servers Connected to the Internet

Our final example covers a situation when you not only have users that need protection while accessing the Internet, but also have servers that need to be accessed by anyone on the Internet, such as Web and mail servers. In this case, it is best to divide your network into two separate entities: an internal network and a DMZ.

The whole purpose of the DMZ is to protect the rest of your network in case one of your servers is compromised. When you have a publicly accessible server, such as your Web server or mail server, you must allow complete access on the port that is being used, such as port 80 for the Web. This increases your chances of being attacked since you cannot limit who is able to access your server. Even if a hacker is able to gain control of your box through the Web port, they still cannot access your internal network, because it is protected from the DMZ. If you had your public Web server on your internal network and someone gained control of it, that person would have complete access to all other hosts on your network. The DMZ serves as a way to isolate your public servers from your private ones.

The network shown in Figure 4.12 has the internal network on Ethernet0, the DMZ network on Ethernet1, and our Internet connection on Serial0. In a case where we have public servers, we definitely need to use the best security available to us, so we will use CBAC to protect this network. The configuration will be somewhat different from the other configurations we have covered, because we will have both inbound and outbound ACLs on both Ethernet interfaces and an inbound list on the serial interface, which gives us a total of five access lists. We are configuring the router this way because once you have more than two interfaces, the easiest approach for securing your networks is to look at each interface and decide what should be allowed through it in each direction. We will cover these lists one by one after we take a look at the configuration that follows.

Figure 4.12 A Network with a DMZ and Internet Connection

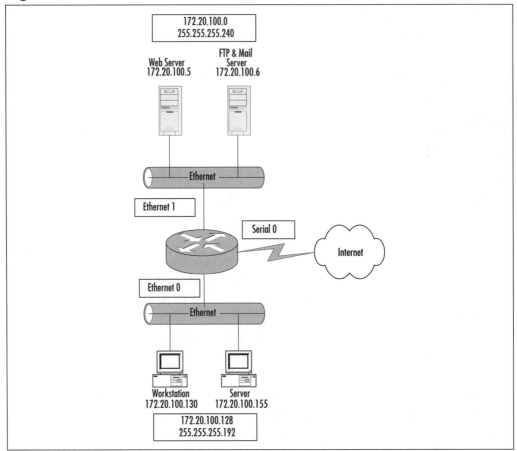

```
ip inspect name DMZ-FW tcp
ip inspect name DMZ-FW ftp
ip inspect name DMZ-FW http
ip inspect name DMZ-FW smtp
ip inspect name Internal-FW tcp
ip inpsect name Internal-FW udp
ip inspect name Internal-FW http
ip inspect name Internal-FW ftp
ip inspect name Internal-FW smtp
ip inspect name Internal-FW realaudio
```

```
interface ethernet 0
 ip address 172.20.100.129 255.255.255.192
 ip access-group Eth0-in in
 ip access-group Eth0-out out
 ip inspect Internal-FW in

interface ethernet 1
ip address 172.20.100.1 255.255.255.240
ip access-group Eth1-in in
ip access-group Eth1-out out
ip inspect DMZ-FW out

interface serial 0
 ip address 192.168.5.1 255.255.255.252
 ip access-group Serial-in in

ip access-list extended Eth0-in
  permit ip 172.20.100.128 0.0.0.63 any
  deny ip any any log-input

ip access-list extended Eth0-out
  permit icmp any 172.20.100.128 0.0.0.63 echo-reply
  permit icmp any 172.20.100.128 0.0.0.63 packet-too-big
  permit icmp any 172.20.100.128 0.0.0.63 time-exceeded
  permit icmp any 172.20.100.128 0.0.0.63 unreachable
  deny ip any any log-input

ip access-list extended Eth1-in
  permit icmp 172.20.100.0 0.0.0.15 any echo-reply
  deny ip any any log-input

ip access-list extneded Eth1-out
  permit tcp any host 172.20.100.5 eq www
  permit tcp any host 172.20.100.6 eq ftp
  permit tcp any host 172.20.100.6 eq smtp
  permit tcp 172.20.100.128 0.0.0.63 host 172.20.100.6 eq pop3
```

```
  permit icmp any 172.20.100.0 0.0.0.15 echo

  permit icmp any 172.20.100.0 0.0.0.15 echo-reply

  permit icmp any 172.20.100.0 0.0.0.15 packet-too-big

  permit icmp any 172.20.100.0 0.0.0.15 time-exceeded

  permit icmp any 172.20.100.0 0.0.0.15 unreachable

  deny ip any any log-input


ip access-list extended Serial-in

  deny ip 172.20.100.0 0.0.0.15 any log-input

  deny ip 172.20.100.128 0.0.0.63 any log-input

  permit ip any any
```

Now we will cover each section of this configuration individually. First, we have the *ip inspect* rules that are configured. We have created two rules: one for the DMZ, and another for our internal network. Both networks could be protected by a single inspect list, but we have tailored each one to fit the types of traffic expected for each network. Our DMZ farm only accepts TCP connections for HTTP, SMTP, and FTP, so those are the only protocols configured for inspection. Our internal network, on the other hand, will need inspection for UDP, and possibly other protocols such as RealAudio, so we have created a separate inspection list for the internal network.

When securing our two networks, we have used a different approach for each one. Our internal network is protected using the same logic as our previous example: Our users are permitted to go anywhere they want, but only responses to our traffic should be let back into our network, as well as a few types of ICMP to allow us to troubleshoot connectivity issues. The only difference between the two examples is the placement of the access lists. On the two-interface router in Figure 4.11, we configured one list on the Ethernet interface, and the second on the Serial interface. On our three-interface router in Figure 4.12, we have put both the inbound and outbound access lists on the Ethernet interfaces. It ends up being much simpler to secure a network with more than two interfaces with this approach because we are applying the security at the choke point. Traffic that is received on our Ethernet0 interface can either be routed to the ethernet1 interface, or the Serial0 interface. Much less administrative work is needed if we have a single list on Ethernet0 to handle the return traffic, instead of two lists: one on Ethernet1 and one on Serial0.

The DMZ network has security applied in the opposite direction. Because these servers are publicly accessible and exposed to more risk than our internal network, we want to be very strict about what traffic is allowed to originate from that network. We are allowing anyone to access the DMZ servers on a list of specific ports (HTTP, FTP, and so on) but we only want to allow response traffic back out from our DMZ. This is the opposite behavior we applied to our internal network, where only response traffic is allowed back in. If someone manages to take control of one of our DMZ servers, they will not be able to initiate any attacks, since only response traffic is allowed from them. Keep in mind that this means our DMZ servers will not have access to the Web, so if you need to download a patch, you will need to use another means of transferring the file, such as having an internal host upload it to the FTP server on the DMZ, or copy it to a floppy disk or CD and loading it directly onto the server.

To help in your understanding of how we are restricting traffic flows through our router, we will cover each access list one by one.

- **Eth0-in** This ACL checks traffic going into our Ethernet0 interface, meaning that it watches traffic sent from our internal hosts. This is a very basic list that allows all traffic from our internal network as long as it is sourced from the appropriate subnet. This will prevent spoof attacks from being launched inside our network, since the router will drop any packets not sourced from our assigned subnet. Any packets allowed through this ACL will be inspected by CBAC and the return traffic will be allowed through the Eth0-out interface.

- **Eth0-out** This ACL filters traffic coming back into our internal network. We have allowed certain types of ICMP to come back into the network, by default, because CBAC is not able to perform state checks on ICMP traffic. We do not want to remove our ability to ping other hosts outside of our network, but we also don't want to be exposed to the entire ICMP suite, so we are only allowing reply packets that can tell us about common problems found on the Internet, such as unreachable destinations and TTL expired packets, which signal a possible routing loop. All other traffic is denied because CBAC will allow response traffic back through by adding temporary entries at the top of this list.

- **Eth1-in** This is the list that decides which traffic should be allowed to originate from the DMZ hosts. As mentioned earlier, we do not want our public servers to be able to initiate connections anywhere because that will prevent our servers from being used as a launch pad if a hacker manages to gain control of it.

- **Eth1-out** This list defines what traffic is allowed to reach our DMZ. This should cover all the services we are providing with these servers. The Web site, FTP site, and mail (SMTP) server should be publicly accessible from anywhere on the Internet. The only restricted service is POP3, which only allows people to download e-mail messages if they are coming from our internal network. Again, we are restricting the types of ICMP that can enter our network, but in this case, we are also allowing echo so that people can ping the servers to test for connectivity. Anything allowed through this list is inspected by CBAC and allowed to return back through the Eth1-in access list.

- **Serial-in** This access list only has one basic function: To prevent certain types of spoofing attacks from outside our network. If any packets enter our serial interface (in the inbound direction), which are sourced from an address that is part of our internal network or DMZ, they will be dropped before they can be forwarded to either network. Hackers may try using one of our addresses as the source for their packets in an attempt to bypass our access lists. For example, if a packet was sourced from our internal network, it will be passed through the POP3 rule on our DMZ network. To prevent hackers from slipping malicious packets through our access lists rules, we must make sure that addresses on our network can only be sourced from one of our Ethernet interfaces.

Security Alert!

Keep in mind that ICMP can be a very useful and very dangerous protocol. You will have to decide if you really want ICMP access allowed within your network. ICMP is very useful for troubleshooting connectivity issues, but hackers can also use ICMP to try and gather information about your network. The more information someone is able to gather about how you are configured, the easier time they will have finding a flaw to exploit. It is also very important to be aware of the fact that a firewall is not the end-all solution for security. In this example, we must allow unrestricted access to port 80 on our Web server. At this point, the firewall will have absolutely no affect on any attacks that exploit flaws in the web server software, since the hackers have open access to your server on port 80. To help reduce this risk, we would need to install an application layer gateway that could filter malformed HTTP requests before they reach the Web server.

Summary

As we have seen, Cisco offers a variety of methods for securing your network at the router. For basic traffic filtering, we have the option to use standard and extended access lists. These can be especially useful in protecting the router itself when a firewall behind the router is protecting your network. For example, you may want to deny all traffic being sent to the router except for the BGP session coming from the next upstream hop.

Lock-and-key and reflexive access lists were designed to help solve some of the shortcomings of the basic access lists by allowing dynamic entries to be placed in the ACL. This is especially useful when you want to protect your network but still allow return traffic back through the router. Although the *established* keyword was meant for this purpose, these new additions provided a much more secure method of performing the same task.

Of course, as people continually find new ways to break through the latest security techniques, networking and security companies continually develop new ways to secure a network. CBAC was created to help bring additional security to the router platform. CBAC is designed to watch the state of all sessions passing through the router so that attackers have a harder time fooling the router into letting a packet through. Although CBAC is not impenetrable, it is one of the most secure methods of protecting a network that is currently offered by Cisco. As time passes, we can be sure that as new vulnerabilities are found, new ways to defend against them will be implemented into the devices that carry the data over our networks.

Solutions Fast Track

Access Lists

☑ Standard access lists only filter on source address, while extended access lists can filter based on much more information, such as source address, destination address, source port, destination port, and protocol number, to name a few.

☑ Access lists can either be named or numbered. Named access lists were created to make access list administration easier by allowing them to be better identified and allowing the deletion of a single line.

☑ When applying access lists, make sure to think about them with respect to the interface they will be applied on. If you are blocking inbound traffic on the serial interface, all other interfaces connected to the router will still have full access to each other. For example, if you block Telnet sessions coming inbound through your serial interface, a host on the Ethernet interface could still Telnet to the router.

Lock-and-key Access Lists

☑ Allows authenticated access through an access list via a Telnet session.

☑ The *autocommand* feature can be used to prevent users from entering the wrong commands. This can be done across all VTY ports, or on a per-user basis.

☑ Remember to use the *host* keyword with the *access-enable* command, or else the entire dynamic ACL will be opened, instead of one particular host address.

☑ Be sure your inbound access list doesn't restrict Telnet access to your router, or else you will not be able to use the lock-and-key feature.

☑ You can only create one dynamic access list per extended access list. Anything beyond the first one will be ignored. You can have multiple entries using the same *dynamic-name* in an extended ACL.

☑ Dynamic access lists must have different names from any other named access lists defined in the router.

Reflexive Access Lists

☑ Allows increased security by only allowing traffic through an ACL if it is a response to a request initiated from inside your network.

☑ Reflexive ACLs can only look at transport layer (Layer 4) information when deciding what traffic should be allowed into the network. This can cause problems with applications such as FTP, if it is not running in passive mode.

☑ There are three separate parts to a reflexive access list: the inbound ACL, outbound ACL, and the reflexive ACL. The reflexive portion of the ACL is not defined like a regular access list, but created within an extended ACL.

☑ Cannot be used with applications that change port numbers during a session or ask a server to initiate a connection back towards the client on a different port.

Context-based Access Control

☑ Provides more protection than reflexive access lists, because it keeps a detailed state table of all connections through the router, while reflexive access lists only add a mirror image of an extended ACL to the reflexive list.

☑ CBAC is able to read the application layer data for certain applications such as FTP and RealAudio. This allows for more flexibility and security in your router because you are not faced with the choice of making large openings in your access lists versus not using a particular application.

☑ Requires you to create an inspect list to specify which applications CBAC should watch for. When using CBAC as an Internet firewall, your minimum configuration should include TCP and UDP inspection to allow basic connectivity to the Internet. Other inspection statements may need to be configured to allow certain applications to function properly.

Configuring Port to Application Mapping

☑ Allows you to configure known services on nonstandard ports for use with CBAC.

☑ PAM can be configured on a per-host basis, which allows only certain hosts to access a service on the configured port. Hosts can also use different services on the same port number if PAM is configured this way.

☑ You cannot assign a service to a system-defined port. For example, you cannot configure Telnet to run on port 25, which is SMTP.

Frequently Asked Questions

The following Frequently Asked Questions, answered by the authors of this book, are designed to both measure your understanding of the concepts presented in this chapter and to assist you with real-life implementation of these concepts. To have your questions about this chapter answered by the author, browse to **www.syngress.com/solutions** and click on the **"Ask the Author"** form.

Q: I have created an access list, but it does not seem to have any affect. Why?

A: Once you've created your access list, be sure you apply it to an interface with the *ip access-group interface* command. Also make sure that you apply your access list at the appropriate interface. If you apply a list inbound on the Serial0 interface, traffic flowing from Ethernet0 to Ethernet1 will not be checked against that access list.

Q: After applying an access list on your enterprise router, there has been a drastic decrease in throughput. What could be a potential problem here?

A: First recall how an access list works. An access list utilizes "top-down" processing when testing traffic. Typically, access lists can get quite lengthy on an enterprise router. A problem here could be that the majority of your traffic is permitted or denied near the end of the access list. When creating an access list, it is important to test the majority of your traffic first.

Q: I am using reflexive access lists and traffic is being allowed back into my network that I am specifically denying with my inbound ACL. How can I fix this?

A: Make sure you have placed your *evaluate* statement correctly. If you want traffic to be denied even when one of your users has initiated the connection, be sure to place that *deny* statement before the *evaluate* statement. Once the first match is found, whether it is in the inbound ACL, or the evaluated ACL, the router will not process any farther.

Q: I forgot to set a timeout on my lock-and-key access list, and now I have entries that will not expire. It is peak usage time for this router and I do not want to reboot it, but I need to remove this entry. How can I do this without bringing down my network?

A: Cisco has added a command specifically to delete temporary entries if they don't have a timeout, or if they need to be removed before a timeout has expired. This command is used in privileged exec mode and has the syntax *clear access-template* [*access-list number* | *name*] [*dynamic-name*] [*source-address*] [*destination-address*].

Q: How do I know CBAC is working properly?

A: You can check to see if CBAC is making any changes by doing a *show ip access-list* command. When you view the ACL with that command, you should see a bunch of entries at the top of the list that you didn't put there. If you view the list under *show running-config*, you will see your access list as you originally wrote it.

## Chapter 5

Network Address Translation/Port Address Translation

Solutions in this chapter:

- **NAT Overview**

- **NAT Architectures**

- **Guidelines for Deploying NAT and PAT**

- **IOS NAT Support for IP Telephony**

- **Configuring NAT on Cisco IOS**

- **Considerations on NAT and PAT**

☑ **Summary**

☑ **Solutions Fast Track**

☑ **Frequently Asked Questions**

233

Introduction

In today's world of enterprise networks, one of the major problems facing IT professionals is the rapidly depleting supply of globally unique Internet network addresses. Measures have been taken to slow the rate at which IP addresses are being allocated—including strategies such as Classless Inter-Domain Routing (CIDR), Network Address Translation (NAT), and Port Address Translation (PAT). This chapter will discuss NAT and PAT and how they can contribute to a security policy, the implications of NAT, and considerations when implementing NAT.

Network Address Translation is designed for IP address simplification and conservation. It enables private IP networks that use non-registered RFC1918 IP addresses to connect to the Internet. NAT operates on a device, usually connecting two networks together, that allows them to communicate. Typically, one network uses RFC1918 IP addresses, which are translated into globally unique IP addresses. Other scenarios in which NAT can be utilized will be discussed later in this chapter.

NAT by itself is not a security measure and should not be implemented in such a fashion. A common misconception is that NAT will allow a company to "hide" its internal network. This can be an added security benefit, but should not be relied upon as the only security measure. Although typical private networks use addresses that are never intended to be publicly issued, a company's ISP may have knowledge of that particular network. If routing between the company and the ISP is not done properly, a route to the company may be leaked throughout the ISP, possibly exposing its network to the public.

NAT Overview

Generally, NAT is used when a company's internal addresses are not globally unique and thus cannot be routed on the Internet (for instance, using RFC1918 private addresses), or because two separate networks which need to communicate are using an overlapping IP address space.

NAT allows (in most cases) hosts in a private network (inside network) to transparently communicate with destination hosts (outside network) in a global or public network. This is achieved by modifying the *source address* portion of an IP packet as it traverses the NAT device. The NAT device will keep track of each translation (conversation) between the source host (inside network) and destination host (outside network), and vice versa. This means that NAT is a stateful technique and devices implementing NAT are stateful devices.

Throughout this chapter and in the Cisco documentation, networks will be described as being either an *inside* network or an *outside* network. An *inside* network is the set of networks subject to translation. All other networks are considered *outside* networks.

One of the variations of NAT is PAT. This solution only works if the application does not rely on an IP address in the data portion of the packet for functionality. In such cases, Application Layer Gateways included inside the NAT (discussed later) may be needed to assist a NAT device.

The following is a list of terms used when referring to NAT and their descriptions. Keep in mind that different vendors may refer to these terms in varying contexts.

Address Realm

An address realm is a network in which the network addresses (IP addresses) are uniquely assigned to hosts so traffic can be routed to them. Routing protocols used within the network are responsible for routing traffic to the destination network. Often referred to as *inside* and *outside* networks, address realms help define zones which are separated and need to communicate with each other. For example, a company's internal network could be seen as one address realm. This realm is under a single administrative authority which needs to communicate with networks outside its jurisdiction. These outside networks, which could be another company's network or even the Internet, are also considered address realms. The definition of realm will vary depending on the context in which it is used.

Designing & Planning…

RFC 1918 Private Addressing

Throughout this chapter, we have discussed private addressing and the mysterious RFC 1918. Now would be a good time to discuss exactly what private addressing is and how RFC 1918 is involved with all of it. To begin, though, we need a brief history lesson.

The Internet, as we know it today, can trace its roots back to the Department of Defense's DARPA Project in the late 1960s and early 1970s. The original Internet was envisioned to consist of only a few organizations with a limited number of hosts utilizing it. As such, efficient

Continued

address allocation was not a primary consideration. The early to mid 1990s saw exponential growth in the utilization of networking. This growth, fueled by the increased home and business use of the Web, caused IP address allocation to grow at an alarming rate, to the point where the limited address space capacity began to be a serious concern. In order to counter this, RFC 1918 was proposed.

RFC 1918 proposed that three groups of IP addresses be set aside for organizations to use on their internal networks. The private address allocation is as follows:

- One Class A network address: 10.0.0.0 with 16277216 possible host addresses
- 16 Class B network addresses: 172.16.0.0 thru 172.31.0.0, each with 65526 possible host addresses
- 256 Class C network addresses: 192.168.0.0 thru 192.168.255.0, each with 256 possible host addresses

These address spaces are available to any organization that wishes to use them. In fact, if your organization is medium to large in size, you are very likely utilizing one of these address spaces already. A couple of key points to remember when utilizing them are:

- These addresses CANNOT be advertised on the Internet or to other outside networks. Although almost every service provider has provisions and safeguards built into there networks to prevent such an occurrence, imagine the traffic that an organization would face if they received all of the traffic destined for these generic private networks
- In order to communicate to outside networks, a NAT device must be incorporated in order to translate private addresses to valid global IP addresses. This can come in the form of a router or firewall device.
- Devices outside of the internal network will not be able to see resources such as Web or e-mail servers, and will require utilization of NAT coming into the network, or utilization of a demilitarized zone (DMZ) between the internal and external networks.

Private addressing is a very useful and efficient solution for a growing network. It allows an administrator to utilize an internal network-addressing scheme exclusive to the addresses given a company by its ISP. Also, it gives organizations a great deal of flexibility in the selection of an

Continued

ISP. By utilizing private addressing space, an organization can easily change from one ISP to another with very little reconfiguration, usually only on the network edge devices. Overall, RFC 1918 private addressing offers scalability and flexibility to organizations of almost every size and, as such, is a viable solution for organizations.

NAT

The basic configuration of NAT operates on a device which connects two networks together. One of these networks (designated as "inside") is addressed with either private RFC 1918 addresses or others which need to be converted into legal addresses before packets are forwarded to their destination network (designated as "outside").

NAT is a method by which IP addresses are mapped from one Address Realm to another. This type of translation provides transparent routing from host to host. There are many variations of address translation that assist in translating different applications; however, all NAT implementations on various devices should share the following characteristics:

- Transparent address assignment

- Transparent routing through address translation (routing refers to forwarding packets and not exchanging routing information)

- ICMP error packet data translation

Transparent Address Assignment

NAT translates addresses from an "inside" network to addresses in an "outside" network, and vice versa. This provides transparent routing for the traffic traversing both networks. The translation in some cases may extend to transport level identifiers such as TCP/UDP ports. Address translation is done at the start of a session. The following describes two types of address assignment:

- **Static address assignment** Static address assignment is a one-to-one address mapping for hosts connecting an "inside" network with an "outside" network for the duration of the NAT session. Static address assignment ensures that the translation table is static and not dynamic. Using static address assignment, your internal host is visible from the outside network since it is always assigned the same global IP address. This can be useful for some applications, but care must also be taken to secure each machine.

- **Dynamic address assignment** Dynamic address assignment is the process in which addresses are translated by the NAT device dynamically based on usage requirements. Once a NAT is no longer being used, it is terminated. NAT then frees that translation so the global address can be used in another translation.

Transparent Routing

Transparent routing refers to routing traffic between separate address realms (from an "inside" network to an "outside" one), by modifying address contents in the IP header to be valid in the address realm into which the traffic is routed to. A NAT device is placed at the border between two address realms and translates addresses in IP headers so that when the packet leaves one realm and enters another, it can be routed properly. Typically, there are three phases to address translation.

- **Address Binding** Address binding is the phase in which an "inside" IP address is associated with an "outside" address, or vice versa. This assumes that dynamic NAT is being used and not static NAT. Address binding is fixed, with a pool of assigned static addresses. These addresses are dynamically assigned on a per-session basis. For example, whenever a host on the "inside" network must reach another host on the "outside" network, it will begin a session with that host. A translation will occur on the NAT device associating a global IP address on the "outside" network with the IP address of the host on the "inside" network. Once a session is created, all traffic originating from the same "inside" host will use an identical translation. The start of each new session will result in the creation of a new translation. A NAT device will support many simultaneous sessions. (Consult the vendor's documentation for specific information.)

- **Address Lookup and Translation** Once a translation is established for a session, all packets belonging to the session will be subject to address lookup and translation.

- **Address Unbinding** Address unbinding is the phase in which an "inside" host IP address is no longer associated with a global address. NAT will perform address unbinding when it believes the last session using an address binding has terminated.

An example of transparent routing is when a Company's "inside" network uses the subnet 192.168.1.0/24, and the "outside" network uses the subnet 207.139.221.0/24. Transparent routing would occur on the device that separates the two subnets. Instead of using a router to route packets based on destination address, NAT alters the source address of an IP packet originating from the "inside" network and changes it to a valid IP address in the "outside" network. The NAT device then builds a table to keep track of the translations that have occurred to maintain communications between a host on the "inside" network and a host on the "outside" network. Figure 5.1 illustrates this example.

Figure 5.1 NAT Translation

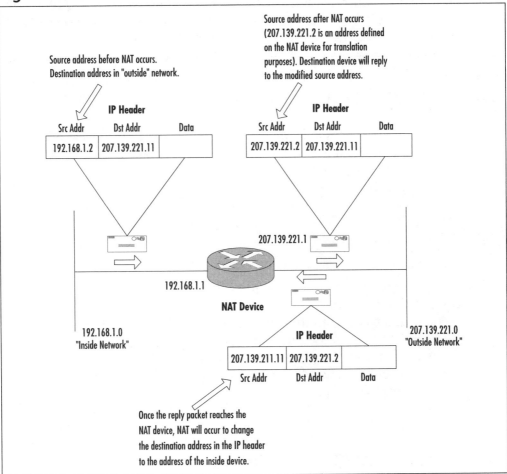

Public, Global, and External Networks

A global, public, or external network is an address realm with a unique network address assigned by the Internet Assigned Numbers Authority (IANA), or an equivalent address registry.

NOTE

Do not confuse public, global, and external networks with the term "outside" network. "Outside" is more of a generic term to describe a destination network in which NAT must occur in order to communicate with that network. "Outside" networks may refer to networks using global IP addresses, but it may also refer to the destination network in a situation where both networks use private IP addresses.

Private and Local Networks

A private or local network is an address realm independent of external network addresses. A private or local network uses IP addresses specified in RFC 1918. These addresses are private and therefore should never be used globally. Transparent routing between hosts in a private realm and external realm is made possible by a NAT device.

NOTE

Do not confuse private and local networks with the term "inside" network. As with the term "outside" network, "inside" network is more of a generic usage to describe the source network in which NAT must occur in order for two hosts to communicate. An "inside" network may refer to a network that uses the private IP addresses (RFC1918), but it may also refer to the source network used by a NAT device to communicate between global IP addresses.

Application Level Gateways

Not all applications are easily translated by NAT devices. This is especially true of those that include IP addresses and TCP/UDP ports in the data portion of the packet. Simple NAT may not always work with certain protocols. This is why most modern implementations of NAT include Application Layer Gateway functionality built in. Application Level Gateways (ALGs) are application-specific translation agents that allow an application on a host in one address realm to connect to another host running a translation agent in a different realm transparently. An ALG may interact with NAT to set up state, use NAT state information, alter application-specific data, and perform whatever else is necessary to get the application to run across different realms.

For example, recall that NAT and PAT can alter the IP header source and destination addresses, as well as the source and destination port in the TCP/UDP header. RealAudio clients on the "inside" network access TCP port 7070 to initiate a conversation with a RealAudio server located on an "outside" network and to exchange control messages during playback such as pausing or stopping the audio stream. Audio session parameters are embedded in the TCP control session as a byte stream. The actual audio traffic is carried in the opposite direction (originating from the RealAudio server, and destined for the RealAudio client on the "inside" network) on ports ranging from 6970 to 7170.

As a result, RealAudio will not work with a traditional NAT device. One workaround is for an ALG to examine the TCP traffic to determine the audio session parameters and selectively enable inbound UDP sessions for the ports agreed upon in the TCP control session. Another workaround could have the ALG simply redirecting all inbound UDP sessions directed to ports 6970 thru 7170 to the client address on the "inside" network.

ALGs are similar to proxies in that both ALGs and proxies aid application-specific communication between clients and servers. Proxies use a special protocol to communicate with proxy clients and relay client data to servers and vice versa. Unlike proxies, ALGs do not use a special protocol to communicate with application clients, and do not require changes to application clients.

NAT Architectures

There are many variations of NAT that aid to different applications. The following is a list of some of the variations of NAT.

Traditional NAT or Outbound NAT

Traditional NAT is a dynamic translation that allows hosts within the "inside" network to transparently access hosts in the "outside" network. In traditional NAT, the initial outbound session is unidirectional (one-way)—outbound from the private network. Once a session has been established with a device on the "outside" network, bidirectional communication will occur for the duration of that session.

IP addresses of hosts in the "outside" network are unique, while IP addresses of hosts in the "inside" network use RFC 1918 private IP addresses. Since the IP addresses of the "inside" network are private and cannot be used globally, they must be translated into global addresses.

A traditional NAT router in Figure 5.2 would allow Host A to initiate a session to Host Z, but not the other way around. Also, the address space from the global address pool used on the "outside" is routable, whereas the "inside" address space cannot be routed globally.

Figure 5.2 Traditional NAT

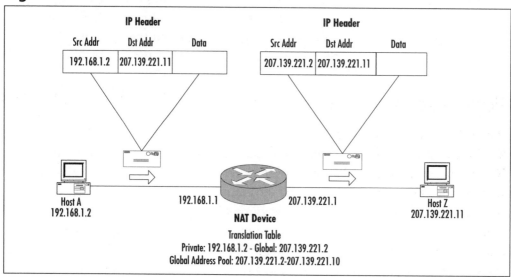

Figure 5.3 shows the reply packets sent by Host Z to Host A. Since Host A originated a session from inside, any packets originating from Host Z in response to Host A will be permitted provided that the security rules on the NAT device permit it. If Host Z attempted to initiate a session with Host A, traditional NAT will not permit this because Host A has a private IP address. This IP address is reserved for private networks and will therefore never be routed globally. From the perspective of Host Z, Host A's IP address is 207.139.221.2 (the translated address). If Host Z attempts to initiate a session with this IP address, the NAT device will not be able to associate 207.139.221.2 with an "inside" IP address with traditional NAT. In order to allow Host Z to initiate a session with Host A, Static NAT (explained later) will need to be configured.

Figure 5.3 A Traditional NAT Reply

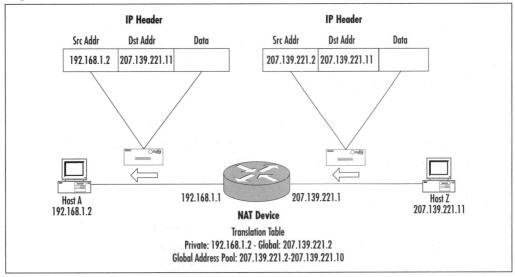

Port Address Translation

Port Address Translation (PAT) extends the concept of translation one step further by also translating transport identifiers like TCP and UDP port numbers, and ICMP query identifiers. This allows the transport identifiers of a number of private hosts to be multiplexed into the transport identifiers of a single global IP address. PAT allows numerous hosts from the "inside" network to share a single "outside" network IP address. The advantage of this type of translation is that only one global IP address is needed, whereas with NAT, each "inside" host must translate to a unique "outside" IP address.

> **NOTE**
>
> Both NAT and PAT can be combined. The advantage being that when NAT exhausts the pool of global IP addresses, PAT can then be used until one of the NAT translations times out. This method ensures that all "inside" hosts can be successfully translated into "outside" global IP addresses.

Figure 5.4 illustrates PAT. Host A on the "inside" network needs to communicate with Host Z on the "outside" network. Because these two hosts are on different networks and the "inside" network uses IP addresses from a private address space, NAT/PAT is needed to allow the two hosts to communicate. Unfortunately, the administrator only has a limited number of global IP addresses, many of which have already been assigned to various devices. Therefore, NAT cannot be used for translations. As an alternative, PAT can be used instead.

Figure 5.4 PAT

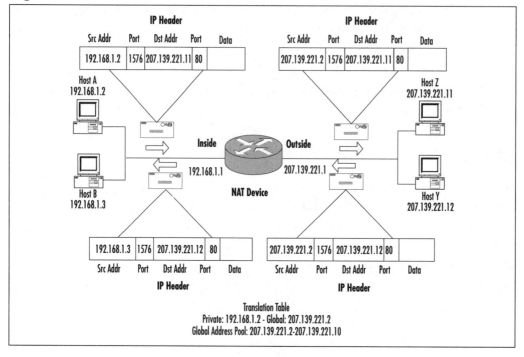

The steps taken in order to perform PAT are:

1. Host A attempts to initiate a session with Host Z. Since Host Z is not on the same network as Host A, Host A must send the packet to the router (default gateway) in order for it to be routed correctly.

2. Once the packet reaches the "inside" interface of the router in which PAT is enabled, the router examines the translation table for an existing translation. Since this is a new session, the router creates a new translation record in the table. Since only one IP address is assigned to the pool of IP addresses to translate to, a unique port number is added to the *source address*. This will allow the router to keep track of the translation for the duration of the session: PAT Global 207.139.221.2(1576) Local 192.168.1.2

The router then alters the IP header and changes the source address to the IP address of the "outside" interface of the router.

3. The packet is then transparently routed to Host Z.

4. Host Z replies to Host A by sending the packet to the "outside" interface of the router (*destination address*).

5. Once the packet reaches the "outside" interface, the router examines the IP header, checks the translation table for an existing translation. Since a translation already exists in the table, the router changes the destination address to the IP address of Host A.

6. The process is repeated until the session between Host A and Host Z is terminated.

Static NAT

With static NAT, sessions can be initiated from hosts in the "inside" or "outside" network. "Inside" addresses are bound to globally unique addresses using static translations since the connections are established in either direction. A translation that occurs from the "inside" network to the "outside" network will be translated with the statically configured address on the NAT device. When a session must be established from an "outside" network to an "inside" network, the static translation must already be manually set up on the router. By creating a static translation, you are translating an "inside" IP address to a fixed "outside" global IP address. This translation will never change and will always remain in the translation table. For example, if there is a resource on the "inside" network that must be made accessible to the "outside" network, the global IP address of the resource can be advertised worldwide through the DNS. Since this resource has been statically translated into a global IP, this IP can be advertised in a DNS record. If the resource is a mail server, an MX record may be created in the company's zone associating the MX record with the global IP that was statically assigned to the resource in the "inside" network. By doing this, even though the mail server is not physically located in the "outside" network, it can still be accessed as if it were.

Figure 5.5 illustrates a static NAT translation. A session is initiated from Host Z on the "outside" network. Since the NAT device has a static translation for Host A's IP address to a global IP address, the NAT device can forward the packet from Host Z to Host A's static NAT public IP address. Recall that with traditional or outbound NAT, a session can only be initiated from the "inside" host, which causes a dynamic translation to occur on the NAT device. Once this translation has been created, only then can the "outside" host reply back to the "inside" host. Once the session times out, the "inside" host will need to start a new session with the "outside" host causing the NAT device to create a new translation and possibly allocating a new global IP address to the "inside" host for the duration of the session (if NAT is used). With a static NAT, the translation is always active; the global IP address will never be allocated dynamically to another host on the "inside" network for translation purposes.

Figure 5.5 Static NAT

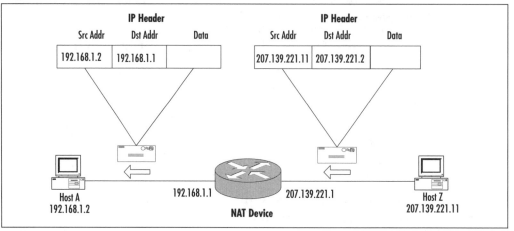

NOTE

Using this type of configuration to allow global access to resources has security-related advantages. If the NAT device is a Cisco PIX firewall or Cisco Router running FW IOS, Access Control Lists can be used to limit the type of traffic permitted to reach the resource. Compare this with having a server that is physically placed in the "outside" network allowing global access. In this case, limiting the type of traffic would be very difficult, if not impossible, creating a security risk.

Twice NAT

Twice NAT is a variation of NAT in that both the source and destination addresses are modified by the NAT device as the packet crosses address realms. Compare this to traditional NAT where only one of the addresses (either source or destination) is translated when traversing the NAT device.

Twice NAT is necessary when both "inside" and "outside" networks have overlapping address space. Although this type of problem does not occur often, a need for Twice NAT would arise when two companies merge their networks together and use overlapping address spaces, or when a company chooses an IP subnet that is already in use on the Internet. Figure 5.6 illustrates Twice NAT.

Figure 5.6 Twice NAT

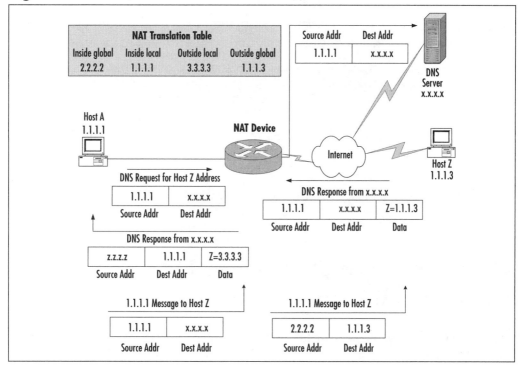

The router performs the following process when translating overlapping addresses:

1. The device Host 1.1.1.1 opens a connection to Host C by DNS name. A name-to-address lookup request is sent to DNS server x.x.x.x.

2. The router intercepts the DNS reply and translates the returned address (data portion of packet) if there is an overlap (that is, the resulting legal address resides illegally in the "inside" network). To translate the return address, the router creates a simple translation entry mapping the overlapping address 1.1.1.3 to an address from a separately configured, outside local address pool.

NOTE

The router examines every DNS reply, ensuring that the IP address is not in the "inside" network. If it is, the router translates the address.

3. Host 1.1.1.1 opens a connection to 3.3.3.3.

4. The router sets up translations mapping inside local and global addresses to each other, and outside global and local addresses to each other.

5. The router replaces the source address with the inside global address and replaces the destination address with the outside global address.

6. Host C receives the packet and continues the conversation.

7. The router does a lookup, replaces the destination address with the inside local address, and replaces the source address with the outside local address.

8. Host 1.1.1.1 receives the packet and the conversation continues, using this translation process.

Guidelines for Deploying NAT and PAT

When deploying NAT and PAT in a network, there are many things to take into consideration. Various factors will contribute to which type of NAT is used, factors such as the number of available global IP addresses for translations, or whether the "inside" network uses global or RFC 1918 IP addresses. The following outlines some general guidelines for deploying NAT.

-   How many public IP addresses are available for translation from "inside" IP addresses? If there are only a limited number of global IP addresses for many "inside" hosts (for example, 8 global addresses for 250 "inside" hosts), PAT, or a combination of dynamic NAT and PAT, may be necessary.

-   Router performance needs to be considered for all types of NAT. NAT increases the time it takes for a packet to arrive at a destination address. When a packet traverses a NAT device, the IP header must be modified. This is currently done using process switching which places considerable load on the system.

- What type of addressing scheme is being used on the "inside" network? Are private RFC 1918 addresses being used? If so, then NAT will need to occur for the "inside" network(s) to be able to reach the "outside" networks.

- Not all applications will work with NAT. Be aware of what type of traffic will be translated and if the functionality of those applications will be affected by NAT. If this is the case, an ALG may need to be implemented to assist in the translation process. Application types that do not need an ALG, or where an ALG is built into Cisco's NAT implementation, are listed later in this chapter. Not all applications can be used with ALGs.

- A disadvantage of NAT is the loss of end-to-end IP connectivity. It becomes much harder to trace packets that undergo numerous IP address changes over multiple NAT hops. On the other hand, an advantage to this is that it becomes difficult if not impossible for hackers to determine a packet's source to trace or obtain the original source or destination addresses.

Designing & Planning...

What Applications Need an ALG?

ALGs (Application Level Gateways) have been mentioned several times throughout this chapter, but the question of what applications may or may not need an ALG has not been answered. The following lists summarize traffic types that may or may not be supported in Cisco IOS NAT.

Some examples of traffic types supported in the Cisco IOS NAT are as follows:

- Any TCP/UDP traffic that does not carry source and/or destination IP addresses in the data portion of an IP packet.
- HTTP
- TFTP
- Telnet
- Archie
- Finger

Continued

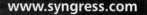
www.syngress.com

- NTP
- NFS
- rlogin, rsh, rcp

Although the following traffic types carry IP addresses in the data portion of an IP packet, Cisco IOS NAT will provide ALG functions for the following applications:

- ICMP
- FTP (including PORT and PASV commands)
- NetBIOS over TCP/IP
- RealAudio
- CuSeeMe
- Streamworks
- DNS name-lookup queries and reverse name-lookup queries.
- H.323/NetMeeting (IOS 12.0(1)/12.0(1)T or later)
- H.323 v2 (IOS 12.1(5) or later)
- Selsius Skinny Client Protocol (IOS 12.1(5) or later)
- VDOLive (IOS 11.3(4), 11.3(4)T or later)
- Vxtreme (IOS 11.3(4), 11.3(4)T or later)
- IP Multicast (IOS 12.0(1)T source address translation only)

The following traffic types are not currently supported by Cisco IOS NAT:

- Routing table updates
- DNS zone transfers
- BOOTP
- Talk, ntalk
- SNMP
- NetShow

Some guidelines to follow for implementing static NAT are:

- How many "inside" devices need to be statically translated? Remember that each global IP used for static translations cannot be used for dynamic translations.

■   A security policy should be in place to limit the type of traffic permitted to reach that statically translated device. When an "inside" device is statically translated into a global IP address, any devices on the "outside" networks can initiate a session with the "inside" device.

IOS NAT Support for IP Telephony

Recent enhancements to the Cisco IOS support for Network Address Translation have allowed the support for several of Cisco's converged and IP telephony product solutions. Some of the technologies that these newly expanded features support include:

■   H.323 v2

■   Call Manager Support

■   Session Initiation Protocol (SIP)

H.323 v2 Support

Previous to IOS release 12.1(5), Cisco IOS NAT support of the H.323 standard was limited solely to the support of H.323 v1 implementation for Microsoft Net meeting. However, with the release of 12.1(5) and later, NAT supports version H.323 v2. Although a detailed discussion of the H.323 protocol is outside the scope of this chapter, a brief introduction is in order. H.323 is an industrywide, open standard for real-time audio, video, and data over packet networks. H.323 is an ITU-T standard and is part of the H.32x family of protocols. Cisco's IP telephony architecture can use H.323 to communicate with IP phones and IP telephony gateways. In addition, because it is an open protocol, it can be used to communicate with dissimilar systems such as PBXs and other vendors' equipment.

This support also includes the H.225 and H.245 message types, as well as Fast Connect and Alerting messages. The support for H.323 v2 NAT does not, however, include support for Registration Admission and Status messages (RAS), which is a messaging format for gateway-to-gateway communications. The IOS version of PAT does not support H.323 in any of its versions, so NAT is the only solution for this technology. However, Version 6.2 of the PIX software will support it. No added configuration is required in order for the IOS to support H.323 NAT; only the correct IOS release is required.

CallManager Support

Cisco CallManager is the IP PBX component of the Cisco Architecture for Voice Video and Integrated Data, or AVVID as it is commonly known. Cisco CallManager communicates connection information with the endpoint IP phones through the use of a protocol known as *Skinny Station Protocol*. Skinny Station Protocol is also often used to connect the CallManager servers with gateway devices; however, its primary use remains that of communicating between IP phones and CallManager servers.

NAT support for CallManager/Skinny Station Protocol also came with the release of the 12.1(5) IOS. This support allows a router running NAT to be placed between the CallManager server(s) and the IP telephone set. When the IP phone performs a session request, the router will detect the Skinny Station Protocol request and automatically perform the port translation. This functionality is present with no configuration on IOS 12.1(5). However, if you wish to use a TCP port other than the default port, you can use the *ip nat skinny service tcp port* command. Once again, this functionality is limited to NAT; PAT cannot support this.

Session Initiation Protocol

Session Initiation Protocol or SIP is an alternative to H.323 messaging for Voice over IP (VoIP) and similar real-time transmission protocols. Like H.323, it provides support for call setup and processing in an IP environment. Session Description protocol (SDP) is a protocol that resides within SIP and is used for control and creation of multimedia sessions.

NAT support for SIP and SDP came with the release of the 12.2(8) IOS software. NAT can allow SIP/SDP messages to pass through the router and encode the messages back to the original at the packet level. In order for NAT to work with SIP and SDP, an Application Level Gateway (ALG) must be incorporated. NAT support for SIP is automatic with IOS 12.2(8), however the port used by NAT for SIP can be changed by use of the *ip nat service* command. PAT support is not available for this solution in the IOS, but it is available in the 6.2 version of the PIX firewall software.

Configuring NAT on Cisco IOS

Cisco's implementation of NAT functionality on a router is fundamentally the same as the implementation of NAT on a PIX firewall (PIX was covered in

Chapter 3). Performance-wise, the NAT session limit on a router depends on the amount of DRAM available on the router, and the load on the router. Each NAT translation consumes approximately 160 bytes of DRAM. As a result, ten thousand translations would consume about 1.6MB. This should not impose a burden on a typical router provided it is not overloaded by other processes. PAT, as described previously, is handled differently. The translations occur with one global IP address. The translation table maintains each translation by assigning a unique port number to each translation. Since TCP/UDP port numbers are encoded in 16 bits, there are theoretically 65,536 possible values, resulting in 65,536 simultaneous sessions for each protocol.

The following section will outline the commands necessary to implement, and verify, NAT operation on a Cisco router. The commands necessary to configure NAT on the Cisco PIX firewall differ from the ones used in the IOS. These commands will be covered in detail in Chapter 3.

Configuration Commands

This section will cover the commands necessary to implement NAT on a Cisco router. The configuration commands necessary to implement NAT on a Cisco Secure PIX firewall will be covered in the next chapter.

Before NAT can be implemented, the "inside" and "outside" networks must be defined. To define the "inside" and "outside" networks, use the *ip nat* command.

```
ip nat inside | outside
```

- **Inside** Indicates the interface is connected to the inside network (the network is subject to NAT translation).
- **Outside** Indicates the interface is connected to the outside network.

Mark the interface as being on the inside or outside realms with the following:

```
interface ethernet0
ip nat inside
```

Enter interface configuration mode and designate *ethernet0* as the "inside" network interface.

```
interface serial1
ip nat outside
```

Enter interface configuration mode and designate *serial0* as the "outside" network interface.

Once the "inside" and "outside" network interfaces have been defined, an access list must be created to define the traffic that will be translated. This will only define the traffic to be translated and will not control any NAT functions by itself. To create an access list, use the *access-list* command:

```
access-list access-list-number permit source [source-wildcard]
```

- **Access-list-number** Number of an access list. This is a decimal number from 1 to 99.

- **Deny** Denies access if the conditions are matched.

- **Permit** Permits access if the conditions are matched.

- **Source** Number of the network or host from which the packet is being sent. Use the keyword *any* as an abbreviation for source 0.0.0.0 and source-wildcard 255.255.255.255.

- **Source-wildcard** (optional) Wildcard bits to be applied to the source. Use the keyword *any* as an abbreviation for source 0.0.0.0 and source-wildcard 255.255.255.255.

```
access-list 10 permit ip 192.168.1.0 0.0.0.255 any
```

This specifies that traffic originating from the 192.168.1.0 subnet destined for any other network should be translated. By itself, the access list will not translate the specified traffic.

A pool of IP addresses must be defined for dynamic NAT translations. To do this, use the *ip nat* command:

```
ip nat pool name start-ip end-ip {netmask netmask | prefix-length
    prefix-length} [type rotary]
```

- **Name** Name of the pool.

- **Start-ip** Starting IP address for range of addresses in address pool.

- **End-ip** Ending IP address for range of addresses in address pool.

- **Netmask** *netmask* Specify the netmask of the network to which the pool addresses belong.

- **Prefix-length** *prefix-length* Number that indicates how many bits of the netmask are ones.

- **Type-rotary** (optional) Indicates that the range of addresses in the address pool identify real, inside hosts where TCP load distribution will occur.

Define a pool of global addresses to be allocated as needed.

```
ip nat pool net-208 207.139.221.10 207.139.221.128 netmask >255.255.255.0
```

Specifies a pool of global IP addresses with the name *net-208* will contain the range of IP addresses 207.139.221.10 thru 207.139.221.128.

To enable NAT for the inside destination address, the *ip nat inside destination* command will be used:

```
ip nat inside destination list {access-list-number | name} pool name
```

- **list** *access-list-number* Standard IP access list number. Packets with destination addresses that pass the access list are translated using global addresses from the named pool.
- **list** *name* Name of a standard IP access list.
- **pool** *name* Name of the pool from which global IP addresses are allocated during dynamic translation.

```
ip nat pool net-208 207.139.221.10 207.139.221.128 netmask >255.255.255.0
```

Define a pool of global IP addresses called *net-208* with the IP addresses 207.139.221.10 thru 207.139.221.128.

```
access-list 10 permit any 204.71.201.0 0.0.0.255
```

Specify that traffic destined for the network address 204.71.201.0 will be translated to global addresses defined in the pool *net-207*.

```
ip nat inside destinationn list 10 pool net-207
```

Enable NAT for traffic defined in access list 10 to be translated to addresses from the *net-207* pool. This will translate the destination address, not the source.

To enable NAT for the inside source address, use the *ip nat inside source* command.

```
ip nat inside source {list {access-list-number | name} pool name
   [overload] | static local-ip global-ip
```

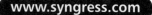

- **List *access-list number*** Standard IP access list number. Packets with source addresses that pass the access list are dynamically translated using global addresses from the named pool.

- **List *name*** Name of the standard IP access list.

- **Pool *name*** Name of the pool from which global IP addresses are allocated dynamically.

- **Overload** (optional) Enables the router to use one global address for many local addresses (PAT).

- **Static *local-ip*** Sets up a single static translation.

- **Global-ip** Sets up a single static translation. This argument establishes the globally unique IP address which an inside host will be translated to.

Establish dynamic source translation using an access list to define the traffic to be translated based on source address.

```
ip nat pool net-207 207.139.221.10  207.139.221.128  netmask 255.255.255.0
```

Define a pool of IP addresses with the name *net-207* and a range of IP addresses from 207.139.221.10 thru 207.139.221.128.

```
access-list 10 permit ip 192.168.1.0 0.0.0.255 any
```

Specify that traffic originating from the 192.168.1.0 network will be translated.

```
ip nat inside source list 10 pool net-207
```

Enable dynamic NAT for traffic defined in access list 10 to be translated to addresses from the *net-207* pool. This will translate the source address and not the destination address. To enable static NAT translation for the "inside" host 192.168.1.10 to the global IP address 207.139.221.10 use the following command:

```
ip nat inside source static 192.168.1.10 207.139.221.10
```

To enable PAT in conjunction with, or instead of, NAT:

```
ip nat pool net-207 207.139.221.10  netmask 255.255.255.0
```

Define a single global IP address with the name *net-207* and an IP address of 207.139.221.10.

```
access-list 10 permit ip 192.168.1.0 0.0.0.255
```

Specify that traffic originating from the 192.168.1.0 network will be translated.

```
ip nat inside source list 10 pool net-207 overload
```

Enable PAT for traffic defined in access list 10 to be translated to the address defined in the *net-207* pool. This will translate the source address. To enable NAT of the outside source address, use the *ip nat outside source* command:

```
ip nat outside source {list {access-list-number | name} pool name | static
    global-ip local-ip}
```

- **List** *access-list-number* Standard IP access list number. Packets with source addresses that pass the access list are translated using the global addresses from the named pool.

- **List** *name* Name of a standard IP access list.

- **Pool** *name* Name of the pool from which global IP addresses are allocated.

- **Static** *global-ip* Sets up a single static translation. This argument establishes the globally unique IP address assigned to an outside host.

- **Local-ip** Sets up a single static translation. This argument establishes the local IP address of an outside host as it appears to the inside world.

```
ip nat translation {timeout | udp-timeout | dns-timeout | tcp-timeout |
    finrst-timeout} seconds
```

- **Timeout** Specifies that the timeout value applies to dynamic translations except for overload translations. Default is 86400 seconds (24 hours).

- **Udp-timeout** Specifies that the timeout value applies to the UDP port. Default is 300 seconds (5 minutes).

- **Dns-timeout** Specifies that the timeout value applies to connections to the Domain Naming System. Default is 60 seconds.

- **Tcp-timeout** Specifies that the timeout value applies to the TCP port. Default is 86400 seconds (24 hours).

- **Finrst-timeout** Specifies that the timeout value applies to Finish and Reset TCP packets, which terminate a connection. Default is 60 seconds.

- **Seconds** Number of seconds the specified port translation times out.

```
ip nat translation timeout 300
```

This example specifies that translations will timeout after 300 seconds (5 minutes) of inactivity.

```
ip nat translation timeout 600
```

This specifies that NAT translations will timeout after 600 seconds (10 minutes) of inactivity.

Verification Commands

The following are commands used to verify the operation of NAT on a Cisco router.

- **show ip nat statistics** Displays NAT statistics.

- **show ip nat translations [verbose]** Displays NAT translations, where *verbose* optionally displays additional information for each translation table entry, including how long ago the entry was created and used.

The following is a sample output from the *show ip nat statistics*. Table 5.1 outlines the significant fields in the sample output.

```
Router#show ip nat statistics
Total translations: 2 (0 static, 2 dynamic; 0 extended)
Outside interfaces: Serial0
Inside interfaces: Ethernet1
Hits: 135  Misses: 5
Expired translations: 2
Dynamic mappings:
— Inside Source
access-list 1 pool net-208 refcount 2
 pool net-208: netmask 255.255.255.240
        start 171.69.233.208 end 171.69.233.221
        type generic, total addresses 14, allocated 2 (14%), misses 0
```

Table 5.1 Explanation of the Significant Fields from the *show ip nat statistics* Sample Output

Field	Description
Total translations	Number of translations active in the system. This number is incremented each time a translation is created and is decremented each time a translation is cleared or times out.
Outside interfaces	List of interfaces marked as outside with the *ip nat outside* command.

Continued

Table 5.1 Continued

Field	Description
Inside interfaces	List of interfaces marked as inside with the *ip nat inside* command.
Hits	Number of times the software does a translations table lookup and finds an entry.
Misses	Number of times the software does a translation table lookup, fails to find an entry, and must try to create one.
Expired translations	Cumulative count of translations that have expired since the router was booted.

Configuring NAT between a Private Network and the Internet

Company XYZ management has decided to allow employees access to the Internet. A leased line to their ISP has been purchased and installed, and a Cisco router has been purchased to route the company's internal traffic to their ISP. The ISP has assigned a range of 128 global IP addresses (207.139.221.0/25) to the company to use as they see fit. Administrators have used a private 192.168.1.0/24 subnet for their internal hosts. Figure 5.7 illustrates the design.

Figure 5.7 NAT and the Internet

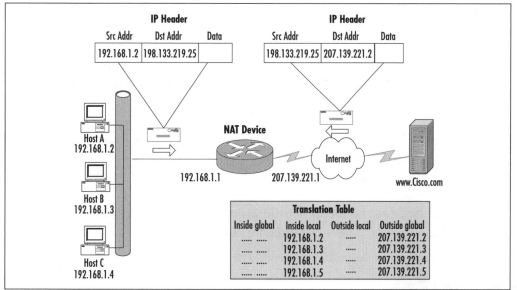

Here are the steps to follow for the configuration example, with explanations for clarification as you go through the commands:

```
configure terminal
interface ethernet0
ip address 192.168.1.1 255.255.255.0
```

This assigns an IP address to *ethernet0 interface*.

```
ip nat inside
```

This designates *ethernet0 interface* as an "inside" network.

```
no shutdown
```

This serves to remove the interface from shutdown state.

```
interface serial0
ip address 207.139.221.1 255.255.255.128
Assign IP address to serial0 interface.ip nat outside
```

This designates *serial0 interface* as an "outside" network.

```
no shutdown
```

This removes the interface from shutdown status.

```
exit
access-list 10 permit ip 192.168.1.0 0.0.0.255
```

This specifies that traffic originating from the 192.168.1.0 network will be translated.

```
ip nat pool net-207 207.139.221.2  207.139.221.126  netmask 255.255.255.128
```

This defines a pool of global IP addresses named *net-207* with an address range of 207.139.221.2 thru 207.139.221.126 to be used for NAT.

```
ip nat pool net-207-PAT  207.139.221.127  netmask 255.255.255.128
```

This defines a single global IP address named *net-207-PAT* with address 207.139.221.127 to be used for PAT.

```
ip nat inside source list 10 pool net-207
```

This specifies that the source IP address of traffic defined in access list 10 will be NAT'd with IP addresses defined in the *net-207* pool.

```
ip nat inside source list 10 pool net-207-PAT  overload
```

Lastly, this specifies that the source IP address of traffic defined in access list 10 will be PATed with IP addresses defined in *net-207-PAT* pool. PAT will occur once NAT has used all available addresses in the *net-207* pool. Once a translation has timed out due to inactivity, that global IP address will be reused for future NAT translations.

Configuring NAT in a Network with DMZ

Company XYZ has decided to host both a Web server and an e-mail server on their LAN. They would like to make these servers publicly available yet provide full security for them. It has been decided that a demilitarized zone (DMZ) will be created to keep the servers separated from the company's local LAN. The Cisco router currently used has an additional Ethernet port which will be designated as the DMZ. The DMZ subnet will use the private IP address space of 192.168.2.0/24, while the Web server and e-mail server will be statically translated into two global IP addresses currently used in the NAT global pool. Figure 5.8 illustrates the new scenario.

Figure 5.8 NAT with DMZ

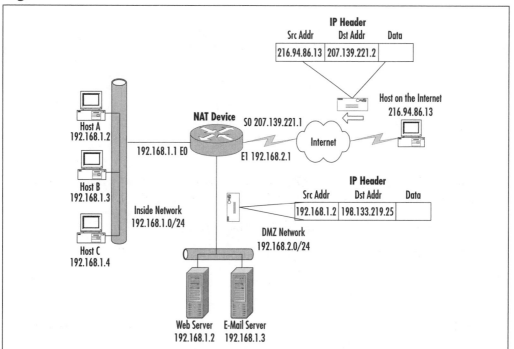

Here are the steps to follow, with explanations of the commands:

```
configure terminal
interface ethernet0
ip address 192.168.1.1 255.255.255.0
```

This assigns an IP address to *ethernet0 interface*.

```
ip nat inside
```

This designates *ethernet0 interface* as an "inside" network.

```
no shutdown
```

This removes the interface from shutdown status.

```
interface serial0
ip address 207.139.221.1 255.255.255.128
```

This assigns the IP address to *serial0 interface*.

```
ip nat outside
```

This designates *serial0 interface* as an "outside" network.

```
no shutdown
```

This removes the interface from shutdown status.

```
interface ethernet1
ip address 192.168.2.1 255.255.255.0
```

This assigns the IP address to *ethernet1 interface*.

```
ip nat inside
```

This designates *ethernet1 interface* as an "inside" network.

```
no shutdown
```

This removes the interface from shutdown status.

```
access-list 10 permit ip 192.168.1.0 0.0.0.255
```

This specifies that traffic originating from the 192.168.1.0 network will be translated.

```
ip nat pool net-207 207.139.221.4  207.139.221.126  netmask 255.255.255.128
```

This defines a pool of global IP addresses named *net-207* with an address range of 207.139.221.4 thru 207.139.221.126 to be used for NAT.

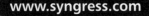

```
ip nat pool net-207-PAT   207.139.221.127  netmask 255.255.255.128
```

This defines a single global IP address named *net-207-PAT* with address 207.139.221.127 to be used for PAT.

```
ip nat inside source list 10 pool net-207
```

This specifies that the source IP address of traffic defined in access list 10 will be NATed with IP addresses defined in the *net-207* pool.

```
ip nat inside source list 10 pool net-207-PAT  overload
```

This specifies that the source IP address of traffic defined in access list 10 will be PATed with the IP address defined in the *net-207-PAT* pool. PAT will occur once NAT has used all available addresses in the *net-207* pool. Once a translation has timed out due to inactivity, that global IP address will be reused for future NAT translations.

```
ip nat inside source static 192.168.2.2 207.139.221.2 netmask 255.255.255.128
```

This creates a static translation for the "inside" IP address 192.168.2.2 to the global IP address 207.139.221.2. Any traffic destined for 207.139.221.2 will be statically translated to 192.168.2.2.

```
ip nat inside source static 192.168.2.3 207.139.221.3 netmask 255.255.255.128
```

Considerations on NAT and PAT

Even though NAT helps get around the problem of scarce globally-routable IP addresses, it does have an impact on the functionality of certain protocols, therefore complicating their deployment. This section outlines some of the problems associated with NAT.

IP Address Information in Data

Numerous applications fail when packets traverse a NAT device. These packets carry IP address or port information in the data portion of the packet. Since NAT only alters the IP header to perform the translation, the data portion is left untouched. With the aid of an ALG, a work around may be provided in some cases. But if the packet data is IPSec secured (or secured by another transport or application level mechanism), the application is going to fail.

Bundled Session Applications

Bundled session applications such as FTP, H.323, SIP, and RTSP, which use a control connection to establish data flow are also usually broken up by NAT devices. This occurs because the applications exchange address and port information within the control session to establish data sessions and session orientations. NAT cannot know the interdependency of the bundled sessions and would therefore treat each session as if they were unrelated to one another. Applications like these can fail for a variety of reasons. Two of the most common reasons for failure are:

- Addressing information in the data portion of the packet is realm-specific and is not valid once the packet crosses the originating realm.

- Control sessions create new data sessions that NAT has no information about. These will fail in many cases.

Peer-to-Peer Applications

Peer-to-peer applications are more prone to failure than client-server-based applications, and can be originated by any of the peers if those peers are located in different realms. NAT translations, however, may not be established because the hosts on the "inside" network are not visible to the host on the "outside" network. This is problematic with traditional NAT (dynamic NAT and PAT) where connections are client to server.

IP Fragmentation with PAT en Route

IP fragmentation with PAT can occur when two hosts send fragmented TCP/UDP packets to the same destination host, and they happen to use the same fragmentation identifier. When the target host receives the two unrelated packets (which carry the same fragmentation ID from the same assigned host address), the target host is unable to distinguish which of the two sessions the packets belong to (due to the translation of the local source address when compared to the global PAT address), causing both sessions to be corrupted.

Applications Requiring Retention of Address Mapping

When a session is established across realms through the use of NAT, the translation for that session will eventually timeout and then be utilized by another session traversing realms. This can be a problem for applications that require numerous sessions to the same external address. NAT cannot know this requirement ahead of time and may reassign the global address between sessions. For example, if Host A on the "inside" network has established a session with Host Z on the "outside" network, the application will function properly. Once the session stops sending traffic and the NAT timer expires, the translation will be terminated and the global IP allocated for that specific translation will be used for another translation. What happens if Host Z requires more data and tries to initiate a session with the IP address that Host A had while it was translated? At this point, the application will no longer function properly.

In order to remedy this problem, keepalive messages need to be sent between hosts to keep the translation active. This can be especially annoying and may not be possible in some situations. An alternative is to use an ALG to keep the address mapping from being discarded by NAT.

IPSec and IKE

NAT operates by modifying source addresses within the IP header while it passes through the NAT device. Due to the nature of IPSec, the AH protocol is designed to detect alterations to IP packet headers. So, when NAT alters the source address information, the destination host receiving the altered packet discards the packet since the IP headers have been altered. The IPSec AH secure packet traversing NAT will simply not reach the target application.

IPSec ESP encrypted packets may be altered by NAT devices only in a limited number of cases. In the case of TCP/UDP packets, NAT would need to update the checksum in the TCP/UDP headers whenever the IP header is changed. However, as the TCP/UDP header is encrypted by the ESP, NAT would not be able to make this checksum update because it is now encrypted. TCP/UDP packets that are encrypted and traverse a NAT device will fail because the TCP/UDP checksum validation on the receiving end will not reach the target application.

Internet Key Exchange Protocol (IKE) can potentially pass IP addresses as node identifiers during the Main, Aggressive, and Quick modes. In order for an IKE negotiation to correctly pass through NAT, these data portions should be modified. However, these payloads are often protected by encryption. For all practical purposes, end-to-end IPSec is almost impossible to accomplish with NAT translation en route.

Summary

NAT solves the problem of the limited supply of global IP addresses available. By implementing a private IP address scheme in a private network, those addresses can then be translated into global IP addresses via a NAT device. This chapter covered various generic terms used by NAT, variations of NAT, how to deploy NAT on a network, and considerations for using NAT. As I stated at the beginning of the chapter, NAT is not a security feature and should not be used for security. It simply allows private IP addresses to be translated into global IP addresses. The myth that NAT "hides" a network is exactly that, a myth. A company's ISP may have knowledge of that private network and can therefore inject a route to that network in their routing tables therefore exposing the private network.

NAT uses the concept of an address realm to separate the "inside" network (a network with private addresses) from the "outside" network (the network outside of the private, or separated, segment of the network). NAT incorporates a system known as transparent address assignment in order to assign outside or global addresses to inside hosts. There are two methods used to accomplish this: static and dynamic address assignment. This system also works with transparent routing in order to route traffic between the inside and outside address realms. There are three phases of transparent routing: *address binding, address lookup and translation,* and *address unbinding.*

Application Level Gateways (ALGs) provide NAT with the ability to translate packets for applications that include TCP/UDP ports in the data portions of the packet. A prime example of such an application is RealAudio. ALGs act as specific translation agents for this information in order to allow the application traffic to pass over NAT. There are four primary architectures for NAT:

- Traditional or outbound NAT
- Port Address Translation (PAT)
- Static NAT
- Twice NAT

The choice of which architecture to deploy depends on the type of applications being supported. When deploying NAT within your enterprise, there are a number of considerations that must be taken into account, including the following:

- Available public addresses
- Router performance capabilities

- The addressing scheme
- The type of applications that will be used

Recent updates to NAT functionality now allow much greater support for IP telephony and converged data solutions for the Cisco IOS. Currently supported protocols include:

- H.323 v2
- CallManager support with support for Skinny Station Protocol
- Session Initiation Protocol (SIP) support for an alternative Voice over IP solution to H.323

NAT is configured on the Cisco IOS through the use of the *ip nat inside | outside* command. Next comes the configuration of access list(s) to allow or disallow hosts access, which is followed by the configuration of address pools for both inside and outside addresses. NAT configuration can be verified by use of the *show ip nat statistics* command as well as the *show ip nat translation* command.

Several factors should be considered before deploying NAT within your network. These include the following:

- Problems with IP address information in data packets. Because of the inherent nature of NAT to translate only the IP address header, IP information in the packets will not be translated. This problem can be generally remedied by use of an ALG.

- Problems with bundled session applications. These arise from the fact that such applications use a control connection in order to establish and maintain data flow. The majority of such issues are resolved in the 12.1(5) and later releases of Cisco IOS.

- Problems with peer-to-peer applications. This occurs because peers that exist in different realms are not visible to peer devices on outside realms. There is little work around for this problem; it is advised that client/server applications be used instead, when possible.

- IP fragmentation with PAT en route. This rare occurrence happens when two hosts originate fragmented TCP/UDP packets to the same destination host, and they happen to use the same fragmentation identifier. This is a very rare occurrence, however, and there is no workaround.

- Problems with applications requiring retention of address mapping. This can be a problem for applications that require numerous sessions to the same external address. NAT cannot know this requirement ahead of time and may reassign the global address between sessions. In order to remedy this problem, keepalive messages need to be sent between hosts to keep the translation active.

- Problems with IPSec and IKE. For all practical purposes, end-to-end IPSec is almost impossible to accomplish with NAT translation en route. This is because of the nature of IPSec. The AH protocol is designed to detect alterations to IP packet header, so when NAT alters the source address information, the destination host receiving the altered packet will discard the packet since the IP headers have been altered.

Solutions Fast Track

NAT Overview

☑ NAT is incorporated by the IOS in order to allow hosts within a private addressing space to communicate to outside networks.

☑ PAT is similar to NAT, however, in that it allows multiple inside addresses to use the same outside address by utilizing several ports on the same IP address.

☑ Transparent address assignment allows inside hosts to communicate with outside addresses transparently. There are two forms of transparent address assignment: static and dynamic.

☑ Transparent routing is the process by which the inside or local address is converted to the outside or global address, and vice versa. There are three stages to transparent routing: address binding, address lookup and translation, and address unbinding.

☑ Application level gateways allow NAT to translate addresses for application that incorporate TCP/UDP information within the data portions of their headers.

NAT Architectures

- ☑ Traditional or outbound NAT is a dynamic translation allowing inside hosts to communicate transparently with outside hosts.

- ☑ Static NAT involves the static mapping of inside addresses to outside addresses. This translation will remain until it is manually changed on the router.

- ☑ Twice NAT involves both the source and the destination address being modified by a NAT device as packets cross address realms. This is most often incorporated when there is overlapping address space between inside and outside networks.

Guidelines for Deploying NAT and PAT

- ☑ The number of available global IP addresses available for NAT must be taken into consideration before incorporating NAT into your network.

- ☑ Router performance is a key element to consider when deploying NAT. Process switching must be incorporated in order to perform NAT translations. Ensure that the router you have selected is capable of handling the added workload.

- ☑ Not all application will work with NAT. In such cases, Application Level Gateways (ALGs) should be incorporated.

IOS NAT Support for IP Telephony

- ☑ H.323 is a protocol used for IP telephony and Voice over IP convergence. As of IOS release 12.1(5), NAT supports H.323 v2.

- ☑ NAT support for CallManager comes in the form of support for Skinny Station Protocol sessions between IP phones and CallManager servers. This support is also available in IOS 12.1(5).

- ☑ Session Initiation Protocol, a protocol that can serve as a substitute for H.323 functionality is also supported by NAT. This functionality is available with version 12.2(8) of the IOS and also requires the use of an Application Level Gateway (ALG).

Configuring NAT on Cisco IOS

☑ NAT configuration begins with the use of the *ip nat inside | outside* command at the interface level.

☑ An access list is used to determine which hosts will have access to NAT resources and the address mappings by use of address pools.

☑ Address pools are used in order to specify the available pool of inside and outside addresses. This is accomplished by use of the *ip nat pool* command.

☑ NAT operation is verified by use of the *show ip nat statistics* and *show ip nat translations* commands.

Considerations on NAT and PAT

☑ Packets that incorporate IP addressing information including TCP and UPD port numbers may encounter problems when traversing a network that incorporates NAT. In order to work around this, an ALG may be incorporated.

☑ Bundled session applications, applications that use a control connection in order to establish data flow, may encounter failures in NAT networks.

☑ Applications that require retention of address mappings will timeout when NAT is used. In order to remedy this, keepalive messages need to be used to keep the session active.

Frequently Asked Questions

The following Frequently Asked Questions, answered by the authors of this book, are designed to both measure your understanding of the concepts presented in this chapter and to assist you with real-life implementation of these concepts. To have your questions about this chapter answered by the author, browse to **www.syngress.com/solutions** and click on the **"Ask the Author"** form.

Q: Should I use NAT or PAT?

A: It is a good idea to implement both depending on how many global addresses are available and how many local hosts need to be translated. If a NAT pool is implemented, PAT can then be used once all of the NAT translations are used up. Once a translation times out, it will then be re-allocated to another local host trying to open a session with a host on the outside. Therefore, NAT is the best practice, if and when enough globally valid IP addresses are available. If not, PAT could be used to provide outside connectivity with a few globally valid IP addresses.

Q: This chapter continually used the term inside and outside addresses. How do I classify these?

A: Inside addresses are those you will need to translate in order to communicate to the outside world. This could be for a variety of reasons, but the most common is the use of private addressing space. Outside addresses are not a part of your private network's address scheme. Therefore, in order for them to communicate to the inside network, they will need to be translated to an internal address. This form of address is needed in order for internal hosts to communicate outside of their address realm.

Q: I have implemented NAT on my network. At different points in time, hosts are no longer being translated. Why is this happening?

A: Check the number of global addresses in your global pool. The number of hosts requiring translation may be out-numbering available addresses. If this is the case, remove one address from the NAT pool and assign that address to PAT.

Q: Static address assignment seems like a lot of administrative work. What possible benefit does it offer?

A: Static address assignment is useful when you want the ability to keep a resource in a private addressing space, but still require outside resources to be able to access it with the same IP address constantly. A good example of this would be a mail server sitting in your DMZ.

Q: Did support for the H.323 specification only begin with IOS release 12.1(5)?

A: Earlier versions of the IOS did support the Microsoft Net meeting version of the H.323 v1 specification. However, IOS 12.1(5) and later releases support the entire H.323 specification except for registration and status messages (RAS) services.

Q: If PAT allows me to map several inside addresses to only one global address, wouldn't it just be better to use that as a solution instead of employing traditional NAT?

A: While PAT does allow that capability, you will encounter several limitations. Specifically, PAT does not support all of the applications you may encounter, and does not, in its current release, support IP telephony applications as well. It also places more load on the system than NAT.

## Chapter 6

Cryptography

Solutions in this chapter:

- **Understanding Cryptography Concepts**

- **Learning about Standard Cryptographic Algorithms**

- **Understanding Brute Force**

- **Knowing When Real Algorithms Are Being Used Improperly**

- **Understanding Amateur Cryptography Attempts**

☑ **Summary**

☑ **Solutions Fast Track**

☑ **Frequently Asked Questions**

Introduction

Cryptography is everywhere these days, from hashed passwords to encrypted mail, to Internet Protocol Security (IPSec) virtual private networks (VPNs) and even encrypted filesystems. Security is the reason why people opt to encrypt data, and if you want your data to remain secure you'd best know a bit about how cryptography works. This chapter certainly can't teach you how to become a professional cryptographer—that takes years of study and practice—but you *will* learn how most of the cryptography you will come in contact with functions (without all the complicated math, of course).

We'll examine some of the history of cryptography and then look closely at a few of the most common algorithms, including Advanced Encryption Standard (AES), the recently announced new cryptography standard for the U.S. government. We'll learn how key exchanges and public key cryptography came into play, and how to use them. I'll show you how almost all cryptography is at least theoretically vulnerable to brute force attacks.

Naturally, once we've covered the background we'll look at how cryptography can be broken, from cracking passwords to man-in-the-middle-type attacks. We'll also look at how other attacks based on poor implementation of strong cryptography can reduce your security level to zero. Finally, we'll examine how weak attempts to hide information using outdated cryptography can easily be broken.

Understanding Cryptography Concepts

What does the word *crypto* mean? It has its origins in the Greek word *kruptos*, which means *hidden*. Thus, the objective of cryptography is to hide information so that only the intended recipient(s) can "unhide" it. In crypto terms, the hiding of information is called *encryption*, and when the information is unhidden, it is called *decryption*. A cipher is used to accomplish the encryption and decryption. Merriam-Webster's Collegiate Dictionary defines *cipher* as "a method of transforming a text in order to conceal its meaning." The information that is being hidden is called *plaintext*; once it has been encrypted, it is called *ciphertext*. The ciphertext is transported, secure from prying eyes, to the intended recipient(s), where it is decrypted back into plaintext.

History

According to Fred Cohen, the history of cryptography has been documented back to over 4000 years ago, where it was first allegedly used in Egypt. Julius Caesar even used his own cryptography called *Caesar's Cipher*. Basically, Caesar's Cipher rotated the letters of the alphabet to the right by three. For example, *S* moves to *V* and *E* moves to *H*. By today's standards the Caesar Cipher is extremely simplistic, but it served Julius just fine in his day. If you are interested in knowing more about the history of cryptography, the following site is a great place to start: www.all.net/books/ip/Chap2-1.html.

In fact, ROT13 (rotate 13), which is similar to Caesar's Cipher, is still in use today. It is not used to keep secrets from people, but more to avoid offending people when sending jokes, spoiling the answers to puzzles, and things along those lines. If such things occur when someone decodes the message, then the responsibility lies on them and not the sender. For example, Mr. G. may find the following example offensive to him if he was to decode it, but as it is shown it offends no one: V guvax Jvaqbjf fhpxf…

ROT13 is simple enough to work out with pencil and paper. Just write the alphabet in two rows; the second row offset by 13 letters:

```
ABCDEFGHIJKLMNOPQRSTUVWXYZ

NOPQRSTUVWXYZABCDEFGHIJKLM
```

Encryption Key Types

Cryptography uses two types of keys: *symmetric* and *asymmetric*. Symmetric keys have been around the longest; they utilize a single key for both the encryption and decryption of the ciphertext. This type of key is called a *secret key*, because you must keep it secret. Otherwise, anyone in possession of the key can decrypt messages that have been encrypted with it. The algorithms used in symmetric key encryption have, for the most part, been around for many years and are well known, so the only thing that is secret is the key being used. Indeed, all of the really useful algorithms in use today are completely open to the public.

A couple of problems immediately come to mind when you are using symmetric key encryption as the sole means of cryptography. First, how do you ensure that the sender and receiver each have the same key? Usually this requires the use of a courier service or some other trusted means of key transport. Second, a problem exists if the recipient does not have the same key to decrypt the ciphertext from the sender. For example, take a situation where the symmetric key for a piece of crypto hardware is changed at 0400 every morning at both ends of a circuit. What happens if one end forgets to change the key (whether it is done with a strip tape, patch blocks, or some other method) at the appropriate time and sends ciphertext using the old key to another site that has properly changed to the new key? The end receiving the transmission will not be able to decrypt the ciphertext, since it is using the wrong key. This can create major problems in a time of crisis, especially if the old key has been destroyed. This is an overly simple example, but it should provide a good idea of what can go wrong if the sender and receiver do not use the same secret key.

Tools & Traps…

Assessing Algorithmic Strength

Algorithmic security can only be proven by its resistance to attack. Since many more attacks are attempted on algorithms which are open to the public, the longer an algorithm has been open to the public, the more attempts to circumvent or break it have occurred. Weak algorithms are broken rather quickly, usually in a matter of days or months, whereas stronger algorithms may be used for decades. However, the openness of the algorithm is an important factor. It's much more difficult to break an algorithm (whether weak or strong) when its complexities are completely unknown. Thus when you use an open algorithm, you can rest assured in its strength. This is opposed to a proprietary algorithm, which, if weak, may eventually be broken even if the algorithm itself is not completely understood by the cryptographer. Obviously, one should limit the trust placed in proprietary algorithms to limit long-term liability. Such scrutiny is the reason the inner details of many of the patented algorithms in use today (such as RC6 from RSA Laboratories) are publicly available.

Asymmetric cryptography is relatively new in the history of cryptography, and it is probably more recognizable to you under the synonymous term *public key cryptography*. Asymmetric algorithms use two different keys, one for encryption and one for decryption—a *public key* and a *private key*, respectively. Whitfield Diffie and Martin Hellman first publicly released public key cryptography in

1976 as a method of exchanging keys in a secret key system. Their algorithm, called the Diffie-Hellman (DH) algorithm, is examined later in the chapter. Even though it is commonly reported that public key cryptography was first invented by the duo, some reports state that the British Secret Service actually invented it a few years prior to the release by Diffie and Hellman. It is alleged, however, that the British Secret Service never actually did anything with their algorithm after they developed it. More information on the subject can be found at the following location: www.wired.com/wired/archive/7.04/crypto_pr.html

Some time after Diffie and Hellman, Phil Zimmermann made public key encryption popular when he released Pretty Good Privacy (PGP) v1.0 for DOS in August 1991. Support for multiple platforms including UNIX and Amiga were added in 1994 with the v2.3 release. Over time, PGP has been enhanced and released by multiple entities, including ViaCrypt and PGP Inc., which is now part of Network Associates. Both commercial versions and free versions (for non-commercial use) are available. For those readers in the United States and Canada, you can retrieve the free version from http://web.mit.edu/network/pgp.html. The commercial version can be purchased from Network Associates at www.pgp.com.

Learning about Standard Cryptographic Algorithms

Just why are there so many algorithms anyway? Why doesn't the world just standardize on one algorithm? Given the large number of algorithms found in the field today, these are valid questions with no simple answers. At the most basic level, it's a classic case of tradeoffs between security, speed, and ease of implementation. Here *security* indicates the likelihood of an algorithm to stand up to current and future attacks, *speed* refers to the processing power and time required to encrypt and decrypt a message, and *ease of implementation* refers to an algorithm's predisposition (if any) to hardware or software usage. Each algorithm has different strengths and drawbacks, and none of them is ideal in every way. In this chapter, we will look at the five most common algorithms that you will encounter: Data Encryption Standard (DES), AES [Rijndael], International Data Encryption Algorithm (IDEA), Diffie-Hellman, and Rivest, Shamir, Adleman (RSA). Be aware, though, that there are dozens more active in the field.

Understanding Symmetric Algorithms

In this section, we will examine several of the most common symmetric algorithms in use: DES, its successor AES, and the European standard, IDEA. Keep in mind that the strength of symmetric algorithms lies primarily in the size of the keys used in the algorithm, as well as the number of cycles each algorithm employs. All symmetric algorithms are also theoretically vulnerable to *brute force attacks*, which are exhaustive searches of all possible keys. However, brute force attacks are often infeasible. We will discuss them in detail later in the chapter.

DES

Among the oldest and most famous encryption algorithms is the Data Encryption Standard, which was developed by IBM and was the U.S. government standard from 1976 until about 2001. DES was based significantly on the Lucifer algorithm invented by Horst Feistel, which never saw widespread use. Essentially, DES uses a single 64-bit key—56 bits of data and 8 bits of parity—and operates on data in 64-bit chunks. This key is broken into 16 separate 48-bit subkeys, one for each round, which are called *Feistel cycles*. Figure 6.1 gives a schematic of how the DES encryption algorithm operates.

Each round consists of a substitution phase, wherein the data is substituted with pieces of the key, and a permutation phase, wherein the substituted data is scrambled (reordered). Substitution operations, sometimes referred to as confusion operations, are said to occur within S-boxes. Similarly, permutation operations, sometimes called diffusion operations, are said to occur in P-boxes. Both of these operations occur in the "F Module" of the diagram. The security of DES lies mainly in the fact that since the substitution operations are non-linear, so the resulting ciphertext in no way resembles the original message. Thus, language-based analysis techniques (discussed later in this chapter) used against the ciphertext reveal nothing. The permutation operations add another layer of security by scrambling the already partially encrypted message.

Every five years from 1976 until 2001, the National Institute of Standards and Technology (NIST) reaffirmed DES as the encryption standard for the U.S. government. However, by the 1990s the aging algorithm had begun to show signs that it was nearing its end of life. New techniques that identified a shortcut method of attacking the DES cipher, such as differential cryptanalysis, were proposed as early as 1990, though it was still computationally unfeasible to do so.

Figure 6.1 Diagram of the DES Encryption Algorithm

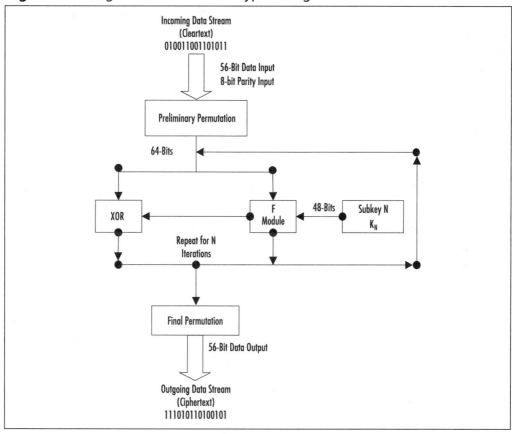

SECURITY ALERT

How can symmetric algorithms such as DES be made more secure? Theoretically, there are two ways: either the key length needs to be increased, or the number of rounds in the encryption process needs to be increased. Both of these solutions tend to increase the processing power required to encrypt and decrypt data and slow down the encryption/decryption speed because of the increased number of mathematical operations required. Examples of modified DES include 3-DES (a.k.a. Triple DES) and DESX. Triple DES uses three separate 56-bit DES keys as a single 168-bit key, though sometimes keys 1 and 3 are identical, yielding 112-bit security. DESX adds an additional 64-bits of key data. Both 3-DES and DESX are intended to strengthen DES against brute force attacks.

Significant design flaws such as the short 56-bit key length also affected the longevity of the DES cipher. Shorter keys are more vulnerable to brute force attacks. Although Whitfield Diffie and Martin Hellman were the first to criticize this short key length, even going so far as to declare in 1979 that DES would be useless within 10 years, DES was not publicly broken by a brute force attack until 1997.

The first successful brute force attack against DES took a large network of machines over 4 months to accomplish. Less than a year later, in 1998, the Electronic Frontier Foundation (EFF) cracked DES in less than three days using a computer specially designed for cracking DES. This computer, code-named "Deep Crack," cost less than $250,000 to design and build. The record for cracking DES stands at just over 22 hours and is held by Distributed.net, which employed a massively parallel network of thousands of systems (including Deep Crack). Add to this the fact that Bruce Schneier has theorized that a machine capable of breaking DES in about six minutes could be built for a mere $10 million. Clearly, NIST needed to phase out DES in favor of a new algorithm.

AES (Rijndael)

In 1997, as the fall of DES loomed ominously closer, NIST announced the search for the Advanced Encryption Standard, the successor to DES. Once the search began, most of the big-name cryptography players submitted their own AES candidates. Among the requirements of AES candidates were:

- AES would be a private key symmetric block cipher (similar to DES).

- AES needed to be stronger and faster then 3-DES.

- AES required a life expectancy of at least 20-30 years.

- AES would support key sizes of 128-bits, 192-bits, and 256-bits.

- AES would be available to all—royalty free, non–proprietary and unpatented.

Within months NIST had a total of 15 different entries, 6 of which were rejected almost immediately on grounds that they were considered incomplete. By 1999, NIST had narrowed the candidates down to five finalists including MARS, RC6, Rijndael, Serpent, and Twofish.

Selecting the winner took approximately another year, as each of the candidates needed to be tested to determine how well they performed in a variety of environments. After all, applications of AES would range anywhere from portable smart cards to standard 32-bit desktop computers to high-end optimized 64-bit computers. Since all of the finalists were highly secure, the primary deciding factors were speed and ease of implementation (which in this case meant memory footprint).

Rijndael was ultimately announced as the winner in October of 2000 because of its high performance in both hardware and software implementations and its small memory requirement. The Rijndael algorithm, developed by Belgian cryptographers Dr. Joan Daemen and Dr. Vincent Rijmen, also seems resistant to power- and timing-based attacks.

So how does AES/Rijndael work? Instead of using Feistel cycles in each round like DES, it uses iterative rounds like IDEA (discussed in the next section). Data is operated on in 128-bit chunks, which are grouped into four groups of four bytes each. The number of rounds is also dependent on the key size, such that 128-bit keys have 9 rounds, 192-bit keys have 11 rounds and 256-bit keys require 13 rounds. Each round consists of a substitution step of one S-box per data bit followed by a pseudo-permutation step in which bits are shuffled between groups. Then each group is multiplied out in a matrix fashion and the results are added to the subkey for that round.

How much faster is AES than 3-DES? It's difficult to say, because implementation speed varies widely depending on what type of processor is performing the encryption and whether or not the encryption is being performed in software or running on hardware specifically designed for encryption. However, in similar implementations, AES is always faster than its 3-DES counterpart. One test performed by Brian Gladman has shown that on a Pentium Pro 200 with optimized code written in C, AES (Rijndael) can encrypt and decrypt at an average speed of 70.2 Mbps, versus DES's speed of only 28 Mbps. You can read his other results at fp.gladman.plus.com/cryptography_technology/aes.

IDEA

The European counterpart to the DES algorithm is the IDEA algorithm, and its existence proves that Americans certainly don't have a monopoly on strong cryptography. IDEA was first proposed under the name *Proposed Encryption Standard* (PES) in 1990 by cryptographers James Massey and Xuejia Lai as part of a combined research project between Ascom and the Swiss Federal Institute of Technology. Before it saw widespread use PES was updated in 1991 to increase its strength against differential cryptanalysis attacks and was renamed Improved PES (IPES). Finally, the name was changed to International Data Encryption Algorithm (IDEA) in 1992.

Not only is IDEA newer than DES, but IDEA is also considerably faster and more secure. IDEA's enhanced speed is due to the fact the each round consists of much simpler operations than the Fiestel cycle in DES. These operations (XOR, addition, and multiplication) are much simpler to implement in software than the substitution and permutation operations of DES.

IDEA operates on 64-bit blocks with a 128-bit key, and the encryption/decryption process uses 8 rounds with 6 16-bit subkeys per round. The IDEA algorithm is patented both in the US and in Europe, but free non-commercial use is permitted.

Understanding Asymmetric Algorithms

Recall that unlike symmetric algorithms, asymmetric algorithms require more than one key, usually a *public* key and a *private* key (systems with more than two keys are possible). Instead of relying on the techniques of substitution and transposition, which symmetric key cryptography uses, asymmetric algorithms rely on the use of massively large integer mathematics problems. Many of these problems are simple to do in one direction but difficult to do in the opposite direction. For example, it's easy to multiply two numbers together, but it's more difficult to factor them back into the original numbers, especially if the integers you are using contain hundreds of digits. Thus, in general, the security of asymmetric algorithms is dependent not upon the feasibility of brute force attacks, but the feasibility of performing difficult mathematical inverse operations and advances in mathematical theory that may propose new "shortcut" techniques. In this section, we'll take a look at RSA and Diffie-Hellman, the two most popular asymmetric algorithms in use today.

Diffie-Hellman

In 1976, after voicing their disapproval of DES and the difficulty in handling secret keys, Whitfield Diffie and Martin Hellman published the Diffie-Hellman algorithm for key exchange. This was the first published use of public key cryptography, and arguably one of the cryptography field's greatest advances ever. Because of the inherent slowness of asymmetric cryptography, the Diffie-Hellman algorithm was not intended for use as a general encryption scheme—rather, its purpose was to transmit a private key for DES (or some similar symmetric algorithm) across an insecure medium. In most cases, Diffie-Hellman is not used for encrypting a complete message because it is 10 to 1000 times slower than DES, depending on implementation.

Prior to publication of the Diffie-Hellman algorithm, it was quite painful to share encrypted information with others because of the inherent key storage and transmission problems (as discussed later in this chapter). Most wire transmissions were insecure, since a message could travel between dozens of systems before reaching the intended recipient and any number of snoops along the way could uncover the key. With the Diffie-Hellman algorithm, the DES secret key (sent along with a DES-encrypted payload message) could be encrypted via Diffie-Hellman by one party and decrypted only by the intended recipient.

In practice, this is how a key exchange using Diffie-Hellman works:

- The two parties agree on two numbers; one is a large prime number, the other is an integer smaller than the prime. They can do this in the open and it doesn't affect security.

- Each of the two parties separately generates another number, which they keep secret. This number is equivalent to a *private key*. A calculation is made involving the private key and the previous two public numbers. The result is sent to the other party. This result is effectively a *public key*.

- The two parties exchange their public keys. They then privately perform a calculation involving their own private key and the other party's public key. The resulting number is the *session key*. Each party will arrive at the same number.

- The session key can be used as a secret key for another cipher, such as DES. No third party monitoring the exchange can arrive at the same session key without knowing one of the private keys.

The most difficult part of the Diffie-Hellman key exchange to understand is that there are actually two separate and independent encryption cycles happening. As far as Diffie-Hellman is concerned, only a small message is being transferred between the sender and the recipient. It just so happens that this small message is the secret key needed to unlock the larger message.

Diffie-Hellman's greatest strength is that anyone can know either or both of the sender and recipient's public keys without compromising the security of the message. Both the public and private keys are actually just very large integers. The Diffie-Hellman algorithm takes advantage of complex mathematical functions known as *discrete logarithms*, which are easy to perform forwards but extremely difficult to find inverses for. Even though the patent on Diffie-Hellman has been expired for several years now, the algorithm is still in wide use, most notably in the IPSec protocol. IPSec uses the Diffie-Hellman algorithm in conjunction with RSA authentication to exchange a session key that is used for encrypting all traffic that crosses the IPSec tunnel.

RSA

In the year following the Diffie-Hellman proposal, Ron Rivest, Adi Shamir, and Leonard Adleman proposed another public key encryption system. Their proposal is now known as the RSA algorithm, named for the last initials of the researchers. RSA shares many similarities with the Diffie-Hellman algorithm in that RSA is also based on multiplying and factoring large integers. However, RSA is significantly faster than Diffie-Hellman, leading to a split in the asymmetric cryptography field that refers to Diffie-Hellman and similar algorithms as Public Key Distribution Systems (PKDS) and RSA and similar algorithms as Public Key Encryption (PKE). PKDS systems are used as session-key exchange mechanisms, while PKE systems are generally considered fast enough to encrypt reasonably small messages. However, PKE systems like RSA are not considered fast enough to encrypt large amounts of data like entire filesystems or high-speed communications lines.

NOTE

RSA, Diffie-Hellman and other asymmetric algorithms use much larger keys than their symmetric counterparts. Common key sizes include 1024-bits and 2048-bits, and the keys need to be this large because factoring, while still a difficult operation, is much easier to perform than the exhaustive key search approach used with symmetric algorithms. The relative slowness of public key encryption systems is also due in part to these larger key sizes. Since most computers can only handle 32-bits of precision, different "tricks" are required to emulate the 1024-bit and 2048-bit integers. However, the additional processing time is somewhat justified, since for security purposes 2048-bit keys are considered to be secure "forever"—barring any exponential breakthroughs in mathematical factoring algorithms, of course.

Because of the former patent restrictions on RSA, the algorithm saw only limited deployment, primarily only from products by RSA Security, until the mid-1990s. Now you are likely to encounter many programs making extensive use of RSA, such as PGP and Secure Shell (SSH). The RSA algorithm has been in the public domain since RSA Security placed it there two weeks before the patent expired in September 2000. Thus the RSA algorithm is now freely available for use by anyone, for any purpose.

Understanding Brute Force

Just how secure are encrypted files and passwords anyway? Consider that there are two ways to break an encryption algorithm—brute force and various cryptanalysis shortcuts. Cryptanalysis shortcuts vary from algorithm to algorithm, or may even be non-existent for some algorithms, and they are always difficult to find and exploit. Conversely, brute force is always available and easy to try. Brute force techniques involve exhaustively searching the given keyspace by trying every possible key or password combination until the right one is found.

Brute Force Basics

As an example, consider the basic three-digit combination bicycle lock where each digit is turned to select a number between zero and nine. Given enough time and assuming that the combination doesn't change during the attempts, just rolling through every possible combination in sequence can easily open this lock. The total number of possible combinations (keys) is 10^3 or 1000, and let's say the frequency, or number of combinations a thief can attempt during a time period, is 30 per minute. Thus, the thief should be able to open the bike lock in a maximum of 1000/(30 per min) or about 33 minutes. Keep in mind that with each new combination attempted, the number of remaining possible combinations (keyspace) decreases and the chance of guessing the correct combination (deciphering the key) on the next attempt increases.

Brute force always works because the keyspace, no matter how large, is always finite. So the way to resist brute force attacks is to choose a keysize large enough that it becomes too time-consuming for the attacker to use brute force techniques. In the bike lock example, three digits of keyspace gives the attacker a maximum amount of time of 33 minutes required to steal the bicycle, so the thief may be tempted to try a brute force attack. Suppose a bike lock with a five-digit combination is used. Now there are 100,000 possible combinations, which would take about 55.5 hours for the thief check by brute force. Clearly, most thieves would move on and look for something easier to steal.

When applied to symmetric algorithms such as DES, brute force techniques work very similarly to the bike lock example. In fact, this happens to be exactly the way DES was broken by the EFF's "Deep Crack." Since the DES key is known to be 56 bits long, every possible combination of keys between a string of 56 zeros and a string of 56 ones is tested until the appropriate key is discovered.

As for the distributed attempts to break DES, the five-digit bike lock analogy needs to be slightly changed. Distributed brute force attempts are analogous to having multiple thieves, each with an exact replica of the bike lock. Each of these replicas has the exact same combination as the original bike lock, and the thieves work on the combination in parallel. Suppose there are 50 thieves working together to guess the combination. Each thief tries a different set of 2,000 combinations such that no two thieves are working on the same combination set (sub-keyspace). Now instead of testing 30 combinations per minute, the thieves are testing 1500 combinations per minute, and all possible combinations will be checked in about 67 minutes. Recall that it took the single thief 55 hours to steal the bike, but now 50 thieves working together can steal the bike in just over an hour. Distributed computing applications working under the same fundamentals are what allowed Distributed.net to crack DES in less than 24 hours.

Applying brute force techniques to RSA and other public key encryption systems is not quite as simple. Since the RSA algorithm is broken by factoring, if the keys being used are sufficiently small (far, far smaller than any program using RSA would allow), it is conceivable that a person could crack the RSA algorithm using pencil and paper. However, for larger keys, the time required to perform the factoring becomes excessive. Factoring does not lend itself to distributed attacks as well, either. A distributed factoring attack would require much more coordination between participants than simple exhaustive keyspace coordination. There are projects, such as the www-factoring project (www.npac.syr.edu/factoring.html), that endeavor to do just this. Currently, the www-factoring project is attempting to factor a 130-digit number. In comparison, 512-bit keys are about 155 digits in size.

Using Brute Force to Obtain Passwords

Brute force is a method commonly used to obtain passwords, especially if the encrypted password list is available. While the exact number of characters in a password is usually unknown, most passwords can be estimated to be between 4 and 16 characters. Since only about 100 different values can be used for each character of the password, there are only about 100^4 to 100^{16} likely password combinations. Though massively large, the number of possible password combinations is finite and is therefore vulnerable to brute force attack.

Before specific methods for applying brute force can be discussed, a brief explanation of password encryption is required. Most modern operating systems use some form of password hashing to mask the exact password. Because passwords are never stored on the server in cleartext form, the password authentication system becomes much more secure. Even if someone unauthorized somehow obtains the password list, he will not be able to make immediate use of it, hopefully giving system administrators time to change all of the relevant passwords before any real damage is caused.

Passwords are generally stored in what is called *hashed* format. When a password is entered on the system it passes through a *one-way hashing function*, such as Message Digest 5 (MD5), and the output is recorded. Hashing functions are one-way encryption only, and once data has been hashed, it cannot be restored. A server doesn't need to know what your password is. It needs to know that *you* know what it is. When you attempt to authenticate, the password you provided is passed through the hashing function and the output is compared to the stored hash value. If these values match, then you are authenticated. Otherwise, the login attempt fails, and is (hopefully) logged by the system.

Brute force attempts to discover passwords usually involve stealing a copy of the username and hashed password listing and then methodically encrypting possible passwords using the same hashing function. If a match is found, then the password is considered cracked. Some variations of brute force techniques involve simply passing possible passwords directly to the system via remote login attempts. However, these variations are rarely seen anymore due to account lockout features and the fact that they can be easily spotted and traced by system administrators. They also tend to be extremely slow.

Appropriate password selection minimizes—but cannot completely eliminate—a password's ability to be cracked. Simple passwords, such as any individual word in a language, make the weakest passwords because they can be cracked with an elementary *dictionary attack*. In this type of attack, long lists of words of a particular language called *dictionary files* are searched for a match to the encrypted password. More complex passwords that include letters, numbers and symbols require a different brute force technique that includes all printable characters and generally take an order of magnitude longer to run.

Some of the more common tools used to perform brute force password attacks include L0phtcrack for Windows passwords, and Crack and John the Ripper for UNIX passwords. Not only do hackers use these tools but security professionals also find them useful in auditing passwords. If it takes a security professional N days to crack a password, then that is approximately how long it will take an attacker to do the same. Each of these tools will be discussed briefly, but be aware that written permission should always be obtained from the system administrator before using these programs against a system.

L0phtcrack

L0phtCrack is a Windows NT password-auditing tool from the L0pht that came onto the scene in 1997. It provides several different mechanisms for retrieving the passwords from the hashes, but is used primarily for its brute force capabilities. The character sets chosen dictate the amount of time and processing power necessary to search the entire keyspace. Obviously, the larger the character set chosen, the longer it will take to complete the attack. However, dictionary based attacks, which use only common words against the password database are normally quite fast and often effective in catching the poorest passwords. Table 6.1 lists the time required for L0phtcrack 2.5 to crack passwords based on the character set selected.

Table 6.1 L0phtcrack 2.5 Brute Force Crack Time Using a Quad Xeon 400 MHz Processor

Test: Brute Force Crack Machine: Quad Xeon 400 MHz	
Character Set	Time
Alpha-Numeric	5.5 Hours
Alpha-Numeric-Some Symbols	45 Hours
Alpha-Numeric-All Symbols	480 Hours

Used with permission of the L0pht

L0pht Heavy Industries, the developers of L0phtcrack, have since sold the rights to the software to @stake Security. Since the sale, @stake has released a program called LC3, which is intended to be L0phtcrack's successor. LC3 includes major improvements over L0phtcrack 2.5, such as distributed cracking and a simplified sniffing attachment that allows password hashes to be sniffed over Ethernet. Additionally, LC3 includes a password-cracking wizard to help the less knowledgeable audit their system passwords. Figure 6.2 shows LC3 displaying the output of a dictionary attack against some sample user passwords.

LC3 reflects a number of usability advances since the older L0phtcrack 2.5 program, and the redesigned user interface is certainly one of them. Both

L0phtCrack and LC3 are commercial software packages. However, a 15-day trial can be obtained at www.atstake.com/research/lc3/download.html.

Figure 6.2 Output of a Simple Dictionary-Based Attack

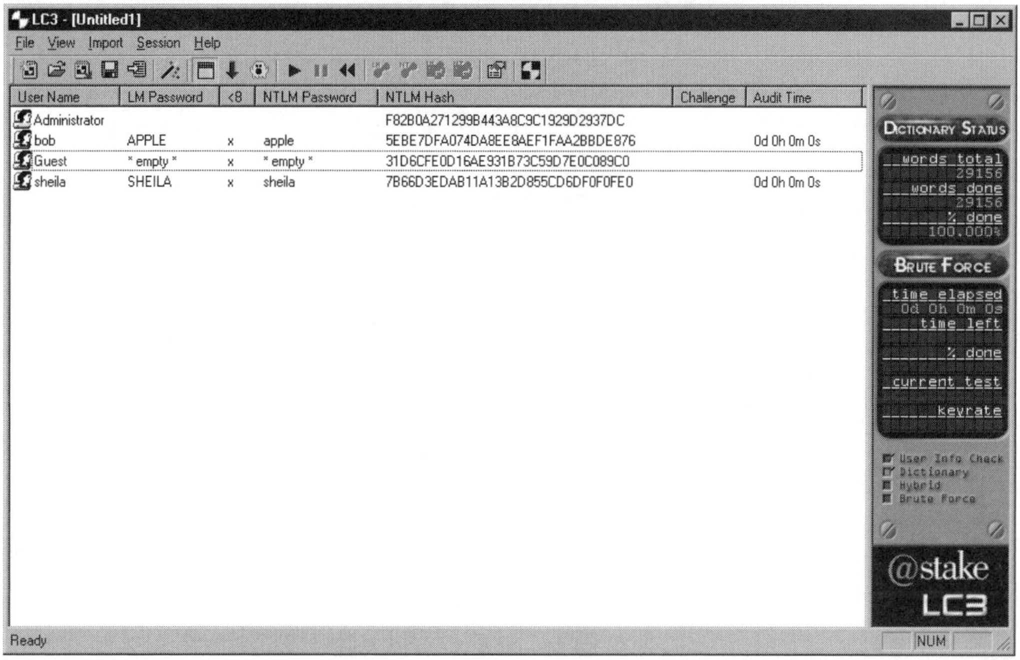

Crack

The oldest and most widely used UNIX password cracking utility is simply called *Crack*. Alec Muffett is the author of Crack, which he calls a password-guessing program for UNIX systems. It runs only on UNIX systems against UNIX passwords, and is for the most part a dictionary-based program. However, in the latest release available (v5.0a from 1996), Alec has bundled Crack7, a brute force password cracker that can be used if a dictionary-based attack fails. One of the most interesting aspects of this combination is that Crack can test for common variants that people use when they think they are picking more secure passwords. For example, instead of "password," someone may choose "pa55word." Crack has user-configurable permutation rules that will catch these variants. More information on Alec Muffett and Crack is available at www.users.dircon.co.uk/~crypto.

John the Ripper

John the Ripper is another password-cracking program, but it differs from Crack in that it is available in UNIX, DOS, and Win32 editions. Crack is great for older systems using crypt(), but John the Ripper is better for newer systems using MD5 and similar password formats. John the Ripper is used primarily for UNIX passwords, but there are add-ons available to break other types of passwords, such as Windows NT LanManager (LANMAN) hashes and Netscape Lightweight Directory Access Protocol (LDAP) server passwords. John the Ripper supports brute force attacks in *incremental mode*. Because of John the Ripper's architecture, one of its most useful features is its ability to save its status automatically during the cracking process, which allows for aborted cracking attempts to be restarted even on a different system. John the Ripper is part of the OpenWall project and is available from www.openwall.com/john.

A sample screenshot of John the Ripper is shown in Figure 6.3. In this example, a sample section of a password file in OpenBSD format is cracked using John the Ripper. Shown below the password file snippet is the actual output of John the Ripper as it runs. You can see that each cracked password is displayed on the console. Be aware that the time shown to crack all four passwords is barely over a minute only because I placed the actual passwords at the top of the "password.lst" listing, which John uses as its dictionary. Real attempts to crack passwords would take much longer. After John has cracked a password file, you can have John display the password file in unshadowed format using the **show** option.

Figure 6.3 Sample Screenshot of John the Ripper

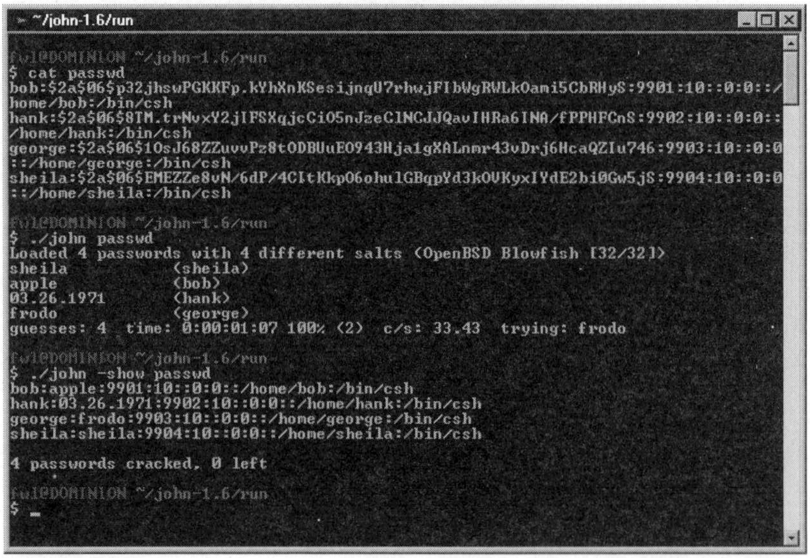

Knowing When Real Algorithms Are Being Used Improperly

While theoretically, given enough time, almost any encryption standard can be cracked with brute force, it certainly isn't the most desirable method to use when "theoretically enough time" is longer than the age of the universe. Thus, any shortcut method that a hacker can use to break your encryption will be much more desirable to him than brute force methods.

None of the encryption algorithms discussed in this chapter have any serious flaws associated with the algorithms themselves, but sometimes the way the algorithm is implemented can create vulnerabilities. Shortcut methods for breaking encryption usually result from a vendor's faulty implementation of a strong encryption algorithm, or lousy configuration from the user. In this section, we'll discuss several incidents of improperly used encryption that are likely to be encountered in the field.

Bad Key Exchanges

Because there isn't any authentication built into the Diffie-Hellman algorithm, implementations that use Diffie-Hellman-type key exchanges without some sort of authentication are vulnerable to man-in-the-middle (MITM) attacks. The most notable example of this type of behavior is the SSH-1 protocol. Since the protocol itself does not authenticate the client or the server, it's possible for someone to cleverly eavesdrop on the communications. This deficiency was one of the main reasons that the SSH-2 protocol was completely redeveloped from SSH-1. The SSH-2 protocol authenticates both the client and the server, and warns of or prevents any possible MITM attacks, depending on configuration, so long as the client and server have communicated at least once. However, even SSH-2 is vulnerable to MITM attacks prior to the first key exchange between the client and the server.

As an example of a MITM-type attack, consider that someone called Al is performing a standard Diffie-Hellman key exchange with Charlie for the very first time, while Beth is in a position such that all traffic between Al and Charlie passes through her network segment. Assuming Beth doesn't interfere with the key exchange, she will not be able to read any of the messages passed between Al and Charlie, because she will be unable to decrypt them. However, suppose that Beth intercepts the transmissions of Al and Charlie's public keys and she responds to them using her own public key. Al will think that Beth's public key is actually

Charlie's public key and Charlie will think that Beth's public key is actually Al's public key.

When Al transmits a message to Charlie, he will encrypt it using Beth's public key. Beth will intercept the message and decrypt it using her private key. Once Beth has read the message, she encrypts it again using Charlie's public key and transmits the message on to Charlie. She may even modify the message contents if she so desires. Charlie then receives Beth's modified message, believing it to come from Al. He replies to Al and encrypts the message using Beth's public key. Beth again intercepts the message, decrypts it with her private key, and modifies it. Then she encrypts the new message with Al's public key and sends it on to Al, who receives it and believes it to be from Charlie.

Clearly, this type of communication is undesirable because a third party not only has access to confidential information, but she can also modify it at will. In this type of attack, no encryption is broken because Beth does not know either Al or Charlie's private keys, so the Diffie-Hellman algorithm isn't really at fault. Beware of the key exchange mechanism used by any public key encryption system. If the key exchange protocol does not authenticate at least one and preferably both sides of the connection, it may be vulnerable to MITM-type attacks. Authentication systems generally use some form of digital certificates (usually X.509), such as those available from Thawte or VeriSign.

Hashing Pieces Separately

Older Windows-based clients store passwords in a format known as LanManager (LANMAN) hashes, which is a horribly insecure authentication scheme. However, since this chapter is about cryptography, we will limit the discussion of LANMAN authentication to the broken cryptography used for password storage.

As with UNIX password storage systems, LANMAN passwords are never stored on a system in cleartext format—they are always stored in a hash format. The problem is that the hashed format is implemented in such a way that even though DES is used to encrypt the password, the password can still be broken with relative ease. Each LANMAN password can contain up to 14 characters, and all passwords less than 14 characters are padded to bring the total password length up to 14 characters. During encryption the password is split into a pair of seven-character passwords, and each of these seven-character passwords is encrypted with DES. The final password hash consists of the two concatenated DES-encrypted password halves.

Since DES is known to be a reasonably secure algorithm, why is this implementation flawed? Shouldn't DES be uncrackable without significant effort? Not exactly. Recall that there are roughly 100 different characters that can be used in a password. Using the maximum possible password length of 14 characters, there should be about 100^{14} or 1.0×10^{28} possible password combinations. LANMAN passwords are further simplified because there is no distinction between upper- and lowercase letters—all letters appears as uppercase. Furthermore, if the password is less than eight characters, then the second half of the password hash is always identical and never even needs to be cracked. If only letters are used (no numbers or punctuation), then there can only be 26^7 (roughly eight billion) password combinations. While this may still seem like a large number of passwords to attack via brute force, remember that these are only theoretical maximums and that since most user passwords are quite weak, dictionary-based attacks will uncover them quickly. The bottom line here is that dictionary-based attacks on a pair of seven-character passwords (or even just one) are much faster than those on single 14-character passwords.

Suppose that strong passwords that use two or more symbols and numbers are used with the LANMAN hashing routine. The problem is that most users tend to just tack on the extra characters at the end of the password. For example, if a user uses his birthplace along with a string of numbers and symbols, such as "MONTANA45%," the password is still insecure. LANMAN will break this password into the strings "MONTANA" and "45%." The former will probably be caught quickly in a dictionary-based attack, and the latter will be discovered quickly in a brute force attack because it is only three characters. For newer business-oriented Microsoft operating systems such as Windows NT and Windows 2000, LANMAN hashing can and should be disabled in the registry if possible, though this will make it impossible for Win9x clients to authenticate to those machines.

Using a Short Password to Generate a Long Key

Password quality is a subject that we have already briefly touched upon in our discussion of brute force techniques. With the advent of PKE encryption schemes such as PGP, most public and private keys are generated using passwords or passphrases, leaving the password generation steps vulnerable to brute force attacks. If a password is selected that is not of significant length, that password can be brute force attacked in an attempt to generate the same keys as the user. Thus PKE systems such as RSA have a chance to be broken by brute force, not because of any deficiency in the algorithm itself, but because of deficiencies in the key generation process. The best way to protect against these types of round-about attacks is to use strong passwords when generating any sort of encryption key. Strong passwords include the use of upper- and lowercase letters, numbers, and symbols, preferably throughout the password. Eight characters is generally considered the minimum length for a strong password, but given the severity of choosing a poor password for key generation, I recommend you use at least twelve characters for these instances.

High quality passwords are often said to have high entropy, which is a semi-finite measurement that attempts to quantify the relative quality of a password. Longer passwords typically have more entropy than shorter passwords, and the more random each character of the password is, the more entropy in the password. For example, the password "albatross" (about 30 bits of entropy) might be reasonably long in length, but has less entropy than a totally random password of the same length such as "g8%=MQ+p" (about 48 bits of entropy). Since the former might appear in a list of common names for bird species, while the latter would never appear in a published list, obviously the latter is a stronger and therefore more desirable password. The moral of the story here is that strong encryption such as 168-bit 3-DES can be broken easily if the secret key has only a few bits of entropy.

Improperly Stored Private or Secret Keys

Let's say you have only chosen to use the strong cryptography algorithms, you have verified that there are not any flaws in the vendors' implementations, and you have generated your keys with great care. How secure is your data now? It is still only as secure as your private or secret key. These keys must be safeguarded at all costs, or you may as well not even use encryption.

Since keys are simply strings of data, they are usually stored in a file somewhere in your system's hard disk. For example, private keys for SSH-1 are stored in the *identity* file located in the .ssh directory under a user's home directory. If the filesystem permissions on this file allow others to access the file, then this private key is compromised. Once others have your private or secret key, reading your encrypted communications becomes trivial. (Note that the SSH identity file is used for authentication, not encryption; but you get the idea.)

However, in some vendor implementations, your keys could be disclosed to others because the keys are not stored securely in RAM. As you are aware, any information processed by a computer, including your secret or private key, is located in the computer's RAM at some point. If the operating system's kernel does not store these keys in a protected area of its memory, they could conceivably become available to someone who dumps a copy of the system's RAM to a file for analysis. These memory dumps are called *core dumps* in UNIX, and they are commonly created during a denial of service (DoS) attack. Thus a successful hacker could generate a core dump on your system and extract your key from the memory image. In a similar attack, a DoS attack could cause excess memory usage on the part of the victim, forcing the key to be swapped to disk as part of virtual memory. Fortunately, most vendors are aware of this type of exploit by now, and it is becoming less and less common since encryption keys are now being stored in protected areas of memory.

Tools & Traps…

Netscape's Original SSL Implementation: How Not to Choose Random Numbers

As we have tried to point out in this section, sometimes it does not matter if you are using an algorithm that is known to be secure. If your algorithm is being applied incorrectly, there will be security holes. An excellent example of a security hole resulting from misapplied cryptography is Netscape's poor choice of random number seeds used in the Secure Sockets Layer (SSL) encryption of its version 1.1 browser. You no doubt note that this security flaw is several years old and thus of limited importance today. However, below the surface we'll see that this particular bug is an almost classic example of one of the ways in which vendors implement broken cryptography, and as such it continues to remain relevant to this day. We will limit this discussion to the vulnerability in the UNIX version of Netscape's SSL implementation as discovered by Ian Goldberg and David Wagner, although the PC and Macintosh versions were similarly vulnerable.

Before I can explain the exact nature of this security hole we will need to cover some background information, such as SSL technology and random numbers. SSL is a certificate-based authentication and encryption scheme developed by Netscape during the fledgling days of e-commerce. It was intended to secure communications such as credit card transactions from eavesdropping by would-be thieves. Because of U.S. export restrictions, the stronger and virtually impervious 128-bit (key) version of the technology was not in widespread use. In fact, even

Continued

domestically, most of Netscape's users were running the anemic 40-bit international version of the software.

Most key generation, including SSL key generation, requires some form of randomness as a factor of the key generation process. Arbitrarily coming up with random numbers is much harder than it sounds, especially for machines. So we usually end up using pseudo-random numbers that are devised from mostly random events, such as the time elapsed between each keystroke you type or the movement of your mouse across the screen.

For the UNIX version of its version 1.1 browser, Netscape used a conglomeration of values, such as the current time, the process ID (PID) number of the Netscape process and its parent's process ID number. Suppose the attacker had access to the same machine as the Netscape user simultaneously, which is the norm in UNIX-based multi-user architectures. It would be trivial for the attacker to generate a process listing to discover Netscape's PID and its parent's PID. If the attacker had the ability to capture TCP/IP packets coming into the machine, he could use the timestamps on these packets to make a reasonable guess as to the exact time the SSL certificate was generated. Once this information was gathered, the attacker could narrow down the keyspace to about 10^6 combinations, which is then brute force attacked with ease at near real-time speeds. Upon successfully discovering Netscape's SSL certificate seed generation values, he can generate an identical certificate for himself and either eavesdrop or hijack the existing session.

Clearly, this was a serious security flaw that Netscape would need to address in its later versions, and it did, providing patches for the 1.x series of browsers and developing a new and substantially different random number generator for its 2.x series of browsers. You can read more details about this particular security flaw in the archives of Dr. Dobbs' Journal at www.ddj.com/documents/s=965/ddj9601h.

Understanding Amateur Cryptography Attempts

If your data is not being protected by one of the more modern, computationally secure algorithms that we've already discussed in this chapter, or some similar variant, then your data is probably not secure. In this section, we're going to discover how simple methods of enciphering data can be broken using rudimentary cryptanalysis.

Classifying the Ciphertext

Even a poorly encrypted message often looks indecipherable at first glance, but you can sometimes figure out what the message is by looking beyond just the stream of printed characters. Often, the same information that you can "read between the lines" on a cleartext message still exists in an enciphered message.

For the mechanisms discussed below, all the "secrecy" is contained in the algorithm, not in a separate key. Our challenge for these is to figure out the algorithm used. So for most of them, that means that we will run a password or some text through the algorithm, which will often be available to us in the form of a program or other black box device. By controlling the inputs and examining the outputs, we hope to determine the algorithm. This will enable us to later take an arbitrary output and determine what the input was.

NOTE

The techniques described in this section are largely ineffective on modern algorithms such as DES and its successors. What few techniques do exist to gain information from modern ciphertext are quite complicated and only work under special conditions.

Frequency Analysis

The first and most powerful method you can employ to crack simple ciphertext is *frequency analysis*, which is based on the idea that certain letters are used more often than others. For example, I can barely write a single word in this sentence that doesn't include the letter *e*. How can letter frequency be of use? You can create a letter frequency table for your ciphertext, assuming the message is of sufficient length, and compare that table to one charting the English language (there are many available). That would give you some clues about which characters in the ciphertext might match up with cleartext letters.

The astute reader will discover that some letters appear with almost identical frequency. How then can you determine which letter is which? You can either evaluate how the letters appear in context, or you can consult other frequency tables that note the appearance of multiple letter combinations such as *sh*, *ph*, *ie* and *the*.

Crypto of this type is just a little more complicated than the Caesar Cipher mentioned at the beginning of the chapter. This was state-of-the-art hundreds of years ago. Now problems of this type are used in daily papers for commuter entertainment, under the titles of "Cryptogram," "CryptoQuote," or similar. Still, some people will use this method as a token effort to hide things. This type of mechanism, or ones just slightly more complex, show up in new worms and viruses all the time.

Ciphertext Relative Length Analysis

Sometimes the ciphertext can provide you with clues to the cleartext even if you don't know how the ciphertext was encrypted. For example, suppose that you have an unknown algorithm that encrypts passwords such that you have available the original password and a ciphertext version of that password. If the length or size of each is the same, then you can infer that the algorithm produces output in a 1:1 ratio to the input. You may even be able to input individual characters to obtain the ciphertext translation for each character. If nothing else, you at least know how many characters to specify for an unknown password if you attempt to break it using a brute force method.

If you know that the length of a message in ciphertext is identical to the length of a message in cleartext, you can leverage this information to pick out pieces of the ciphertext for which you can make guesses about the cleartext. For example, during WWII while the Allies were trying to break the German Enigma codes, they used a method similar to the above because they knew the phrase "Heil Hitler" probably appeared somewhere near the end of each transmission.

Similar Plaintext Analysis

A related method you might use to crack an unknown algorithm is to compare changes in the ciphertext output with changes in the cleartext input. Of course, this method requires that you have access to the algorithm to selectively encode your carefully chosen cleartext. For example, try encoding the strings "AAAAAA," "AAAAAB" and "BAAAAA" and note the difference in the cipher-text output. For monoalphabetic ciphers, you might expect to see the first few characters remain the same in both outputs for the first two, with only the last portion changing. If so, then it's almost trivial to construct a full translation table for the entire algorithm that maps cleartext input to ciphertext output and vice versa. Once the translation table is complete, you could write an inverse function that deciphers the ciphertext back to plaintext without difficulty.

What happens if the cipher is a polyalphabetic cipher, where more than one character changes in the ciphertext for single character changes in cleartext? Well, that becomes a bit trickier to decipher, depending on the number of changes to the ciphertext. You might be able to combine this analysis technique with brute force to uncover the inner workings of the algorithm, or you might not.

Monoalphabetic Ciphers

A monoalphabetic cipher is any cipher in which each character of the alphabet is replaced by another character in a one-to-one ratio. Both the Caesar Cipher and ROT13, mentioned earlier in the chapter, are classic examples of monoalphabetic ciphers. Some monoalphabetic ciphers scramble the alphabet instead of shifting the letters, so that instead of having an alphabet of *ABCDEFGHIJKLMNOPQRSTUVWXYZ*, the cipher alphabet order might be *MLNKBJVHCGXFZDSAPQOWIEURYT*. The new scrambled alphabet is used to encipher the message such that M=A, L=B…T=Z. Using this method, the cleartext message "SECRET" becomes "OBNQBW."

You will rarely find these types of ciphers in use today outside of word games because they can be easily broken by an exhaustive search of possible alphabet combinations and they are also quite vulnerable to the language analysis methods we described. Monoalphabetic ciphers are absolutely vulnerable to frequency analysis because even though the letters are substituted, the ultimate frequency appearance of each letter will roughly correspond to the known frequency characteristics of the language.

Other Ways to Hide Information

Sometimes vendors follow the old "security through obscurity" approach, and instead of using strong cryptography to prevent unauthorized disclosure of certain information, they just try to hide the information using a commonly known reversible algorithm like UUEncode or Base64, or a combination of two simple methods. In these cases, all you need to do to recover the cleartext is to pass the ciphertext back through the same engine. Vendors may also use XOR encoding against a certain key, but you won't necessarily need the key to decode the message. Let's look at some of the most common of these algorithms in use.

XOR

While many of the more complex and secure encryption algorithms use XOR as an intermediate step, you will often find data obscured by a simple XOR operation. XOR is short for *exclusive or*, which identifies a certain type of binary operation with a truth table as shown in Table 6.2. As each bit from A is combined with B, the result is "0" only if the bits in A and B are identical. Otherwise, the result is 1.

Table 6.2 XOR Truth Table

A	B	A XOR B
0	0	0
0	1	1
1	0	1
1	1	0

Let's look at a very simple XOR operation and how you can undo it. In our simple example, we will use a single character key ("a") to obscure a single character message ("b") to form a result that we'll call "ciphertext" (see Table 6.3).

Table 6.3 XOR of "a" and "b"

Item	Binary Value
a	01100001
b	01100010
ciphertext	00000011

Suppose that you don't know what the value of "a" actually is, you only know the value of "b" and the resulting "ciphertext." You want to recover the key so that you can find out the cleartext value of another encrypted message, "cipher2," which is 00011010. You could perform an XOR with "b" and the "ciphertext" to recover the key "a," as shown in Table 6.4.

Table 6.4 XOR of "ciphertext" and "b"

Item	Binary Value
ciphertext	00000011
b	01100010
a	01100001

Once the key is recovered, you can use it to decode "cipher2" into the character "z" (see Table 6.5).

Table 6.5 XOR of "cipher2" and "a"

Item	Binary Value
cipher2	00011010
a	01100001
z	01111010

Of course, this example is somewhat oversimplified. In the real world, you are most likely to encounter keys that are multiple characters instead of just a single character, and the XOR operation may occur a number of times in series to obscure the message. In this type of instance, you can use a null value to obtain the key—that is, the message will be constructed such that it contains only 0s.

Abstract 1 and 0 manipulation like this can be difficult to understand if you are not used to dealing with binary numbers and values. Therefore, I'll provide you with some sample code and output of a simple program that uses a series of 3 XOR operations on various permutations of a key to obscure a particular message. This short Perl program uses the freely available IIIkey module for the backend XOR encryption routines. You will need to download IIIkey from www3.marketrends.net/encrypt/ to use this program.

```perl
#!/usr/bin/perl
# Encodes/Decodes a form of XOR text
# Requires the IIIkey module
# Written specifically for HPYN 2nd Ed.
# by FWL 01.07.02


# Use the IIIkey module for the backend
# IIIkey is available from http://www3.marketrends.net/encrypt/
use IIIkey;


# Simple input validation
sub validate() {
        if (scalar(@ARGV) < 3) {
        print "Error: You did not specify input correctly!\n";
```

```
            print "To encode data use ./xor.pl e \"Key\" \"String to
                Encode\"\n";
            print "To decode data use ./xor.pl d \"Key\" \"String to
                Decode\"\n";
            exit;
            }
}


validate();


$tmp=new IIIkey;
$key=$ARGV[1];
$intext=$ARGV[2];


if ($ARGV[0] eq "e") {   # encode text
        $outtext=$tmp->crypt($intext, $key);
        print "Encoded $intext to $outtext";
} elsif ($ARGV[0] eq "d") { # decode text
        $outtext=$tmp->decrypt($intext, $key);
        print "Decoded $intext to $outtext";
} else { # No encode/decode information given!
        print "To encode or decode? That is the question.";
        exit;
}
```

Here's some sample output:

```
$ ./xor.pl e "my key" "secret message"
Encoded secret message to 8505352480^0758144+510906534

$ ./xor.pl d "my key" "8505352480^0758144+510906534"
Decoded 8505352480^0758144+510906534 to secret message
```

UUEncode

UUEncode is a commonly used algorithm for converting binary data into a text-based equivalent for transport via e-mail. As you probably know, most e-mail systems cannot directly process binary attachments to e-mail messages. So when you attach a binary file (such as a JPEG image) to an e-mail message, your e-mail client takes care of converting the binary attachment to a text equivalent, probably through an encoding engine like UUEncode. The attachment is converted from binary format into a stream of printable characters, which can be processed by the mail system. Once received, the attachment is processed using the inverse of the encoding algorithm (UUDecode), resulting in conversion back to the original binary file.

Sometimes vendors may use the UUEncode engine to encode ordinary printable text in order to obscure the message. When this happens, all you need to do to is pass the encoded text through a UUDecode program to discern the message. Command-line UUEncode/UUDecode clients are available for just about every operating system ever created.

Base64

Base64 is also commonly used to encode e-mail attachments similar to UUEncode, under Multipurpose Internet Mail Extensions (MIME) extensions. However, you are also likely to come across passwords and other interesting information hidden behind a Base64 conversion. Most notably, many Web servers that implement HTTP-based basic authentication store password data in Base64 format. If your attacker can get access to the Base64 encoded username and password set, he or she can decode them in seconds, no brute force required. One of the telltale signs that a Base64 encode has occurred is the appearance of one or two equal signs (=) at the end of the string, which is often used to pad data.

Look at some sample code for converting between Base64 data and cleartext. This code snippet should run on any system that has Perl5 or better with the MIME::Base64 module from CPAN (www.cpan.org). We have also given you a couple of usage samples.

```
#!/usr/bin/perl
# Filename: base64.pl
# Encodes/Decodes Base-64 text
# Requires the MIME::Base64 module
# Written specifically for HPYN 2nd Ed.
```

```perl
# by FWL 01.07.02


# Use the MIME module for encoding/decoding Base-64 strings
use MIME::Base64;


# Simple input validation
sub validate() {
        if (scalar(@ARGV) < 2) {
        print "Error: You did not specify input correctly!\n";
        print "To encode data use ./base64.pl e \"String to Encode\"\n";
        print "To decode data use ./base64.pl d \"String to Decode\"\n";
        exit;
        }
}


validate();


$intext=$ARGV[1];


if ($ARGV[0] eq "e") {   # encode text
        $outtext=encode_base64($intext);
        print "Encoded $intext to $outtext";
} elsif ($ARGV[0] eq "d") { # decode text
        $outtext=decode_base64($intext);
        print "Decoded $intext to $outtext";
} else { # No encode/decode information given!
        print "To encode or decode? That is the question.";
        exit;
}
```

Here's some sample output:

```
$ ./base64.pl e "Secret Password"
Encoded Secret Password to U2VjcmV0IFBhc3N3b3Jk
```

```
$ ./base64.pl d "U2VjcmV0IFBhc3N3b3Jk"
Decoded U2VjcmV0IFBhc3N3b3Jk to Secret Password
```

Compression

Sometimes you may find that compression has been weakly used to conceal information from you. In days past, some game developers would compress the size of their save game files not only to reduce space, but also to limit your attempts to modify it with a save game editor. The most commonly used algorithms for this were SQSH (Squish or Squash) and LHA. The algorithms themselves were somewhat inherited from console games of the 1980s, where they were used to compress the ROM images in the cartridges. As a rule, when you encounter text that you cannot seem to decipher via standard methods, you may want to check to see if the information has been compressed using one of the plethora of compression algorithms available today.

Notes from the Underground...

Consumer-Oriented Crypto— The SDMI Hacking Challenge

Sometimes organizations decide to use cryptography that isn't necessarily amateur, but shouldn't really be considered professional grade either. For example, the Secure Digital Music Initiative (SDMI) is trying to develop a watermarking scheme for digital music that carries an extra-encoded signal that prevents the music from being played or copied in an unauthorized manner. In developing its watermarking scheme, the SDMI proposed six watermarking schemes to the hacking community and offered up a $10,000 prize to whoever could break the watermarking technology, producing a song without any watermark from a sample song with a watermark. Only samples of the watermarked songs were made available; the SDMI did not release any details about how the watermarking schemes themselves worked. A before-and-after sample of a different song was provided for each of the watermarking schemes, so that differences could be noted.

Two of the six watermarking schemes were dropped shortly after the contest began, and the remaining four were ultimately broken

Continued

within weeks by a team of academic researchers led by Princeton Professor Edward W. Felten. Felten and his associates chose not to accept the $10,000 bounty, opting instead to publicly publish the results of their research. It seems there was a small loophole in the agreement that was presented to challengers before they would be given the files. It said that they had to agree to keep all information secret in order to collect the $10,000. It didn't say anything about what would happen if the challenger wasn't interested in the money. Shortly thereafter, the seemingly upset SDMI threatened a lawsuit under the provisions of the Digital Millennium Copyright Act (DMCA) that prevented the sharing of knowledge that could be used to circumvent copyright protection schemes. Ultimately the SDMI chose not to pursue the matter, and Felten and his associates presented their findings at the 10th USENIX Security Symposium. Felten's conclusion, which is generally shared by the security community at large, was that any attempts at watermarking-type encryption would ultimately be broken. Also of interest is the fact that Felten's team identified that no special knowledge in computer science was needed to break the watermarking schemes; only a general knowledge of signal processing was required.

You might view this story as yet another example of a vendor attempting to employ what they proclaim to be "highly secure proprietary algorithms," but it is also an example of the continuing evolution of cryptography and its applications in new ways. Even if these new applications of cryptography don't lend themselves well to the use of conventional algorithms, you would be wise to remain skeptical of newly proposed unproven algorithms, especially when these algorithms are kept secret.

Summary

This chapter looked into the meaning of cryptography and some of its origins, including Caesar's Cipher. More modern branches of cryptography are *symmetric* and *asymmetric* cryptography, which are also known as *secret key* and *public key* cryptography, respectively.

The most common symmetric algorithms in use today include DES, AES, and IDEA. Since DES is showing its age, we looked at how NIST managed the development of AES as a replacement, and how Rijndael was selected from five finalists to become the AES algorithm. From the European perspective, we saw how IDEA came to be developed in the early 1990s and examined its advantages over DES.

The early development of asymmetric cryptography was begun in the mid-1970s by Diffie and Hellman, who developed the Diffie-Hellman key exchange algorithm as a means of securely exchanging information over a public network. After Diffie-Hellman, the RSA algorithm was developed, heralding a new era of public key cryptography systems such as PGP. Fundamental differences between public key and symmetric cryptography include public key cryptography's reliance on the factoring problem for extremely large integers.

Brute force is an effective method of breaking most forms of cryptography, provided you have the time to wait for keyspace exhaustion, which could take anywhere from several minutes to billions of years. Cracking passwords is the most widely used application of brute force; programs such as L0phtcrack and John the Ripper are used exclusively for this purpose.

Even secure algorithms can be implemented insecurely, or in ways not intended by the algorithm's developers. Man-in-the-middle attacks could cripple the security of a Diffie-Hellman key exchange, and even DES-encrypted LANMAN password hashes can be broken quite easily. Using easily broken passwords or passphrases as secret keys in symmetric algorithms can have unpleasant effects, and improperly stored private and secret keys can negate the security provided by encryption altogether.

Information is sometimes concealed using weak or reversible algorithms. We saw in this chapter how weak ciphers are subject to frequency analysis attacks that use language characteristics to decipher the message. Related attacks include relative length analysis and similar plaintext analysis. We saw how vendors sometimes conceal information using XOR and Base64 encoding and looked at some sample code for each of these types of reversible ciphers. We also saw how, on occasion, information is compressed as a means of obscuring it.

Solutions Fast Track

Understanding Cryptography Concepts

- ☑ Unencrypted text is referred to as *cleartext*, while encrypyted text is called *ciphertext*.

- ☑ The two main categories of cryptography are *symmetric key* and *asymmetric key* cryptography. Symmetric key cryptography uses a single secret key, while asymmetric key cryptography uses a pair of public and private keys.

- ☑ Public key cryptography was first devised as a means of exchanging a secret key securely by Diffie and Hellman.

Learning about Standard Cryptographic Algorithms

- ☑ The reason why so many cryptographic algorithms are available for your use is that each algorithm has its own relative speed, security and ease of use. You need to know enough about the most common algorithms to choose one that is appropriate to the situation to which it will be applied.

- ☑ Data Encryption Standard (DES) is the oldest and most widely known modern encryption method around. However, it is nearing the end of its useful life span, so you should avoid using it in new implementations or for information you want to keep highly secure.

- ☑ Advanced Encryption Standard (AES) was designed as a secure replacement for DES, and you can use several different keysizes with it.

- ☑ Be aware that asymmetric cryptography uses entirely different principles than symmetric cryptography. Where symmetric cryptography combines a single key with the message for a number of cycles, asymmetric cryptography relies on numbers that are too large to be factored.

- ☑ The two most widely used asymmetric algorithms are Diffie-Hellman and RSA.

Understanding Brute Force

☑ Brute force is the one single attack that will always succeed against symmetric cryptography, given enough time. You want to ensure that "enough time" becomes a number of years or decades or more.

☑ An individual machine performing a brute force attack is slow. If you can string together a number of machines in parallel, your brute force attack will be much faster.

☑ Brute force attacks are most often used for cracking passwords.

Knowing When Real Algorithms Are Being Used Improperly

☑ Understand the concept of the man-in-the-middle attack against a Diffie-Hellman key exchange.

☑ LANMAN password hashing should be disabled, if possible, because its implementation allows it to be broken quite easily.

☑ Key storage should always be of the utmost importance to you because if your secret or private key is compromised, all data protected by those keys is also compromised.

Understanding Amateur Cryptography Attempts

☑ You can crack almost any weak cryptography attempts (like XOR) with minimal effort.

☑ Frequency analysis is a powerful tool to use against reasonably lengthy messages that aren't guarded by modern cryptography algorithms.

☑ Sometimes vendors will attempt to conceal information using weak cryptography (like Base64) or compression.

Frequently Asked Questions

The following Frequently Asked Questions, answered by the authors of this book, are designed to both measure your understanding of the concepts presented in this chapter and to assist you with real-life implementation of these concepts. To have your questions about this chapter answered by the author, browse to **www.syngress.com/solutions** and click on the **"Ask the Author"** form.

Q: Are there any cryptography techniques which are 100 percent secure?

A: Yes. Only the One Time Pad (OTP) algorithm is absolutely unbreakable if implemented correctly. The OTP algorithm is actually a Vernam cipher, which was developed by AT&T way back in 1917. The Vernam cipher belongs to a family of ciphers called *stream ciphers*, since they encrypt data in continuous stream format instead of the chunk-by-chunk method of block ciphers. There are two problems with using the OTP, however: You must have a source of truly random data, and the source must be bit-for-bit as long as the message to be encoded. You also have to transmit both the message and the key (separately), the key must remain secret, and the key can *never* be reused to encode another message. If an eavesdropper intercepts two messages encoded with the same key, then it is trivial for the eavesdropper to recover the key and decrypt both messages. The reason OTP ciphers are not used more commonly is the difficulty in collecting truly random numbers for the key (as mentioned in one of the sidebars for this chapter) and the difficulty of the secure distribution of the key.

Q: How long is DES expected to remain in use?

A: Given the vast number of DES-based systems, I expect we'll continue to see DES active for another five or ten years, especially in areas where security is not a high priority. For some applications, DES is considered a "good enough" technology since the average hacker doesn't have the resources available (for now) to break the encryption scheme efficiently. I predict that DES will still find a use as a casual eavesdropping deterrent, at least until the widespread adoption of IPv6. DES is also far faster than 3-DES, and as such it is more suitable to older-style VPN gear that may not be forward-compatible with the new AES standard. In rare cases where legacy connections are required, the government is still allowing new deployment of DES-based systems.

Q: After the 9/11 attacks I'm concerned about terrorists using cryptography, and I've heard people advocate that the government should have a back door access to all forms of encryption. Why would this be a bad idea?

A: Allowing back-door access for anyone causes massive headaches for users of encryption. First and foremost, these back door keys are likely to be stored all in one place, making that storage facility the prime target for hackers. When the storage facility is compromised, and I have no doubt that it would be (the only question is how soon), everyone's data can effectively be considered compromised. We'd also need to establish a new bureaucracy that would be responsible for handing out the back door access, probably in a manner similar to the way in which wiretaps are currently doled out. We would also require some sort of watchdog group that certifies the deployment group as responsible. Additionally, all of our encryption schemes would need to be redesigned to allow backdoor access, probably in some form of "public key + trusted key" format. Implementation of these new encryption routines would take months to develop and years to deploy. New cracking schemes would almost certainly focus on breaking the algorithm through the "trusted key" access, leaving the overall security of these routines questionable at best.

Q: Why was CSS, the encryption technology used to protect DVDs from unauthorized copying, able to be broken so easily?

A: Basically, DVD copy protection was broken so easily because one entity, Xing Technologies, left their key lying around in the open, which as we saw in this chapter is a cardinal sin. The data encoded on a DVD-Video disc is encrypted using an algorithm called the Content Scrambling System (CSS) which can be unlocked using a 40-bit key. Using Xing's 40-bit key, hackers were able to brute force and guess at the keys for over 170 other licensees at a rapid pace. That way, since the genie was out of the bottle, so to speak, for so many vendors, the encryption for the entire format was basically broken. With so many keys to choose from, others in the underground had no difficulty in leveraging these keys to develop the DeCSS program, which allows data copied off of the DVD to be saved to another media in an unencrypted format. Ultimately, the CSS scheme was doomed to failure. You can't put a key inside millions of DVD players, distribute them, and not expect someone to eventually pull it out.

## Chapter 7

Cisco LocalDirector and DistributedDirector

Solutions in this chapter:

- **Improving Security Using Cisco LocalDirector**

- **LocalDirector Security Features**

- **Securing Geographically Dispersed Server Farms Using Cisco DistributedDirector**

- **DistributedDirector Security Features**

☑ **Summary**

☑ **Solutions Fast Track**

☑ **Frequently Asked Questions**

Introduction

When it was first deployed, Cisco Systems' LocalDirector was positioned as a replacement solution for the "round-robin" redundancy and load-balancing methods used on the Internet. The networking and computing trade sheets referred to these devices as *load balancers*. However, when applied to LocalDirector, the load balancing term is actually a misnomer. While load balancers are able to equally distribute traffic loads across multiple servers, LocalDirector is capable of additional functions like scalability, high availability, server connection management, and server security.

Even with a highly secure network, one also needs to be certain there is some level of redundancy built into the network. This will ensure that attacks intended to suck up your bandwidth meet with a minimum of success.

LocalDirector can help you with this. On the other hand, there are many other devices that can complete this job more efficiently. The LocalDirector technology is somewhat outdated, and even Cisco is beginning to suggest other devices to perform these same functions. The replacement for LocalDirector is now Cisco Content Services Switch (detailed information on CSSs can be found in Chapter 10). Therefore, if you are only starting to add redundancy and distribution features to your server network, you might be interested in looking into CSS solutions first.

DistributedDirector is also a load-balancing solution used to distribute traffic between geographically distant servers. Again, these features were improved and further developed in the CSS product line.

Improving Security Using Cisco LocalDirector

Cisco's LocalDirector allows you to load-balance Internet resource requests among multiple local servers. One would typically use this solution to front-end a Web server farm, based in the same location, and thus load-balance Web traffic to the most appropriate server.

Using this technology, LocalDirector allows you to publish a Web address, along with a single Internet Protocol (IP) address associated with that address, and yet have one of many Web servers respond to that resource request. Redundancy, introduced by this feature, allows for increased availability and stability of the server network in case of attacks (especially in regards to denial of service (DoS) attacks).

LocalDirector Technology Overview

Cisco's LocalDirector uses the Open System Interconnection (OSI) Layers 3 and 4 (Network and Transport Layers respectively) as a load-balancing technology that allows you to publish a single Uniform Resource Locator (URL) and a single IP address for an entire server farm. From a technical point of view, it acts as a transparent TCP/IP bridge within the network.

The LocalDirector determines which server is most appropriate by tracking network sessions and server load conditions in real time.

Such technology helps decrease the response time of your service while increasing service reliability. Service response time is decreased because resource requests for a URL or IP address are directed to the most appropriate server (the least busy server, for example) within the server farm. Likewise, service reliability is increased because LocalDirector monitors individual servers in the server farm and forwards resource requests only to servers that are operating correctly.

Before the inception of this technology, you would have to know the name or IP address of every individual Web server in the server farm, or you would have to make use of multiple IP addresses associated with a single DNS name (the so-called DNS round-robin load balancing). Neither of these techniques were user friendly, nor did they result in appropriate load distribution. They were also unreliable, because no attempt was made to verify the servers' availability in real time.

Cisco's LocalDirector can be compared to an Automatic Call Distributor (ACD) in the telephony world. LocalDirector is similar to an ACD in that incoming telephone calls are routed to a pool of agents and answered as soon as an agent is available. It works as a front-end for a Web server farm and redirects resource requests to the most appropriate server. Figure 7.1 depicts a typical LocalDirector implementation.

LocalDirector Product Overview

The LocalDirector product is available in three different ranges:

- **LocalDirector 416** This is both the entry-level product as well as the medium-size product. It supports up to 90 Mbps throughput and 7,000 connections per second.

- **LocalDirector 430** This is the high-end product. It supports up to 400 Mbps throughput and 30,000 connections per second.

- **LocalDirector 417** Newer platform with different mounting features. It is even more productive than 430 series and has more memory—two Fast Ethernet and one Gigabit Ethernet interfaces.

Figure 7.1 A Typical LocalDirector Implementation

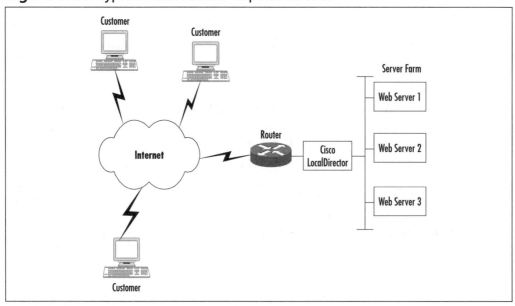

For additional performance, LocalDirector can be used with the Accelerated Server Load Balancing (ASLB) feature of the Catalyst 6000 series switches to increase throughput to 15 million packets per second (mpps).

LocalDirector Security Features

The following information about the security features of LocalDirector will allow you to better understand the security mechanisms it uses and enable you to configure or change these features. Although there are not many of them, correct usage of those present will help you protect the server farm from attacks and network hiccups.

Filtering of Access Traffic

Since LocalDirector maintains and tracks the state of communications for all clients and server hosts, it can control access to specific servers based on various conditions—for example, by source IP address or service port number. This allows you to increase security by restricting which resources the client is allowed to access.

LocalDirector protects your network by only allowing specific traffic to pass between virtual and real servers, restricting both external and internal access to

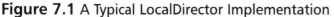

servers. It does not have full Access Control List (ACL) features, but several options are provided:

- **SecureAccess** Allows you to manipulate a connection based on the source IP address of the client. Traffic from certain clients can be directed to a specific virtual server or dropped altogether.

- **SecureBind** Allows you to restrict traffic to a specific port using port-bound (as opposed to IP-bound) servers. Incoming TCP traffic to a port that is not specified as available is terminated by a reset packet (TCP RST). This feature is not available for UDP-based traffic.

- **SecureBridging** Because LocalDirector acts as a transparent TCP/IP bridge, it will pass traffic to the real server's IP addresses. Thus, clients who know the real server's IP address can access it directly if the server is configured to be bridged (the default setting). Bridging can be turned off, thereby forcing client traffic through the LocalDirector virtual address.

- **Secure IP Address** This is similar to static NAT. It allows LocalDirector to translate the IP address of a real server to a virtual IP address, thereby hiding the IP address of the real server while still allowing the physical server to connect to the outside world.

The following is an example of a configuration using SecureAccess, SecureBind, and SecureBridging features. Suppose in Figure 7.1 that LocalDirector is on the local network 192.168.2.0, which has two Web servers: 192.168.2.1 and 192.168.2.2. These hosts run public Web services on port 80 and intranet services (which have to be available only to internal clients from the 192.168.2.0 network) on port 8080. We will create one virtual server—server 192.168.2.10—and using the SecureAccess feature, redirect external clients to 192.168.2.1:80 and 192.168.2.2:80, while redirecting clients from the internal network to 192.168.2.1:8080 and 192.168.2.2:8080.

```
secure 0
secure 1
virtual 192.168.2.10:80:0:tcp is
virtual 192.168.2.10:80:1:tcp is
real 192.168.2.1:80:tcp is
real 192.168.2.2:80:tcp is
```

```
real 192.168.2.1:8080:tcp is
real 192.168.2.2:8080:tcp is
bind 192.168.2.10:80:0:tcp 192.168.2.1:80:tcp
bind 192.168.2.10:80:0:tcp 192.168.2.2:80:tcp
bind 192.168.2.10:80:1:tcp 192.168.2.1:8080:tcp
bind 192.168.2.10:80:1:tcp 192.168.2.2:8080:tcp
assign 192.168.2.10:80:1:tcp 192.168.2.0 255.255.255.0
```

The first two lines turn off transparent bridging on both interfaces (the SecureBridging feature). The next two lines are used to define two virtual servers, both running on port 80 at IP address 192.168.2.10. Four real port-bound servers are described after that (the SecureBind feature). Then (*bind* commands) four real servers are assigned to instances of the virtual server. Lastly, the *assign* command is used to redirect internal clients to a specific instance of the virtual server, the one that is redirected to intranet servers on 192.168.2.1:8080 and 192.168.2.2:8080. This is an example of the SecureAccess feature.

Using *synguard* to Protect Against SYN Flood Attacks

The SYN flood attack is a form of DoS strike that occurs when a server receives many SYN packets (which are used for connection initiation in TCP) without any follow-up. By definition, these potential connections have to be put on hold for some time before they are considered expired. This causes connection queues to fill up, preventing any other TCP connections from being established until the backlog is cleared.

On host systems (for example, on Web servers), you will need to employ techniques for minimizing the effect of a SYN attack. One of these techniques is to increase the size of the connection queue so the attacker needs more time and resources to cause problems—a condition that will apply to the host itself as well, causing it to consume more resources than normal. Another technique is to determine whether or not your host software vendor has any patches that help protect against SYN attacks. Many products, including IBM's AIX, Microsoft's NT, and Sun's Solaris now have these types of patches, although they generally do not eliminate the cause of the problem, but instead only try to ease the consequences. LocalDirector, on the other hand, has a *synguard* feature which is used to protect servers from excessive SYN packets. It counts incoming SYNs and SYN-ACK replies from the server. Once the number of unanswered SYNs reaches a certain limit, all incoming SYN packets to this virtual server are dropped.

By default, this feature is disabled, making the default value 0. The maximum number of SYNs allowed needs to be configured before the feature is enabled.

The following syntax is used to configure the *synguard* feature (from configuration mode):

```
synguard virtual_id count
```

where *virtual_id* is the virtual server IP address or name and port (if a server is port-bound), and *count* is the maximum number of unanswered SYNs allowed to this virtual server.

To disable *synguard*, either set the count back to zero, or use the *no* command:

```
no synguard virtual_id count
```

Note that the *synguard* command provides limited protection against SYN attacks to the virtual server. One of its uses is to notify a system administrator that something bad is happening—LocalDirector always sends a syslog message when it enters protection mode (that is, when the number of unanswered SYN packets exceeds the threshold). After the feature is activated, LocalDirector begins protecting the real network and servers from SYN flood attacks.

The following example illustrates the use of *synguard*:

```
LocalDirector(config)# show synguard
        Machine      Port    SynGuard      Status
    www.test.com   default          0
```

No threshold is set for server www.test.com, so we'll set it to 500 SYN packets.

```
LocalDirector(config)# synguard www.test.com 500
LocalDirector(config)# show synguard
        Machine      Port    SynGuard      Status
    www.test.com   default        500
LocalDirector(config)# show syn
        Machine      Port     Conns   Syn Count
    www.test.com   default      648         176
```

The *show syn* command displays the total number of active connections and current number of active TCP handshakes (unanswered SYN packets).

The following example shows *synguard* in active mode. Notice how the status changes to Active after the number of unanswered SYNs has increased to the threshold.

```
LocalDirector(config)# show synguard
          Machine      Port    SynGuard        Status
     www.site.com   default         500        Active
LocalDirector(config)# show syn
          Machine      Port      Conns   Syn Count
     www.site.com   default        892         500
LocalDirector(config)#
```

Using NAT to Hide Real Addresses

LocalDirector supports Network Address Translation (NAT). This allows you to use unregistered IP addresses on your inside network (usually the server farm) and prevents hackers from being able to directly target the real server's IP address.

RFC 1918 reserves three address ranges—often referred to as *private, internal,* or *unregistered* address ranges—for internal use. These address ranges are not routed on the Internet and packets need to be converted to registered IP addresses before they can be sent to the Internet. NAT performs this conversion from private IP addresses to registered IP addresses, and vice versa, allowing devices access to and from the Internet. This also conserves registered IP addresses.

Increased security is provided through NAT by hiding the internal IP address range and making it more difficult for potential hackers to access as well as learn about the internal structure of your network.

Figure 7.2 shows an example of a device performing NAT. The 10.0.0.x IP address range is not accessible via the Internet, without first going through the NAT conversion process where the registered IP address range is converted to the private IP address range.

Figure 7.2 The NAT Conversion Process

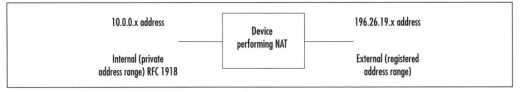

Incoming connections to virtual servers are not subject to NAT, as forwarding and load balancing is performed on the Ethernet level by manipulating MAC addresses in packets, with LocalDirector working as a bridge. There is a possibility of making it translate IP addresses instead, although it is not recommended.

Other NAT capabilities of LocalDirector can be used to statically translate IP addresses of outgoing connections from the real server to the outside world. For example, you can translate this IP to the IP of the virtual server, so the actual IP address of the real server is never revealed, even if the server connects to the hosts outside LocalDirector.

Restricting Who Is Authorized to Have Telnet Access to LocalDirector

You can specify who is authorized to have Telnet access to the LocalDirector. This can be entered either in the form of an IP address or a network address. Limiting who can Telnet into the LocalDirector is an easy and highly effective way of keeping unauthorized persons from trying to gain access to, or cause the disruption of, your systems.

The following syntax is used to configure who has Telnet access (from configuration mode):

```
telnet ip mask
```

Here, *ip* is the IP address or network of the host that is authorized to access the LocalDirector Telnet management interface, and *mask* is the subnet mask for the network specified in this command. Use 255.255.255.255 if you specified a single IP address.

To disable this feature, use the *no* command:

```
no telnet ip mask
```

You can use the following syntax to view allowed IP addresses or networks:

```
show telnet
```

Password Protection

Like most Cisco devices, LocalDirector supports two levels of password protection: *privileged* and *nonprivileged*. The *enable* password is used to enter the privileged level and allows you to view settings, as well as make configuration changes. The *telnet* password is used for the nonprivileged level that allows you to view certain settings but not change them. Passwords can consist of up to 16 alphanumeric symbols and are not case-sensitive; they are converted into lowercase and stored in an encrypted MD5 form.

The *enable* Password

The *enable* password is the privileged-level password. There is no default *enable* password. Be sure to set one before you deploy LocalDirector. The following syntax is used to create an *enable* password (from configuration mode):

```
enable password password
```

The *telnet* Password

The *telnet* password is a user-level password. The default *telnet* password is *cisco.*

The following syntax is used to change the default *telnet* password (from configuration mode):

```
password password
```

Here, *password* is a password of up to 16 alphanumeric characters.

Configuring & Implementing...

Password Protection

For maximum protection, configure Telnet access restriction to allow only a minimal amount of IP addresses to access LocalDirector. One is ideal, although this is not always possible—for example, if you have several management stations.

Always use a different password for each of the password levels. Having the same password for each security level is a frequently encountered misconfiguration and is strongly discouraged.

A common security mistake is failing to change the default *telnet* password (*cisco*) before deploying LocalDirector.

Syslog Logging

Often, knowing when your network is under attack is as important as taking steps to protect yourself against the attack. This is where logging plays an important role.

If a syslog server is configured, LocalDirector will log error and event messages to an external syslog server. For example, a syslog message will be generated if LocalDirector enters synguard protection mode.

The following syntax is used to configure the syslog feature (from configuration mode):

```
syslog {host ip |console}
```

Here the word *host* defines that syslog messages should be sent to a syslog server with IP address *ip*, while *console* specifies that syslog messages will be displayed on the local console (connected to the console port).

To disable syslog messaging, use the *no* command:

```
no syslog {host ip |console}
```

You can use the following syntax to view previously sent syslog messages:

```
show syslog
```

Securing Geographically Dispersed Server Farms Using Cisco DistributedDirector

Cisco's DistributedDirector is a product that allows you to load-balance Internet resource requests among geographically dispersed servers. Its typical application is for a corporation to make use of Web servers, or Web server farms, in multiple locations to service Web requests.

DistributedDirector achieves this by redirecting resource requests to servers located closest to the customer requesting that service. This feature was greatly developed and improved in the Cisco Content Services Switch product—a sophisticated device for Web traffic distribution (see Chapter 10 for additional details about the CSS product line).

DistributedDirector Technology Overview

Cisco's DistributedDirector uses routing table intelligence in the network infrastructure to transparently redirect a customer's service requests to the closest server, as determined by the client-to-server proximity or client-to-server latency.

By using this technology, you can decrease the service response time and increase the service reliability, as well as reduce the cost of long distance communication. The service response time is decreased, and the cost of long distance communications reduced because resource requests to a URL or IP address are redirected to the server closest to the customer requesting the service. The service reliability is increased because DistributedDirector monitors individual servers and does not direct resource requests to servers that are not operating correctly.

Designing & Planning...

Using LocalDirector and DistributedDirector Together

These two products are complimentary in the sense that they can be used together to provide both global scalability of topologically (and geographically) distant server farms and local scalability for redundant clusters. In this scenario, DistributedDirector is responsible for global traffic distribution between virtual servers, where each in its turn is represented by LocalDirector, which provides the local load balancing, ensuring traffic is directed to the highest-available physical server at each distribution site.

DistributedDirector doesn't know anything about the structure of the sites it distributes traffic to. It simply treats them as single servers. When its server availability check fails, it means no physical server behind the corresponding LocalDirector is available or that LocalDirector itself is unavailable at that site. So, provided LocalDirector is itself functioning (this can be ensured by using the failover features), the site will be considered operational by a DistributedDirector as long as it has at least one physical server working. This is a serious availability enhancement—as long as at least one physical server in one geographical location is operational, people will be able to reach your site without knowing of your problems.

Director Response Protocol (DRP) is a protocol that allows DistributedDirector to query routers (DRP server agents) for routing table topological metrics. (DRP agent functionality has been available in IOS releases since 11.3(2)T.) Various Internal Gateway Protocols can be used—RIP, OSPF, IGRP, EIGRP, Integrated, IS-IS, and so on DistributedDirector uses this information to calculate the distance from the client to the servers and redirect the customer's service requests to the closest server. DistributedDirector can function in two modes—Caching DNS mode and HTTP Session Redirect mode. In the first instance, it acts as a caching DNS server, resolving DNS requests for a Web server's name to the IP address of the closest server. In the second mode, it acts as a Web server itself, issuing HTTP redirect messages to the client (HTTP status code 302), and providing the IP address of the nearest real Web server.

Cisco's DistributedDirector can be compared to a regionalized 1-800 number in the telephony world, where incoming calls to a toll-free number are routed to agents located in the same region the call originated, saving on long-distance charges that would otherwise be incurred if the call were answered at a centralized location.

Figure 7.3 depicts a typical DistributedDirector implementation. Web requests are sent to the DistributedDirector, which redirects them to the most appropriate Web server. Often, this is the nearest server from a geographical standpoint. For example, the Web server in San Francisco might best service a Web request from Customer 1 and Customer 2 (who are in the U.S.), whereas the Web server in London might better service a Web request from Customer 3 (who is in Ireland, for example).

Figure 7.3 A Typical DistributedDirector Implementation

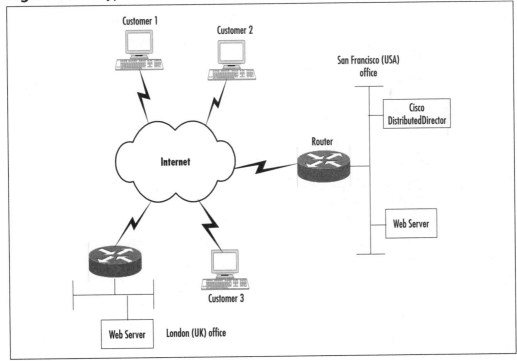

DistributedDirector Product Overview

The DistributedDirector product is available in three different ranges:

- **DistributedDirector 2501/2502** This is the entry-level product. DistributedDirector 2501 has an Ethernet interface, and DistributedDirector 2502 has a Token Ring.

- **DistributedDirector 4700M** This is the medium-level product and comes in models that have Ethernet, Fast Ethernet, Token Ring, and FDDI interfaces.

- **The Cisco 7200 Series Router** This is the high-end product, and is based on the modular Cisco 7200 router, with the DistributedDirector feature set.

DistributedDirector Security Features

The following information about the security features of DistributedDirector will allow you to better understand the security mechanisms they use, and enable you to configure or change these features. DistributedDirector does not provide many security features for the network. Its use in security architecture is based on the enhanced redundancy it provides. Therefore, this section describes securing the product itself from various attacks.

Limiting the Source of DRP Queries

Security of the whole system can be increased by limiting DRP server agents' access to devices having specific source IP addresses. This is done using standard Cisco Access Control Lists (ACLs) together with the *ip drp access-group* command.

If this feature is not implemented, intruders can exploit this vulnerability by creating forged DRP queries and disrupting the normal DRP process by providing incorrect DRP information, thus creating DoS attacks or redirecting clients to false servers. The possibility of a DoS attack against DistributedDirector itself also exists—it can be flooded with illegitimate DRP packets. Protection against this attack is provided by the same feature, because DRP queries that do not originate from authorized DRP sources are discarded even before they can be processed.

The following syntax is used to configure this feature (from global configuration mode):

```
ip drp access-group access-list-number
```

Here *access-list-number* is the standard IP access list describing agents' permissions to connect to the device.

Authentication between DistributedDirector and DRP Agents

In order to increase security and help prevent DoS attacks based on DRP, authentication of DRP queries and responses between the DistributedDirector and the Director Response Protocol (DRP) agents is supported.

By using DRP authentication, DistributedDirector stops intruders from forging DRP queries and disrupting or interfering with the service request redirection function. The authentication feature is based on Keyed-Hashing for Message Authentication Code (HMAC) – Message Digest 5 (MD5) digital signatures. The following syntax is used to configure this feature (from global configuration mode):

```
ip drp authentication key-chain key-chain-name
```

Here *key-chain-name* is the name of the key chain (a string of characters without spaces) containing one or more authentication keys.

To disable this feature, use the *no* command:

```
no ip drp authentication key-chain key-chain-name
```

> **SECURITY ALERT!**
>
> For additional security, use multiple keys on a key chain so you can set key lifetimes using the *accept-lifetime* and *send-lifetime* commands.

You will also need to configure a key chain itself, including actual keys and key-strings, using the *key chain*, *key*, and *key-string* commands.

The *key chain* Command

The *key chain* command is the structure that holds the authentication keys and key-strings together. The following syntax is used to configure this feature (from global configuration mode):

```
key chain name-of-chain
```

Here *name-of-chain* is the name of the key chain.
To disable this feature, use the *no* command:

```
no key chain name-of-chain
```

Use the following syntax to verify key chain information:

```
show key chain
```

The *key* Command

The *key* is a number used to identify the authentication key on a key chain. The following syntax is used to configure this feature (from the key chain configuration):

```
key number
```

Here *number* is the identification number of an authentication key on a key chain. The range of keys is 0 to 2147483647. The key numbers do not have to be consecutive.
To disable this feature, use the *no* command:

```
no key number
```

The *key-string* Command

The *key-string* command is used to identify the authentication string for the key. The following syntax is used to configure this feature (from the key configuration):

```
key-string text
```

Here, *text* is the authentication string, which can contain from 1 to 80 upper-case and lowercase alphanumeric characters (the first character cannot be a number, however). This string must be contained in the DRP packets received in order for them to be authenticated.
To disable this feature, use the *no* command:

```
no key-string text
```

There are two options *accept-lifetime* and *send-lifetime* that define when this specific string will be used for authentication.
The following is an example of DRP authentication using a *key chain*, *keys*, *key-strings*, and *accept-lifetime*, as well as *send-lifetime*. In this example, the password *xonix* will always be a valid key for accepting and receiving. The *tetris* key, on the other hand, will be accepted from 15:30 to 17:30 (7,200 seconds) on May 14, 2002 and

be sent from 16:00 to 17:00 (3,600 seconds) on May 14, 2002. The overlap allows for a migration of keys or a discrepancy in the router's time. The *klingons* key-string works in the same way but with different times.

```
ip drp authentication key-chain gameboy
!
key chain gameboy
 key 1
  key-string xonix
 key 2
  key-string tetris
  accept-lifetime 15:30:00 May 14 2002 duration 7200
  send-lifetime 16:00:00 May 14 2002 duration 3600
 key 3
  key-string klingons
  accept-lifetime 16:30:00 May 14 2002 duration 7200
  send-lifetime 17:00:00 May 14 2002 duration 3600
```

Password Protection

Because DistributedDirector runs a modified copy of Cisco's Internet-working Operating System (IOS), the procedure for changing passwords on DistributedDirector is the same as for regular IOS. DistributedDirector supports three different levels of password protection: *enable secret*, *enable*, and *telnet*.

Security Alert!

For maximum protection, use a different password for the three different password levels that DistributedDirector supports. Although IOS allows you to make all the passwords the same, this is strongly discouraged for security reasons.

The *enable secret* Password

The *enable secret* password is the most secure, encrypted privileged-level password, and can be used even if an *enable* password is configured. The following syntax is used to create an *enable secret* password (from configuration mode):

```
enable secret password password
```

Here, *password* is the *enable secret* password.

The *enable* Password

The *enable* password is a less secure, non-encrypted privileged-level password. It's used when the *enable secret* password does not exist. The following syntax is used to create an *enable* password (from configuration mode):

```
enable password password
```

Here, *password* is the *enable* password.

The *telnet* Password

The *telnet* password is a user-level password that allows you to look at some of the configuration information, but not change any configuration. By default, Telnet is not allowed and there is no default *telnet* password. You will need to configure both the *telnet* password as well as an *enable* password for you to be able to Telnet into DistributedDirector. The following syntax is used to configure a *telnet* password (from vty configuration mode):

```
password password
```

Here, *password* is the *telnet* password.

Syslog Logging

As already noted, knowing that an attack is occurring is an important way to protect against it. Logging plays an imperative role in this.

Again, because DistributedDirector runs a modified copy of Cisco's IOS, the procedure for configuring logging to an external syslog server is the same as with regular IOS.

The following syntax is used to configure the *syslog* feature (from configuration mode):

```
logging ip
```

Here, *ip* is the IP address of the log host.

To disable syslog, use the *no* command:

```
no logging ip
```

Use the following syntax to view syslog messages in the buffer:

```
show logging
```

Summary

Load-balancing solutions provide extra redundancy and availability for network servers—both Web and generic TCP servers—by distributing traffic destined for one virtual server between several physical servers. Cisco LocalDirector and DistributedDirector can be used for this purpose. LocalDirector acts as a front-end for a local server farm, while DistributedDirector provides traffic distribution among geographically distant servers.

The LocalDirector product range consists of three appliances, from entry-level to high-level devices. The high-level product, LocalDirector 417, is able to support Gigabit Ethernet speeds. There is also a possibility of cooperation with Catalyst 6000 switches for increase of throughput (to 15 million packets per second).

LocalDirector features various security-related technologies: SecureAccess, which provides for traffic filtering by source of connection; SecureBind, which allows port-bound servers (instead of only IP-based redirection); and SecureBridging, which helps to protect real servers from direct connections from the outside world. It also has static NAT features, and the capability to protect against SYN flood attacks.

The device itself has common Cisco-style password protection and is capable of sending syslog messages to remote servers.

DistributedDirector works together with Cisco routers, which provides it with IGP metrics of corresponding networks. This allows it to select the server nearest to each specific client, thus saving on long-distance communications and decreasing delays in service. Product range consists of two appliances that run modified Cisco IOS software and one device based on a modular 7200 series router.

Security features of DistributedDirector are limited to authentication of its communications with routers (DRP agents). This authentication is based on the HMAC-MD5 hashing algorithm. It also has the Cisco common password system (non-privileged mode and enable mode) and syslog subsystem.

Solutions Fast Track

Improving Security Using Cisco LocalDirector

☑ Security-related use of LocalDirector mainly comes from its increased reliability and redundancy features.

☑ LocalDirector also serves to protect against SYN flood attacks.

☑ It can balance stateless TCP and UDP servers.

☑ The LocalDirector product range consists of three series—the 416, 430, and 417 product lines.

☑ The 417 series, in addition to two Fast Ethernet interfaces, has a one Gigabit Ethernet interface.

☑ When used together with the Catalyst 6000 Accelerated Server Load Balancing feature, LocalDirector can achieve throughput of up to 15 million packets per second.

LocalDirector Security Features

☑ LocalDirector has some restricted traffic filtering abilities.

☑ It can also perform static NAT for outgoing connections, helping hide an internal server's IP address.

☑ The LocalDirector command interface is password protected in a manner similar to other Cisco devices. It has the capability to restrict Telnet access to a device based on its IP address.

Securing Geographically Dispersed Server Farms Using Cisco DistributedDirector

☑ Cisco's DistributedDirector is a product that allows load balancing of Internet resource requests among geographically dispersed servers.

☑ DistributedDirector achieves this by redirecting resource requests to servers located closest to the customer requesting that service.

☑ DistributedDirector works in cooperation with Cisco routers, which provide information on network topology and distance.

☑ DistributedDirector can function in two modes—Caching DNS mode and HTTP Session Redirect mode.

☑ The DistributedDirector product line includes two appliances—entry-level and medium-level devices—plus a high-end product based on the 7200 series modular Cisco router.

☑ In the process of calculating network distances, DistributedDirector can use various IGP protocols, such as RIP, OSPF, IGRP, EIGRP, Integrated IS-IS, and so on.

DistributedDirector Security Features

☑ Security of the system is achieved by limiting the source/destination of DRP communications of DistributedDirector with participating routers.

☑ DRP communications can be also authenticated using MD5 keyed hashing algorithms.

☑ Command-line interface is protected in the same way as all IOS devices. This is because DistributedDirector runs a modified copy of Cisco IOS software.

Frequently Asked Questions

The following Frequently Asked Questions, answered by the authors of this book, are designed to both measure your understanding of the concepts presented in this chapter and to assist you with real-life implementation of these concepts. To have your questions about this chapter answered by the author, browse to **www.syngress.com/solutions** and click on the **"Ask the Author"** form.

Q: How are SSL connections supported by LocalDirector?

A: When load-balancing SSL connections (HTTPS servers), LocalDirector has to ensure that once a connection is established, all requests from the same client are redirected to the same server since this encrypted connection uses a unique key that is established during session setup. To achieve this, the device supports the so-called "sticky" mode for connections. A connection can be made sticky based on the client source IP address or SSL session ID (which is provided by the client's browser).

Q: What is the major problem with stickiness based on source IP address?

A: The major problem in such cases is that all connections from the same source IP address are redirected to the same physical server. This does not work well when several clients behind a firewall try to connect to the same server. If a firewall performs while hiding NAT (so all source IPs are translated to the same address), then from the point of view of a LocalDirector they come from the same client. When one of these clients finishes the connection, tearing it up in a proper way (by exchanging FIN packets with the server), LocalDirector loses its state, and packets from other clients who did not finish their session yet can be redirected to another physical server, causing disruption of the SSL connection. This is not an implementation error since all IP-based stickiness solutions suffer from the same problem.

Q: What is the major problem with SSL ID-based stickiness?

A: With SSL ID-based stickiness, LocalDirector forwards packets based on their SSL ID, which is provided by the client's browser inside a TCP packet. This works well even when there are many clients with the same IP address since persistence of the connection is not based on IP address. Unfortunately, Microsoft Internet Explorer 5 users experience problems with this mode because the browser randomly clears this field approximately once every 30 to 120 seconds, which causes LocalDirector to redirect the connection randomly to one of the physical servers. This problem appears to be fixed in IE 6.0. Netscape Navigator does not suffer from it either.

Q: Does DistributedDirector experience problems with SSL connections?

A: No, because it uses DNS or HTTP redirect to inform the client of the IP address of a real server, so all communications after redirection are performed between client and server directly, without interference from the DistributedDirector.

Q: Can DistributedDirector work without DRP agents?

A: Not always. However, the device has some balancing modes that do not require any external information. They share equally load balancing, primary/backup server balancing, and random server balancing.

## Chapter 8

Virtual Private Networks and Remote Access

Solutions in this chapter:

- **Overview of the Different VPN Technologies**

- **Layer 2 Transport Protocol**

- **IPSec**

☑ **Summary**

☑ **Solutions Fast Track**

☑ **Frequently Asked Questions**

Introduction

When you think about the world today, with hackers everywhere, you need something to reassure you that you have a little privacy. The Virtual Private Network (VPN) provides that—on a LAN, WAN, and Remote Access scale for many different types of people.

If you think about it, you can have people anywhere in the world using a VPN on a WAN, sending secure messages over a service provider's network in the middle. Also, you could have people working on the road or from home using a VPN to securely connect to the company infrastructure over an Internet Service Provider (ISP). The latest, and possibly best, way is to use a VPN over some wireless device such as a Cisco Aironet Card or other type of wireless device.

All network administrators are focused on securing their network from the outside world. With the implementation of a VPN from a PC to a Cisco piece of equipment (in other words, a Cisco VPN Concentrator) using IPSec, you are able to securely send information to and from both sides of the VPN. This makes for a very secure environment for remote access users to perform work on a WAN. VPNs can be utilized on different levels of the OSI model, depending on what they are being used for at that time.

In the following chapter, you will learn how IPSec works within a VPN to help prevent security breaches on a network. Also, you will understand the different types of VPNs used today, and discover how IPSec works from end-to-end. To describe it simply, a VPN is a network deployed on a shared infrastructure, employing the same security, management, and throughput policies applied in a private network. Figure 8.1 shows how VPN works in the real world.

Overview of the Different VPN Technologies

As discussed in the introduction, VPNs can take many different forms and be implemented in various ways. Not only can a VPN be classified by the OSI Reference model layer it is implemented on, but also by which VPN model it employs.

The Peer Model

A *peer* VPN model is one in which the path determination at the network layer is done on a hop-by-hop basis. The edge nodes (customer sites) form a network layer peering relationship with the VPN service provider network and use the best route through the network, rather than connecting to other edge nodes (customer sites) via a predetermined path though the network.

Figure 8.1 A Typical VPN

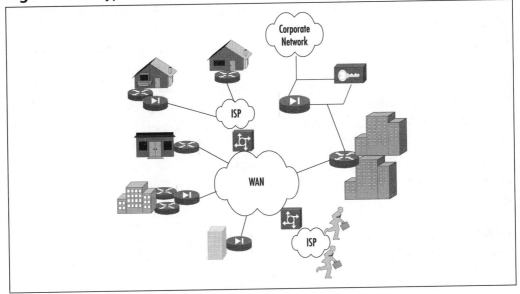

One of the major drawbacks of this model is that all network layer addressing must be unique within the VPN service provider network and the individual VPNs. A traditional routed network is an example of a *peer* model.

In Figure 8.2, a packet from Network 1, destined for Network 2, is first sent to router A. Router A determines that the best path for this packet to follow is via router B. Router B determines that the best path for this packet to follow is via router C. Router C determines that the best path for this packet to follow is via router D, which in turn delivers the packet to Network 2.

Figure 8.2 A Typical Peer Model

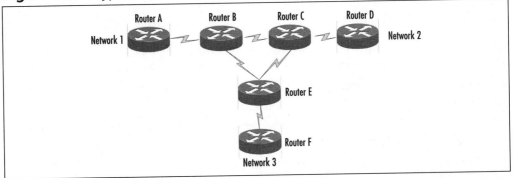

The Overlay Model

An *overlay* VPN model is one in which path determination at the network layer is done on a "cut-through" basis to another edge node (customer site). The network layer has no knowledge of the underlying infrastructure. All edge nodes (customer sites) are effectively one hop away from each other, no matter how many physical hops are between them.

An advantage of this type of VPN is that network addressing between the different VPNs and the VPN service provider networks does not have to be unique, except for within a single VPN.

It is generally accepted that the *overlay* model results in suboptimal routing in larger networks and that full mesh *overlay* topologies have scalability problems, since they create large numbers of router adjacencies. Examples include ATM, Frame Relay, and tunneling implementations. In Figure 8.3, Network 1 is one hop away from Network 2, no matter how many physical hops are between them.

Figure 8.3 A Typical Overlay Model

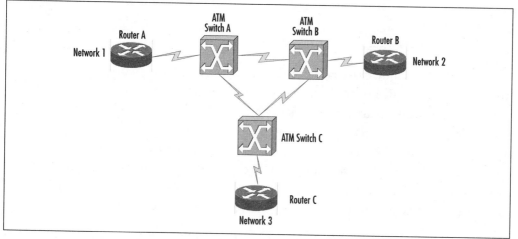

Link Layer VPNs

Link layer VPNs are implemented at the link layer (Layer 2) of the OSI Reference model. The link layer provides the networking platform, while discrete networks are built at the network layer. The different VPNs share the same infrastructure, but have no visibility of one another. The difference between this model and that of dedicated circuits is that there is no synchronized data clock shared by the sender and receiver, as well as no dedicated transmission path provided by the underlying network. Frame Relay and ATM networks are examples of link layer VPNs.

Network Layer VPNs

Network layers are VPNs implemented at the network layer (Layer 3) of the OSI Reference model. We will now look at the two types of VPNs that work within the network layer: Tunneling and Virtual Private Dial Networks (VPDN).

Tunneling VPNs

Tunneling VPNs are becoming increasingly popular and most VPN growth is expected in this area. Tunnels can be created either between a source and destination router, router-to-router, or host-to-host. Tunneling can be point-to-point or point-to-multipoint, but point-to-point tunneling is much more scaleable than point-to-multipoint. This is due to point-to-point tunneling requiring substantially less management overhead, both from an establishment as well as a maintenance point of view.

One of the major advantages of tunneling is that the VPN backbone and the VPN connected subnets do not have to have unique network addresses. This is particularly important when you consider that the majority of organizations today use private address space.

A VPN using tunneling could be constructed with or without the knowledge of the network provider, and could span multiple network providers. Obviously, performance might be a problem if the service provider is not aware of the tunneling and does not provide adequate Quality of Service (QoS).

Cisco's Generic Routing Encapsulation (GRE) is used for tunneling between source and destination router, or router-to-router. GRE tunnels provide a specific pathway across a shared WAN and encapsulate traffic with new packet headers to ensure delivery to a specific destination. A GRE tunnel is configured between the source (*ingress*) router and the destination (*egress*) router. Packets designated to be forwarded across the tunnel are encapsulated with a GRE header, transported across the tunnel to the tunnel end-point address, and stripped of their GRE header.

The IETF's Layer 2 Tunneling Protocol (L2TP) and Microsoft's Point-to-Point Tunneling Protocol (PPTP) are used for host-to-host tunneling. PPTP should not be used without additional security features, such as those provided by IPSec, as it is known to have several security vulnerabilities. Some of these vulnerabilities have been addressed by the strengthening of PPTP's authentication mechanism, MS-CHAP, in the revised MS-CHAP version 2. Even with these changes, PPTP's security mechanisms provide only weak security and are vulnerable to attack.

Host-to-host tunneling is considerably more secure than router-to-router tunneling due to the fact that with host-to-host tunneling the entire "conversation" can be encrypted. This is not the case in router-to-router tunneling, since only the tunnel can be encrypted while the host-to-router and router-to-host parts on both sides of the "conversation" remain in cleartext. Tunneling is considered an *overlay* VPN model.

Virtual Private Dial Networks

VPDNs that utilize the Internet as a carrier for remote access (RAS) traffic are becoming very popular.

Not only do they offer substantial cost savings compared to traditional RAS solutions, they also provide substantial flexibility. Any ISP point of presence (PoP) could be used to provide secure RAS access services at a fraction of traditional costs.

L2TP and PPTP are fundamental to VPDN design and provide the tunneling features through which the RAS traffic reaches the desired services. A VPDN could be considered an *overlay* VPN model.

Controlled Route Leaking

This method uses route filtering to control route propagation to only the members of a particular VPN. Multiple VPNs sharing the same network layer infrastructure are only separated from one another by the fact that routes to the other VPNs are blocked from each other. This is a rather simple and unsophisticated method of implementing a VPN, but it might be very effective for extranets or smaller network applications. Controlled route leaking is considered a *peer* VPN model.

Transport and Application Layer VPNs

These are VPNs implemented at the transport and application layer (Layers 4 and 5) of the OSI Reference model. These implementations require the application to be VPN-aware and hence need to be written with this in mind. While certainly possible, this form of VPN is not common.

With the IETF developing their Transport Layer Security (TLS) protocol, this form of VPN might become more important in the future. TLS 1.0 is at the proposed standard stage as RFC 2246.

Intranet VPNs

An intranet VPN links enterprise customer headquarters, remote offices, and branch offices to an internal network over a shared infrastructure using dedicated connections. Intranet VPNs differ from extranet VPNs in that they only allow access to the enterprise customer's employees. In Figure 8.4, we see a typical VPN dial-up scenario.

Figure 8.4 VPN Client to Router VPN via Dial-up

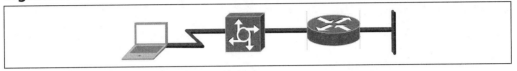

Extranet VPNs

An *extranet* VPN links outside customers, suppliers, partners, or communities of interest to an enterprise customer's network over a shared infrastructure using dedicated connections (see Figure 8.5). Extranet VPNs differ from intranet VPNs in that they allow access to users outside the enterprise.

Figure 8.5 Router-to-Router VPN Gateway

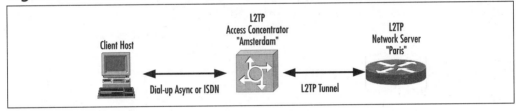

Access VPNs

An *access* VPN provides remote access to an enterprise customer's intranet or extranet over a shared infrastructure (see Figure 8.6). Access VPNs use analog, dial, ISDN, digital subscriber line, mobile IP, and various cable technologies. They securely connect mobile users, telecommuters, and branch offices.

Figure 8.6 Other Vendors to the Router VPN

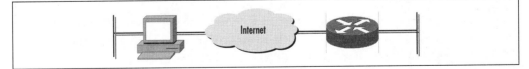

Layer 2 Transport Protocol

L2TP is an Internet Engineering Task Force (IETF) standard that combines the best features of two existing tunneling protocols: Cisco's Layer 2 Forwarding Protocol (L2F) and PPTP. L2TP has replaced Cisco's own proprietary L2F protocol.

L2TP is a key building block for VPNs in the dial access space. Using L2TP tunneling, an ISP, or other access provider, can create a virtual tunnel to link customer's remote sites or remote users with corporate networks. L2TP allows organizations to provide connectivity to remote users by leveraging a service provider's existing infrastructure. This can often be achieved at a lower cost and without the delays caused by establishing your own infrastructure.

The L2TP access controller (LAC) located at the ISP's PoP exchanges messages with remote users and communicates by way of L2TP requests and responses with the customer's L2TP network server (LNS) to set up tunnels (see Figure 8.7). L2TP passes packets through the virtual tunnel between end points of a point-to-point connection. Frames from remote users are accepted by the ISP's PoP, stripped of any linked framing or transparency bytes, encapsulated in L2TP, and forwarded over the appropriate tunnel. The customer's home gateway accepts these L2TP frames, strips the L2TP encapsulation, and processes the incoming frames for the appropriate interface. L2TP is an extension of Point-to-Point Protocol (PPP) and is vendor interoperable.

Figure 8.7 L2TP Architecture

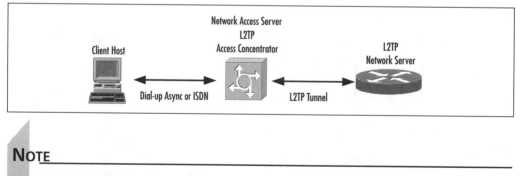

NOTE

L2TP is *not* a security protocol. It is, however, crucial to the operation of VPNs—in particular, to dial VPNs. Security for L2TP is provided through IPSec.

L2TP uses a *compulsory* tunneling model, which means that the tunnel is created without any action from the user, and without giving the user a choice in the matter.

In this scenario, a user dials into a Network Access Server (NAS), authenticates either against a locally configured profile or against a policy server, and after successful authentication, a L2TP tunnel is dynamically established to a predetermined endpoint, where the user's PPP session is terminated.

L2TP is supported in IOS from version 11.3(5)AA on limited platforms such as the Cisco AS5200, AS5300, AS5800, and the 7200 series. Platform support was extended to the 1600, 2500, 2600, 3600, 4000, 4500, 7500, and UAC 6400 in version 12.0(5)T.

Configuring Cisco L2TP

The following example illustrates how L2TP can be used to provide enterprise connectivity to remote users using a shared network such as a service provider. In this example, the user's domain name is very important, as this is what the LAC uses to determine which L2TP tunnel it needs to send the packet through.

It is also important to understand that the client host gets an IP address from the remote network. The connection between the LAC and the LNS can typically be a series of IP networks, such as the Internet. Figure 8.8 shows a typical L2TP scenario, displaying LAC as well as the LNS.

Figure 8.8 L2TP Configuration

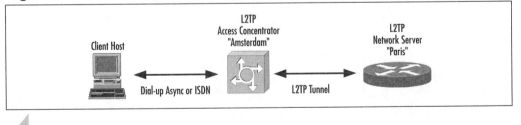

NOTE

Within this chapter, the asterisks (*) within the code listings represent a password being entered. Be sure you do not use simple passwords, as this is the most common security mistake made by network and security administrators. Either pick some good random password or mask the password, since this is a simple way to improve your security.

An LAC Configuration Example

The following is a basic LAC configuration for the scenario shown previously in Figure 8.8.

```
aaa new-model
```

Enables AAA.

```
aaa authentication ppp default local
```

Enables AAA authentication for PPP.

```
username Amsterdam password 7 **********
```

Defines the username as "Amsterdam."

```
vpdn enable
```

Enables VPDN.

```
vpdn-group 1
```

Defines VPDN group number 1.

```
request dialin l2tp ip 172.25.1.19 domain test.com
```

Allows the LAC to respond to dial in requests using L2TP from the IP address 172.25.1.19 domain test.com.

A LNS Configuration Example

The following is a basic LNS configuration for the scenario shown previously in Figure 8.8.

```
01:   aaa new-model
```

Enables AAA.

```
02:   aaa authentication ppp default local
```

Enables AAA authentication for PPP.

```
03:   username Paris password 7 **********
```

Defines the username as "Paris."

```
04:   interface Virtual-Template1
```

Creates virtual-template 1 and assigns all values for virtual access interfaces.

```
05:   ip unnumbered Ethernet0
```

Uses the IP address from interface Ethernet 0.

```
06:    no ip mroute-cache
```

Disables multicast fast switching.

```
07:  ppp authentication chap
```

Uses CHAP to authenticate PPP.

```
08:  vpdn enable
```

Enables VPDN.

```
09:  vpdn-group 1
```

Creates vpdn-group number 1.

```
10:    accept dialin l2tp virtual-template 1 remote Amsterdam
```

Accepts all dial-in l2tp tunnels from virtual-template from remote peer Amsterdam.

IPSec

IPSec, or Internet Protocol Security as it is known by its full name, was developed by the IETF to address the issue of network layer security. It is not a single protocol or specification, but rather a framework of open standards for ensuring secure private communications over public IP networks. IPSec is documented in a series of RFCs. The overall IPSec implementation is guided by RFC 2401, "Security Architecture for the Internet Protocol."

NOTE

IPSec's strength lies in the fact that it allows organizations to implement strong security, without the need to change any of their applications. Only network layer infrastructures change, such as routers, firewalls, and cases where a software client is required. As with IP, IPSec is completely transparent from the end-user perspective.

The IETF maintains an official depository for its work on IPSec. This information can be found at www.ietf.org/html.charters/ipsec-charter.html.

While IP dwarfs all other network protocols in sheer deployment numbers and has been more successful than its inventors could ever imagine, it was not designed to be secure. IP has long been vulnerable to many forms of attack, including spoofing, sniffing, session hijacking, and man-in-the-middle attacks.

Initial security standards focused on application level protocols and software, such as Secure Sockets Layer (SSL) which is used mainly for securing Web traffic, Secure Shell (SSH) which is used for securing Telnet sessions and file transfers, and Pretty Good Privacy (PGP) which is used for securing e-mail. These forms of security can be limiting, as the application itself needs to support them. However, in some cases application layer security provides additional features not supported by network layer security. Open PGP's digital signature is an example of such a feature.

Another way of implementing security is at the network layer, as the applications are secured, even if they are not themselves aware of the security mechanisms. IPSec is based on this model.

Cisco has made IPSec support available since IOS release 11.3(3)T. It also supports IPSec in its PIX firewall product range as well as its Cisco Secure VPN Client software available for the Microsoft Windows operating systems. It uses the approach that no matter what application is used, all packet level information has to travel through the network layer. By securing the network layer, the applications can automatically benefit from the security offered by that layer.

Due to its flexibility and strong security, as well as its vendor interoperability feature, IPSec has found favour with all of the major networking and operating systems vendors. Most of these vendors have replaced, or at least supplemented, their own proprietary network layer security mechanism with IPSec.

Before the development of IPSec, the acceptance and large scale deployment of VPNs was often hampered by security concerns. Existing solutions were either proprietary or used weak security algorithms.

The strength of proprietary solutions is often difficult to assess, since little information about them is made available and their deployment is usually limited to a specific vendor.

Multivendor interoperability was also a problem. This requirement was spurred on by the new economy, where mergers and acquisitions and unlikely partnerships are becoming commonplace. IPSec addresses these concerns.

IPSec Architecture

In simplified terms, IPSec provides three main functions:

- Authentication only, provided through the Authentication Header (AH) protocol

- Authentication and confidentiality (encryption), provided through the Encapsulating Security Payload (ESP) protocol

- Key exchange, provided either manually or through the Internet Key Exchange (IKE) protocol

Table 8.1 and 8.2 show the standards and features of IPSec on Cisco IOS. These tables provide a basic understanding of how IPSec works through each standard.

Table 8.1 IPSec Standards Supported by Cisco IOS and PIX Firewall

Standard	Description
IPSec	AH provides data authentication and integrity for IP packets passed between two different systems. AH does not provide data confidentiality (such as encryption) of packets. Authentication is achieved by applying a keyed one-way hash function to the packet to create a message digest.
	ESP is a security protocol used to provide confidentiality (such as encryption), data origin authentication, integrity, and optional anti-replay. It also provides confidentiality by performing encryption at the IP packet layer. It supports a variety of symmetric encryption algorithms. (The default algorithm for IPSec is DES.)
DES	DES employs a 56-bit key used for ensuring high encryption. DES is used to encrypt and decrypt packet data. It also turns cleartext into ciphertext through an encryption algorithm.
Triple DES (3DES)	3DES is an encryption protocol for use in IPSec on Cisco products. The 3DES algorithm is a variant of the 56-bit DES. 3DES operates similarly to DES but in that data is broken into 64-bit blocks. 3DES then processes each block three times (that would be one time within each 56-bit key).
Diffie-Hellman (DH)	DH is a public key cryptography protocol. It allows two parties to establish a shared secret key used by encryption algorithms over some type of insecure channel.

Continued

Table 8.1 Continued

Standard	Description
Message Digest 5 (MD5) and Secure Hash Algorithm (SHA1)	These are both hash algorithms used to authenticate packet data.
RSA Signatures: Rivest, Shamir, and Adelman Signatures (RSA)	RSA is a public-key cryptographic system used for authentication.
Internet Key Exchange (IKE)	IKE is a protocol that provides authentication of the IPSec peers, negotiation of IKE and IPSec security associations (SA). Also, it establishes keys for encryption algorithms used by IPSec.
Certificate Authorities (CA)	Provides a so-called digital identification card to each querying device.

Table 8.2 IPSec-VPN Features on Cisco IOS

Feature	Description
Data confidentiality	The IPSec sender can encrypt packets before transmitting them across a network; this improves security.
Data integrity	The IPSec receiver can authenticate packets sent by the IPSec sender; this ensures the data has not been altered during transmission.
Data origin authentication	The IPSec receiver can authenticate the source of the IPSec packets sent.
Anti-replay	The IPSec receiver can detect and reject replayed packets.

IPSec provides secure communications between two end-points, called IPSec peers. These communications are essentially sets of security associations (SAs) and define which protocols should be applied to sensitive packets, as well as the keying between the two peers. Multiple IPSec tunnels can exist between two peers, securing different data streams, with each communication having a separate set of security associations.

In Figure 8.9, IPSec is used in tunnel mode to protect the traffic between the two private networks connected via the public network.

Figure 8.9 IPSec Deployed across a Public Network

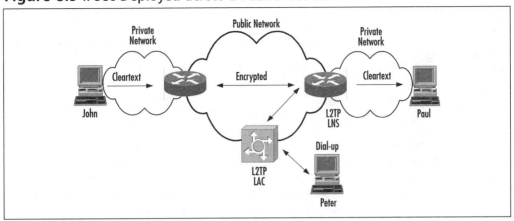

In this scenario, the end hosts (John and Paul) do not need to support IPSec. Only the routers that connect the private networks to the public network need to support IPSec. Traffic on the private network is not encrypted (cleartext) and only gets encrypted when it has to pass over the public network.

IPSec over L2TP is also shown to provide secure remote access support for Peter, via PSTN dial-up, to access the corporate network. In this case, the end host (Peter) must also support IPSec.

Security Associations

IPSec SAs define how two or more IPSec parties will use security services in the context of a particular security protocol (AH or ESP) to communicate securely on behalf of a particular flow. Amongst other information, SAs contain the shared secret keys used to protect data in a particular flow, as well as their lifetimes.

SAs are unidirectional connections and are unique per security protocol (AH or ESP). This means that if both AH and ESP services are required, two or more SAs have to be created.

SAs can be created manually, or automatically by using IKE. If created manually, the SAs are established as soon as they are created and do not expire. When created through IKE, SAs are established when needed and expire after a certain amount of time, or after a certain volume of traffic, whichever is reached first. The default Cisco IOS lifetimes are 3600 seconds (one hour) and 4,608,000 KB. An additional level of security is provided by this, as it forces a periodic security association renegotiation, thus periodically renewing the encryption key material.

An SA is identified by three parameters:

- **Security Parameter Index (SPI)** A pseudo-arbitrary 32-bit value that is assigned to an SA when it is first created. Together with an IP address and security protocol (either AH or ESP) it uniquely identifies a particular SA. Both AH and ESP always contain a reference to an SPI. When SAs are manually created (for example, IKE is not used), the SPI has to be manually specified for each SA.

- **IP Destination Address** The destination endpoint of the SA. This could be a host or network device such as a router or firewall.

- **Security Protocol Identifier** This could be either AH or ESP. SAs specify whether IPSec is used in *transport* or *tunnel* mode.

  - A *transport* mode SA is a security association between two hosts.

  - A *tunnel* mode SA is essentially an SA applied to an IP tunnel. Whenever either end of a security association is a security gateway, the SA is a tunnel mode SA. Thus tunnel mode is always used between two gateways or between a gateway and a host.

Use the *show crypto IPSec security-association-lifetime* syntax to view the lifetimes.

```
show crypto ipsec security-association-lifetime
Security association lifetime: 4608000 kilobytes/3600 seconds
```

Anti-replay Feature

Anti-replay is an important IPSec feature that uses sequence numbers together with data authentication to reject old or duplicate packets that could be used in an attack.

Replay attacks occur when an attacker intercepts an authenticated packet and later transmits it in order to disrupt service or use it with some other malicious intent in mind.

Cisco IOS always uses anti-replay protection when it provides data authentication services, except when security associations are manually established without the use of IKE.

A Security Policy Database

Security Associations are used by IPSec to enforce a security policy. A higher level Security Policy Database (SPD) specifies what security services are to be applied to IP packets and how.

An SPD discriminates between traffic that is to be IPSec-protected and traffic allowed to bypass IPSec. If the traffic is to be IPSec-protected, it also determines which specific SA the traffic should use.

Each SPD entry is defined by a set of IP and upper-layer protocol field values, called selectors. In effect, these selectors are used to filter outgoing traffic in order to map it into a particular SA.

Authentication Header

The AH is an important IPSec security protocol that provides packet authentication and anti-replay services. AH is defined in RFC 2402 and uses IP Protocol 51. AH can be deployed in either *transport* or *tunnel* mode.

Transport mode is generally used when the client host initiates the IPSec communication. It provides protection for upper-layer protocols, in addition to selected IP header fields. In transport mode, the AH is inserted after the IP header and before an upper-layer protocol (such as TCP, UDP, and ICMP), or before any other previously inserted IPSec headers.

In Figure 8.10 and Figure 8.11, the mutable fields referred to are fields like time-to-live, which cannot be included in authentication calculations because they change as the packet travels.

Figure 8.10 AH in *Transport* Mode

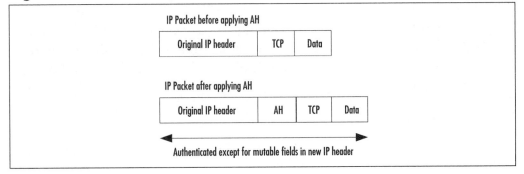

Figure 8.11 AH in *Tunnel* Mode

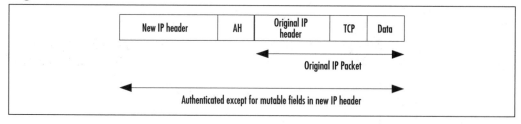

Encapsulating Security Payload

ESP is an important IPSec security protocol that provides data encryption, data authentication, and optional anti-replay services. ESP can be used on its own or with AH packet authentication. ESP encapsulates the data that is to be protected and can be deployed in either transport or tunnel mode. ESP is defined in RFC 2406 and uses IP Protocol number 50.

Transport mode provides protection for upper layer protocols, but not for the IP header. This means that the ESP is inserted after the IP header and before an upper-layer protocol or any other IPSec header. With IPv4, this means the ESP is placed after the IP header (and any options that it contains), and before the upper layer protocol. This makes ESP and AH compatible with non-IPSec-compliant routers.

Tunnel mode ESP may be employed in either hosts or security gateways. In tunnel mode, the "inner" IP header carries the ultimate source and destination addresses, while an "outer" IP header may contain distinct IP addresses (of security gateways, for example). In tunnel mode, ESP protects the entire inner IP packet, including the entire inner IP header. The position of ESP in tunnel mode relative to the outer IP header, is the same as for ESP in transport mode.

In order to use NAT, you need to configure static NAT translations. This is due to AH being incompatible with NAT because NAT changes the source IP address. This, in turn, will break the AH header and cause the packets to be rejected by the IPSec peer or peers.

Manual IPSec

In manual IPSec, the device keys, plus those of the systems it will be communicating with are manually configured. This makes manual IPSec very configuration intensive and prone to misconfiguration. This method is generally only practical for small, relatively static environments.

In manual IPSec, security associations need to be manually defined, a function that is automated when IKE is used. For larger, more complex environments, the use of IKE is strongly advised to automate key management.

Internet Key Exchange

IKE is a key management protocol used in IPSec to create an authenticated, secure communication channel between two entities and then negotiate the security associations for IPSec. This process requires that the two entities authenticate themselves to each other and exchange the required key material.

IPSec assumes that a security association is in place, but does not itself have a mechanism for creating this association. IPSec uses IKE to automatically create and maintain these security associations.

IKE is defined in RFC 2409 and is a hybrid protocol which implements Oakley and SKEME key exchanges inside the Internet Security Association Key Management Protocol (ISAKMP) framework, which, in turn, is defined by RFC 2408.

IKE offers several advantages over manually defined keys (manual keying):

- Eliminates manual configuration of keys

- Allows you to specify a lifetime for IPSec security association

- Allows encryption keys to change during IPSec sessions

- Supports the use of public key-based authentication and CAs, making IPSec scalable

- Allows dynamic authentication of peers

IKE negotiation has two phases:

1. **Phase One** The two peers negotiate and set up a bidirectional ISAKMP SA which they then use to handle phase-two negotiation. One such SA between a pairs of peers can handle negotiations for multiple IPSec SAs.

2. **Phase Two** Using the ISAKMP SA, the peers negotiate IPSec (ESP and/or AH) as required. IPSec SAs are unidirectional (a different key is used in each direction) and are always negotiated in pairs to handle two-way traffic. There may be more than one pair defined between two peers.

Both of these phases use the UDP protocol and port 500 for their negotiations. The actual IPSec SAs use the ESP or AH protocols.

In selecting a suitable key management protocol for IPSec, the IETF considered several different protocols and eventually chose IKE. Sun's Simple Key management for Internet Protocols (SKIP) seemed to be a favorite, but was eventually not chosen. In an effort to be standards-compliant, Sun is now also offering IKE support. Another protocol, Photorus, described in RFC 2522 and RFC 2523, was considered too experimental.

NOTE

Don't confuse IPSec SAs with IKE SAs. IKE SAs create the tunnel used by IPSec SAs. There is only one IKE SA between two devices, but there can be multiple IPSec SAs for the same IKE SA.

Authentication Methods

IPSec peers must be authenticated to each other. The peers must agree on a common authentication protocol through a negotiation process.

Multiple authentication methods are supported.

- **Preshared keys** The same key is preconfigured in each device. The peers authenticate each other by computing and sending a keyed hash of data that includes the preshared key. If the receiving side can independently recreate the same hash using its preshared key, it knows that both parties must share the same key.

- **Public key encryption** Each party generates a pseudo-random number (nonce) and encrypts it in the other party's public key. The parties authenticate each other by computing a keyed hash containing the other peer's nonce, decrypted with the local private key as well as other publicly and privately available information.

- **Digital signatures** Each device digitally signs a set of data and sends it to the other party. This method is similar to the public key cryptography one, except that it provides nonrepudiation (the ability for a third-party to prove that a communication between the two parties took place).

IKE and Certificate Authorities

Even with IKE, the keys for enabling the strong security offered by IPSec become difficult to manage in larger secure networks. Digital certificates together with trusted third-party CAs offer a mechanism to scale IPSec to the Internet.

IKE interoperates with the X.509 certificate standard. X.509 certificates, are the equivalent of digital ID cards and are the building block with which CAs like Verisign and Entrust authenticate IPSec connections.

Cisco and VeriSign, Inc. co-developed a certificate management protocol called Certificate Enrollment Protocol (CEP). CEP is an early implementation of Certificate Request Syntax (CRS), an emerging standard proposed by the IETF. CEP specifies how a device communicates with a CA, including how to retrieve the CA's public key, how to enroll a device with the CA, and how to retrieve a Certificate Revocation List (CRL). CEP uses RSA's PKCS (public key cryptography standards) 7 and 10 as key technologies. The IETF's Public Key Infrastructure Working Group is working to standardize a protocol for these functions.

Figure 8.12 shows an example of multiple routers in a mesh topology where key management is not performed via a CA. Every time a new router is added, keys need to be created between each of the participating IPSec routers.

Figure 8.12 Key Management without CA

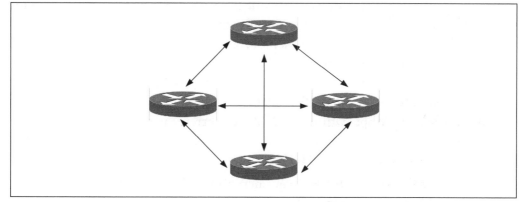

As an example, if you wanted to add an additional router to Figure 8.12, four additional two-part keys would be required to add just a single encryption router. The key's numbers grow exponentially as you add more routers and the configuration and management of these keys becomes problematic. CAs offer an ideal solution to such an environment.

Figure 8.13 shows a typical scenario where key management is performed through a CA.

Figure 8.13 Key Management with CA

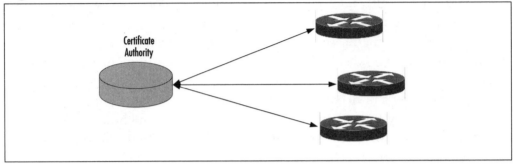

Certificate
Authority

IPSec limitations

One of the few limitations of IPSec is that it only supports unicast IP datagrams. No support for multicasts or broadcasts is currently provided.

Network Performance

IPSec can have a significant impact on your network performance. The degree to which it does so is dependant on the specific implementation. Ensuring that the routers and firewalls have sufficient memory and processor capacity helps in minimizing performance degradation.

For larger implementations, hardware-based IPSec acceleration provided by the Integrated Services Adapter (ISA) adapter is strongly advised. The ISA can encrypt traffic at 90 Mbps with up to 2000 concurrent sites or users.

Network Troubleshooting

One of the drawbacks of network layer encryption is that it does complicate network troubleshooting and debugging.

Intrusion detection, such as that offered by the Cisco Secure Intrusion Detection System (IDS) is also affected by IPSec. In order to determine if suspicious activity is occurring, the Cisco Secure IDS sensor analyzes both the packet header information and packet data information. If these are encrypted by IPSec, then the sensor cannot analyze the packet and determine if the packet contains any suspicious information.

IPSec and Cisco Encryption Technology

Prior to IPSec's development and standardization, Cisco developed a proprietary network layer encryption technology called Cisco Encryption Technology (CET). CET was first introduced in IOS release 11.2 and was based on the 40- and 56-bit DES encryption algorithm.

CET has now largely been replaced by the standards-based IPSec, although Cisco still maintains support for it. While specific CET images will no longer be available in release 12.1, CET will continue to be included as part of the IPSec images (CET End-of-Life announced in Cisco Product Bulletin, No. 1118).

In many aspects, CET is very similar to IPSec. IPSec does however have some major advantages over CET, namely:

- **Multivendor interoperability** Since IPSec is standardized, it interoperates not only with other vendors' equipment, but also on a variety of platforms such as routers, firewalls, and hosts.

- **Scalability** IPSec deploys the IKE key management technique, and includes support for CAs that allow virtually unlimited scalability.

- **Data authentication** CET provides only for data confidentiality.

- **Anti-replay** CET does not support this important feature and is vulnerable to this form of attack.

- **Stronger encryption** CET only supports 40- and 56-bit DES, which is now considered unsecure.

- **Host implementations** CET only supports router-to-router implementations. It does, however, have an advantages over IPSec:

  - **Speed** It's faster than IPSec; however, this is mainly because it isn't as thorough. For instance, CET does not offer per-packet data authentication, nor packet expansion.

Like L2F and many other technologies developed by Cisco, CET is another prime example of where Cisco has developed a technology, worked with the Internet community to standardize it and then replaced it's own proprietary solution with the standardized version.

Configuring Cisco IPSec

The following examples show how IPSec can be used to encrypt and protect network traffic between two networks. The first example demonstrates IPSec manual keying, while the second shows IPSec over a GRE Tunnel.

NOTE

When using access-lists or any form of filtering, remember that IKE uses UDP port 500 and IPSec ESP and AH use protocol numbers 50 and 51. These ports and protocols must not be blocked.

In very simplified terms IPSec is configured by:

1. Creating a SA (either manually or by using IKE)
2. Defining the SPD (access-lists which specify which traffic is to be secured)
3. Applying these access lists to an interface by way of crypto map sets

IPSec Manual Keying Configuration

The following example illustrates the use of IPSec Manual Keying to encrypt TCP/IP traffic between the 10.1.1.0/24 and 10.1.3.0/24 networks.

If a host on network 10.1.1.x wants to send a packet to a host on network 10.1.3.x, the packet from host 10.1.1.x is sent in cleartext to the Capetown router. The Capetown router uses the IPSec tunnel between the Capetown and London router to encrypt the packet and sends it to the London router that decrypts the packet and sends it to the host on network 10.1.3.x in cleartext. Cisco 3640s with IOS release 11.3(8)T1 (Enterprise Plus IPSec 56 feature set) were used for this example.

NOTE

In IOS release 12.0, the crypto map statement *set security-association inbound...* has changed to *set session-key inbound...*

In this example (Figure 8.14), DES was used as the encryption cipher. This was mainly done to accommodate an international audience, where export restrictions might limit the availability of strong encryption. Please note that DES is no longer considered secure and, wherever possible, a stronger cipher such as 3DES should be used.

Figure 8.14 Network Diagram for IPSec Manual Keying

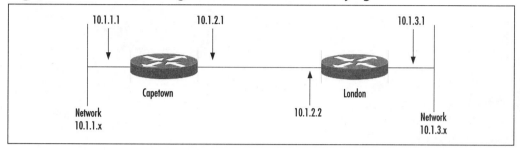

Here is the configuration of the Capetown router:

```
version 11.3
service timestamps debug uptime
service timestamps log uptime
no service password-encryption
!
hostname capetown
!
enable password a
!
ip subnet-zero
!
!
no crypto isakmp enable
!
!
crypto ipsec transform-set encrypt-des esp-des
!
 !
 crypto map test 8 ipsec-manual
 set peer 10.1.2.2
 set security-association inbound esp 1000 cipher ****************
     authenticator 01
```

```
  set security-association outbound esp 1001 cipher ****************
       authenticator 01
  set transform-set encrypt-des
  match address 100
!
!
!
interface Serial0/0
 ip address 10.1.2.1 255.255.255.0
 no ip route-cache
 no ip mroute-cache
 crypto map test
!
interface Serial0/1
 no ip address
 shutdown
!
interface Serial0/2
 no ip address
 shutdown
!
interface Serial0/3
 no ip address
 shutdown
!
interface Ethernet1/0
  ip address 10.1.1.1 255.255.255.0
!
ip classless
ip route 0.0.0.0 0.0.0.0 10.1.2.2
!
access-list 100 permit ip 10.1.1.0 0.0.0.255 10.1.3.0 0.0.0.255
!
!
line con 0
line aux 0
line vty 0 4
```

```
 login
!
end
```

The following is the configuration of the London router:

```
version 11.3
service timestamps debug uptime
service timestamps log uptime
no service password-encryption
!
hostname london
!
enable password a
!
ip subnet-zero
!
!
no crypto isakmp enable
!
!
crypto ipsec transform-set encrypt-des esp-des
!
  !
 crypto map test 8 ipsec-manual
 set peer 10.1.2.1
 set security-association inbound esp 1001 cipher ***************
     authenticator 01
 set security-association outbound esp 1000 cipher ***************
     authenticator 01
 set transform-set encrypt-des
 match address 100
!
!
!
interface Ethernet0/0
 ip address 10.1.3.1 255.255.255.0
!
```

```
interface Serial0/0
 ip address 10.1.2.2 255.255.255.0
 no ip route-cache
 no ip mroute-cache
 no fair-queue
 crypto map test
!
interface Serial0/1
 no ip address
 shutdown
!
ip classless
ip route 0.0.0.0 0.0.0.0 10.1.2.1
!
access-list 100 permit ip 10.1.3.0 0.0.0.255 10.1.1.0 0.0.0.255
!
!
line con 0
line aux 0
line vty 0 4
 login
!
end
```

To verify and debug the preceding example, use the *show crypto engine connections active* and *show crypto ipsec sa* commands.

```
capetown#show crypto engine connections active
ID   Interface   IP-Address   State   Algorithm     Encrypt   Decrypt
1    Serial0/0   10.1.2.1     set     DES_56_CBC    235       0
2    Serial0/0   10.1.2.1     set     DES_56_CBC    0         236
capetown#
```

The command *show crypto engine connections active* shows active encryption connections for all crypto engines. Of particular interest are the encrypt counters that show encryption is working.

```
capetown#show crypto ipsec sa

interface: Serial0/0
```

```
 Crypto map tag: test, local addr. 10.1.2.1

local  ident (addr/mask/prot/port): (10.1.1.0/255.255.255.0/0/0)
remote ident (addr/mask/prot/port): (10.1.3.0/255.255.255.0/0/0)
current_peer: 10.1.2.2
  PERMIT, flags={origin_is_acl,}
 #pkts encaps: 235, #pkts encrypt: 235, #pkts digest 0
 #pkts decaps: 236, #pkts decrypt: 236, #pkts verify 0
 #send errors 0, #recv errors 0

  local crypto endpt.: 10.1.2.1, remote crypto endpt.: 10.1.2.2
  path mtu 1500, media mtu 1500
  current outbound spi: 3E9

  inbound esp sas:
   spi: 0x3E8(1000)
     transform: esp-des ,
     in use settings ={Tunnel, }
     slot: 0, conn id: 2, crypto map: test
     no sa timing
     IV size: 8 bytes
     replay detection support: N



  inbound ah sas:



  outbound esp sas:
   spi: 0x3E9(1001)
     transform: esp-des ,
     in use settings ={Tunnel, }
     slot: 0, conn id: 1, crypto map: test
     no sa timing
     IV size: 8 bytes
     replay detection support: N
```

```
outbound ah sas:
```

```
capetown#
```

The *show crypto ipsec sa* command shows the settings used by current security associations. Of particular interest are local and remote crypto endpoints, the transform set used (encryption algorithm), as well as statistics of the packets encrypted and decrypted.

IPSec over GRE Tunnel Configuration

Figure 8.15 illustrates the use of IPSec over a GRE Tunnel to encrypt non-IP-based traffic. In this example, Novell's Internetwork Packet Exchange (IPX) was used, but the same example holds true for other non-IP-based protocols such as AppleTalk.

Cisco 3640s with IOS release 11.3(8)T1 (Enterprise Plus IPSec 56 feature set) were used for this example. DES was used as the encryption cipher. This was mainly done to accommodate an international audience, where export restrictions might limit the availability of strong encryption. Please note that DES is no longer considered secure and wherever possible, a stronger cipher such as 3DES or AES should be used.

Figure 8.15 Network Diagram for IPSec over a GRE Tunnel

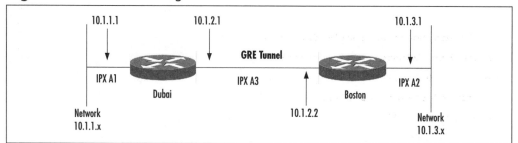

Cisco 3640s with IOS release 11.3(8)T1 (Enterprise Plus IPSec 56 feature set) were used for this example. DES was used as the encryption cipher. This was mainly done to accommodate an international audience, where export restrictions might limit the availability of strong encryption. Please note that DES is no longer considered secure and wherever possible, a stronger cipher such as 3DES or AES should be used.

The following is the configuration of the Dubai router:

```
version 11.3
service timestamps debug uptime
service timestamps log uptime
no service password-encryption
!
hostname dubai
!
!
ip subnet-zero
ipx routing 0001.425f.9391
!
!
!
crypto isakmp policy 10
 authentication pre-share
 group 2
 lifetime 3600
crypto isakmp key ****** address 10.1.5.1
!
!
crypto ipsec transform-set tunnelset esp-des esp-md5-hmac
!
  !
  crypto map toBoston local-address Loopback0
  crypto map toBoston 10 ipsec-isakmp
  set peer 10.1.5.1
  set transform-set tunnelset
  match address 101
!
!
!
interface Loopback0
 ip address 10.1.4.1 255.255.255.0
!
interface Tunnel0
 no ip address
 no ip route-cache
```

```
 no ip mroute-cache
 ipx network A3
 tunnel source Serial0/0
 tunnel destination 10.1.2.2
 crypto map toBoston
!
interface Serial0/0
 ip address 10.1.2.1 255.255.255.0
 no ip route-cache
 no ip mroute-cache
 no fair-queue
 crypto map toBoston
!
interface Serial0/1
 no ip address
 shutdown
!
interface Serial0/2
 no ip address
 shutdown
!
interface Serial0/3
 no ip address
 shutdown
!
interface Ethernet1/0
 ip address 10.1.1.1 255.255.255.0
 ipx network A1
!
ip classless
ip route 0.0.0.0 0.0.0.0 10.1.2.2
!
access-list 101 permit gre host 10.1.2.1 host 10.1.2.2
!
!
!
!
```

```
!
line con 0
line aux 0
line vty 0 4
 login
!
end
```

Here is the configuration of the Boston router:

```
version 11.3
service timestamps debug uptime
service timestamps log uptime
no service password-encryption
!
hostname boston
!
!
ip subnet-zero
ipx routing 0001.42a5.79a1
!
!
!
crypto isakmp policy 10
 authentication pre-share
 group 2
 lifetime 3600
crypto isakmp key ****** address 10.1.4.1
!
!
crypto ipsec transform-set tunnelset esp-des esp-md5-hmac
!
 !
 crypto map toDubai local-address Loopback0
 crypto map toDubai 10 ipsec-isakmp
 set peer 10.1.4.1
 set transform-set tunnelset
 match address 101
```

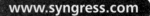

```
!
!
!
interface Loopback0
 ip address 10.1.5.1 255.255.255.0
!
interface Tunnel0
 no ip address
 no ip route-cache
 no ip mroute-cache
 ipx network A3
 tunnel source Serial0/0
 tunnel destination 10.1.2.1
 crypto map toDubai
!
interface Ethernet0/0
 ip address 10.1.3.1 255.255.255.0
 ipx network A2
!
interface Serial0/0
 ip address 10.1.2.2 255.255.255.0
 no ip route-cache
 no ip mroute-cache
 no fair-queue
 crypto map toDubai
!
interface Serial0/1
 no ip address
 shutdown
!
ip classless
ip route 0.0.0.0 0.0.0.0 10.1.2.1
!
access-list 101 permit gre host 10.1.2.2 host 10.1.2.1
!
!
!
```

```
!
!
line con 0
line aux 0
line vty 0 4
 login
!
end
```

To verify and debug the preceding example, use the *show crypto engine connections active*, *show ipx route ping ipx* …, and *show crypto ipsec sa* commands.

```
dubai#show crypto engine connections active
ID    Interface     IP-Address    State  Algorithm               Encrypt  Decrypt
17    no idb        no address    set    DES_56_CBC                 0         0
22    Tunnel0       unassigned    set    HMAC_MD5+DES_56_CB 0                 20
23    Tunnel0       unassigned    set    HMAC_MD5+DES_56_CB 20                0
dubai#
```

The command *show crypto engine connections active* displays all active encryption connections for all crypto engines. Of particular interest are the encrypt counters that show that the encryption is working.

```
dubai#show ipx route
Codes: C - Connected primary network,
       c - Connected secondary network
       S - Static
       F - Floating static
       L - Local (internal)
       W - IPXWAN
       R - RIP
       E - EIGRP
       N - NLSP
       X - External
       A - Aggregate
       s - seconds
       u - uses
       U - Per-user static
```

```
3 Total IPX routes. Up to 1 parallel paths and 16 hops allowed.

No default route known.


C          A1 (NOVELL-ETHER),    Et1/0
C          A3 (TUNNEL),          Tu0
R          A2 [151/01] via       A3.0001.42a5.79a1,    27s, Tu0
dubai#
```

The *show ipx route* command displays the ipx routing table and shows that network A2 is known via RIP through Tunnel 0. IPX traffic between network A1 and A2 is being encapsulated in TCP/IP and tunneled through the network.

```
dubai#ping ipx a2.0001.42a5.79a1
Type escape sequence to abort.
Sending 5, 100-byte IPX cisco Echoes to A2.0001.42a5.79a1, timeout is
    2 seconds:
!!!!!
Success rate is 100 percent (5/5), round-trip min/avg/max = 8/8/8 ms
dubai#
```

The *ping ipx …* command proves that the remote IPX device is accessible through the encrypted IPSec Tunnel interface. The output of *show crypto engine connections active* and *show crypto ipsec sa* will confirm that five packets have been encrypted—the five IPX ping packets.

```
dubai#show crypto ipsec sa

interface: Tunnel0
    Crypto map tag: toBoston, local addr. 10.1.4.1


    local   ident (addr/mask/prot/port): (10.1.2.1/255.255.255.255/47/0)
    remote ident (addr/mask/prot/port): (10.1.2.2/255.255.255.255/47/0)
    current_peer: 10.1.5.1
      PERMIT, flags={origin_is_acl,}
     #pkts encaps: 57, #pkts encrypt: 57, #pkts digest 57
     #pkts decaps: 57, #pkts decrypt: 57, #pkts verify 57
     #send errors 1, #recv errors 0
```

```
        local crypto endpt.: 10.1.4.1, remote crypto endpt.: 10.1.5.1
        path mtu 1514, media mtu 1514
        current outbound spi: 71313FA

        inbound esp sas:
         spi: 0x111214EE(286397678)
            transform: esp-des esp-md5-hmac ,
            in use settings ={Tunnel, }
            slot: 0, conn id: 22, crypto map: toBoston
            sa timing: remaining key lifetime (k/sec): (4607992/2989)
            IV size: 8 bytes
            replay detection support: Y


        inbound ah sas:


        outbound esp sas:
         spi: 0x71313FA(118690810)
            transform: esp-des esp-md5-hmac ,
            in use settings ={Tunnel, }
            slot: 0, conn id: 23, crypto map: toBoston
            sa timing: remaining key lifetime (k/sec): (4607992/2989)
            IV size: 8 bytes
            replay detection support: Y


        outbound ah sas:



interface: Serial0/0
      Crypto map tag: toBoston, local addr. 10.1.4.1

     local  ident (addr/mask/prot/port): (10.1.2.1/255.255.255.255/47/0)
     remote ident (addr/mask/prot/port): (10.1.2.2/255.255.255.255/47/0)
     current_peer: 10.1.5.1
```

```
     PERMIT, flags={origin_is_acl,}

 #pkts encaps: 57, #pkts encrypt: 57, #pkts digest 57

 #pkts decaps: 57, #pkts decrypt: 57, #pkts verify 57

 #send errors 1, #recv errors 0


  local crypto endpt.: 10.1.4.1, remote crypto endpt.: 10.1.5.1

  path mtu 1514, media mtu 1514

  current outbound spi: 71313FA


  inbound esp sas:

   spi: 0x111214EE(286397678)

      transform: esp-des esp-md5-hmac ,

      in use settings ={Tunnel, }

      slot: 0, conn id: 22, crypto map: toBoston

      sa timing: remaining key lifetime (k/sec): (4607992/2989)

      IV size: 8 bytes

      replay detection support: Y



  inbound ah sas:



  outbound esp sas:

   spi: 0x71313FA(118690810)

      transform: esp-des esp-md5-hmac ,

      in use settings ={Tunnel, }

      slot: 0, conn id: 23, crypto map: toBoston

      sa timing: remaining key lifetime (k/sec): (4607992/2989)

      IV size: 8 bytes

      replay detection support: Y



  outbound ah sas:


dubai#
```

Here, the *show crypto ipsec sa* shows the settings used by current security associations. Of particular interest are local and remote crypto endpoints, the transform set used (encryption algorithm), as well as the statistics of the packets encrypted and decrypted.

Connecting IPSec Clients to Cisco IPSec

A common design is to use IPSec between an IPSec-aware host client (such as a remote PC) and an IPSec router or firewall.

This means that the host client needs to be IPSec-aware. This can be achieved though either the host client's operating system being IPSec-aware or through a third-party IPSec software client.

Cisco Secure VPN Client

The Cisco VPN Client is a software program that runs on Windows, Linux, and Mac OS X-based PCs. The Cisco VPN Client on a remote PC communicates with a Cisco VPN device on an enterprise network, or with an ISP creates a secure connection over the Internet. Through this connection, you can access a private network as if you were an onsite user, hallmarks of a virtual private network.

Cisco Secure VPN Client is a software program that provides IPSec support to Windows 95, Windows 98, and Windows NT operating systems which do not have native IPSec support. It does this by integrating into the existing IP stack.

The latest Windows release is Cisco Secure VPN Client 3.5.1 which is a component of the Cisco Secure VPN software. Version 3.5.1 also supports Linux, Solaris, and Mac OS X.

New Feature in Release 3.5.1

There is only one new feature in Release 3.5.1:

- **Zone Lab Support** This feature maintains policies for the firewall on remote VPN Client PCs.

New Features in Release 3.5

The following are new features in Release 3.5:

- **Integrated Firewall** The VPN Client on the Windows platform will include a stateful firewall integrated within. This firewall will be transparent to the user.

- **Centralized Protection Policy (CPP) on a VPN Concentrator** The Concentrator may be configured for CPP, in which an administrator

may set up firewall rules on the Concentrator then send them to the
VPN Clients.

- **Support for Personal Firewalls** If there were rules configured on the
firewall that are on the VPN Client PC, the VPN Client polls the firewall
to determine whether the firewall software is still running on the PC.

- **Smart Card** The VPN Client does support authentication using digital
certificates. This is by way of electronic tokens and smart cards.

- **IPSec over TCP** IPSec over TCP encapsulates encrypted data traffic
in each TCP packet. This will allow the VPN Concentrator to operate in
a way in which ESP and IKE cannot.

Windows 2000

The Microsoft Windows 2000 operating system (Server, Professional, Advanced
Server, and Datacenter Server versions) now has native support for IPSec, without
the use of any third-party software. Full support of industry IETF standards is
provided.

Microsoft makes available a tool called IP Security Monitor that administrators can use to confirm whether IPSec communications are successfully secured.
The tool shows how many packets have been sent over the AH or ESP security
protocols and how many security associations and keys have been generated since
the computer was last started.

IP Security Monitor also indicates whether or not IPSec is enabled in a
given computer. This information is located in the lower-right corner of the
window. To start IP Security Monitor, click **Start | Run**, type **ipsecmon** and
then click **OK**.

For remote Windows 2000 clients to use IPSec across a public IP network on
a dial-up basis, the use of L2TP or Microsoft's PPTP protocol are required to
establish a tunnel through the public IP network. Once the tunnel is established,
IPSec can be used in transport mode to secure communications through the
tunnel.

Linux FreeS/WAN

The Secure Wide Area Network project or FreeS/WAN aims to make IPSec
freely available on Linux platforms. It does so by providing free source code for
IPSec. The project's official Web site can be found at www.freeswan.org.

It all started with John Gilmore, the founder and main driving force behind FreeS/WAN, who wanted to make the Internet more secure and protect traffic against wiretapping.

To avoid export limitations imposed by the U.S. Government of cryptographic products, FreeS/WAN has been completely developed and maintained outside of the United States of America. As a result, the strong encryption supported by FreeS/WAN is exportable.

Those interested in large scale FreeS/WAN implementations should read a paper called "Moat: a Virtual Private Network Appliance and Services Platform" that discusses a large VPN deployment using FreeS/WAN. It was written by John S. Denker, Steven M. Bellovin, Hugh Daniel, Nancy L. Mintz, Tom Killian, and Mark A. Plotnick, and is available for download from www.research.att.com/~smb/papers/index.html.

Summary

VPN will help scale network security in a way that will be more manageable and reliable. With the use of IPSec within the VPN, you are addressing the concerns of network security from end to end. This provides a secure means for the transmission of data to and from your intended source.

Since VPNs are so widely used now by companies for WANs to Remote Access, we should soon see them in all wireless devices. Wireless is quickly becoming as secure as a remote user using a VPN to connect to a corporate LAN.

With Cisco leading the way in the use of IPSec with their line of IOS Routers, PIX firewalls, and VPN Concentrators, network security breaches should be reduced. With the multivendor interoperability possibilities that Cisco is currently working on, you will see VPNs being widely used by all network administrators.

Solutions Fast Track

Overview of the Different VPN Technologies

☑ A *peer* VPN model is one in which the path determination at the network layer is done on a hop-by-hop basis.

☑ An *overlay* VPN model is one in which path determination at the network layer is done on a "cut-through" basis to another edge node (customer site).

☑ Link layer VPNs are implemented at link layer (Layer 2) of the OSI Reference model.

Layer 2 Transport Protocol

☑ Layer 2 Transport Protocol (L2TP) is a key building block for VPNs in the dial access space.

☑ It is important to understand that the client host gets an IP address from the remote network.

☑ L2TP is an extension to Point-to-Point Protocol (PPP) and is vendor interoperable.

IPSec

☑ IPSec, or Internet Protocol Security as it's known by its full name, was developed by the IETF to address the issue of network layer security.

☑ Authentication only is provided through the Authentication Header (AH) protocol.

☑ Authentication and confidentiality (encryption) are provided through the Encapsulating Security Payload (ESP) protocol.

☑ Key exchange is provided either manually or through the Internet Key Exchange (IKE) protocol.

☑ IPSec Security Associations (SAs) define how two or more IPSec parties will use security services in the context of a particular security protocol (AH or ESP) to communicate securely on behalf of a particular flow.

Frequently Asked Questions

The following Frequently Asked Questions, answered by the authors of this book, are designed to both measure your understanding of the concepts presented in this chapter and to assist you with real-life implementation of these concepts. To have your questions about this chapter answered by the author, browse to **www.syngress.com/solutions** and click on the **"Ask the Author"** form.

Q: In which IOS release was IPSec first made available?

A: IPSec was first introduced in IOS version 11.3(3)T.

Q: Which two main protocols does IPSec consist of?

A: Authentications Header (AH) and Encapsulating Security Protocol (ESP). AH provides data authentication and integrity for IP packets passed between two different systems. ESP is a security protocol used to provide confidentiality (such as encryption), data origin authentication, integrity and optional anti-replay.

Q: I need to provide authentication between two IPSec peers. What negotiates the IPSec Security Associations between those two peers?

A: IKE is a protocol that provides authentication of the IPSec peers, negotiation of IKE and IPSec Security Associations (SA). It also establishes keys for encryption algorithms used by IPSec.

Q: If I am asked to enable IKE while on a Cisco Router or PIX firewall, which command should I use?

A: *crypto isakmp enable*

Q: In which phase does IKE negotiate IPSec SA parameters and set up matching IPSec SAs in the peer?

A: IKE Phase Two.

Q: I am designing a VPN for my company. What are the different types of VPNs and what do they do?

A: The three types of VPNs are:

- **Access VPN** Provides remote access to an enterprise customer's intranet or extranet over a shared infrastructure. Access VPNs use analog, dial, ISDN, digital subscriber line, mobile IP, and different cable technologies.

- **Intranet VPN** Links enterprise customer headquarters, remote offices, and branch offices to an internal network over a shared infrastructure using dedicated connections.

- **Extranet VPN** Links outside customers, suppliers, partners, or communities of interest to an enterprise customer's network over a shared infrastructure using dedicated connections.

## Chapter 9

Cisco Authentication, Authorization, and Accounting Mechanisms

Solutions in this chapter:

- Cisco AAA Overview
- Cisco AAA Mechanisms
- Authentication Proxy

- ☑ Summary
- ☑ Solutions Fast Track
- ☑ Frequently Asked Questions

Introduction

Authentication, authorization, and accounting (AAA) is an architectural framework for providing the independent but related functions of authentication, authorization, and accounting, and is critical to providing secure remote access to both network devices and resources. The AAA framework typically consists of both a client and a server. The AAA client (for example, a router or network access server (NAS)) requests authentication, authorization, and/or accounting services from a AAA server (for instance, a UNIX or Windows server with appropriate software) that maintains databases containing the relevant AAA information.

Typically, an AAA framework is effective in three ways:

1. It provides centralized authentication for the administration of a large number of routers. An example is a small- to medium-sized business that has a relatively high ratio of routers to network administrators. Centralized authentication would ease the administrative burden of the routers, but because the number of administrators is low, centralized authorization and accounting would not be beneficial.

2. It provides flexible authorization capabilities. An example is a global enterprise that has a large number of both routers and administrators. Administrative duties might be divided along operational and configuration lines such that the implementation of centralized authorization would be an effective addition to centralization authentication.

3. It provides relevant usage or billing information. An example is a service provider that charges customers based on network usage statistics. In this case, the centralized authentication and authorization would be an effective means of supporting the router and NAS administration, while centralized accounting would provide the business with network usage information for billing.

Examples of AAA happen in every day life outside of computers and Cisco devices. For instance, when you go to an ATM machine to withdraw money, you must first insert your bank card and enter your personal identification number (PIN). At this point, you are now authenticating yourself as someone who has the authority to withdraw money. If both your card and PIN are valid, you are successfully authenticated and can now continue the task of withdrawing money. If you have entered an incorrect PIN number, or your card has been damaged (or stolen) and the criteria cannot be validated, you will not be able to continue.

Once authenticated you will be permitted to perform certain actions, such as withdraw, deposit, check your balance on various accounts, and so on. Based on your identity (your bank card and your PIN), you have been preauthorized to perform certain functions, which include withdrawing your hard-earned money. Finally, once you have completed the tasks in which you are authorized to perform, you are then provided with a statement describing your transactions, as well as the remaining balance in your account. The bank will also record your transactions for accounting purposes.

This chapter provides an overview of AAA and its benefits, a description of the RADIUS, TACACS+, and Kerberos security protocols, and a discussion (with examples) of how to configure each of the AAA services on Cisco IOS devices.

Cisco AAA Overview

AAA is comprised of the three independent but related functions of authentication, authorization, and accounting, defined in the following:

- Authentication is the process of identifying and authenticating a user prior to allowing access to network devices and services. User identification and authentication is critical for the accuracy of the authorization and accounting functions.

- Authorization is the process of determining a user's privileges and access rights after they have been authenticated.

- Accounting is the process of recording user activities for accountability, billing, auditing, or reporting purposes.

In some cases, it may not be necessary to implement all AAA mechanisms. For example, if a company simply wishes to authenticate users when they access a certain resource, authentication would be the only element needed. If a company wishes to create an audit trail to reference which users logged in to the network at what times, authentication and accounting will be needed. Typically, AAA is used in remote access scenarios such as end users dialing into an Internet service provider (ISP) to access the Internet, or dialing into their company LAN to access resources. Figure 9.1 illustrates a common implementation of AAA.

In Figure 9.1, Client A is attempting to access the Web site, www.syngress.com. Client A must first connect to their local ISP to gain access to the Internet. When Client A connects to the ISP, they are then prompted for a set of logon credentials (authentication) by the NAS before they can fully access the Internet.

Figure 9.1 An AAA ISP Implementation Example

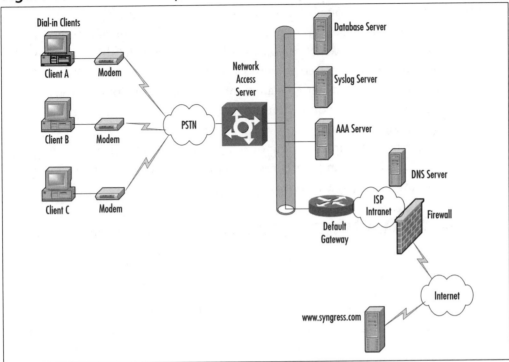

A NAS is a device that usually has interfaces connected to both the backbone and to the Telco (analog or ISDN modems) and receives calls from remote clients who wish to access the backbone via dial-up services. A security server is typically a device such as a Windows NT, UNIX, or Solaris server that is running TACACS+, RADIUS, or another service that enforces security. In Figure 9.1, the AAA server and the syslog server are examples of security servers. Once they have entered their credentials and the AAA server has validated them, if the security policy permits them to use the Internet (authorization), they can now connect to the desired Web site (www.syngress.com). As a policy, the ISP has decided to log all their customer connections on a syslog server (Accounting). This example illustrates all the elements of AAA: Authentication, Authorization, and Accounting.

AAA Authentication

Authentication is the process of identifying and authenticating a user, and typically relies on one or more of the following general methods:

- **Something the user knows** This approach is authentication by knowledge, where the identity is verified by something known only by the user. This is both the most common approach being used today and the weakest method of authentication. Examples include both the UNIX and Windows NT login process, where the user is prompted to enter a password. The integrity of this authentication process depends on the "something" being both secret and hard to guess, which is not something that is easily ensured.

- **Something the user possesses** This approach is authentication by possession, where the identity is verified by something possessed only by the user. This is becoming a more common authentication approach, and is used in most people's daily lives in the form of credit cards and ATM cards. The integrity of this authentication process depends on the "something" being unique and possessed only by the user. If it is lost or stolen, the authentication process is compromised. This form of authentication is typically stronger than something the user knows.

- **Something the user is** This approach is authentication by user characteristic, where the identity is verified by something that is unique *about* the user. This is known as the field of biometrics, and there are many products currently being developed and produced that use techniques such as fingerprint scans, retina scans, and voice analysis. ATM machines are beginning to be deployed with biometric authentication. This is the strongest approach to authentication that avoids the common problems with the other approaches (for example, the password being guessed, a card being lost or stolen); however, it is more difficult to implement.

Two-factor authentication uses a combination of two of the previous approaches to authenticate user identities. Typically, it is a combination of something the user possesses and something the user knows. A common example is the use of an ATM card (something possessed) and an associated PIN (something known) to access an account via an ATM machine.

Within the AAA framework, authentication occurs when a AAA client passes appropriate user credentials to a AAA server, and requests that the server authenticate the user. The AAA server will attempt to validate the credentials, and respond with either an accept or deny message. AAA authentication is typically used in the following scenarios:

- To control access to a network device such as a router or NAS
- To control access to network resources by remote users

Configuring & Implementing...

Remote Administration: Telnet versus Secure Shell

While the use of AAA authentication can provide centralized and robust authentication services for the management of network devices, there is still a risk related to authentication if remote administration is permitted. Many people use Telnet, which is a remote access protocol that allows you to have a "virtual terminal" (vty) over the network, to connect to the vty ports on a network device to administer and manage it remotely. The risk of using Telnet to remotely manage devices across a network is that all data is transmitted across the network in cleartext. There is no encryption protecting the passwords, so anyone with a network sniffer connected to the network in the right manner could capture them.

An alternative to Telnet is secure shell (SSH), which is a Telnet-like protocol that provides traffic encryption and authentication. Both the PIX firewall and Cisco IOS 12.1 (and later) support SSH (version 1). The IOS supports both a SSH server and an integrated SSH client. This means you can use SSH to connect to a SSH server on a network device to perform remote administration tasks, then use a SSH client on that network device to connect to the SSH server on another network device.

In order to use SSH to manage an IOS device, you need to:

- Ensure you have an image that supports it.

- Configure a host name and host domain on your device using the *hostname* and *ip domain-name* global configuration commands.

- Generate an RSA key pair for your device, which automatically enables SSH, using the *crypto key generate rsa* global configuration command.

- Configure the SSH server using the *ip ssh* global configuration command.

In addition, you need to download and install an SSH client onto the workstation you use to perform remote administration. The following sites let you download an SSH v1 client. Make sure you download a v1 client, not a v2 client:

- Windows 3.1, Windows CE, Windows 95, and Windows NT 4.0—download the free Tera Term Pro terminal emulator

Continued

from the following site: hp.vector.co.jp/authors/VA002416/
teraterm.html. Download the SSH extension for Tera Term Pro
from the following site: www.zip.com.au/~roca/ttssh.html.

- Linux, Solaris, OpenBSD, AIX, IRIX, HP/UX, FreeBSD, and
  NetBSD—download the SSH v1 client from the following site:
  www.openssh.com.

- Macintosh (international users only)—download the Nifty
  Telnet 1.1 SSH client from the following site:
  www.lysator.liu.se/~jonasw/freeware/niftyssh/.

AAA Authorization

Authorization can be described as the act of permitting predefined rights or privileges to a user, group of users, system, or a process. Within the AAA framework,
the client will query the AAA server to determine what actions a user is authorized to perform. The AAA server will then return a set of attribute-value (AV)
pairs that defines the user's authorization. The client is then responsible for
enforcing user access control based on those AV pairs. AAA authorization is typically used in the following scenarios:

- To provide authorization for actions attempted while logged into a
  network device.

- To provide authorization for attempts to use network services.

AAA Accounting

Accounting is a method which records (or accounts) the who, what, when, and
where of an action that has taken place. Accounting enables you to track both the
services that users are accessing and the amount of resources they are consuming.
This data can later be used for accountability, network management, billing,
auditing, and reporting purposes. Within the AAA framework, the client sends
accounting records that consist of accounting AV pairs to the AAA server for
centralized storage. An accounting record consists of accounting AV pairs

AAA Benefits

AAA provides a security mechanism to protect a company's resources by authenticating entities (such as individuals or system processes) prior to permitting

access to those resources, determining and controlling what those entities can do once they have authenticated, and logging the actions that were performed for accountability, billing, auditing, reporting, or troubleshooting purposes.

AAA provides several benefits when implemented correctly. Picture a very large network consisting of over one hundred Cisco devices (routers, PIX firewalls) located around the world. By default, each Cisco device requires a password to access EXEC mode (if configured on the console or vty lines) as well as a password to enter privileged EXEC mode. In addition, if any of those devices function as a NAS, individual user accounts will require management as well. If good security practices are implemented, such as different passwords (changed regularly) on each device, then this quickly becomes an administrative nightmare.

Instead of configuring and managing accounts and passwords individually on each device, imagine if there was a centralized database in which user accounts were established, access rights defined, and logging information maintained. AAA is the framework that allows dynamic configuration of the type of authentication, authorization, and accounting that can be done on a per-entity (user, group, system, or system process) basis. You have the ability to define the type of authentication, authorization, and accounting you want by creating lists which define the method by which those functions will be performed, then applying those lists to specific services or interfaces. Cisco documentation refers to these lists as *method lists*. For the purpose of clarity, these lists will be referred to method lists throughout this chapter to avoid confusion.

AAA provides many benefits, such as increased flexibility and control, the ability to scale as networks grow larger, the use of standard protocols such as RADIUS, TACACS+, and Kerberos for authentication, and the ability to define backup AAA servers in case the primary one fails.

Cisco AAA Mechanisms

The previous section provided a high-level overview of AAA and identified the benefits of using it. This section describes how to implement AAA services on Cisco network devices.

As discussed previously, AAA is an architectural framework for providing the independent but related functions of authentication, authorization, and accounting. The AAA framework typically consists of both a client and a server. The AAA client (typically a router or NAS) requests authentication, authorization, and/or accounting services from an AAA server (typically a UNIX or

Windows server with appropriate software) that maintains databases containing the relevant AAA information.

You can configure most Cisco devices, including routers, access servers, firewalls, and virtual private network (VPN) gateways to act as an AAA client. You can configure network devices such as routers to request AAA services to protect the router itself from unauthorized access. You can configure network devices such as access servers and VPN gateways to request AAA services to protect the network itself from unauthorized access by users attempting to utilize the device as an access point. For most of these devices, you configure the desired AAA services through the creation of method lists that define both the AAA mechanisms to be used, and the order in which they should be used. You then apply the method lists to the desired interface or line.

NOTE

Cisco Secure Access Control Server (ACS) is an AAA server that runs on Windows and Solaris platforms, and supports protocols such as RADIUS and TACACS+. For more information about Cisco Secure ACS, please refer to Chapter 14.

To configure AAA on a Cisco network device, you need to perform the following high-level tasks:

1. Enable AAA by using the *aaa new-model* global configuration command.

2. If you are using a separate AAA server, configure the appropriate protocol parameters (for example, RADIUS, TACACS+, or Kerberos). These security protocols are discussed in the next section.

3. Define the appropriate method lists for the desired service (authentication, authorization, accounting).

4. Apply the method lists to the desired interface or line, if required.

Supported AAA Security Protocols

After you have enabled AAA on the device by using the *aaa new-model* global configuration command, you then need to configure the appropriate protocol parameters on the device. Cisco devices generally support the RADIUS, TACACS+, and Kerberos security protocols for use within an AAA mechanism. In the following paragraphs, each of these protocols is briefly described, and the relevant Cisco configuration commands for that protocol are identified and described.

As today's networks grow larger and larger, the need for remote dial-in access increases. In a company such as an ISP, managing NASs with modem pools for a large number of users can be an administrative headache. Since a pool of modems are typically how remote users will gain access to the Internet, great care and attention must be taken to secure them. In a company such as an ISP, their business revolves around granting access to the Internet for remote users. If the method in which remote users access the Internet is compromised, the ISP could lose a lot of money due to their customers being unable to use the services for which they have paid. Typically, users accounts will be stored in a single database which is then queried for authentication requests by a NAS or router.

RADIUS

The Remote Access Dial-In User Service (RADIUS) protocol was developed by Livingston Enterprises, Inc. as an access server authentication and accounting protocol. The RADIUS specification (RFC 2138 was made obsolete by RFC 2865 and updated in RFC 2868) is a proposed standard security protocol and RADIUS accounting standard (RFC 2139 was made obsolete by RFC2866 and updated in RFC2867) is informational and for accounting purposes.

From large enterprise networks such as ISPs to small networks consisting of a few users requiring remote access, RADIUS can be used as a security protocol on any size network. RADIUS uses less CPU overhead, and consumes less memory than TACACS+.

RADIUS is a client/server protocol. The RADIUS client is typically a NAS, router or switch, which requests a service such as authentication or authorization from the RADIUS server. A RADIUS server is usually a daemon running on a UNIX machine or service running on a Windows NT/2000 server machine. The daemon is the software, such as Cisco Secure ACS or another RADIUS or TACACS+ server program, that fulfills requests from RADIUS clients.

When authorization information is needed by the client, it queries the RADIUS server and passes the user credentials to the designated RADIUS server. The server then acts on the configuration information necessary for the client to deliver services to the user. A RADIUS server can also act as a proxy client to other RADIUS servers or other kinds of authentication servers. Figure 9.2 illustrates what happens when a user attempts to log in and authenticate to a NAS or router using RADIUS.

Figure 9.2 Authenticating with RADIUS

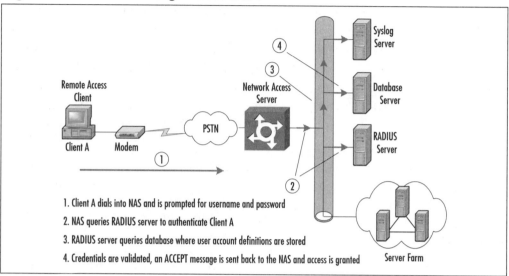

1. Client A dials into NAS and is prompted for username and password
2. NAS queries RADIUS server to authenticate Client A
3. RADIUS server queries database where user account definitions are stored
4. Credentials are validated, an ACCEPT message is sent back to the NAS and access is granted

1. The remote user dials into a NAS and is prompted for credentials such as a username and password by the NAS.

2. The username and encrypted password are sent from the RADIUS client (NAS) to the RADIUS server via the network.

3. The RADIUS server queries the database where user account definitions are stored.

4. The RADIUS server evaluates the credentials and replies with one of the following responses:

    ■ **REJECT** The user is not authenticated; they are prompted to re-enter the username and password, otherwise access is denied.

    ■ **ACCEPT** The user is authenticated.

    ■ **CHALLENGE** A challenge is issued by the RADIUS. The challenge may request additional information from the user.

    ■ **CHANGE PASSWORD** A request from the RADIUS server specifying that the user must change their current password.

Configuring RADIUS on Cisco

To use RADIUS as an AAA mechanism, you must specify the host running the RADIUS server software, and a secret text string that it shares with the RADIUS client. Table 9.1 identifies and describes the global configuration commands needed to define a RADIUS server and its parameters.

Table 9.1 RADIUS Global Configuration Commands

Command	Task
radius-server host {*hostname* | *ip-address*} [auth-port *port-number*] [acct-port *port-number*] [timeout *seconds*] [retransmit *retries*] [key *string*] [alias {*hostname* | *ip-address*}]	Specifies the IP address or host name of the remote RADIUS server, and optionally specifies additional parameters identified in the following. Use the *no* form of the command to delete a specified RADIUS server. *hostname* – enters the host name of the server to which RADIUS requests will be directed. -or- *ip-address* – enters the IP address of the server to which RADIUS requests will be directed. (optional) auth-port *port-number* – enters the UDP port for authentication requests (default is 1645). (optional) acct-port *port-number* – enters the UDP port for accounting requests (default is 1646). (optional) timeout *seconds* – designates the time interval to wait for the RADIUS server reply before retransmitting (1 to 1000). This setting overrides the global value of the *radius-server timeout* command. If no timeout value is specified, the global value is used. (optional) key *string* – the authentication and encryption key used between the router and the RADIUS daemon running on this RADIUS server. This key overrides the global setting of the *radius-server key* command. If no key string is specified, the global value is used. (optional) alias {*hostname* | *ip-address*} – allows up to eight aliases per line for any given RADIUS server.

Continued

Table 9.1 Continued

Command	Task
radius-server key {0 *string* | 7 *string* | *string*}	Sets the authentication and encryption key for all RADIUS communications between the device and the RADIUS server. To disable the key, use the *no* form of this command. 0 *string* – the 0 specifies that an unencrypted (*string*) key will follow. 7 *string* – the 7 specifies that a hidden key (*string*) will follow. *string* – the unencrypted (cleartext) shared key. The specified key must be the same on both the RADIUS client and RADIUS server.
radius-server retransmit *retries*	Specifies the number of times the router transmits each RADIUS request to the server before giving up (default is 3). To disable retransmission, use the *no* form of this command.
radius-server timeout *seconds*	Specifies the number of seconds a router waits for a reply to a RADIUS request before retransmitting the request (default is 5). To restore the default, use the *no* form of this command.
radius-server deadtime *minutes*	Specifies the number of minutes a RADIUS server, which is not responding to authentication requests, is passed over by requests for RADIUS authentication. To set deadtime to 0, use the *no* form of this command.
aaa group server radius *group-name*	By default, all RADIUS servers are considered part of one group with respect to method lists. In other words, the device will request services from all defined RADIUS servers in the order in which they are listed. This command allows you to group different RADIUS server hosts into distinct lists and distinct methods. Use the *no* form of the command to remove a group server from the configuration.

Continued

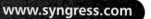

Table 9.1 Continued

Command	Task
	group-name – the character string used to name the group of servers. Employ the server command to specify a server that belongs in the group server.
server ip-address [auth-port port-number] [acct-port port-number]	After using the aaa group server command to define a RADIUS group server, use this command to specify the IP address of a RADIUS server that belongs in the group server. Use the no form of the command to remove a server from the server group. ip-address – enters the IP address of the RADIUS server (optional) auth-port port-number – the UDP port for authentication requests (default is 1645). (optional) acct-port port-number – the UDP port for accounting requests (default is 1646).

> **NOTE**
>
> If you specify the key in the *radius-server host* command, you must make sure the text string matches the encryption key defined on the RADIUS server. In addition, because leading spaces are ignored, but spaces within and at the end of the key are used, you should always configure the key as the last item in the command. If you use spaces in your key, do not enclose the key in quotation marks.

The following example enables AAA and defines multiple RADIUS servers with different IP addresses, different ports for authentication requests, and timeout or retry settings that are different from the default. If RADIUS authentication is specified in a method list, then the defined RADIUS servers will be queried in their order of definition.

```
aaa new-model
radius-server host 192.168.1.10 auth-port 4645 timeout 10 retries 5 key
```

```
      RadiusPassword1
radius-server host 192.168.2.10 auth-port 5645 timeout 10 retries 5 key
      RadiusPassword2
```

NOTE

You can use multiple *radius-server host* commands to specify multiple hosts. The software searches for hosts in the order in which you specify them. If no host-specific timeout, retransmit, or key values are specified, the global values apply to each host

TACACS+

Another available security protocol is Terminal Access Controller Access System (TACACS). TACACS provides a method to validate users attempting to gain access to a service through a router or NAS. The original Cisco TACACS was modeled after the original Defense Data Network (DDN) application. Similar to RADIUS, a centralized server running TACACS software responds to client requests in order to perform AAA requests.

TACACS+ allows an administrator to separate the authentication, authorization, and accounting AAA mechanisms, therefore providing the ability to implement each service independently. Each of the AAA mechanisms can be tied into separate databases.

Currently, the Cisco IOS software supports three versions of the TACACS security protocol. They are:

- **TACACS** The original specification of TACACS. This version has the ability to perform authentication requests only.

- **XTACACS** In addition to authentication, extended TACACS has the ability to perform the accounting element of AAA.

- **TACACS+** The latest version of TACACS is TACACS+. This version enhances the previous versions by providing all elements of AAA. Packets rely on TCP as the transport protocol, therefore making the connection reliable. TACACS+ can also encrypt the body of traffic traveling between the TACACS+ server and client. Only the TACACS+ header is left unencrypted.

TACACS and XTACACS are now deprecated and are not compatible with the AAA security features in Cisco. This section will focus on the operation and configuration of TACACS+.

TACACS+ separates each of the functions of AAA by allowing configurations of each element independently of one another.

Figure 9.3 illustrates the process that occurs when a user attempts to log in by authentication to a NAS using TACACS+.

Figure 9.3 Logging on Using TACAS+

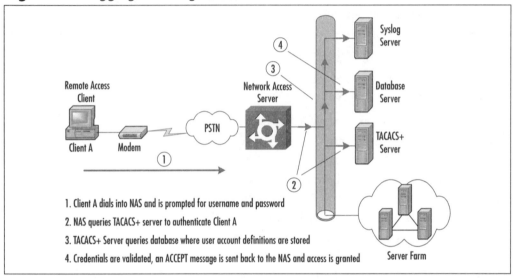

1. Client A dials into NAS and is prompted for username and password
2. NAS queries TACACS+ server to authenticate Client A
3. TACACS+ Server queries database where user account definitions are stored
4. Credentials are validated, an ACCEPT message is sent back to the NAS and access is granted

1. When the connection is established, the network access server will contact the TACACS+ server to obtain an authentication prompt, which is then displayed to the user. The user enters their username and the NAS then contacts the TACACS+ server to obtain a password prompt. The NAS displays the password prompt to the user, and the user enters their password.

2. These credentials are then sent to the TACACS+ daemon running on a server.

3. The TACACS+ server will query either a user database and compare Client A's credentials with those stored in the database server.

4. The NAS will eventually receive one of the following responses from the TACACS+ daemon:

- **ACCEPT** The user is authenticated and the service may begin.

- **REJECT** The user failed authentication. The user may be denied further access, or will be prompted to retry the login sequence depending on the TACACS+ daemon.

- **ERROR** An error occurred at some time during authentication. This can be either at the daemon or in the network connection between the daemon and the network access server. If an ERROR response is received, the network access server will typically try to use an alternative method for authenticating the user.

- **CONTINUE** The user is prompted for additional authentication information.

If the user is employing PPP to authenticate to a NAS, either PAP (Password Authentication Protocol) or CHAP (Challenge Handshake Authentication Protocol) can be used for authentication. Both PAP and CHAP automatically and transparently send authentication credentials (e.g., username and password) through the PPP link instead of prompting the user for the information. For example, when a user connects to an ISP with their modem, PPP is used to encapsulate the traffic to and from the remote user and the NAS. PPP can send authentication information in the form of PAP and CHAP to the NAS for authentication and authorization purposes. PAP sends passwords in cleartext that can easily be viewed using a packet sniffer. CHAP uses a three-way handshake process to validate each side of the point-to-point link, and also encrypts the username and password exchanged during that handshake. CHAP is a much more secure protocol than PAP and should be used whenever possible.

Configuring TACAS+ on Cisco

To configure TACACS+ as your security protocol for AAA, you must specify the host running the TACACS+ server software, and a secret text string that it shares with the TACACS+ client. Table 9.2 identifies and describes the global configuration commands needed to define a TACACS+ server and key.

Table 9.2 TACACS+ Global Configuration Commands

Command	Task
tacacs-server host *name* [single-connection] [port *integer*] [timeout *integer*] [key *string*]	Specifies the IP address or host name of the remote TACACS+ server host, as well as the assigned authentication and accounting destination port numbers. *name* – enters the host name or IP address of the server in which TACACS+ requests will be directed. (optional) single-connection – specifies that the client should maintain a single open connection when exchanging information with the TACACS+ server. (optional) port *integer* – specifies the TCP port in which the TACACS+ client will send TACACS+ requests. This value should match the configuration of the TACACS+ server (default is 49). (optional) timeout integer – specifies the time (in seconds) that the TACACS+ client will wait for the TACACS+ server to respond. This setting overrides the default timeout value set with the tacacs-server timeout command for this server only. (optional) key *string* – specifies the shared secret text string used between the TACACS+ client and server. The specified key must be the same on both devices. The key specified here will override the key specified in the tacacs-server key command.
tacacs-server key *key*	Specifies the shared secret text string used between the TACACS+ client and server.
aaa group server tacacs+ *group-name*	By default, all TACACS+ servers are considered part of one group with respect to method lists. In other words, the device will request services from all defined TACACS+ servers in the order in which they are listed. This command allows you to group different TACACS+ server hosts into distinct lists and distinct methods. Use the *no* form of the command to remove a

Continued

Table 9.2 Continued

Command	Task
	group server from the configuration. *group-name* – specifies the character string name used by the group of servers. Use the *server* command to specify a server that belongs in the group server.
server *ip-address*	After using the *aaa group server* command to define a TACACS+ group server, use this command to specify the IP address of a TACACS+ server that belongs in the group server. Use the *no* form of the command to remove a server from the server group. *ip*-address – specifies the IP address of the TACACS+ server.

NOTE

Specifying the *key* string with the *tacacs-server host* command overrides the default key set by the global configuration *tacacs-server key* command.

The following example enables AAA and defines multiple TACACS+ servers with different IP addresses, different ports for authentication requests, and timeout or retry settings different from the default. If RADIUS authentication is specified in a method list, then the defined RADIUS servers will be queried in their order of definition.

```
aaa new-model
tacacs-server host 192.168.1.11 port 1149 timeout 10 key TacacsPassword1
tacacs-server host 192.168.2.11 port 2149 timeout 10 key TacacsPassword 2
```

Kerberos

A major security concern for today's networks is the usage of network monitoring tools to capture packets traversing a network. Contained in these packets is sensitive information such as a users login ID and password. Protocols such as Telnet, FTP, POP3, and many others, send the information in cleartext. What this means, is that anyone who looks at the contents of the packet (data portion), will be able to see everything in plaintext.

Firewalls have been put in place to protect a network from intrusion that originates from the "outside," this assumption does not protect a network from attacks that originate from the "inside." An often overlooked security measure is having users on the "inside" network prove their identity to the services they are accessing.

The name "Kerberos" originates from Greek mythology, and describes the three-headed dog that guards the entrance to Hades. It was developed by MIT as a solution to the aforementioned security problems. Kerberos uses strong cryptography protocol, which means that a client must prove their identity to a server or service, and a server or service must prove its identity to the client across an insecure network (such as the Internet). After a client has used Kerberos to prove their identity, data exchanged between the client and server will be encrypted, thereby making network monitoring tools useless when capturing packets that contain sensitive data.

How does Kerberos work? Well, Kerberos works similar to how your driver's license works as identification. For example, in a situation where you need to prove your identity, your driver's license contains enough unique information on it (photo, name and address, birth date) to prove who you are without any other ID. In addition to the unique information, your driver's license is issued by a single recognized authority—in the U.S., the DMV. It must be renewed periodically (typically on your birthday), and once it has expired, it's no longer valid. In the Kerberos world, the governing agency would be the Kerberos *authentication server* (AS), and your driver's license would be called a *ticket*. The following steps outline the process in which Kerberos authenticates a client so it can use a service. Before the process actually occurs, both the user and service are required to register keys with the AS. The user's key is derived from a password they choose. The service key, on the other hand, is a randomly chosen key since no user is required to type in a password for the service.

1. First, the user sends a message to the AS requesting that the "user would like to talk to server."

2. When the AS receives this message, it makes two copies of a brand new key. This key is called the *session* key, and will be used in the exchange between user and service.

3. It then places one of the session keys in a packet (for clarity, the packet will be called *packet1*), along with the name of the service—for example,

sessionkey@email. It then encrypts this packet with the user's key (recall that the user's key is derived from the password they choose).

4. It places the other session key in another packet (for clarity, the packet will be called *packet2*), along with the name of the user—for example, *sessionkey@rlusignan*. It then encrypts this packet with the services key.

5. Both packet1 and packet2 are then returned to the user.

6. The user decrypts packet1 with their key, extracting the session key and the name of the service in it—for example, *email*.

7. The user will be unable to decrypt packet2 (since it is encrypted with the service's key). Instead, they place a note with the current time in another packet (for clarity, the packet will be called *packet3*), and encrypts this packet with the session key and then passes both packet2 and packet3 to the service.

8. The service decrypts packet2 with its own key, extracting the session key and note with the user on it. It then decrypts packet3 with the session key to extract the note with the current time on it. This process identifies the user.

The timestamp on packet3 is to prevent another individual from copying pacekt2 and using it to impersonate the user at a later time. What happens if the clocks on both machines are slightly off? A little leeway is given between the two computers (five minutes is a common time interval).

In Kerberos language, packet2 is called the *ticket*, and packet3 is called the *authenticator*. The authenticator usually contains more information than what is listed in the example, some of this which comes from other fields in the packet such as the checksum.

In the previous example, there is a small problem. This process must occur every time a user attempts to use a service. The user must enter a password each time this occurs (to decrypt packet1). The most obvious way around this problem is to cache the key that was derived from the user's password. This poses another security problem, caching keys and having them around is very dangerous. An attacker can used a copy of this cached key to impersonate the user at anytime (or until the password was changed by the user).

The solution is for Kerberos to introduce a new agent, called the *ticket granting server* (TGS). The TGS is logically separated from the AS; in other words, even though both agents may be running on the same machine, they remain separate entities. These two entities are commonly referred to as the *key distribution center* (KDC). The KDC's purpose is as follows; before accessing any service, the user requests a ticket to contact the AS. This ticket is called the *ticket granting ticket* (TGT). After receiving the TGT, any time the user wishes to contact a service, they request a ticket not from the AS, but from the TGS. In addition, the reply is encrypted not with the user's key, but with the session key that the AS provided for use with the TGS. Inside that packet is a new session key for use with the regular service. The rest of the process continues as explained previously.

If this extra process confuses you (how could it not?), think about it in this manner. When a visitor arrives at a company to take a tour, that visitor typically exchanges their regular ID (such as a driver's license) for a guest ID. During the tour, in order to get into the various areas of the company, the visitor will show their guest ID each time it's needed. If this guest ID was dropped or stolen, since it is only valid for a limited time (until the visitor realizes that they have lost their guest ID, and in order to get their driver's license back, they report the guest ID as being lost or stolen), a new guest ID would be issued.

Kerberos 5 is used in Windows 2000 as the default authentication protocol. This allows for the "single logon" concept that permits a user to enter their user-name and password only once. From that point on (assuming authorization has been granted) they will be able to access services available in foreign realms.

In the AAA model, Kerberos only fulfills the authentication mechanism. It does not provide any authorization or accounting functionality. If Kerberos is used for authentication, TACACS+ may be used in conjunction with Kerberos to provide authorization or accounting mechanisms.

Configuring Kerberos

In order to configure a Cisco router or NAS to authenticate users using the Kerberos 5 protocol, the following steps must first be taken:

1. Define a Kerberos Realm in which the router or NAS resides in.
2. Copy SRVTAB file from the KDC to the router or NAS.
3. Specify Kerberos authentication on the router or NAS.
4. Enable credential forwarding on the router or NAS.

NOTE

SRVTAB (also known as KEYTAB) is a password that a network service shares with the KDC.

Note that the previous steps assume that a Kerberos server is running and configured. Configuration of a Kerberos server is outside the scope of this chapter. For more information on configuration of a Kerberos server, refer to the relevant vendor documentation. To configure the router to authenticate to a specified Kerberos realm, perform the following tasks in Table 9.3 in global configuration mode.

Table 9.3 Configuring the Router to a Kerberos Realm

Command	Task
kerberos local-realm *kerberos-realm*	Define the default realm for the router.
kerberos server *kerberos-realm* [*hostname* | *ipaddress*] [*port-number*]	Specifies the KDC the router or NAS will use in a given realm. *hostname* – hostname of the KDC. -or- *ipaddress* – IP address of the KDC. (optional) *port-number* – specifies the port number Kerberos will use. The default port is 88.
kerberos realm [dns-domain | host] kerberos-realm	Optionally, map a host name or DNS domain to a Kerberos realm. dns-domain – name of the DNS domain. -or- host – name of the DNS host. kerberos-realm – name of the Kerberos realm to which the specified domain belongs to.

In order for users to authenticate to the router or NAS using Kerberos, the device must share a secret key with the KDC. In order to accomplish this, the device needs a copy of the SRVTAB file located on the KDC. To copy the SRVTAB file, it should be transferred over the network via the Trivial File Transfer Protocol (TFTP).

NOTE

A TFTP server must be running on a network host in order for the router to successfully download the SRVTAB. A copy of a Cisco's version of a TFTP server is available at www.cisco.com.

To copy the SRVTAB files from the KDC to the router or NAS, use the *kerberos srvtab remote* command in global configuration mode, as shown in Table 9.4.

Table 9.4 The kerberos srvtab remote Command

Command	Task
kerberos srvtab remote [*hostname* | *ip-address*] [*file name*]	Retrieve a SRVTAB file from the KDC. *hostname* – specifies the host name of the KDC that the SRVTAB files will be downloaded from. -or- *ip-address* – specifies the IP address of the KDC that the SRVTAB files will be downloaded from. *file name* – specifies the name of the SRVTAB file to download from the KDC.

WARNING

The SRVTAB is the core of Kerberos security. Using TFTP to transfer this key is an IMPORTANT security risk! Be very careful about the networks in which this file crosses when transferred from the server to the router. To minimize the security risk, use a cross-over cable that is directly connected from a PC to the router's Ethernet interface. Configure both interfaces with IP addresses in the same subnet. By doing this, it is physically impossible for anyone to capture the packets as they are transferred from the Kerberos server to the router.

Once the SRVTAB file has been copied, Kerberos must now be specified as the authentication protocol using the *aaa authentication* command. For example:

```
aaa authentication login default krb5
```

Optionally, you can configure the router or NAS to forward users' TGTs with them as they authenticate from the router to another host that uses Kerberos for authentication. For example, if a user Telnets to the router, and Kerberos is used for authentication, their credentials can be forwarded to a host they are attempting to access (from the router). This host must also be using Kerberos as its authentication protocol. To have all clients forward users' credentials as they connect to other hosts in the Kerberos realm, use the command shown in Table 9.5.

Table 9.5 Forwarding Credentials

Command	Task
kerberos credential forward	Forward user credentials upon successful Kerberos authentication.

To use Kerberos to authenticate users when they connect to a router or NAS using Telnet, use the following command shown in Table 9.6 in global configuration mode.

Table 9.6 Authenticating Users

Command	Task
aaa authentication login [default | *list-name*] krb5_telnet	Set login authentication to use Kerberos 5 Telnet authentication protocol when using Telnet to connect to the router. *default* – keyword to modify the *default* method list which will automatically be applied to all interfaces. *list-name* – name of the method list to be referenced when applying the method list to an interface. krb_telnet –keyword to specify Kerberos as the authentication protocol when users establish telnet sessions to the router or NAS. This is different than using krb5 keyword which specifies that Kerberos will be used for any login authentication, not just Telnet authentication.

Users have the ability to open Telnet sessions to other hosts from the router or NAS they are currently logged in on. Kerberos can be used to encrypt the Telnet session using 56-bit Data Encryption Standard (DES) with 64-bit Cipher Feedback (CFB). To enable this when a user opens a Telnet session to another host, use the command shown in Table 9.7.

Table 9.7 Enabling 56-bit DES with 64-bit CFB

Command	Task
connect *host* [*port*] /encrypt kerberos or telnet *host* [*port*] /encrypt kerberos	Establishes an encrypted Telnet session. *host* – specifies the host name or IP address of the host to establish a Telnet session to. (optional)*port* – specifies the port in which the Telnet session will be established. /encrypt kerberos – specifies that data transferred during the Telnet session will be encrypted.

The following configuration example shows how to enable user authentication on a router via the Kerberos database. Remember that in order to enable Kerberos on a router, the necessary steps for configuring a Kerberos server must be done before configuring the router.

```
aaa new-model
```

Enable the AAA security services.

```
kerberos local-realm syngress.com
```

Set the Kerberos local realm to *syngress.com*.

```
kerberos server syngress.com krbsrv
Translating "krbsrv"...domain server (192.168.1.10) [OK]
```

Specify the KDC for the *syngress.com* realm.

```
kerberos credentials forward
```

Enable the forwarding of credentials when initiating sessions from the router or NAS to another device using Kerberos authentication when the */encrypt kerberos* command is specified.

```
kerberos srvtab remote krbsrv srvtab
[output ommitted]
```

Specify the server in which the file *srvtab* will be downloaded from via TFTP.

```
aaa authentication login default krb5
```

Specify that the *default* method list will use Kerberos as the authentication protocol.

Choosing RADIUS, TACAS+, or Kerberos

The two most widely used security protocols are RADIUS and TACACS+. Which one should be implemented in your enterprise?

Several factors will influence your decision on which protocol to implement. Vendor interoperability and how the protocols are structured are typical factors that lead to the final decision.

Designing & Planning...

Security Protocol Considerations

Selecting a security protocol can be a daunting task for administrators. Many factors have to be taken into consideration. For example, will this security protocol facilitate only Cisco routers? Should I dedicate only one server or use two servers in case of failure? What services should I configure any of the AAA mechanisms on? Or simply: Which protocol is easier to configure then the others.

Remember the key differences between RADIUS and TACACS+. At the transport layer of the OSI model TACACS+ uses TCP while RADIUS uses UDP. TCP is a connection-oriented protocol, therefore RADIUS does not have the ability to resend lost or corrupted packets, RADIUS packets are sent on a "best effort" basis.

TACACS+ follows the AAA architecture by separating each of the AAA elements. This can be taken advantage of in an environment where Kerberos is already used as an authentication protocol. In such cases, TACACS+ can be used as an authorization or accounting protocol.

Transport Protocol Considerations

Like the title states, RADIUS uses User Datagram Protocol (UDP) as the transport layer protocol, whereas TACACS+ uses Transport Control Protocol (TCP) as its transport layer protocol. What this means is that TACACS+ traffic is more reliable than RADIUS traffic. If any disruption occurs (such as corrupted or dropped packets), TACACS+ will retransmit those unacknowledged packets, while RADIUS will not.

Packet Encryption

RADIUS only encrypts the password portion of the access–request packet from the client to the server. The rest of the packet is sent in cleartext, which can be captured and viewed by a network monitoring tool.

TACACS+ encrypts the entire body of the packet, but does not encrypt the TACACS+ header. The header contains a field that indicates whether the body of the packet is encrypted or not.

Authentication and Authorization

RADIUS combines both the AAA elements of authentication and authorization. The *access-accept* packet exchanged by the RADIUS client and server contain authorization information. This makes it difficult to separate the two elements.

TACACS+ uses the AAA architecture. This architecture separates authentication, authorization, and accounting allowing for advantages such as multiprotocol use. For example, TACACS+ could provide the authorization and accounting elements, and Kerberos may be used for the authorization element.

Protocol Support

RADIUS does not support the following protocols, but TACAS+ does:

- AppleTalk Remote Access (ARA) protocol
- NetBIOS Frame Protocol Control protocol
- Novell Asynchronous Services Interface (NASI)
- X.25 PAD connection

Designing & Planning...

AAA Server Protection and the Loopback Interface

Because AAA servers are critical components of any organization's security infrastructure, they need to be protected accordingly. Whether they are used for only one of the AAA services or all three, the information they contain and the services they provide need to be protected. The AAA authentication service and data provide the mechanisms to reliably establish the identities of users connecting to the network devices or

Continued

using network resources. The AAA authorization service and data provide the mechanism for ensuring that authenticated users are prevented from unauthorized access to resources. The AAA accounting service and data provide critical usage information, especially for an ISP that uses the information for billing purposes.

Because the AAA services need to be available and the AAA data needs to be accurate, protection of the servers is critical and can be achieved using a defense-in-depth approach. In addition, hardening the platform configurations of AAA servers, firewalls or packet-filtering routers can be used to ensure that only authorized devices (valid AAA clients) communicate with servers. Because this protection is based on the IP addresses of the AAA clients, ensuring that the source IP address of AAA clients is standard and consistent can reduce the administration of the packet-filtering protection. By assigning all IP addresses used for loopback interfaces from one address block and by using the *ip tacacs source-interface* and *ip radius source-address* commands on AAA clients to use the loopback interface of AAA communications, the maintenance of the packet-filtering protection is reduced. The packet-filtering rules can be established to only allow communication with the AAA servers from the defined loopback interface block. As new devices are added, the packet-filtering rules do not need to be modified.

While this approach may not be required for small organizations, it can be effective for larger ones with complex networks (ISPs).

Configuring AAA Authentication

Authentication on Cisco devices comes in many forms. There are many features that Cisco devices (especially PIX and routers) perform which authentication would benefit. For example, accessing a router either through the console or vty (Telnet) lines in order to perform configuration, diagnostics, or troubleshooting tasks. In an ISP environment, users dialing in to a NAS must be authenticated before access will be granted to the Internet. Depending on how the device has been configured, authentication may be provided by security protocols such as RADIUS, TACACS+, Kerberos, or a local user database on the device.

A basic form of authentication is, by default, already provided on Cisco devices. During the initial configuration of a router, you will be asked to enter an *enable* password. This password will allow access to a privileged EXEC mode where modifications and diagnostics (which were not available in EXEC mode) may be done. The default authentication on these devices only requires one set of credentials (a password) in order to continue. Worse yet, the Telnet protocol sends data in cleartext over the network. If a user Telnets into a device, the login and enable passwords will be readily available to anyone who captures the packets.

In order to configure authentication on Cisco devices, you must first define a method list of authentication methods, and then apply that list to the various interfaces. A method list defines the various types of authentication (network, login, or privileged EXEC mode authentication) to be performed, and the order in which they will occur.

Once the list has been defined, it must then be applied to a specified interface such as vty lines (Telnet), console lines, or groups of asynchronous interfaces (modems) and services such as the ability to use HTTP through a router or PIX before it will become active. There is also a default method list which may be altered. This default list is automatically applied to interfaces or services which require a login unless another method list is applied to that interface or service, overriding the default method list. For example, a method list named *admin* is created and then applied to the vty lines. This done, the default method list will no longer apply to that interface because the *admin* method list was explicitly applied.

The purpose of a method list is to identify one or more authentication methods and the order in which they will be attempted to authenticate a user. This is where the security protocols (RADIUS, TACACS+, and Kerberos) may be specified. For example, a method list can be configured to query a RADIUS server first in order to validate a username and password. If the RADIUS server is nonresponsive, the method list could specify that a TACACS+ server be queried next to validate that same username and password. If the TACACS+ server is nonresponsive, the method list could specify that the local user database on the device be queried to validate the same username and password as a last resort. This process only occurs in the event that a security server has failed and is unable to perform validation. If the RADIUS server denies the credentials of the user (an incorrect password or invalid username), the TACACS+ server and local user database would never be queried in this case.

The next few sections discuss how to enable AAA authentication for the three primary scenarios you will encounter:

- Configuring Login Authentication Using AAA
- Configuring PPP Authentication Using AAA
- Enabling Password Protection for Privileged EXEC Mode

Configuring Login Authentication Using AAA

Login authentication using AAA controls login access to the device itself. The steps you need to follow to enable login authentication using AAA are identified and described next. The commands used in these steps are identified and described in Table 9.8.

1. Enable AAA on the device by issuing the *aaa new-model* command while in global configuration mode.

    ```
    aaa new-model
    ```

2. Once AAA has been enabled, you then need to specify security protocol parameters such as the IP address of the AAA authentication server and the secret key that the device will exchange with it. To specify the parameters for a RADIUS server within global configuration mode, use the following commands:

    ```
    radius-server host 192.168.1.10
    radius-server key RadiusPassword1
    ```

3. To specify the parameters for a TACACS+ server, use these commands:

    ```
    tacacs-server host 192.168.1.11
    tacacs-server key TacacsPassword1
    ```

4. You must then define a login authentication method list that specifies one or more authentication mechanisms and the order in which they will be attempted. Use the *aaa authentication login* command to define a method list. The following command example creates a named method list called *login_auth_example*, and specifies that the default group of RADIUS servers be queried first, then the default group of TACACS+ servers, followed by the local database.

    ```
    aaa authentication login login_auth_example group radius group
    tacacs+ local
    ```

5. Finally, apply the method lists to a particular interface, line, or service if required.

    ```
    line vty 0 4
        login authentication auth_example
    ```

Table 9.8 Login Authentication Commands

Command	Task
aaa new-model	Enables AAA globally on the device.
aaa authentication login {default	*list-name*} *method1* [*method2…*]	Creates a login authentication method list. *default* – enters keyword to modify the *default* method list which will automatically be applied to all interfaces that do not have a method list explicitly applied to them. *list-name* – name of the method to be referenced when applying the method list to an interface. *method1* [*method2…*] – one or more keywords to specify authentication mechanisms. See Table 9.9 for a list of method keywords that can be used in this command.
line [aux	console	tty	vty] *line-number* [*end-line-number*]	Enter interface configuration mode for the interface to which you want to apply the authentication list. aux – enters configuration mode for the aux port. console – enters configuration mode for the console port. tty – enters configuration mode for tty line. vty – enters configuration mode for vty (Telnet) line. *line-number* – enters the starting line number. *end-line-number* – enters the end line number.
login authentication [default	*list-name*]	Applies the authentication list to a line or set of lines. default – specifies that the default method list should be used for authentication. *list-name* – specifies the method list to use for authentication.

WARNING

When AAA is enabled, then authentication will use the local database, by default, on all lines. To avoid being locked out of a device, make sure you add an administrator account to the local username database *prior* to enabling AAA. In addition, be certain the default method list for authentication includes a local method that guarantees access to the device.

A login authentication method list defined using the *aaa authentication login* command must specify one or more of the *method* keywords identified and described in Table 9.9.

Table 9.9 AAA Authentication Login Methods

Method Keyword	Description
enable	Uses the enable password for authentication.
krb5	Uses Kerberos 5 for authentication.
krb5-telnet	Uses Kerberos 5 Telnet authentication protocol when using Telnet to connect to the device.
line	Uses the line password for authentication.
local	Uses the local username database for authentication.
local-case	Uses case-sensitive local username authentication.
none	Uses no authentication.
group radius	Uses the list of all RADIUS servers for authentication.
group tacacs+	Uses the list of all TACACS+ servers for authentication.
group group-name	Uses a subset of RADIUS or TACACS+ servers for authentication, as defined by the *aaa group server radius* or *aaa group server tacacs+* command.

WARNING

Be careful when stating that no password is necessary for login authentication. This option defeats the purpose of a security policy entirely.

```
aaa authentication login local
```

This specifies that the local database on the device will be queried to perform authenticated requests.

```
aaa authentication login krb5
```

This specifies that a Kerberos 5 server will be queried to perform authentication requests.

```
aaa server group radius radiuslogin
server 192.168.1.1
server 192.168.1.2
server 192.168.1.3
aaa authentication login group radiuslogin none
```

This specifies that servers at IP addresses 192.168.1.1, 192.168.1.2, and 192.168.1.3 are members of the *radiuslogin* group. Login authentication will use this group of servers to perform authentication requests. If the RADIUS server at IP address 192.168.1.1 is unavailable to perform the authentication request, the next server (192.168.1.2) will be queried, if the server at IP address 192.168.1.2 is unavailable, the next server (192.168.1.3) will be queried to perform the authentication request. If all of the RADIUS servers are unavailable, then no authentication will be required.

```
aaa server group tacacs+ logintacacs
server 172.16.1.1
server 172.16.1.2
server 172.16.1.3
aaa authentication login group logintacacs local
```

This specifies that servers at IP addresses 172.16.1.1, 172.16.1.2, and 172.16.1.3 are members of the *logintacacs* group. Login authentication will use this group of servers to perform authentication requests. If the TACACS+ server at IP address 172.16.1.1 is unavailable to perform the authentication request, the next server (172.16.1.2) will be queried. If the server at IP address 172.16.1.2 is unavailable, the next server (172.16.1.3) will be queried to perform the authentication request. If all of the TACACS+ servers are unavailable, the local user database will be used to perform authentication requests.

Configuring PPP Authentication Using AAA

In an environment such as an ISP, users often access network resources through dialup via async (analog modem) or ISDN. When this occurs, a network protocol (such as PPP) takes charge of the network connection setup and authentication. PPP authentication is very similar to login authentication. When a user configures a workstation to dial up to their ISP, they must enter their login ID and password (as well as the phone number of the ISP). When the user connects to the NAS, the login ID and password is transmitted over the phone line. If they are successfully authenticated, they will then be able to access the Internet (or other services in which they are authorized to access).

The steps you need to follow to enable PPP login authentication using AAA are identified and described next. The commands used in these steps are identified and described in Table 9.10.

1. Enable AAA on the device by issuing the *aaa new-model* command while in global configuration mode.

   ```
   aaa new-model
   ```

2. Once AAA has been enabled, you then need to specify security protocol parameters such as the IP address of the AAA authentication server and the secret key that the device will exchange with it. To specify the parameters for a RADIUS server within global configuration mode, use the following commands:

   ```
   radius-server host 192.168.1.10
   radius-server key RadiusPassword1
   ```

   To specify the parameters for a TACACS+ server, use the following commands:

   ```
   tacacs-server host 192.168.1.11
   ```

3. You must then define a PPP authentication method list that specifies one or more authentication mechanisms and the order in which they will be attempted. Use the *aaa authentication ppp* command to define a method list. The following example of the command creates a named method list called *ppp_auth_example*, and specifies that the default group of RADIUS servers be queried first, followed by the default group of TACACS+ servers, and then the local database.

   ```
   aaa authentication ppp ppp_auth_example group radius group
       tacacs+ local
   ```

4. Finally, apply the method lists to a particular interface, line, or service if required.

```
interface async 4
    encapsulation ppp
    ppp authentication chap ppp_auth_example
```

Table 9.10 PPP Authentication Commands

Command	Task
aaa new-model	Enables AAA globally on the device.
aaa authentication ppp {default | *list-name*} *method1* [*method2...*]	Creates a local authentication list. default – enters a keyword to modify the *default* method list which will automatically be applied to all interfaces. *list-name* – enters the name of the method list to be referenced when applying the method list to an interface. *method1* [*method2...*] – one or more keywords to specify authentication mechanisms. See Table 9.11 for a list of method keywords that can be used in this command.
ppp authentication {chap | pap | chap pap} [if-needed] [default | *list-name*] [callin] [one-time]	Applies the authentication list to a line or set of lines selected on the previous command. chap – selects the challenge handshake authentication protocol when exchanging login credentials. pap – selects the password authentication protocol when exchanging login credentials. chap pap – selects CHAP first, if the client does not support CHAP, then use PAP when exchanging login credentials. if-needed – if specified, users will not need to authenticate if user has already provided authentication (used on async interfaces). This is useful if a user has already authenticated via normal login procedure, and keeps the user from entering their username and password twice.

Continued

Table 9.10 Continued

Command	Task
	default – keyword to modify *default* method list which will automatically be applied to all interfaces.
	list-name – name of the method to be referenced when applying the method list to an interface.
	callin – specifies that authentication will be performed on incoming calls only.
	one-time – designates use of one-time passwords such as token card passwords. Note that one-time passwords are not supported by CHAP.

A PPP authentication method list defined using the *aaa authentication ppp* command must specify one or more of the *method* keywords identified and described in Table 9.11.

Table 9.11 AAA Authentication PPP Methods

Method Keyword	Description
if-needed	Does not authenticate if the user has already been authenticated on a TTY line.
krb5	Uses Kerberos 5 for authentication.
Local	Uses the local username database for authentication.
local-case	Uses case-sensitive local username authentication.
none	Uses no authentication.
group radius	Uses the list of all RADIUS servers for authentication.
group tacacs+	Uses the list of all TACACS+ servers for authentication.
group *group-name*	Uses a subset of RADIUS or TACACS+ servers for authentication, as defined by the *aaa group server radius* or *aaa group server tacacs+* command.

NOTE

You can use the AAA Scalability feature to specify the number of background processes that will be used within the device to handle AAA authentication and authorization requests. Because previous IOS releases only had one background process to handle all requests, the parallelism of AAA servers could not be exploited fully. Because increasing the number of background processes can be expensive for the AAA client (router or NAS), you should be careful when using this feature and ensure the device is appropriately configured with respect to memory and CPU. To specify the number of processes, use the following global configuration command:

 aaa processes number

 where *number* is the number of background processes you want to handle the AAA authentication and authorization requests.

Enabling Password Protection for Privileged EXEC Mode

When a user successfully authenticates on a device via the console (if configured) or via Telnet, they are in EXEC mode. In order to enter privileged EXEC mode, the user must use the *enable* command. Typically, the *enable* password is stored locally on the device, by using the *aaa authentication enable default* command, a method list can be used to specify the authentication mechanisms that will be used for anyone attempting to enter privileged EXEC mode. Table 9.12 describes the command you should use to specify a method list that will be used with the *enable* command.

Table 9.12 The Enable Authentication Command

Command	Task
aaa authentication enable default *method1 [method2...]*	Enables user ID and password checking for users attempting to enter privileged EXEC mode. *method [method2...]* – one or more keywords to specify authentication mechanisms. See Table 9.13 for a list of method keywords that can be used in this command.

 An enable default authentication method list defined using the *aaa authentication enable default* command must specify one or more of the *method* keywords identified and described in Table 9.13.

Table 9.13 AAA Authentication Enable Default Methods

Method Keyword	Description
enable	Uses the enable password for authentication.
line	Uses the line password for authentication.
none	Uses no authentication.
group radius	Uses the list of all RADIUS servers for authentication.
group tacacs+	Uses the list of all TACACS+ servers for authentication.
group *group-name*	Uses a subset of RADIUS or TACACS+ servers for authentication as defined by the *aaa group server radius* or *aaa group server tacacs+* command.

The following example creates a named method list called *admin-enable*. When users attempt to enter privileged EXEC mode, the TACACS+ group server will be queried to authenticate the user. If the TACACS+ server is unavailable, the previously configured enable password will be used for authentication.

```
aaa authentication enable admin-enable group tacacs+ enable
```

Authorization

The second mechanism in AAA is authorization. Authorization can be defined as the act of granting permission to a user, group of users, a system, or system process. For example, if a user logs in to a server, their user account will be preauthorized to use certain services such as file access or printing. On a router or NAS, authorization may include the ability to access the network when logging in via PPP, or the ability to use a certain protocol such as FTP.

A Cisco device can be used to restrict user access to the network so that users can only perform certain functions after they have successfully authenticated. Like authentication, a remote or local database can be used to define the ability of a user once they have authenticated.

An example of authorization that is enabled by default on Cisco devices is the ability to enter privileged EXEC mode. Once a user types **enable** at the EXEC prompt, they are prompted for a password (if the router or NAS is configured with an enable password). If the correct enable password is entered, the user is now authorized to use privileged EXEC mode. Instead of the enable password, a database of users may be used that previously defines whether a user may or may not access privileged EXEC mode. If a RADIUS or TACACS+ server is configured for use with authorization, then the ability to enter privileged EXEC mode will be defined on the security server, and may not rely on the configured enable password, or may rely on it in a fail-safe configuration on the Cisco device.

The following list defines the authorization types that may be used on a router or NAS:

- **EXEC** Applies to the attributes associated with a user EXEC terminal session.

- **Command** Applies to EXEC mode commands that a user issues. Command authorization attempts authorization for all EXEC mode commands, including global configuration commands associated with a specific privilege level.

- **Network** Applies to network connections. This can include a PPP, SLIP, or ARAP connection.

- **Reverse Access** Applies authorization to reverse-Telnet sessions.

The following list defines the methods in which a user may be authorized:

- **TACACS+** As with authentication, a TACACS+ server is queried to authorize a user to perform a certain action. TACACS+ authorization defines specific rights for users by associating the appropriate user with the authorized services.

- **If-Authenticated** The user is allowed to access the requested function provided the user has been authenticated successfully.

- **Local** Similar to authentication, the router or NAS consults its local database, as defined by the *username* command, to authorize specific rights for users. Only a limited set of functions can be controlled via the local database.

- **RADIUS** As with authentication, a RADIUS server is queried to authorize a user to perform a certain action. RADIUS authorization defines specific rights for users by associating the appropriate user with the authorized services.

- **Kerberos Instance Map** The router or NAS uses the instance defined by the *kerberos instance map* command for authorization.

- **None** No authorization will occur.

Configure Authorization

The steps you need to follow to configure authorization using AAA are identified and described next. The commands used in these steps are identified and described in Table 9.14.

1. Enable AAA on the device by issuing the *aaa new-model* command while in global configuration mode.

    ```
    aaa new-model
    ```

2. Because authorization relies on authentication and occurs after it, you must configure AAA authentication as described in the previous section.

3. As discussed in the preceding section, you need to specify security protocol parameters such as the IP address of the AAA authorization server and the secret key that the device will exchange with it. To specify the parameters for a RADIUS server within global configuration mode, use the following commands:

    ```
    radius-server host 192.168.1.10
    radius-server key RadiusPassword1
    ```

    To specify the parameters for a TACACS+ server, use these commands:

    ```
    tacacs-server host 192.168.1.11
    tacacs-server key TacacsPassword1
    ```

4. You must then define a AAA authorization method list that specifies one or more authorization mechanisms and the order in which they will be attempted. Use the *aaa authorization* command to define a method list. The following examples specify that for both EXEC and network attempted actions, the default method list will send authorization requests first to the default group of TACACS+ servers, and then to the local database.

    ```
    aaa authorization exec default group tacacs+ local
    aaa authorization network default group tacacs+ local
    ```

Table 9.14 identifies and describes the commands used to specify and apply an AAA authorization method list.

Table 9.14 AAA Authorization Commands

Command	Task
aaa authorization {network | exec | commands *level* | reverse-access | configuration} {default | *list-name*} *method1* [*method2*...]	Sets parameters that restrict a user's network access. network – enters keyword to specify that authorization will run for all network-related service requests. -or- exec – keyword to specify that authorization will run to determine if the user is permitted to run an EXEC shell. -or- commands *level* – keyword to specify that authorization will run for all commands at the specified privilege *level*. Valid *level* entries are 0 – 15. -or- reverse-access – keyword to specify that authorization will run for reverse access connections, such as reverse Telnet. -or- configuration – keyword to specify that the configuration will be downloaded from the AAA server. default – keyword to modify the *default* method list which will automatically be applied to all interfaces. *list-name* – name of the method list to be referenced when applying the method list to an interface. *method1* [*method2*...] – one or more keywords to specify authorization mechanisms. See Table 9.15 for a list of method keywords that can be used in this command.
aaa authorization config-commands	If aaa authorization command's *level method* command is enabled, all commands, including configuration commands, are authorized by AAA using the method specified. Because there are configuration commands that are identical to some EXEC-level commands, there can be some confusion in the authorization process. Using the no aaa authorization

Continued

Table 9.14 Continued

Command	Task
	config-commands command stops the network access server from attempting configuration command authorization.
authorization {arap	commands *level*	exec	reverse-access} [default	*list-name*]	In line configuration mode, this enables authentication, authorization, and accounting (AAA) for a specific line or group of lines. To disable authorization, use the *no* form of this command. Arap – enables authorization for lines configured for AppleTalk Remote Access (ARA) protocol. commands *level* – enables authorization on the selected lines for all commands at the specified privilege *level*. Valid entries are 0 through 15. exec – enables authorization to determine if the user is allowed to run an EXEC shell on the selected lines. reverse-access – enables authorization to determine if the user is allowed reverse access privileges. (optional) default	*list-name* – enables the default method list created with the aaa authorization command or specifies the name of a list of authorization methods to use.
ppp authorization [default	*list-name*]	In interface configuration mode, enables authentication, authorization, and accounting (AAA) authorization on the selected interface. To disable authoriza-tion, use the *no* form of this command. (optional) default	*list-name* – enters the default method list created with the aaa authorization command or specify the name of a list of authorization methods to use.

An authorization method list defined using the *aaa authorization* command must specify one or more of the *method* keywords identified and described in Table 9.15.

Table 9.15 AAA Authorization Methods

Method Keyword	Description
if-authenticated	Allows the user to access the requested function if the user is authenticated.
krb5-instance	Uses the instance defined by the *kerberos instance map* command.
local	Uses the local username database for authorization.
none	Uses no authorization.
group radius	Uses the list of all RADIUS servers for authorization.
group tacacs+	Uses the list of all TACACS+ servers for authorization.
group *group-name*	Uses a subset of RADIUS or TACACS+ servers for authorization as defined by the *aaa group server radius* or *aaa group server tacacs+* command.

NOTE

AAA authorization does not apply to the console line, even if a named method list is created and applied to it, the method list will be ignored.

TACACS+ Configuration Example

The following example defines two TACACS+ servers that provide both authentication and authorization services. The example does the following:

1. Enables AAA.

2. Defines two TACACS+ servers and defines the key they will use for communication with clients.

3. Defines the login authentication named method list called *admins*.

4. Defines the PPP authentication named method list called *remote*.

5. Defines the *default* authorization method list for users attempting to enter privileged EXEC mode. The TACACS+ group server will be queried first, then the local database.

6. Defines the *default* AAA authorization method list for users attempting to use network services. Only the TACACS+ group server will be queried.

7. Applies the *remote* named method for PPP authentication.

8. Applies the *admins* named method list to the console.

9. Applies the *admins* named method list to the vty (Telnet) lines 0 through 4.

```
aaa new-model
tacacs-server host 192.168.1.11
tacacs -server host 192.168.2.11
tacacs-server key TacacsPassword
aaa authentication login admins group tacacs+ local
aaa authentication ppp remote group tacacs+ local
aaa authorization exec default group tacacs+ local
aaa authorization network default group tacacs+
interface group-async1
 ppp authentication chap remote
group-range 1 16
line console 0
  login authentication admins
line vty 0 4
login authentication admins
```

WARNING

Be extremely careful when specifying authentication to the console. It is very easy to lock yourself out of the device. The *admins* method list specifies that a TACACS+ server will be queried for authentication. If that TACACS+ is not available, the local user database on the device will be used. If *local* was not specified and the TACACS+ server was unavailable, you would then be locked out of the device until the TACACS+ was again available.

Accounting

Finally, the last mechanism of AAA is accounting. Accounting provides the method for collecting and sending information used for billing, auditing, and reporting, such as user identities, start and stop times, commands executed, number of packets sent and received, and the number of bytes sent and received.

Accounting enables you to track the services users are accessing as well as the amount of network resources they are consuming. When accounting is activated, the router or NAS reports user activity to the TACACS+ or RADIUS security server (depending on which security method you have implemented) in the form of accounting records. Each accounting record consists of accounting attribute value (AV) pairs, meaning that an attribute will have a specific value. For example, for the pair "address=192.168.2.1", address is the attribute and 192.168.2.1 is the value. These AV pairs are stored on the accounting server, which may be analyzed for network management, client billing, and/or auditing purposes.

All accounting methods must be defined through AAA. When accounting is activated, it is globally applied to all interfaces on the router or NAS; therefore, you do not have to specify whether accounting is enabled or not on an interface-by-interface or line-by-line basis. The following lists the different types of accounting available on the Cisco IOS:

- **Network Accounting** Provides information for all network sessions (PPP, SLIP, or ARAP) such as packet and byte counts.

- **Connection Accounting** Provides information about all outbound connections originating from the router or NAS, such as Telnet.

- **EXEC Accounting** Provides information about user EXEC terminal sessions (user shells) on the NAS or router, including username, date, start and stop times, the NAS or router IP address, and (for dial-in users) the telephone number the call originated from if caller ID is enabled.

- **System Accounting** Provides information about all system-level events such as system reboots.

- **Command Accounting** Provides information about EXEC shell commands being used for a specific privilege level on a NAS or router. Each accounting record will include a list of the commands executed for that privilege level, as well as the date and time the command was executed, and the user who executed it.

Configuring Accounting

In order to enable accounting on a router or NAS, you must first issue the *aaa accounting* command.

Table 9.16 describes the command you should use to specify a method list that will be used for accounting.

Table 9.16 The Enable Accounting Command

Command	Description
aaa accounting {auth-proxy | system | network | exec | connection | commands *level*} {default | *list-name*} {start-stop | stop-only | wait-start | none} [broadcast] *group groupname*	In global configuration mode, this enables AAA accounting of requested services for billing or security purposes when using RADIUS or TACACS+. To disable AAA accounting, use the *no* form of this command.
	auth-proxy – enters the keyword to provide information about all authenticated-proxy user events.
	-or-
	system – designates keyword to perform accounting for all system-level events.
	-or-
	network – enters keyword to perform accounting for all network-related service requests such as PPP,. SLIP, and ARAP.
	-or-
	exec – enters keyword to perform accounting for EXEC sessions (user shells).
	-or-
	connection – enters keyword to provide information about all outbound connections from the router or NAS.
	-or-
	commands – enters keyword to perform accounting for all commands at the specified privilege *level*. Valid entries are 0 thru 15 in increasing level of privilege.
	default – enters keyword to specify that the listed accounting methods that follow will be used as the default list of methods for accounting services.

Continued

Table 9.16 Continued

Command	Description
	-or-
	list-name – specifies a named method list of accounting methods that can be applied to an interface or line.
	start-stop – specifies that accounting notices be sent at both the beginning and the end of a process. The requested user process begins regardless of whether the "start" accounting notice was received by the accounting server.
	-or-
	wait-start – specifies that accounting notices be sent at both the beginning and the end of a process. In this case the user process can continue only if the "start" accounting notice was received and acknowledged by the accounting server. If not, the user process will be terminated.
	-or-
	stop-only – specifies that accounting notices be sent only at the end of a process.
	-or-
	none – specifies that accounting services be disabled on this line or interface. (optional) broadcast – keyword that enables sending accounting records to multiple AAA servers. Simultaneously sends accounting records to the first server in each group. If the first server is unavailable, fail over occurs using the backup servers defined within that group. *group groupname* – one or more keywords to specify accounting mechanisms. See Table 9.17 for a list of method keywords that can be used in this command.
aaa accounting update [newinfo] [periodic *number*]	In global configuration mode, enables periodic interim accounting records to be sent to the accounting server. To disable interim accounting updates, use the *no* form of this command.

Continued

Table 9.16 Continued

Command	Description
	(optional) newinfo – specifies that an interim accounting record be sent to the accounting server whenever there is new accounting information to report. (optional) periodic *number* – specifies that an interim accounting record be sent to the accounting server periodically, as defined by the argument *number*, which specifies the number of minutes.
accounting {arap | commands *level* | connection | exec} [default | *list-name*]	In line configuration mode, enables AAA accounting services to a specific line or group of lines. To disable AAA accounting services, use the *no* form of this command. arap – specifies that accounting be enabled on lines configured for AppleTalk Remote Access Protocol (ARAP). -or- commands *level* – specifies that accounting be enabled on the selected lines for all commands at the specified privilege *level*. Valid privilege level entries are 0 thru 15. -or- connection – specifies both CHAP and PAP be enabled, and that PAP authentication be performed before CHAP. -or- exec – specifies that accounting be enabled for all system-level events not associated with users. (optional) default – specifies the default method list. -or- (optional) *list-name* – specifies a named accounting methods list (*list-name*).
ppp accounting [default | *list-name*]	In interface configuration mode, enables AAA accounting services on the selected interface. To disable AAA accounting

Continued

Table 9.16 Continued

Command	Description
	services, use the *no* form of this command.
	(optional) default – specifies the default method list.
	-or-
	(optional) *list-name* – specifies a named accounting methods list (*list-name*).

WARNING

Be careful when specifying wait-start accounting on an interface or line. If none of the accounting servers are available for receiving the accounting record, then the user process associated with that interface or line will be locked out. Because of this, make sure you don't use wait-start accounting on the console line. A reasonable general practice would be to use wait-start accounting for remote users, start-stop accounting for local users, and stop-only accounting for any command accounting; however, you should make sure these recommendations satisfy your requirements before implementing them.

An accounting method list defined using the *aaa accounting* command must specify one or more of the *method* keywords identified and described in Table 9.17.

WARNING

Because it can cause congestion when many users are logged in to the network, be careful when using the *aaa accounting update periodic* command.

Table 9.17 AAA Accounting Methods

Method Keyword	Description
group radius	Uses the list of all RADIUS servers for accounting.
group tacacs+	Uses the list of all TACACS+ servers for accounting.
group *group-name*	Uses a subset of RADIUS or TACACS+ servers for accounting as defined by the *aaa group server radius* or *aaa group server tacacs+* command.

WARNING

Be careful when enabling command accounting using the *aaa accounting command*, especially for higher privilege levels such as 15, because all keystrokes sent to the device during a privileged EXEC session will be logged in the AAA accounting database. For example, when changing sensitive configurations on the device (for instance, enable secret), the changes will be recorded in the AAA accounting database (for example, new enable secret).

Suppress Generation of Accounting Records for Null Username Sessions

There may be a situation in which authentication is set to *none*. This means that users who connect to lines (vty, tty, or con) are not required to authenticate. If accounting is activated, an accounting record will be created with NULL as their username. To avoid seeing these records, you can disable accounting of records with a username of NULL. To do this, use the command:

```
aaa accounting suppress null-username
```

This will prevent accounting records from being generated for users whose username string is NULL.

RADIUS Configuration Example

The following example uses RADIUS to implement AAA accounting, including implementing wait-start accounting for remote users, start-stop accounting for local users, and stop-only accounting for any commands. The example does the following:

1. Enables AAA.

2. Defines two RADIUS servers and the key they will use for communication with clients.

3. Defines the login authentication named method list called *admins*. The RADIUS group server will be used for authentication, then the local database.

4. Defines the *default* PPP authentication method list. The RADIUS group server will be used for authentication, then the local database.

5. Defines the EXEC authorization named method list called *adminauth* for all EXEC sessions. The RADIUS group server will be used for authorization. If the RADIUS servers are not available, then it will allow the user to perform the function if they have been successfully authenticated.

6. Defines the *default* authorization method list for network-related service requests. The RADIUS group server will be used for authorization. If the RADIUS servers are not available, then it will allow the user to perform the function as if they had been successfully authenticated.

7. Defines the *default* accounting method list for all exec sessions. Start–stop accounting records will be sent to the RADIUS group server.

8. Defines the exec accounting named method list called *remoteacc*. Wait-start accounting records will be sent to the RADIUS group server.

9. Defines the default accounting method list for all network-related service requests. Wait-start accounting records will be sent to the RADIUS group server.

10. Applies the *admins* named method list to the console.

11. Applies the login authentication named method list called *admins* to the vty (Telnet) lines 0 thru 4.

12. Applies the EXEC authorization named method list called *adminauth* to the vty (Telnet) lines 0 thru 4.

13. Applies the EXEC accounting named method list called *remoteacc* to vty (Telnet) lines 0 thru 4.

```
aaa new-model
radius-server host 192.168.1.10
radius -server host 192.168.2.10
radius-server key RadiusPassword
```

```
aaa authentication login admins group radius local
aaa authentication ppp default group radius local
aaa authorization exec adminauth group radius if-authenticated
aaa authorization network default group radius if-authenticated
aaa accounting exec default start-stop group radius
aaa accounting exec remoteacc wait-start group radius
aaa accounting network default wait-start group radius
line console 0
     login authentication admins
line vty 0 4
     login authentication admins
     authorization exec adminauth
     accounting exec remoteacc
```

Typical RAS Configuration Using AAA

In the following example, an ISP is using a Cisco AS5200 access server to enable remote analog customers to dial in to the AS5200 (NAS) and access the Internet. The ISP has decided that authentication and accounting will be enabled and the security protocol of choice will be RADIUS. Login authentication will occur on each of the asynchronous interfaces (modems), vty lines on the NAS (Telnet), and the console. The AAA configuration examples are outlined in bold. Figure 9.4 illustrates this configuration.

Figure 9.4 An AAA ISP Example

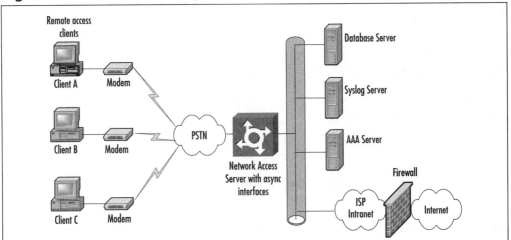

```
!
version 11.3
service timestamps debug datetime msec
service timestamps log datetime msec
service password-encryption
no service udp-small-servers
no service tcp-small-servers
!
hostname NAS
!
```
aaa new-model
```
Enable AAA globally
```
aaa server group radius loginradius
server 172.16.1.200
server 172.16.1.210

Define a group of RADIUS servers which will be used for authentication and accounting. If the server is at IP address 172.16.1.200, RADIUS will query the server at 172.16.1.210 as a backup.

```
aaa authentication login console enable
```

Enable login authentication for users accessing the AS5200 by the console port. The authentication uses the enable password:

```
aaa authentication login vty group loginradius.
```

Enable RADIUS authentication when accessing the AS5200 by Telnet.

```
aaa authentication login dialin group loginradius
```

Create a method list named **dialin** which will query a RADIUS server for authentication.

```
aaa authentication ppp default loginradius
```

Set RADIUS authentication for the *default* method list for PPP sessions.

```
aaa authentication ppp dialin if-needed loginradius
```

Create a method list named **dialin** which will query a RADIUS server for authentication unless the user has already been authenticated (if-needed).

```
aaa accounting login isp-accounting start-stop group loginradius
```

Create a method list named **isp-accounting** which will execute accounting during login attempts and the accounting servers will be defined in the *loginradius* server group.

```
enable secret secretpass
!
async-bootp dns-server 172.16.1.5 172.16.1.6
isdn switch-type primary-5ess
!
controller T1 0
 framing esf
 clock source line primary
 linecode b8zs
 pri-group timeslots 1-24
!
controller T1 1
 framing esf
 clock source line secondary
 linecode b8zs
 pri-group timeslots 1-24
!
interface Loopback0
 ip address 172.16.1.254 255.255.255.0
!
interface Ethernet0
 ip address 172.16.1.2 255.255.255.0
!
interface Serial0
 no ip address
 shutdown
!
interface Serial1
 no ip address
 shutdown
!
interface Serial0:23
 no ip address
```

```
 encapsulation ppp
 isdn incoming-voice modem
!
interface Serial1:23
 no ip address
 isdn incoming-voice modem
!
interface Group-Async1
 ip unnumbered Loopback0
 encapsulation ppp
 async mode interactive
 peer default ip address pool dialin_pool
 no cdp enable
 ppp authentication chap pap dialin
```

Set the authentication method for *Group-Async1* to be CHAP, then PAP (if the connecting party does not support CHAP) using the *dialin* method-list for authentication.

```
ppp accounting isp-accounting
```

Enable the accounting method defined in the *isp-accounting* method list on all async interfaces defined by *Group-Async1*.

```
 group-range 1 48
!
router eigrp 10
 network 172.16.1.0
 passive-interface Dialer0
 no auto-summary
!
ip local pool dialin_pool 172.16.1.10 172.16.1.250
ip default-gateway 172.16.1.1
ip classless
!
dialer-list 1 protocol ip permit
!
line con 0
 login authentication console
line 1 48
```

```
   autoselect ppp
   autoselect during-login
  login authentication dialin
```

Set the authentication method for lines 1 to 48 to that specified in the *dialin* method list.

```
   modem DialIn
  line aux 0
  login authentication console
```

Set the authentication method for the console to that specified in the *console* method list.

```
  line vty 0 4
  login authentication vty
```

Set the authentication method for Telnet to that specified in the *vty* method list.

```
   transport input telnet rlogin
  !
  end
```

Typical Firewall Configuration Using AAA

The following sample configuration displays how authentication and authorization can be used on a Cisco Secure PIX firewall. In this example, the following services will be permitted when authentication and authorization are enabled:

- **Telnet** When the user connects to a host on the outside network via Telnet, they will see a username and password prompt before the connection to the host is established. This is the PIX perform authorization (for the use of Telnet). If the authentication succeeds, a connection will be established to the target host and another prompt will appear from the host beyond the PIX.

- **FTP** When the user initiates an FTP session to a remote host, a username prompt will appear. The user needs to enter **local_username@ remote_username** for username and **local_password@remote_ password** for password. The PIX sends the *local_username* and *local_password* to the security server, and if the authentication (and authorization) succeeds at the PIX, the *remote_username* and *remote_password* are passed to the destination FTP server beyond.

- **HTTP** A window is displayed in the browser requesting a username and password. If authentication (and authorization) succeeds, the user arrives at the destination Web site beyond the PIX. Keep in mind that browsers cache usernames and passwords.

Figure 9.5 illustrates AAA on a Cisco Secure PIX firewall. For more information on the Cisco Secure PIX firewall, see Chapter 3.

Figure 9.5 An AAA PIX Example

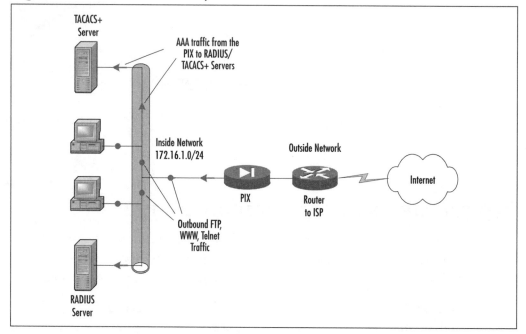

If it appears that the PIX should be timing out an HTTP connection but is not doing so, it is likely that reauthentication is taking place with the browser sending the cached username and password to the PIX, which then forwards this to the authentication server. If this problem occurs, clear the cache in the Web browser settings.

```
PIX Version 5.2
nameif ethernet0 outside security0
nameif ethernet1 inside security100
nameif ethernet2 dmz security10
```

```
enable password 8Ry2YjIyt7RRXU24 encrypted

passwd 2KFQnbNIdI.2KYOU encrypted

hostname firewall

fixup protocol ftp 21

fixup protocol http 80

fixup protocol smtp 25

fixup protocol h323 1720

fixup protocol rsh 514

fixup protocol sqlnet 1521

names

pager lines 24

no logging timestamp

no logging standby

logging console debugging

no logging monitor

no logging buffered

no logging trap

no logging history

logging facility 20

logging queue 512

interface ethernet0 auto

interface ethernet1 auto

interface ethernet2 auto

mtu outside 1500

mtu inside 1500

mtu dmz 1500

ip address outside 207.139.221.2 255.255.255.0

ip address inside 172.16.1.1 255.255.255.0

ip address dmz 127.0.0.1 255.255.255.255

no failover

failover timeout 0:00:00

failover ip address outside 0.0.0.0

failover ip address inside 0.0.0.0

failover ip address dmz 0.0.0.0

arp timeout 14400

global (outside) 1 207.139.221.10-207.139.221.50 netmask 255.255.255.0

nat (inside) 1 172.16.1.0 255.255.255.0 0 0
```

```
static (inside,outside) 207.139.221.5 172.16.0.22 netmask 255.255.255.255 >0
0
conduit permit icmp any any
conduit permit tcp any any
conduit permit udp any any
route outside 0.0.0.0 0.0.0.0 207.139.221.1
timeout xlate 3:00:00 conn 1:00:00 half-closed 0:10:00 udp 0:02:00
timeout rpc 0:10:00 h323 0:05:00
timeout uauth 0:05:00 absolute
access-list 100 permit tcp any any eq telnet
access-list 100 permit tcp any any eq ftp
access-list 100 permit tcp any any eq www
```

Create an access list that defines the traffic that will trigger authentication. This access list will be referenced by the *aaa authentication match* command.

```
aaa-server TACACS+ protocol tacacs+
aaa-server RADIUS protocol radius
aaa-server AuthInbound protocol tacacs+
```

Specify that TACACS+ will be used to authenticate inbound traffic.

```
aaa-server AuthInbound (inside) host 171.68.118.101 cisco timeout 5
```

Specify the TACACS+ server IP address to query for authentication requests.

```
aaa-server AuthOutbound protocol radius
```

Specify that RADIUS will be used to authenticate outbound traffic.

```
aaa-server AuthOutbound (inside) host 171.68.118.101 cisco timeout 5
```

Specify the RADIUS server IP address to query for authentication requests.

```
aaa authentication match 100 outside AuthInbound
```

Perform an inbound authentication on any traffic defined in access list 100.

```
aaa authentication match 100 inside AuthOutbound
```

Perform outbound authentication on any traffic defined in access list 100.

```
no snmp-server location
no snmp-server contact
snmp-server community public
no snmp-server enable traps
```

```
floodguard enable

telnet timeout 5

terminal width 80

Cryptochecksum:b26b560b20e625c9e23743082484caca

: end

[OK]
```

Authentication Proxy

Authentication proxy (auth-proxy), which is available in Cisco IOS Software Firewall version 12.0.5.T and later, allows administrators to apply security policies on a per-user basis. Typically, authorization was associated with a user's IP address, or a subnet. For example, if an administrator wanted to restrict access to the FTP protocol, they would create an access list denying (or permitting) use of a single IP address or specific range of IP addresses. This is difficult to implement, especially if a DHCP server is dynamically assigning IP addresses to workstations. Careful IP management is needed to make sure that a group of workstations is assigned an IP from the correct pool; otherwise, use of FTP may be denied because of their IP address.

Instead of implementing access control lists based on the IP address only, the authentication proxy allows the enforcement of a security policy on a per-user basis. Users can be identified by their username (instead of IP address), and based on their username, access profiles are automatically retrieved and applied from a Cisco Secure ACS server or some other RADIUS or TACACS+ authentication server. These profiles are only in use while traffic is being passed to and from the specific user. For example, if a user initiates an HTTP connection to a Web site, the profile will be in use, after a certain amount of time where no HTTP traffic unique to that profile passes through the firewall, the profile will no longer apply to that user.

How the Authentication Proxy Works

The authentication proxy works like this:

1. A user initiates an HTTP session via a Web browser through the IOS Software Firewall and triggers the authentication proxy.

2. The authentication proxy checks if the user has already been authenticated. If the user has been authenticated, the connection is completed. If

the user has not been authenticated, the authentication proxy prompts the user for a username and password.

3. After the user has entered their username and password, the authentication profile is downloaded from the AAA (RADIUS or TACACS+) server. This information is used to create dynamic access control entries (ACEs) which are added to the inbound access control list (ACL) of an input interface, and to the outbound ACL of an output interface (if an output ACL exists). For example, after successfully authenticating by entering my username and password, my profile will be downloaded to the firewall and ACLs will be dynamically altered and then applied appropriately to the inbound and outbound interfaces. If my profile permits me to use FTP, then an outbound ACL will be dynamically added to the outbound interface (typically, the *outside* interface) allowing this. If the authentication fails, then the service will be denied.

4. The inbound and/or outbound ACL is altered by replacing the source IP address in the access list downloaded from the AAA server with the IP address of the authenticated host (in this case, the workstation's IP address).

5. As soon as the user has successfully authenticated, a timer begins for each user profile. As long as traffic is being passed through the firewall, the user will not have to reauthenticate. If the authentication timer expires, the user must reauthenticate before traffic is permitted through the firewall again.

Comparison with the Lock-and-key Feature

Another feature which utilizes authentication and dynamic access control lists is the *lock-and-key access lists*, described in Chapter 4. Table 9.18 provides a quick comparison of the features of the authentication proxy and *lock-and-key*.

Table 9.18 Authentication Proxy versus Lock-and-key

Authentication Proxy	Lock-and-key
Triggers on HTTP connection requests.	Triggers on Telnet connection requests.
TACACS+ or RADIUS authentication and authorization.	TACACS+, RADIUS, or local authentication.

Continued

Table 9.18 Continued

Authentication Proxy	Lock-and-key
Access lists are retrieved from AAA server only.	Access lists are configured on the router only.
Access privileges are granted on a per-user and host IP address basis.	Access privileges are granted based on the user's host IP address.
Access lists can have multiple entries as defined by the user profiles on the AAA server.	Access lists are limited to one entry for each host IP address.
Allows DHCP-based host IP addresses, meaning that users can log in from any host location and obtain authentication and authorization.	Associates a fixed IP address with a specific user. Users must log in from the host with that IP address.

Benefits of Authentication Proxy

Every policy or networking concept has its advantages and disadvantages, the following are some of the benefits provided by the authentication proxy:

- Provides dynamic, per-user AAA authentication and authorization using either TACACS+ or RADIUS security protocols.

- Does not require static IP addresses to authenticate and authorize users. This makes it easier for administrators who use DHCP assigned IP addresses.

- Since authentication and authorization are being used, it aids in the overall security policy of a company.

- User profiles can be configured on a case-by-case basis, permitting varying levels of authorization based on the duties of the user.

- No special client software is needed. Only an HTTP browser (which is typically installed on clients anyhow) is needed, therefore making this completely transparent to the client (apart from entering their username and password).

WARNING

The authentication proxy will not operate correctly with network address translation unless context-based access control (CBAC) has been configured. To ensure the compatibility of authentication proxy with any configuration, ensure you have configured CBAC.

Restrictions of Authentication Proxy

As stated earlier, there are always some minor restrictions when implementing a protocol or policy. The restrictions of the authentication proxy are as follows:

- Only HTTP connections will trigger the authentication proxy.

- HTTP services must be running on the IOS firewall on the default (well-known) port 80.

- The authentication proxy does not yet support accounting.

- JavaScript must be enabled in the client browsers.

- The authentication proxy access lists apply to traffic passing through the IOS firewall. Traffic destined to the router is authenticated by the existing authentication methods defined in the IOS software.

- The authentication proxy does not support concurrent usage. For example, if two separate users attempt to log in from the same workstation, authentication and authorization will only apply to the first user who is successfully authenticated. The second user will fail to be authenticated and will be unable to pass traffic through the IOS firewall until the user is authenticated.

- Load balancing through multiple AAA servers is currently not supported.

Configuring Authentication Proxy

To configure the authentication proxy, you must perform the following high-level tasks:

1. Configure AAA for the authentication proxy.

2. Configure the HTTP server on the IOS firewall.

3. Configure the Authentication Proxy itself.

The following sections describe how to perform these tasks.

This section identifies and describes the steps necessary to configure AAA for the authentication proxy on the IOS firewall:

1. Enable AAA functionality on the router.

    ```
    aaa new-model
    ```

2. Identify the AAA server (e.g., RADIUS or TACACS+) and specify its related parameters.

    ```
    tacacs-server host hostname
    tacacs-server key sting
    ```

3. Define the AAA authentication login methods.

    ```
    aaa authentication login default
    ```

4. Enable the authentication proxy for AAA methods.

    ```
    aaa authorization auth-proxy default [method1 [method2...]]
    ```

5. Create an ACL entry to allow the AAA server return traffic to the firewall.

    ```
    access-list access-list-number permit tcp host source eq tacacs
    host destination
    ```

Configuring the HTTP Server

In order to use the authentication proxy, the HTTP server must be enabled on the IOS firewall, and the authentication method should be set to use AAA. To do this, perform these commands, which are described in Table 9.19:

1. Enable the HTTP server. The authentication proxy uses the HTTP server to communicate with the client for user authentication.

    ```
    ip http server
    ```

2. Set the HTTP server authentication method to AAA.

    ```
    ip http authentication aaa
    ```

3. Specify the access list for the HTTP server. Use the access list number that was configured previously.

```
ip http access-class access-list-number
```

Table 9.19 Configuring the HTTP Server

Command	Description
ip http server	In global configuration mode, this enables the http server on the device. To disable the http server, use the *no* form of this command.
ip http authentication {aaa | enable | local | tacacs}	In global configuration mode, this specifies the authentication method for HTTP server users. To disable a configured authentication method, use the *no* form of this command. aaa – specifies that the AAA facility is used for authentication. -or- enable – specifies that the enable password method is used for authentication (default). -or- local – specifies that the local user database is used for authentication -or- tacacs – specifies that a TACACS or XTACACS server is used for authentication.
ip http access-class *{access-list-number | access-list-name}*	In global configuration mode, assigns an access list to the HTTP server. To remove the assigned access list, use the *no* form of this command *access-list-number* – specifies a standard IP access list number in the range 0 to 99. -or- *access-list-name* – specifies the name of a standard IP access list.

Configuring the Authentication Proxy

Finally, to configure the authentication proxy, use the following commands, described in Table 9.20, in global configuration mode:

1. Set the global authentication proxy idle timeout value in minutes.

```
ip auth-proxy auth-cache-time min
```

2. (Optional) Display the name of the firewall router in the authentication proxy login page. The banner is disabled by default.

```
ip auth-proxy auth-proxy-banner
```

3. Create authentication proxy rules.

```
ip auth-proxy name auth-proxy-name http [auth-cache-time min] [list
std-access-list
```

4. Enter interface configuration mode by specifying the interface type on which to apply the authentication proxy.

```
interface type
```

5. In interface configuration mode, apply the named authentication proxy rule at the interface.

```
ip auth-proxy auth-proxy-name
```

Table 9.20 Configuring the Authentication Proxy

Command	Description
ip auth-proxy auth-cache-time *min*	Sets the global authentication proxy idle timeout value in minutes. If the timeout expires, user authentication entries are removed, along with any associated dynamic access lists. Enter a value in the range 1 to 2,147,483,647. The default value is 60 minutes.
ip auth-proxy auth-proxy-banner	(Optional) Displays the name of the firewall router in the authentication proxy login page. The banner is disabled by default.
Ip auth-proxy name *auth-proxy-name* http [auth-cache-time *min*] [list *std-access-list*]	Creates authentication proxy rules. These rules define how you apply authentication proxy. This command associates connection initiating HTTP protocol traffic with an authentication proxy name. You can associate the named rule with an access control list, providing control over which hosts use the authentication proxy feature. If no standard access list is defined, the named authentication proxy rule intercepts HTTP

Continued

Table 9.20 Continued

Command	Description
	traffic from all hosts whose connection initiating packets are received at the configured interface. *auth-proxy-name* – name of the authentication proxy. (optional) auth-cache-time – keyword to override the global authentication proxy cache timer. This provides more control over timeout values. If no value is specified, the proxy assumes the value set with the ip auth proxy auth-cache=time command. (optional) list – designates keyword to specify the standard access list to apply to a named authentication proxy rule. HTTP connections initiated from hosts defined in the access list are intercepted by the authentication proxy. *std-access-list* – specify the standard access list for use with the list keyword.
interface *type*	Enter interface configuration mode by specifying the interface type on which to apply the proxy. For example, interface *Ethernet0*.
ip auth-proxy *auth-proxy-name*	In interface configuration mode, apply the named authentication proxy rule at the interface. This command enables the authentication proxy with that name.

Authentication Proxy Configuration Example

The following examples highlight the specific authentication proxy configuration entries. These examples do not represent a complete router configuration. Complete router configurations using the authentication proxy are included later in this document.

AAA Configuration

```
aaa new-model
aaa authentication login default tacacs+ radius
```

```
!Set up the aaa new model to use the authentication proxy.
aaa authorization auth-proxy default tacacs+ radius
!Define the AAA servers used by the router
tacacs-server host 172.31.54.143
tacacs-server key cisco
radius-server host 172.31.54.143
radius-server key cisco
```

HTTP Server Configuration

```
! Enable the HTTP server on the router:
ip http server
! Set the HTTP server authentication method to AAA:
ip http authentication aaa
!Define standard access list 61 to deny any host.
access-list 61 deny any
! Use ACL 61 to deny connections from any host to the HTTP server.
ip http access-class 61
```

Authentication Proxy Configuration

```
!set the global authentication proxy timeout value.
ip auth-proxy auth-cache-time 60
!Apply a name to the authentication proxy configuration rule.
ip auth-proxy name HQ_users http
```

Interface Configuration

```
! Apply the authentication proxy rule at an interface.
interface e0
ip address 10.1.1.210 255.255.255.0
ip auth-proxy HQ_users
```

Summary

In this chapter, we provided an overview of AAA and its benefits, described the RADIUS, TACACS+, and Kerberos security protocols, and discussed (with examples) how to configure each of the AAA services on Cisco IOS devices.

AAA is comprised of the three independent but related functions of authentication, authorization, and accounting, which are defined in the following:

- Authentication is the process of identifying and authenticating a user prior to allowing access to network devices and services. User identification and authentication is critical for the accuracy of the authorization and accounting functions.

- Authorization is the process of determining a user's privileges and access rights after they have been authenticated.

- Accounting is the process of recording user activities for accountability, billing, auditing, or reporting purposes.

The benefits of implementing AAA include scalability, increased flexibility and control, standardized protocols and methods, and redundancy. Cisco devices generally support the RADIUS, TACACS+, and Kerberos security protocols for use within an AAA mechanism. Each protocol has its advantages and disadvantages, so which protocol is right for you will depend on your situation and requirements.

On Cisco IOS devices, you enable one or more of the AAA services on a device by:

1. Enable AAA by using the *aaa new-model* global configuration command.

2. If you are using a separate AAA server, configure the appropriate protocol parameters (for example, RADIUS, TACACS+, or Kerberos).

3. Define the appropriate method lists for the desired service (authentication, authorization, accounting).

4. Apply the method lists to the desired interface or line, if required.

Solutions Fast Track

Cisco AAA Overview

☑ AAA is an architectural framework comprised of the three independent but related functions of authentication, authorization, and accounting.

☑ Authentication is the process of identifying and authenticating a user prior to allowing access to network devices and services. Authorization is the process of determining a user's privileges and access rights after they have been authenticated. Accounting is the process of recording user activities for accountability, billing, auditing, or reporting purposes.

☑ The benefits of implementing AAA can include scalability, increased flexibility and control, standardized protocols and methods, and redundancy.

Cisco AAA Mechanisms

☑ Cisco devices generally support the RADIUS, TACACS+, and Kerberos security protocols for use within an AAA mechanism. Each protocol has its advantages and disadvantages, so which protocol is right for you will depend on your situation and requirements.

☑ Within the AAA framework, authentication occurs when an AAA client passes appropriate user credentials to an AAA server, and requests that the server authenticate the user. The AAA server attempts to validate the credentials, and responds with either an accept or a deny message. AAA authentication is typically used in the following scenarios: To control access to a network device such as a router or NAS, or to control access to network resources by remote users.

☑ Within the AAA framework, authorization occurs when an AAA client queries the AAA server to determine what actions a user is authorized to perform. The AAA server returns a set of attribute-value (AV) pairs that defines the user's authorization. The client then enforces user access control based on those AV pairs. AAA authorization is typically used in the following scenarios: To provide authorization for actions attempted while logged in to a network device, or to provide authorization for attempts to use network services.

☑ Within the AAA framework, the client sends accounting records that consist of accounting AV pairs to the AAA server for centralized storage. An accounting record consists of accounting AV pairs.

☑ On Cisco IOS devices, you enable one or more of the AAA services on a device by: (1) Enabling AAA by using the *aaa new-model* global configuration command, (2) Configuring the appropriate protocol parameters (for example, RADIUS, TACACS+, or Kerberos) for your AAA servers, (3) Defining the appropriate method lists for the desired services (authentication, authorization, accounting), and (4) Applying the method lists to the desired interface or line, if required.

Authentication Proxy

☑ Authentication proxy (auth-proxy) is available in Cisco IOS Software Firewall version 12.0.5.T and later, and allows administrators to apply security policies on a per-user basis.

☑ Instead of implementing access control lists based on the IP address only, the authentication proxy allows the enforcement of a security policy on a per-user basis. It allows DHCP-based host IP addresses, meaning that the users can log in from any host location and obtain authentication and authorization.

☑ Authentication proxy is triggered only on HTTP connection requests, and can use either TACACS+ or RADIUS authentication and authorization. For authorization, it retrieves access lists from the AAA server, modifies them based on the user's IP address, and applies then dynamically to the necessary interfaces.

☑ To configure the authentication proxy, the following high-level tasks must be performed: (1) configure AAA for the authentication proxy, (2) configure the HTTP server on the IOS firewall, and (3) configure the authentication proxy itself.

Frequently Asked Questions

The following Frequently Asked Questions, answered by the authors of this book, are designed to both measure your understanding of the concepts presented in this chapter and to assist you with real-life implementation of these concepts. To have your questions about this chapter answered by the author, browse to **www.syngress.com/solutions** and click on the **"Ask the Author"** form.

Q: What is AAA?

A: Authentication, authorization, and accounting (AAA) is an architectural framework for providing the independent but related functions of authentication, authorization, and accounting, and is critical to provide secure remote access to both network devices and resources. The AAA framework typically consists of both a client and server. The AAA client (for example, a router or network access server (NAS)) requests authentication, authorization, and/or accounting services from an AAA server (for example, a UNIX or Windows server with appropriate software) that maintains databases containing the relevant AAA information.

Q: What are the functions authentication, authorization, and accounting?

A: Authentication is the process of identifying and authenticating a user prior to allowing access to network devices and services. Authorization is the process of determining a user's privileges and access rights after they have been authenticated. Accounting is the process of recording user activities for accountability, billing, auditing, or reporting purposes.

Q: What are the benefits of using AAA?

A: The benefits of implementing AAA can include scalability, increased flexibility and control, standardized protocols and methods, and redundancy.

Q: How do I configure AAA services on a Cisco device?

A: To configure AAA on a Cisco network device, you need to perform the following high-level tasks:

1. Enable AAA by using the *aaa new-model* global configuration command.

2. Configure the appropriate protocol parameters (for example, RADIUS, TACACS+, or Kerberos) for the AAA server you are using.

3. Define the appropriate method lists for the desired service (authentication, authorization, accounting).

4. Apply the method lists to the desired interface or line, if required.

Q: What are the three primary scenarios for using AAA authentication with Cisco devices?

A: For Cisco devices, AAA authentication can be used for login authentication, PPP authentication, or for enabling password protection. AAA login authentication controls login access to the device itself. PPP authentication controls access to network resources async interfaces, and enables password protection controls access to privileged EXEC mode using the *enable* command.

Q: What types of AAA authorization can be defined for Cisco devices?

A: For Cisco devices, AAA authorization can be used to control access to EXEC shells (exec), specific command privilege levels (command *level*), network related services (network), and reverse access connections (reverse-access) such as reverse Telnet. Exec and command apply to router access control and are applied to lines, while network and reverse-access primarily deal with dial-in and dial-out access control and are applied to interfaces. Also, note that AAA authentication must be configured in order to use AAA authorization.

Q: What types of AAA accounting can be defined for Cisco devices?

A: For Cisco devices, AAA accounting can be used to record network session information (network), outbound connection information (connection), EXEC shells (exec), system level events (system), and command usage (command). The collected information can be used for a variety of purposes, including accountability, resource usage tracking, and billing.

Q: Should I use RADIUS or TACACS+ as my AAA protocol?

A: Various factors come into play on this question. If encryption and a connection-oriented authorization request is important, then TACACS+ would be the best choice. Recall that TACACS+ uses TCP as its transport protocol and encrypts the entire body of the packet when sending information back and forth, while RADIUS uses UDP for its transport protocol, and only encrypts the password in the access-request packet when sending information back and forth.

Q: Where can I find a RADIUS or TACACS+ server/daemon?

A: There are several programs available for use as a RADIUS or TACACS+ server, for example:

- Cisco Secure ACS, which can be found at www.cisco.com
- Lucent RADIUS, which can be found at www.livingston.com
- RADIUS-VMS server, which can be found at www.radiusvms.com

A listing of available RADIUS and TACACS+ servers can be found at http://ing.ctit.utwente.nl/WU5/backgrounds/products/index.html.

## Chapter 10

Cisco Content Services Switch

Solutions in this chapter:

- Overview of Cisco Content Services Switch

- Cisco Content Services Switch Product Information

- Security Features of Cisco Content Services Switch

☑ Summary

☑ Solutions Fast Track

☑ Frequently Asked Questions

Introduction

The Internet has grown to the point where its value transcends IP connectivity for the support of Web pages, e-mail, and other applications. Businesses now look to the Web for high-performance, reliable transport for bandwidth-intensive applications, and multimedia content such as everything over IP (XoIP), e-commerce transactions, special events, news, and even entertainment services. Content switching is a method to remove delays that might occur in the transport of data across a network. This chapter deals with the technology that allows this to occur and with the dangers the user may face with corruption of data, and why, by using the products described in the following pages, they should be protected from such corruption.

Overview of Cisco Content Services Switch

The *Content Services Switch* (CSS) uses content switching to intelligently redirect service requests to the most appropriate server. The key difference between load balancing and content switching is that content switching makes decisions based on information from Layers 4 through 7 (including URLs, host tags, and cookies) instead of just Layer 4 information (IP addresses and port numbers) such as LocalDirector and DistributedDirector.

Some of you might know this product as the ArrowPoint Content Smart Switch (the CCS login screen still mentions ArrowPoint). Cisco Systems acquired ArrowPoint Communications in June 2000 and incorporated their products and technology into Cisco's product range.

A common implementation of this technology is for a service provider to have two types of Web services. The first service is for contracted Service Level Agreement (SLA) customers and the second for non-SLA customers. In this way, customers with SLAs can be guaranteed a faster Web response time than non-contract customers. This is typically be done using cookies. The CSS recognizes the cookie and processes that flow via the SLA policy to the most appropriate server. Given its priorities, the SLA policy might specify more Web servers than the non-SLA policy.

Cisco Content Services Switch Technology Overview

At first glance, the CSS appears to have similar features to those of LocalDirector or DistributedDirector (if you add the enhanced feature set to the CSS).

Although this observation is partly correct, Web content switching uses a completely different technology compared to load balancing, which is what both LocalDirector and DistributedDirector are based on. Load balancing uses OSI Layer 4 (transport layer) technology while content switching is based on OSI Layers 5 through 7 (session, presentation, and application layers) technology.

Content switching optimizes Web traffic by utilizing information from OSI Layers 5 through 7 to better direct the Web request to the most appropriate server. In this way, content switching can make use of URLs, host tags, and cookies to optimize content delivery.

OSI Layer 3 and 4 (network and transport) switching is simply not optimized for Web-based traffic. For a start, Web traffic is largely asymmetric, with much larger flows back out to the customer from the Web servers than inward-bound flows. It is also very different in the way sessions are constantly brought up and torn down, often with little data involved but many concurrent connections.

Figure 10.1 depicts a typical CSS implementation. The Content Services Switch redirects the Web request to the most appropriate server. The enhanced feature set is required to give the CSS the ability to load-balance geographically distributed servers.

Cisco Content Services Switch Product Information

The CSS product is available in three different ranges:

- **CSS 11050** This is the entry-level product and is suitable for small Web sites as well as points of presence (PoPs). It was designed for throughput of up to 5 Gbps and has a fixed port configuration. Use for up to eight Web servers or caches.

- **CSS 11150** This is the medium-level product and is suitable for small-to-medium-sized Web sites. It was designed for throughput of up to 5 Gbps and has a fixed port configuration. Use for up to 16 Web servers or caches.

- **CSS 11800** This is the high-end product, suitable for large, high-traffic Web sites and Web-hosting infrastructures. It was designed for throughput of up to 20 Gbps and has a modular port configuration.

Figure 10.1 Typical Content Services Switch Implementation

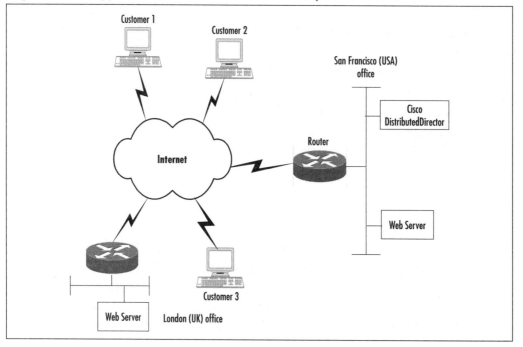

Software that runs on these switches is called Cisco Web Network Services (WebNS). A copy of the basic feature set is bundled with the switches. This software allows network managers to configure load balancing based on SLAs, and provide delivery services for various Web-related services, including streaming video and audio. It also supports "sticky" connections based on IP addresses, Secure Socket Layer IDs (SSL IDs), and cookies. "Stickiness," in short, means that once the connection is made, all other connections from this client will be redirected to the same physical server. This helps CSS ensure reliability of services for e-commerce transactions. An enhanced feature set is also available. The key difference is that the enhanced feature set also includes multisite content routing and site selection, all content replication features, and content distribution as well as delivery services. The current WebNS software version is 5.x.

Because CSS products are tailored to load-balance Web services, these devices include more sophisticated algorithms of application availability testing. Local server selection can be based on server load and application response time, as well as simpler connections and round-robin algorithms. There are global server load-balancing features based on DNS and proximity by source IP address of connection. The CSS can also load-balance any other application that uses TCP or UDP for communication, much like LocalDirector does.

Monitoring and management tools include command-line interface (CLI), Web-based graphical interface, SNMP and RMON capabilities, plus an extensive logging system. It also includes various security-related features, which will be described later, together with some recommendation on securing the device itself.

Security Features of Cisco Content Services Switch

The following information about the security features of the CSS will allow you to better understand the security mechanisms it uses and enable you to configure or change these features. Main security features of CSS include:

- **Denial of service (DoS) attack prevention** The switch checks each session flow at initial flow setup time, eliminating connection-based DoS attacks such as SYN floods. The device also drops all abnormal connections with minimal impact on performance.

- **FlowWall Security** CSS products provide firewall services, which include high-speed Access Control Lists (ACL), that control connections by IP address, TCP port, host tags, URLs, or file types.

- **Network Address Translation (NAT)** Address translation capabilities of CSS help hide the real IP addresses of devices located behind the switch. This prevents direct attacks on Web servers protected by the switch.

- **Firewall load balancing** CSS can work as a load-sharing device for complex firewall structures, preventing bottlenecks and eliminating single points of failure.

FlowWall Security

FlowWall is an integrated firewall that provides wire-speed-per-flow-based filtering of content requests, with no performance penalty. It provides firewall services such as ACLs and flow admission control. These conditions are checked as a part of the flow (session) setup process and after they are validated, packet forwarding for this flow is permitted with wire speed.

FlowWall provides intelligent flow inspection technology that screens for all common DoS attacks, such as SYN floods, ping floods, smurfs, and abnormal or malicious connection attempts.

It does this by discarding packets that have the following characteristics:

- Frame length is too short.

- Frame is fragmented.

- Source IP address = IP destination (LAND attack).

- Source address = Cisco address, or the source is a subnet broadcast.

- Source address is not a unicast address.

- Source IP address is a loop-back address.

- Destination IP address is a loop-back address.

- Destination address is not a valid unicast or multicast address.

If the flow is HTTP flow, then it is considered valid if CSS receives a valid content frame within 16 seconds of starting the flow. It this does not happen, switch will discard all frames and tear the flow down. A real physical server will be contacted only after the flow is validated, so there is no danger that its TCP state tables overflow even if the switch is under SYN flood attack or other state table overflow attack.

Other TCP flows (not HTTP) are considered valid if CSS receives a return ACK for the three-way TCP handshake during the first 16 seconds after the initial SYN packet. If any flow sends an initial SYN packet more than eight times, CSS discards this flow and does not process any SYN packets from the same source/ destination addresses or from port numbers with the same initial sequence numbers.

Using ACLs, policies can be created based on actions (deny/permit/bypass) for traffic matching some or all of the following:

- Source IP address

- Destination IP address

- TCP port

- Host tag

- URL

- File extension

SECURITY ALERT!

FlowWall does not scan for Java and ActiveX traffic, although it is possible to configure for the filtering of Java or ActiveX code by file name or extension.

ACL rules on CSS can be of three types:

- **Deny** These rules prevent any request for matching content from being forwarded to the original server or cache. These rules can be used to block access to specific content or access from specific networks.

- **Permit** These rules do the opposite. They permit traffic that matches the rule. If something is not permitted in ACL, then it is denied by default.

- **Bypass** This rule also permits traffic that matches this rule, but as an addition, all content rules for this traffic are ignored. This is more useful for cache control functions than security—for example, it can be used for specifying that matching traffic is not cached.

The commands used to manage ACLs are a bit different from Cisco IOS or PIX firewall commands. The main difference is that clauses (rules) in an ACL are numbered, so it is possible to insert a new rule between any other two rules without re-creating the whole ACL. An example of ACL configuration is provided next.

```
acl 1
clause 20 permit any 1.2.3.0 255.255.255.0 destination 1.2.3.4
clause 30 permit any 1.2.3.0 255.255.255.0 destination 1.2.3.5
clause 50 permit ICMP any destination any
clause 70 deny any any destination any
apply circuit-(VLAN1)
```

This simple access-list allows access from network 1.2.3.0 thru 1.2.3.255 to the servers 1.2.3.4 and 1.2.3.5 (virtual servers implemented by CSS). It also permits all ICMP traffic and finally denies all that is not permitted. The last line is used to apply this ACL number 1 to a specific circuit (IP interface) with the name VLAN1.

To enable ACL processing, you need to enter a global command *acl enable* in configuration mode.

Configuring & Implementing...

Access Control Lists

It is important you configure ACLs before enabling them, otherwise all traffic will be disabled because an empty access list will implicitly deny all traffic. If you do this by mistake, you can recover using console port only. Console port is not affected by ACL filtering.

The normal sequence of steps when configuring access lists would be the following:

1. Configure access lists for filtering content and apply them, either as one process or by configuring them first and applying them afterwards.

2. Configure access lists for management traffic and apply them.

3. Enable ACL.

For a more in-depth look at Access Lists, refer to Chapter 4. Note that CSS Access Lists are slightly different in configuration and functionality than IOS Access Lists

ACL configuration is described in detail in The Advanced Configuration Guide for CSS.

Example of Nimda Virus Filtering without Access Control Lists

ACL processing on CSS requires extra processor power, and because of this, sometimes it is more convenient to use content rules to provide filtering of the traffic. This filtering essentially redirects "bad" traffic to a non-existent server. It is better to redirect traffic to an existing machine, which does not run any Web server, so it will promptly respond with reset (RST) packets. If the redirection is performed to the non-existent IP address, this introduces extra time-outs while CSS waits for a server's reply and requires more resources. The following description of rules, which will filter all Nimda worm requests, assumes that a reader has some knowledge of CSS configuration commands.

As a first step, a dummy server is configured. It has IP address 10.10.0.1 and will reply with RST packets for all connection attempts.

```
service dummy
  ip address 10.10.0.1
  keepalive type none
  active
```

Now various rules are created that allow CSS to inspect incoming requests for HTTP header fields:

```
header-field-group .ida
  header-field .ida request-line contain ".ida"
header-field-group cmd.exe
  header-field cmd.exe request-line contain "cmd.exe"
header-field-group default.ida
  header-field default.ida request-line contain "default.ida"
header-field-group root.exe
  header-field root.exe request-line contain "root.exe"
header-field-group x.ida
  header-field x.ida request-line contain "x.ida"
```

Each pair of lines in this snippet defines a new group that matches specific content in the HTTP request. For example, first group matches each request that has .ida contained within it.

After that, this configuration is applied to content rules as follows:

```
owner nimdarules
  content block_.ida
    protocol tcp
    port 80
    url "/*"
    header-field-rule .ida weight 0
    add service dummy
    active
  content block_cmd.exe
    protocol tcp
    port 80
    url "/*"
    header-field-rule cmd.exe weight 0
    add service dummy
    active
```

```
content block_default.ida
    protocol tcp
    port 80
    url "/*"
    header-field-rule default.ida weight 0
    add service dummy
    active
content block_root.exe
    protocol tcp
    port 80
    url "/*"
    header-field-rule root.exe weight 0
    add service dummy
    active
content block_x.ida
    protocol tcp
    port 80
    url "/*"
    header-field-rule x.ida weight 0
    add service dummy
    active
```

Each block of content rules in this example defines a rule, which will inspect incoming traffic for connections to port 80/tcp, looking for Nimda-specific headers, and when they are found, the connection is redirected to the dummy server, which tears it down. The *show rules* command will show the number of hits for each rule, giving you a number of attack attempts. The same approach can be used in the defense against CodeRed and similar HTTP-oriented worms.

Using Network Address Translation to Hide Real Addresses

CSS supports wire-speed Network Address Translation (NAT). As described in the LocalDirector chapter, this allows you to use unregistered IP addresses on your inside network (usually the server farm) and prevents hackers from being able to directly target the real server's IP address. Cisco CSS 11000 series switches provide full two-way translation on any Ethernet port at wire speed. The device also supports source group NAT, which allows translation for server-initiated flows going back to the client (for example, as in active FTP sessions) or server-initiated flows, going to other locations.

Firewall Load Balancing

CSS can enhance security by load-balancing traffic among multiple firewalls. This not only eliminates performance bottlenecks but also guards against having a single point of failure.

This is typically done by deploying a CSS in front, and at the back, of the firewalls being load balanced. In this way, traffic for a given flow will traverse the same firewall.

Figure 10.2 depicts a typical CSS implementation to load balance multiple firewalls. This design provides not only firewall load balancing, but also redundancy, while maintaining all the usual firewall security features.

Figure 10.2 A Typical Content Services Switch Implementation to Load-Balance Multiple Firewalls

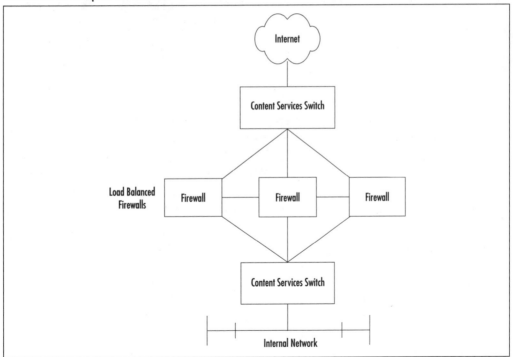

CSS firewall load balancing can be used for distribution of traffic among stateful firewalls, which have their own IP addresses. Firewall load balancing acts as a Layer 3 device. Each link between CSS and firewalls is a separate IP subnet.

CSS ensures that all flows between the same endpoints (pair of IP addresses) will pass through the same firewall in both directions. Firewall load balancing performs only routing functions. No content rules are matched during this process and it is not possible for firewalls in this scenario to perform NAT. If address translation is needed, it can be configured on CSS itself or on another device placed before CSS.

Firewall load balancing configuration essentially consists of defining firewalls' parameters and routing information by either using static routes or an OSPF routing protocol. It is rather easy and requires a minimum of commands. The redundancy of load-balancing solutions can be increased even more by using a pair of switches instead of one on each side of the firewall's array.

Designing & Planning…

Firewall Load Balancing with CSS

CSS can support up to 15 firewalls, distributing traffic between them. It is always better to use dedicated CSS switches in case of heavy traffic load, although it is technically possible to use their free ports for some content switching purposes.

Technically speaking, it is possible to use various firewall platforms at the same time—for example, you can have CSS distributing traffic between PIX and the Check Point firewall. Nevertheless, it is recommended to use the same software platform and, if possible, use firewall state synchronization of separate modules.

Example of Firewall Load Balancing with Static Routes

The following is an example of CSS configuration with two firewalls (which may be connected with a state synchronization link) using static routing.

Suppose you have two content switches—one on client (Internet) side—switch CSS1. It is connected to the Internet via an IP circuit with address 1.2.3.254/24. The circuit connected to the firewalls has IP address 192.168.1.10. Two of the firewalls' external interfaces are on the same subnet 192.168.1.0/24 and have IP addresses 192.168.1.1 and 192.168.1.2. Second switch CSS2 is on servers' side and has IP address 192.168.2.10. Internal interfaces of firewalls are 192.168.2.1 and 192.168.2.2 correspondingly. Lastly, CSS2 is connected to the server network via a circuit with IP address 10.100.1.254/24. Figure 10.3 illustrates this setup.

Figure 10.3 Firewall Load Balancing with Static Routes

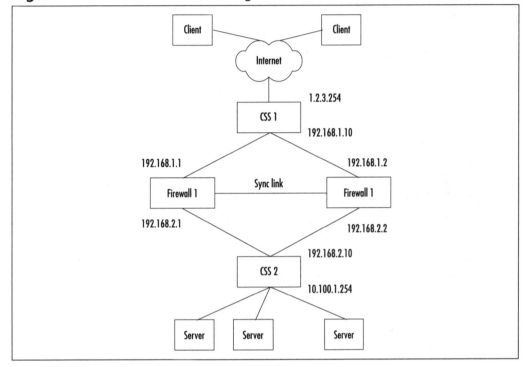

In this case, the relevant part of the configuration for CSS1 will look like the following:

```
ip firewall 1 192.168.1.1 192.168.2.1 192.168.2.10
ip firewall 2 192.168.1.2 192.168.2.2 192.168.2.10
ip route 10.100.1.0/24 firewall 1
ip route 10.100.1.0/24 firewall 2
```

The first two lines describe the configuration of two firewalls—the parameters here are the firewall index (an arbitrary number from 1 to 254), the address of the firewall interface connected to this switch, the address of the firewall interface connected to the switch on the other side, and the IP address of the second CSS. The last two lines describe static routes to the server network 10.100.1.0.24 via both firewalls. Parameters here are the network itself and the index of firewalls through which it can be reached. Second switch CSS2 will be configured in a similar way:

```
ip firewall 1 192.168.2.1 192.168.1.1 192.168.1.10
ip firewall 2 192.168.2.2 192.168.1.2 192.168.1.10
ip route 0.0.0.0/0 firewall 1
ip route 0.0.0.0/0 firewall 2
```

Here, the first two lines mean the same as in the CSS1 case with the interfaces interchanged. The last two lines describe a default route passing through both of the available firewalls.

For an example of firewall load balancing with dynamic route distribution (OSPF), see the Cisco CSS Advanced Configuration Guide.

Password Protection

Content Services Switches support two types of access levels, *User* and *SuperUser,* and up to 32 usernames, including administrator and technician.

The User Access Level

This is the user-level user. This type of access level allows you to have access to a limited set of commands that permit you to monitor and display parameters but not change them (for example, no configuration mode access is provided). The following syntax is used to create a user account (the *global configuration* command):

```
username name [des-password|encrypted-password|password] password
```

Here, *name* is the username you want to create or change (a text string with a maximum of 16 characters is supported), while des-password specifies that the provided password is encrypted with Data Encryption Standard, or DES (use this option only when you are creating a file for use as a script or a startup configuration file; the password is case sensitive and between 6 and 64 characters long). The parameter *encrypted-password* specifies that the password is encrypted (this option is also useful when creating a file for use as a script or a startup configuration file). If the *password* parameter is specified, it means the following password is unencrypted. The last mode is used when creating users online utilizing the console mode. The parameter *password* is the password itself, which must be between 6 and 16 characters long.

The SuperUser Access Level

This is the privileged-level user. This type of access level allows you to both monitor and display parameters, as well as change them. The default privileged-user username is *admin* and the default password is *system*.

The following syntax is used to create a SuperUser account (*global configuration* command):

```
username name [des-password|encrypted-password|password] password superuser
```

Here, *name* is the username you want to create or change (a text string with a maximum of 16 characters is supported). Password encryption options are the same as for other users and the word *superuser*, which is optional, specifies that the user has SuperUser rights. If this word is not present, then the user is created as a normal user.

CSS supports up to 32 different users, including SuperUser. It also has capabilities of defining more gradual access rights to parts of a device's file structure. To use this feature, you have to add to the user's definition one more parameter.

For example:

```
username User1 password mypassword dir-access BBNBNBB
```

The last parameter, *dir-access XXXXXXX,* specifies a user's access rights to the following CSS file areas:

- CSS script
- Log
- Root (contains installed CSS software)
- Archive
- Release root (contains configuration files)
- Core
- MIB directories

Each letter specifies a type of access for the corresponding directory: "N" means no access; "B" means read/write access; "W" means write; and "R" means read access. So, in the preceding example, the user has no access to the root and release root directories but does have read/write access to all other directories.

For increased security, it is also better to issue the command (in configuration mode):

```
restrict user-database
```

It will prevent users without SuperUser rights from clearing running-config and modifying or creating usernames.

The syntax to list existing usernames is:

```
username ?
```

The syntax to remove users is:

```
no username username
```

SECURITY ALERT!

A security mistake that is often made is not to change the default admin password for the Content Services Switch. CSS ships with the default SuperUsername *admin* and the password *system*. Be sure to change this before you deploy the CSS.

Disabling Telnet Access

Although it may be not be feasible for many customers with CSS deployed in more than one location, disabling Telnet access to these switches greatly increases security. Access would then be via the physical console or SSH (recommended) connection.

The syntax to disabling Telnet access is:

```
restrict telnet
```

It is also recommended to check that there is no Web management access enabled. It is disabled by default, but if it is enabled, then the following command will disable it.

```
restrict web-mgmt
```

SSH daemon allows Secure Shell connections to the CSS. It is enabled by default and has some parameters that can be changed in global configuration mode. These parameters are SSH keepalives (enabled by default), the port number for incoming connections (default is 22), and the number of bits in the server key (default is 768 bits).

Syslog Logging

Often, knowing about an attack is as important as taking steps to protect yourself against it. This is where logging plays an important role. If a syslog server is configured, the CSS will log error and event messages to an external syslog server (called *host*).

The following syntax is used to configure the syslog feature (from configuration mode):

```
logging host ip facility number
```

Here *ip* is the IP address of the log host and *number* is the syslog facility number (0 thru 7). This is discussed in greater detail in Chapter 4.

To disable syslog, use the *no* command:

```
no logging host
```

The following command will include logging of all commands entered on CSS:

```
logging commands enable
```

One of the CSS logging subsystems can log all hits for ACL rules. To enable ACL logging (it is disabled by default), you need to do the following (assume you need to enable the logging of hits for clauses 10 and 20 of access list 5, which is applied to circuit VLAN1):

```
acl 5
remove circuit-(VLAN1)
clause 10 log enable
clause 20 log enable
apply circuit-(VLAN1)
```

Unfortunately, logging settings are not saved in running-config, so you will need to reapply them after reboot. For logging commands to become active, you also need to enable the ACL logging subsystem globally. The command to be used in configuration mode is:

```
logging subsystem acl level debug-7
```

Known Security Vulnerabilities

Last year, new vulnerabilities were discovered in various Cisco products, including CSS. Detailed documentation about these and other vulnerabilities is available on

Cisco's Web site at www.cisco.com/warp/public/707/advisory.html. We will briefly list them here.

Cisco Bug ID CSCdt08730

Cisco Bug ID CSCdt08730 allows someone with a nonprivileged user level account to prompt an abnormal event that can cause the switch to reboot, which will prevent normal functioning for up to five minutes. This vulnerability can be continuously reproduced, resulting in a DoS attack.

This vulnerability has been resolved in Cisco WebNS software revision 4.01(12s) and revision 3.10(71s).

Cisco Bug ID CSCdt12748

Cisco Bug ID CSCdt12748 allows someone with a nonprivileged user level account to gain access to files on the CSS that that should not have access to. This vulnerability has been resolved in Cisco WebNS software revision 4.01(23s) and revision 4.10(13s).

Cisco Bug ID CSCdu20931

If users bookmark the URL they are redirected to after a successful authentication on the CSS 11000 series switches, they can later access the Web management interface without having to reauthenticate. This allows users to bypass access control of the Web management interface. This vulnerability has been fixed in Cisco WebNS software revisions 4.01(29s) and 4.10(17s).

Cisco Bug ID CSCdt32570

Cisco Bug ID CSCdt32570 allows someone with user-level access to escalate their privileges to superuser level by issuing a series of keystrokes, which enter the CSS in debug mode. This vulnerability has been fixed in Cisco WebNS software revisions 4.01(19s).

Cisco Bug ID CSCdt64682

A nonprivileged user (user account without administrative privileges) can open an FTP connection to a CSS 11000 series switch and use *GET* and *PUT FTP* commands, without any user-level restrictions enforced. This allows nonprivileged users to access files they normally couldn't.

Cisco Bug ID CSCdt64682 has been fixed in Cisco WebNS software revisions 4.01(23s) and 4.10(13s).

CSS devices did not escape the industrywide bugs discovered recently, nor the SSH v1.5 vulnerabilities, SNMP implementation problems, and CodeRed impact.

Multiple SSH Vulnerabilities

Like many other Cisco devices that were using SSH version 1.5 at the time, CSS contained the following SSH vulnerabilities:

- **CRC-32 integrity check vulnerability** Allows insertion of arbitrary commands in the session once it has been established. (Cisco bug ID CSCdv34668)

- **Traffic analysis** This vulnerability exposes the exact lengths of the passwords used for login authentication. (Cisco bug ID CSCdv34676)

- **Key recovery** This vulnerability may lead to the compromise of the session key. Once the session key is determined, the attacker can decrypt the stored session using any implementation of the crypto algorithm used. (Cisco bug ID CSCdv34679)

These vulnerabilities were fixed in WebNS software versions R4.01 B42s, R4.10 B22s, R5.0 B11s, and R5.01 B6s.

Malformed SNMP Message Handling Vulnerabilities

Again, many Cisco and non-Cisco products are affected by this vulnerability. It allows the attacker to conduct a denial of service by sending malformed SNMP packets to the CSS, causing it to crash and reload. (Cisco bug ID CSCdw64236)

All SNMP related vulnerabilities were fixed in WebNS releases 4.01.053s, 5.00.037s, 5.01.013s, and 5.02.005s.

CodeRed Impact

Although CSS does not contain Microsoft IIS (Internet Information Server), it was also affected by large traffic generated from hosts infected with CodeRed. When the traffic from the worm reaches a significant level, a Cisco CSS 11000 series may suffer a memory allocation error that leads to memory corruption and requires a reboot. This is documented in Cisco bug ID CSCdu76237. This vulnerability was fixed in WebNS releases R3.10 B78s, R4.01 B41s, R4.10 B21s, R5.0 B8s, and R5.01 B5.

Summary

Cisco Content Services Switch (CSS) is a device specifically designed to provide load sharing for Web-related services. It uses information from Layers 4 thru 7 of the ISO/OSI network model (from destination port numbers to browser cookies) in order to decide where to forward each request for content.

The CSS 11000 product line consists of three different models—CSS 11050 (entry-level product), CSS 11150 (medium-level), and CSS 11800 (high-end device with modular port extensions).

Security features of CSS include health checks for each new flow, Access Control Lists (ACLs), and Network Address Translation (NAT). Another application of CSS in security architecture is to provide load balancing for firewalls.

ACL features filtering of connections by their source IP address, destination IP address, TCP port, host tag, URL, or file extension. Another way of filtering can be configuring content rules so that undesired requests are forwarded to a dummy server and dropped there. Worms such as CodeRed or Nimda can be filtered out this way.

CSSs support wire-speed NAT. This allows you to use unregistered IP addresses on your inside network (usually the server farm) and prevents hackers from being able to directly target the real server's IP address.

CSS firewall load balancing can be used for distribution of traffic among stateful firewalls, which have their own IP addresses. Firewall load balancing acts as a Layer 3 device. The function of CSS is to ensure all flows between the same endpoints (pair of IP addresses) will pass through the same firewall in both directions.

Command-line interface (CLI) of CSS supports up to 32 different users and allows for configuration of access privileges, as well as distinction of privileged and nonprivileged users.

An extensive logging system can be configured to provide necessary information in the form of syslog messages, or to store data on the local hard drive.

As many other network devices, CSS has had security vulnerabilities. In particular, it was vulnerable to such industrywide problems as the incorrect handling of malformed SNMP messages and SSH 1.5 bugs.

Solutions Fast Track

Overview of Cisco Content Services Switch

☑ CSS is designed to provide effective load sharing for Web-oriented services and uses information up to the application layer of communications to find the optimal way of doing this.

☑ Information used by CSS in making decisions on forwarding requests includes browser cookies, URLs, host tags, HTTP header fields, and SSL connection IDs.

☑ The enhanced feature set of WebNS management software, which runs on CSS, allows load balancing of geographically distributed server farms.

Cisco Content Services Switch Product Information

☑ The CSS product line includes three devices for all sizes of server farms—from entry-level CSS 11050 through mid-level CSS 11150 to the high-end CSS 11800.

☑ The newest version of WebNS software is 5.x.

☑ Application availability tests (used for making decisions during the load balancing process) include server load, application response time, and global load balancing based on DNS and the proximity of the source IP address. Simpler algorithms resembling those of LocalDirector are also available.

Security Features of Cisco Content Services Switch

☑ CSS performs various checks during the initial phase of flow setup, helping to prevent denial of service attacks.

☑ FlowWall security features include traffic filtering based on various conditions.

☑ The NAT capabilities of CSS help hide real IP addresses of devices located behind the switch.

☑ CSS can work as a load-sharing device for complex firewall structures, preventing bottlenecks and eliminating single points of failure.

Frequently Asked Questions

The following Frequently Asked Questions, answered by the authors of this book, are designed to both measure your understanding of the concepts presented in this chapter and to assist you with real-life implementation of these concepts. To have your questions about this chapter answered by the author, browse to **www.syngress.com/solutions** and click on the **"Ask the Author"** form.

Q: My browser does not work with Web-based management interfaces on CSS. I cannot connect to it. What is going on?

A: First of all, it is better to disable Web-based management and use only command line configuration. If you need to use it, make sure that connections to http and https ports on CSS are allowed from your computer and hot blocked somewhere along the way. The most common problem with the Web interface is that it uses only 128-bit encryption, and browsers that do not support it (for example, Microsoft Internet Explorer earlier than version 4.0), will be refused during the SSL session establishing process. You will need to upgrade the browser.

Q: What are standard, enhanced, and optional feature sets of CSS?

A: The Enhanced feature set contains everything in the Standard feature set plus Network Address Translation (NAT) Peering, Domain Name Service (DNS), Demand-Based Content Replication (Dynamic Hot Content Overflow), Content Staging and Replication, and Network Proximity DNS. Proximity Database and SSH are optional features. In order to activate optional features such as the SSH server, you will need a special license provided with the software when you purchase this optional set.

Q: Where can I find more information on CSS?

A: On the Cisco Web site at http://cisco.com/warp/public/cc/pd/si/11000/prodlit/index.shtml. It includes configuration manuals for all product versions.

Q: Does CSS have any tools for performing automated tasks, such as log rotation?

A: CSS has a built-in scripting language, which resembles UNIX scripting languages.

Q: I forgot the administrative password for my CSS. How can I change it?

A: This procedure is easier than for Cisco routers. You need to connect to the CSS via the console cable. When the device boots, it displays a message: Press any key to access the Offline Diagnostic Monitor menu. If you press a key during the five-second period after this message is displayed, an Offline DM menu will appear. In the main menu, select option number **3** (to enter the advanced options menu), then option **2** in the submenu that appears (the selecting security options menu), then **2** again ("Set administrative user name and password"). After that, just enter the username and password of your choice at the prompt, and reboot the device (option **4** in the main menu).

## Chapter 11

Cisco Secure Scanner

Solutions in this chapter:

- **Minimum System Specifications for Secure Scanner**

- **Searching the Network for Vulnerabilities**

- **Viewing the Results**

- **Keeping the System Up-to-Date**

☑ Summary

☑ Solutions Fast Track

☑ Frequently Asked Questions

Introduction

Cisco Secure Scanner is a vulnerability scanner that maps network devices, identifies device operating systems and versions, open ports and applications listening on them, and vulnerabilities associated with those applications.

Some of the key features of Cisco Secure Scanner include the following:

- It can actively probe the open ports and attempt to confirm vulnerabilities in order to reduce false positives.

- Once you have mapped and scanned your network, the unique Grid Browser enables you to view the results of your scan from many different perspectives and at varying levels of detail. This not only provides you with the capability to identify and drill into the data that you need to implement corrective actions, but also provides you with the flexibility to generate management charts and reports that will communicate the necessary information focus management attention and resources where it is needed.

- Unlike other vulnerability scanners, since Cisco Secure Scanner is licensed without any ties or restrictions based on IP address, there is no requirement to modify your license as your network changes. Nor is its license based on platform types to be scanned; all network devices are mapped and scanned, including UNIX servers, Windows servers, firewalls, routers, switches, and printers.

Designing & Planning...

Risk Management and Vulnerability Scanning

Vulnerability scanning performed without a risk management process can provide tactical value at best. To truly leverage the value of vulnerability scanning, it should actually be a key component of a risk management process. Risk management is the process of assessing risk, implementing countermeasures to reduce the risk to an acceptable level, and maintaining that level of risk. A lifecycle process that is the core of a comprehensive information security program, risk management typically includes two primary subprocesses: *risk assessment* and *risk mitigation*.

Continued

- **Risk assessment** is the process of identifying, analyzing, and interpreting risk. Although the risk assessment process will vary among organizations, it typically includes the steps of identifying critical assets, identifying threats, and identifying vulnerabilities. These factors are analyzed to calculate a quantitative or qualitative risk level for a given system or network. Vulnerability scanning using the Cisco Secure Scanner can automatically identify the technical vulnerabilities within the vulnerability identification step of the process; management and operational vulnerabilities would still need to be identified via other mechanisms. Not only can Secure Scanner identify potential vulnerabilities and attempt to confirm their existence, but it also provides capabilities for the analyst to manipulate the data presentation into a form that is meaningful to the assessment.

- **Risk Mitigation** is the process of selecting and implementing security controls to reduce risk to a level acceptable to management. Typically, the risk level identified as an output of the risk assessment process is analyzed to determine if that level of risk is acceptable to the business. If not, then a risk mitigation plan is developed and executed to reduce the risk to an acceptable level. A key aspect of the risk mitigation plan is the prioritization of security controls and countermeasures so that resources are applied appropriately and efficiently. Because the Cisco Secure Scanner identifies vulnerability severity, attempts confirmation, and provides relevant graphic and reporting capabilities, it can provide key input for the risk mitigation plan development.

This chapter focuses on informing you about how to use Cisco Secure Scanner to scan your network for vulnerabilities, manipulate the display of the results to identify the information you need to better secure your network and communicate the desired information, and generate graphics and reports that will communicate the desired information to management.

Minimum System Specifications for Secure Scanner

Cisco Secure Scanner runs on both Windows NT and Solaris. The minimum requirements for running Secure Scanner on Windows NT are:

- Pentium II 450MHz processor

- Windows NT 4.0 Workstation/Server or Windows 2000 Professional/ Server

- Service Pack 5 or later

- 64MB RAM (96MB RAM recommended)

- Disk Space: 20MB (application), 100MB (session data), 400MB (paging file)

- TCP/IP network interface

- CD-ROM drive

- Microsoft Internet Explorer 4.0 or later (or Netscape Navigator 2.0 or later)

- Microsoft Virtual Machine 5.00.3167 (provided with Cisco Secure Scanner)

- Screen resolution of 800×600 or greater

- Local or domain administrative privileges

NOTE

Cisco Secure Scanner operates normally without Microsoft Internet Explorer; however, you must have Internet Explorer 4.0 or later installed to use Cisco Secure Scanner Help.

The minimum requirements for running Secure Scanner on Solaris are:

- Pentium 266MHz processor or Sun SPARC 5

- Solaris x86 2.5.x, 2.6, 2.7, 2.8 (for Pentium) or Solaris 2.5.x, 2.6, 2.7, 2.8 (for SPARC)

- 64MB RAM (96MB RAM recommended)

- Disk Space: 20MB (application), 100MB (session data), 400MB (paging file)

- TCP/IP network interface

- CD-ROM drive

- Netscape Navigator 2.0 or later

- Screen resolution of 800×600 or greater

- Root privileges

Searching the Network for Vulnerabilities

Once you have installed Cisco Secure Scanner, you can create and initiate a session to search your network for vulnerabilities. The session can be designated as either a passive scan or an active probe (used to confirm any vulnerabilities found). A scan is a non-intrusive session that discovers network devices, identifies open ports on those devices, and attempts to identify applications and versions listening on those ports. By collecting and analyzing banner information associated with a port, the scanner often can identify the application and its version. In order to accurately identify the application and version, the scanner also utilizes a non-intrusive and user-transparent technique called nudges. Where banner information is not provided by the server when connecting to a port, the scanner issues protocol-specific commands (nudges) to collect additional information to identify the application and version. Once the relevant information has been collected, the scanner then uses the Cisco Network Security Database (NSDB) to identify all of the potential vulnerabilities associated with that version of the application. A probe is an intrusive session that attempts to discover additional vulnerabilities and confirm potential ones through actual exploitation attempts. Sessions can also be scheduled to start on recurring or specific dates and times, or at random.

WARNING

Because it is possible to render a service or device unavailable by initiating an active and intrusive probe, you should conduct probe sessions outside peak network usage hours or omit sensitive devices from the probe to prevent loss of service. In addition, you should coordinate with the appropriate systems administrators to ensure that any lost service can be restored as quickly as possible.

In general, users should be unaware that a session is in progress; however, a performance drop may occur, especially if a probe has been selected with a heavy Active Probe Profile (see Figure 11.3 for more details).

There are three primary steps in creating a session to search your network for vulnerabilities:

1. Identifying the network addresses to scan

2. Identifying vulnerabilities to scan by specifying the TCP and UDP ports (and any active probe settings)

3. Scheduling the session

To create a session, select the **page icon** from the Cisco Secure Scanner main screen, as shown in Figure 11.1.

Figure 11.1 Cisco Secure Scanner Main Screen

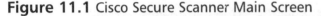

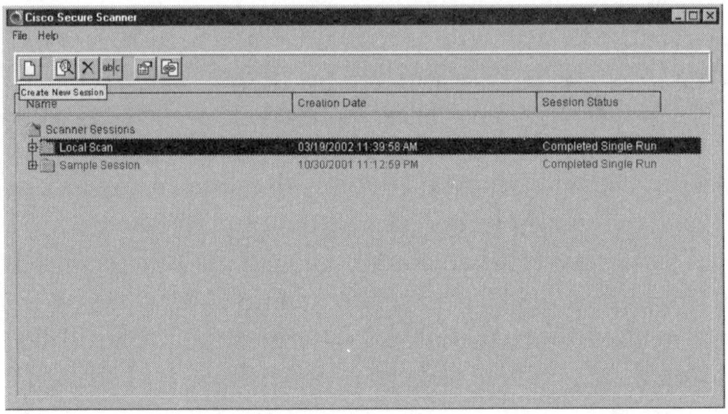

Designing & Planning…

Vulnerability Assessment versus Penetration Testing

As we stated earlier, a vulnerability scanner such as the Cisco Secure Scanner can be a useful tool in an organization's continuous risk management process. Specifically, the scanner can be used to identify and assess technical vulnerabilities as part of the risk assessment portion of the risk management process. But what exactly is vulnerability assessment, and how does it differ from penetration testing?

The differences between the phrases may not always be clear, and may convey different meanings depending on the context within which they are used. However, generally a vulnerability assessment is a systematic review of the security environment and controls of a system or network to identify the degree to which it is at risk. Its goal is to provide

Continued

more comprehensive management guidance on where and how to reduce risk. A penetration test is an attempt to circumvent the security environment and controls of a system or network to identify one or more system weaknesses. Its goal is to exploit vulnerabilities tactically and locally to demonstrate weakness. Because its intent is to circumvent the system controls, a penetration test is typically more intrusive than a vulnerability assessment, and has a higher probability of resulting in a loss of data or service.

Both vulnerability assessments and penetration tests are valuable security checks for evaluating the security of a system or network. Vulnerability assessments can be particularly important both in the pre-deployment lifecycle phases of a system to validate security controls prior to deployment and in the production lifecycle phase to ensure the security posture of the system is maintained. Penetration tests can also be valuable prior to deployment, but can also be used if a particularly reluctant system or network manager needs convincing of the need for specific security control.

Identifying Network Addresses

Once you have selected the **Create New Session** icon, the Session Configuration window appears with the Network Addresses tab selected as shown in Figure 11.2.

Figure 11.2 Session Configuration Window (Network Addresses Tab)

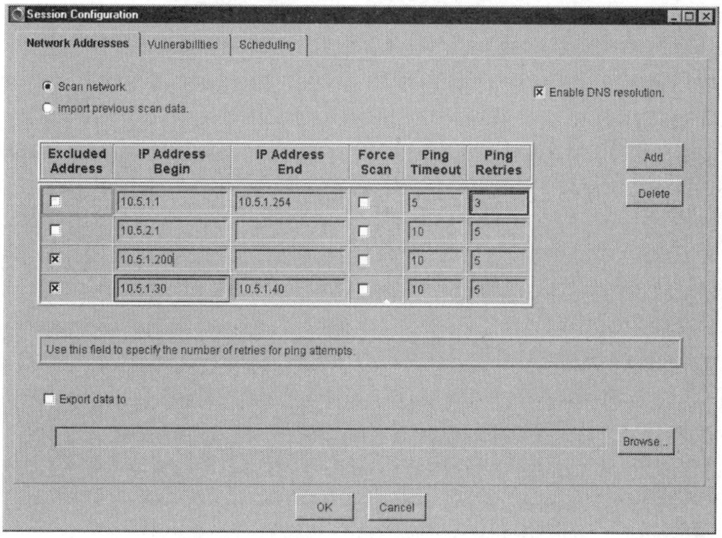

You use this screen to specify the addresses that should be included in the scan session. By default, the Scan Network check box is selected. As shown in the multiple entries in Figure 11.2, you can specify address ranges and single addresses to be included or excluded from the scan. Addresses are included unless the Excluded Address check box is selected. To add or delete a data line containing IP address entries, select either the **Add** or **Delete** buttons. If you want the scan results to include any hostnames associated with the IP addresses, select the **Enable DNS Resolution** check box.

Wᴀʀɴɪɴɢ

Cisco Secure Scanner does not respond to descending address ranges within a data line, so make sure you enter the lowest IP address in a range in the **IP Address Begin** field and the highest IP address in the **IP Address End** field.

Configuring & Implementing...

Firewalls and Cisco Secure Scanner

If some of the target addresses you are attempting to scan are located behind a firewall or packet filtering router, you may not obtain a complete scan of the addresses. If the packet filtering device blocks incoming ICMP Echo Requests, you will not discover the target hosts on the other side of the device if you use the default scan session configuration. The reason is the Secure Scanner uses ping sweeps (ICMP Echo Requests) to discover hosts on the network. If a packet filtering device blocks the ping, it will never reach the host, which will not know to respond, so Secure Scanner will not know that the host exists. If it does not know that the host exists, Secure Scanner will not attempt any port scans or probes of the host.

The good news is that you still may be able to discover hosts behind a packet-filtering device; however, your scan and probe results will be limited by the policy that is being enforced by the packet filter. In other words, you will only be able to identify ports and related vulnerabilities if the packet filter allows that particular traffic to reach the target host. In order to accomplish this, you will need to enable the **Force Scan**

Continued

> option within the **Network Addresses** tab of the **Create Session** window for the appropriate addresses (see Figure 11.2). This option instructs the Secure Scanner to conduct a port scan of the IP addresses in the specified range without performing the ping sweep first. Because Secure Scanner will attempt to connect to all of the ports configured for the session for the specified addresses, the disadvantage of enabling this option is that the session will take longer to complete because the scanner will be attempting to repeatedly connect to ports on some hosts that do not exist. Therefore, make sure you limit the number of addresses for which you enable the **Force Scan** option.

The *Ping Timeout* and *Ping Retries* parameters specify the length of time (in seconds) that the scanner waits for a response from an IP address and the number of times the scanner will ping an IP address before identifying it as not alive, respectively.

NOTE

> Cisco Secure Scanner may appear to hang during the ping session, particularly if the defined scan range is large compared to the number of active devices. It is functioning properly, but attempts to ping each address included in the session, and must wait for a response and retry as appropriate. You can adjust the length of time for a ping session through the *Ping Timeout* and *Ping Retries* parameters within the **Session Configuration** window.

Identifying Vulnerabilities

Once you have identified the address range(s) to be scanned, you must then specify the vulnerabilities to be scanned. Selecting the **Vulnerabilities** tab within the **Session Configuration** window displays the screen shown in Figure 11.3.

You use this screen to specify which TCP and UDP ports to scan, and the degree to which the scanner should attempt to confirm potential vulnerabilities through probes. Within the **Discovery Settings** area of the screen, you can specify the TCP or UDP ports by selecting the relevant tab, then selecting one of the predefined options in the list box on the right. You will then see the list of ports included in that option cataloged in the **Assess vulnerabilities for TCP ports** field on the left.

Figure 11.3 Session Configuration Window (Vulnerabilities Tab)

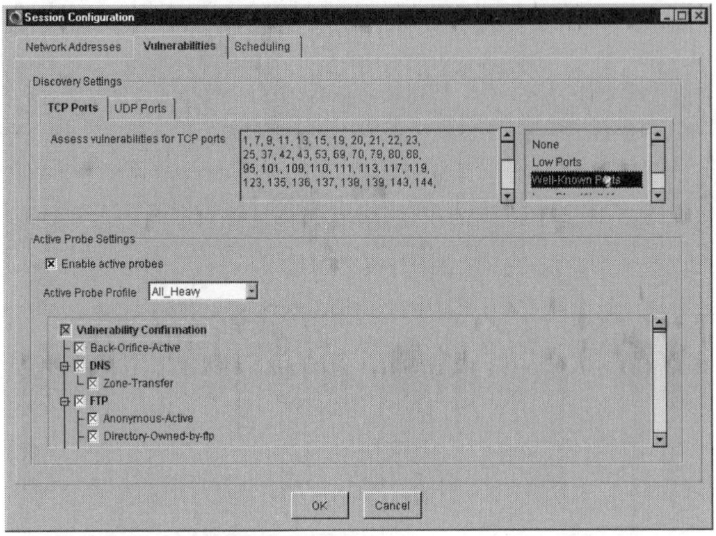

For the TCP ports, the predefined options are:

- **None** No TCP ports will be scanned
- **Low Ports** TCP ports 1 through 1024 will be scanned
- **Well-Known Ports (Default)** Specific TCP ports where common services typically listen will be scanned (for example, Telnet, FTP, SMTP, DNS, HTTP)
- **Low Plus Well-Known** TCP ports 1 through 1024 and any ports above that range where common services typically listen will be scanned
- **All Ports** TCP ports 1 through 65535 will be scanned

For UDP ports, the predefined options are:

- **None** No UDP ports will be scanned
- **Well-Known Ports (Default)** Specific UDP ports where common services typically listen will be scanned (for instance, DNS, TFTP, SNMP, NFS)

You can edit the list of predefined ports within an option by clicking within the ports list, and adding ports or ranges of ports separated by commas. In addition, you can copy lists of ports from one option to another, or from one session to another, by right-clicking the ports list and using the listed options of **Cut**, **Paste**, **Copy**, **Delete**, and **Select All**.

> **WARNING**
>
> Change the default UDP port configuration with care. Because of the connectionless nature of UDP and the implementation of ICMP error message rate limiting by many hosts, scanning a large number of UDP ports can greatly increase the scan time.

You can also configure active and intrusive probing from the **Vulnerabilities** tab of the **Session Configuration** window to confirm potential vulnerabilities identified through the port scan. As shown in Figure 11.3, check the **Enable Active Probes** check box within the **Active Probe Settings** area of the screen. This will allow you to choose a predefined profile from the **Active Probe Profile** drop-down list. The available profiles are defined based on platform type (All, UNIX, Windows) and decreasing intrusiveness (Heavy, Severe, Lite), and are listed next:

- All Heavy
- All Lite
- All Severe
- Unix Heavy
- Unix Lite
- Unix Severe
- Windows Heavy
- Windows Lite
- Windows Severe

When you select a probe profile, the actual probes that are included in that profile are checked in the list below it. You can modify the probes included in the session by selecting or deselecting the individual probes. To obtain information about a particular probe, right-click the probe, and select **Help** from the pop-up menu. This will launch a browser window with information on the vulnerability of the NSDB. The probes are grouped into the following high-level categories:

- Back-Orifice-Active
- DNS
- FTP
- Finger
- HTTP
- MSSQL
- NFS
- NT
- NetBIOS
- RPC
- Rlogin
- Rsh
- SMTP
- SNMP
- TFTP
- Telnet
- Xwindows

NOTE

It is possible to configure user defined/custom vulnerability rules. This could be useful if you are scanning for unique devices or non-standard port numbers. Once a custom rule has been defined, you should distribute that rule throughout the enterprise to ensure consistency across the scanners. Further details on how to create user-defined rules can be found at: www.cisco.com/univercd/cc/td/doc/product/iaabu/csscan/csscan2/csscug/userrule.htm.

Scheduling the Session

Once you have identified the address range(s) and ports to be scanned, and specified the vulnerabilities to be probed, you must then schedule the session. Selecting the **Scheduling** tab within the **Session Configuration** window displays the screen shown in Figure 11.4.

Figure 11.4 Session Configuration Window (Scheduling Tab)

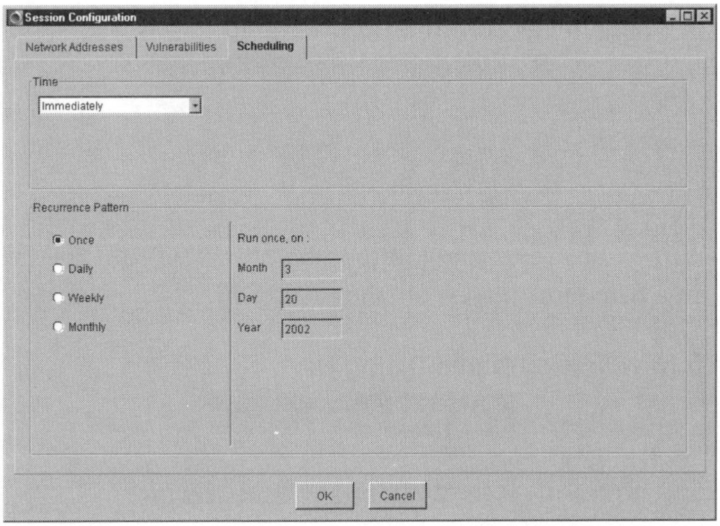

As shown in the **Recurrence** area of the screen, you can schedule a session to be run once, daily, weekly, or monthly. As you can see, the default scheduling configuration has the session being run immediately. Depending on which recurrence pattern you select, you will need to fill out the appropriate information in the area to the right of the pattern selected. For instance, for a daily recurrence pattern, you can specify that the session be run every weekday, or repeated every X number of days. Once this information has been selected, you need to select the time for the scan to run. The options include immediately, every hour of the day, or a random execution within one of four six-hour time windows:

- Midnight – 6:00 A.M.
- 6:00 A.M. – Noon
- Noon – 6:00 P.M.
- 6:00 P.M. – Midnight

Once you have configured the addresses, vulnerabilities, and scheduling, you can click the **OK** button within the **Session Configuration** window. If you have the session configured to perform active probing, you may receive a warning prompt similar to the one shown in Figure 11.5. You should choose whether or not to perform the exploit based on warning information, the criticality of the hosts being scanned, the day and time of the scan, and the degree of administrative support that you have coordinated prior to initiating the scan.

Figure 11.5 Vulnerability Confirmation Warning

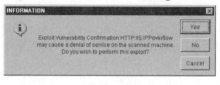

As shown in Figure 11.6, you will then be prompted to name the session. You should type in a name for the session and click **OK**.

Figure 11.6 New Session Name Dialog Box

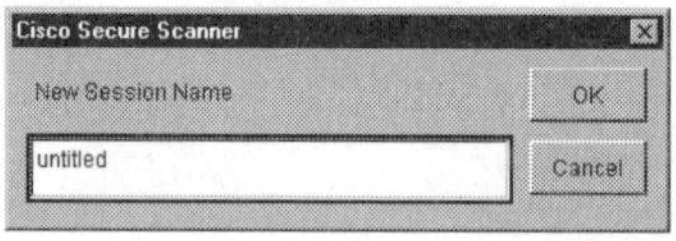

Once you have initiated the session, you will see a progress window that looks similar to the one shown in Figure 11.7.

Figure 11.7 Session Status Window

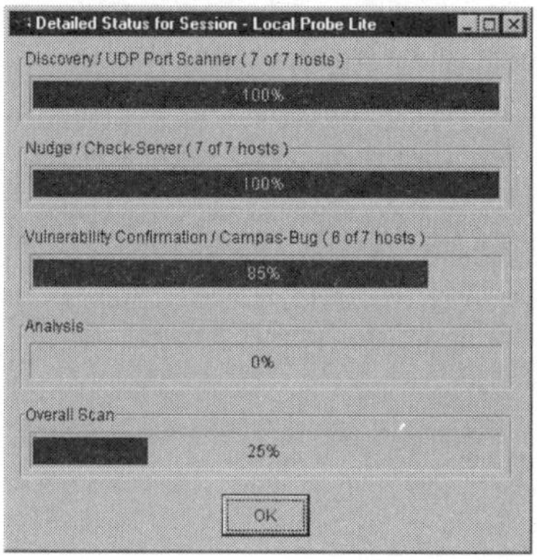

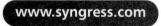

Configuring & Implementing...

Cisco Secure Scanner – General Usage Tips

Like any tool, Cisco Secure Scanner is most effective when used properly. Here are some general tips you can use for maximum benefit.

- The same person or people should perform the scan each time; this may even lead to the creation (or enhancement) of a central team in your organization responsible for security. They should be the ones to take action on the results; this will have the additional effect of creating or enforcing security standards in your organization.

- The session should be run when the network traffic levels are low, as well as during busy hours when all devices are powered up in order to give you a more comprehensive set of results.

- Run unscheduled scans to increase the likelihood of catching devices that may only be active occasionally. An example might be a traveling sales representative who only comes to the office once a week.

- As soon as new devices are added to the network, a scan should be run. Ideally, this should be integrated into both the company change management system and the company system development lifecycle.

- Report any anomalies or new vulnerabilities you have found to Cisco Systems using the NSDB reporting mechanism. As a responsible user of the system, you could help protect other companies from similar attacks. However, be sure you obey your company's policies and don't provide information which may be used against your company, or information which is illegal to provide.

Viewing the Results

Following the completion of a session, the message "Completed Single Run" appears in the Session Status column, and a Result Set subfolder is created within the session folder in the main Secure Scanner screen, as shown in Figure 11.8. The Result Set contains additional subfolders for charts, grids and reports that you create as you analyze the session results. To begin analyzing your data, right click the **Result Set** subfolder and then select **View Grid Data**.

Figure 11.8 Opening the Grid Browser

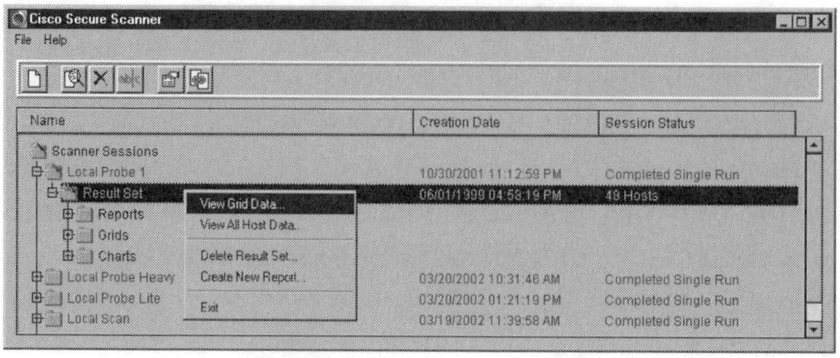

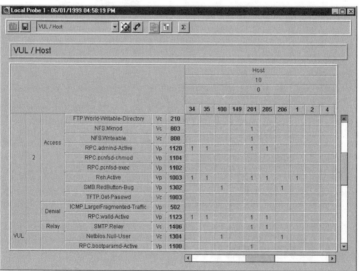

The Grid Browser, shown in Figure 11.9, is a two-dimensional hyperlinked spreadsheet that is used to view session results. You can change the information displayed on the *x* and *y* axes, drill down into selected data cells, perform "data pivoting," view different levels of detail by zooming in or out, show/hide totals or percentages for rows or columns, and create charts. Once you have created grid browser views and charts, you can save them for later use.

Figure 11.9 The Grid Browser

In Figure 11.9, the IP addresses of the hosts are displayed along the *x*-axis, and the vulnerabilities are displayed along the *y*-axis.

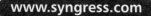

The leading six columns on the left provide the vulnerability details. Let's examine a row from left to right. Column one identifies the data displayed along the *y*-axis (vulnerabilities). Column two shows a value that represents the severity level of the vulnerability (the higher the number, the worse the vulnerability). Column three classifies the type of exploit. Column four identifies the name of the exploit. Column five identifies whether the vulnerability is potential (Vp) or confirmed (Vc). Column six identifies the corresponding ID in the NSDB database.

The top six rows provide the host details. The first row identifies the data that is displayed along the *x*-axis (host). The second row displays the first octet of the host IP address, the third row displays the second octet of the host IP address, the fourth row identifies the third octet of the host IP address, and the fifth row identifies the fourth octet of the host IP address.

Within the grid area, the numbers in the cells represent the number of intersections of a row and column value. For this particular view, the value is always 1; however, the number can vary within other views.

Changing Axis Views

As shown in Figure 11.10, you can change the information displayed along the axes by selecting the **Axis** drop-down menu and selecting a new pair.

Figure 11.10 Changing the Axis Pair

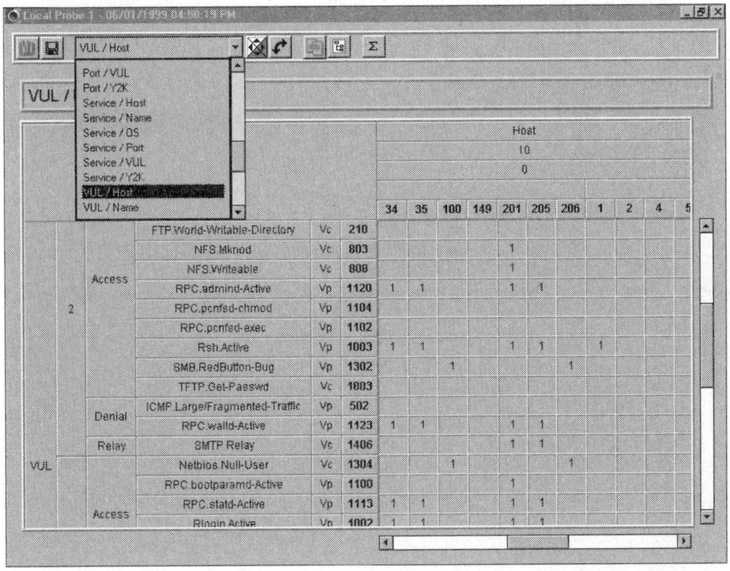

For example, changing the axis pair from Vul / Host to OS / Host results in the view shown in Figure 11.11. This view displays the operating system and version that the scanner identified for each host.

Figure 11.11 OS / Host Grid View

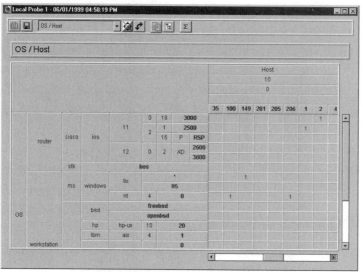

You can swap the axes display by clicking the **Swap Axis** icon on the toolbar, as shown in Figure 11.12.

Figure 11.12 Swapping the Axes

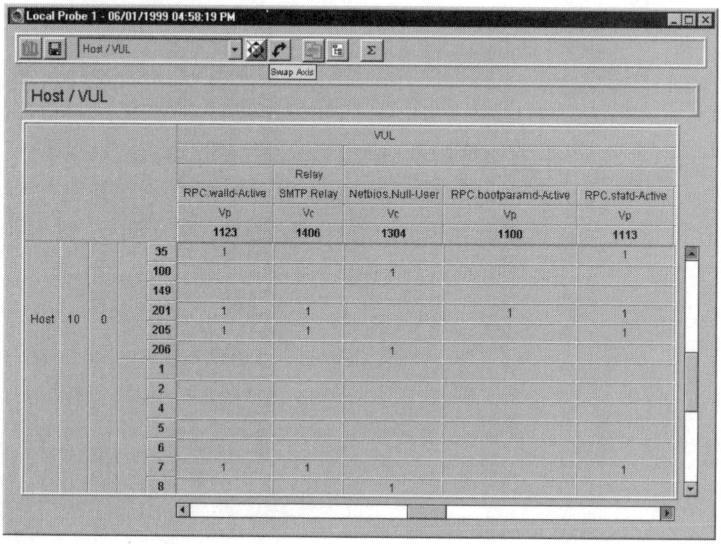

You can change an individual axis within the a view by right-clicking the axis you want to change, selecting **Change Y Axis** (or **Change X axis**), and then selecting the information you want to display, as shown in Figure 11.13.

Figure 11.13 Changing an Individual Axis

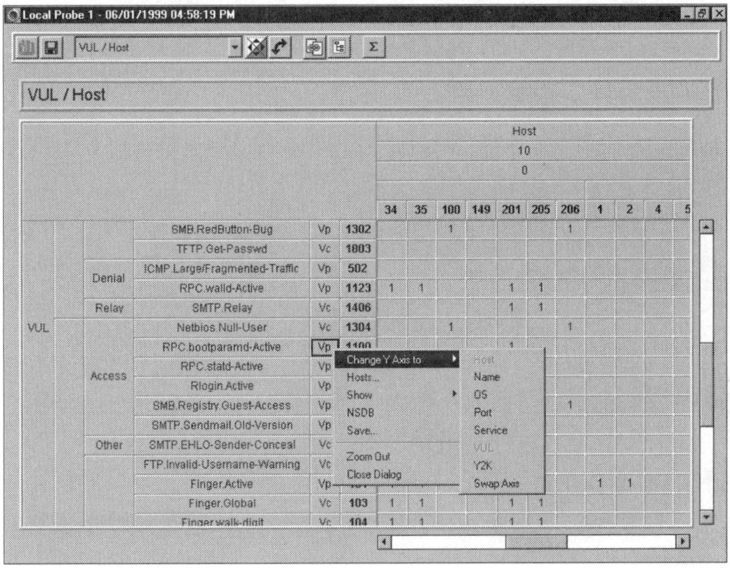

Drilling into Data

Within the Grid Browser, you can also drill down into the data to identify all of the hosts that share a particular attribute such as operating system, specific vulnerability, vulnerability type, open TCP or UDP port, or listening service. This can be valuable in identifying which hosts require a particular patch or countermeasure. To drill into data, you simply select the attribute you are interested in, right-click it, and select **Hosts**. Figure 11.14 illustrates the process of drilling into the hosts that share a particular vulnerability.

After drilling into the data, you will see a window similar to the one shown in Figure 11.15. Notice that the title within the window is the name of the attribute you selected to drill into. All of the hosts that share the particular attribute, in this case a vulnerability, as listed in the window. In addition, Figure 11.15 shows that by clicking on the + next to the host, you will see a listing of all the services and vulnerabilities for that host.

Figure 11.14 Drilling into Data

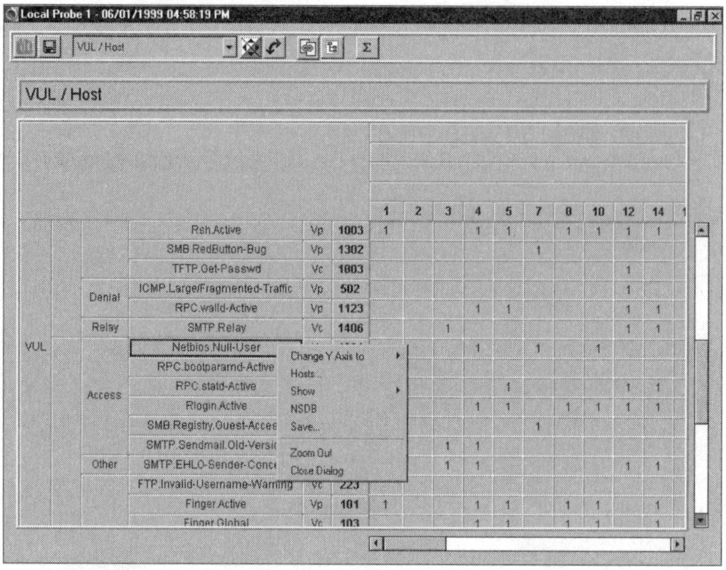

Figure 11.15 Host Detail

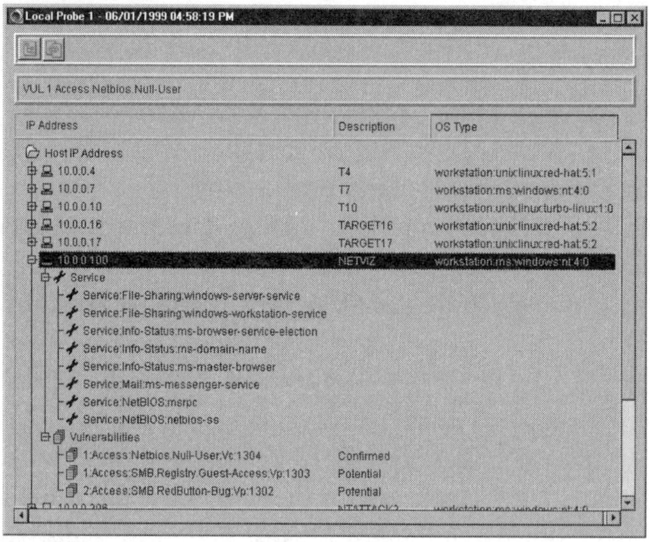

Pivoting Data

Once you have drilled into data and are viewing the services and vulnerabilities associated with a particular host, as shown in the previous figure, you can also perform a manipulation called *data pivoting*. If you see a particular service or vulnerability listed under a host entry, and want to know what other hosts share that service or vulnerability, simply right-click the entry and select **Hosts** as shown in Figure 11.16. You have now pivoted on the data to obtain another view.

Figure 11.16 Pivoting on Data

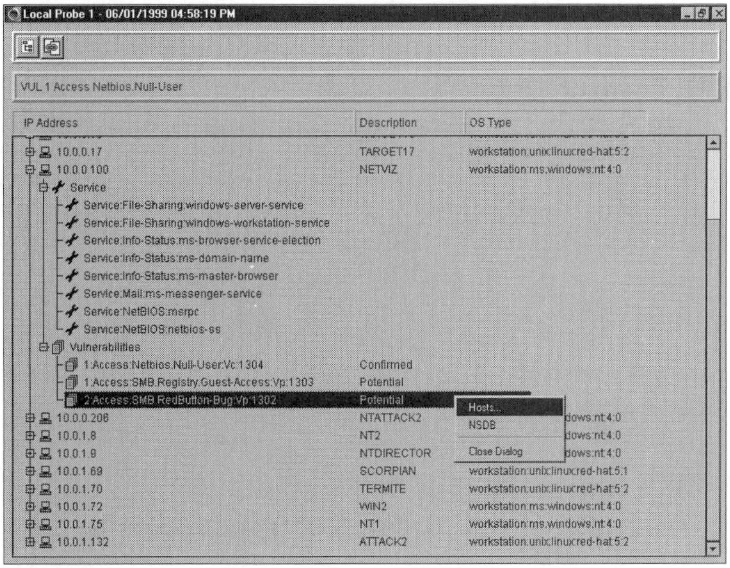

The preceding pivot results in the view illustrated in Figure 11.17. Notice that the format is the same as that shown in Figure 11.15, but the title within the window reflects the attribute selected for pivoting.

Figure 11.17 Pivoted Data View

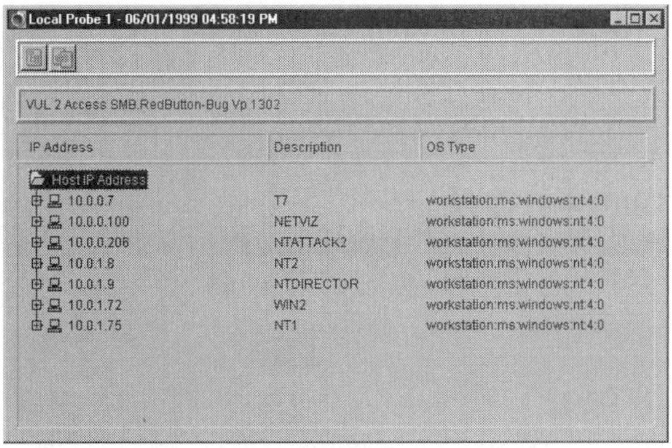

Zooming In and Out

You can also change the level of detail displayed within the Grid Browser through the zooming capability. Let's say you want to change the grid to display the number of vulnerabilities of each severity level for the hosts. As shown in Figure 11.18, simply right-click anywhere within column 2 and then select **Zoom Out**.

Figure 11.18 Zooming Out

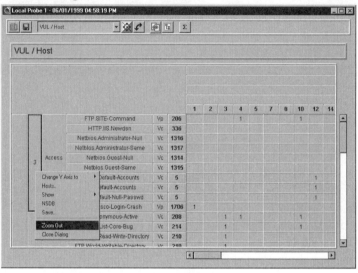

As you can see in Figure 11.19, the cell values change to the total number of vulnerabilities of each severity level for each host. You could also use the zooming capability to view more or less details about operating system types, services, and open ports on the network. You could view the number of hosts running a particular operating system, the number of hosts running a particular service, or the number of hosts with a particular port open.

Figure 11.19 Zoomed-in Data

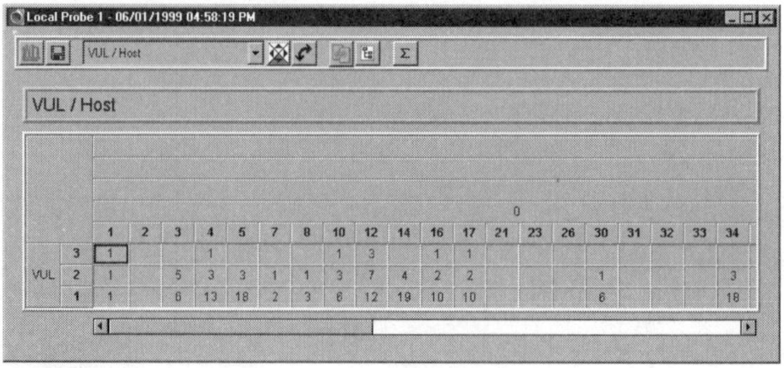

Creating Charts

From within the Grid Browser, you can create charts to represent the data graphically. This is particularly useful for communicating assessment results to management. The Chart Wizard enables you to create many different types of charts, including 2D and 3D, line, area, pie, bar, and stacked charts. You can then use the chart in the generation of a report, or export it for use in a Microsoft PowerPoint slide show. You create a chart by selecting the desired cells and clicking the **Chart** button on the tool bar, as shown in Figure 11.20.

Figure 11.20 Creating a Chart

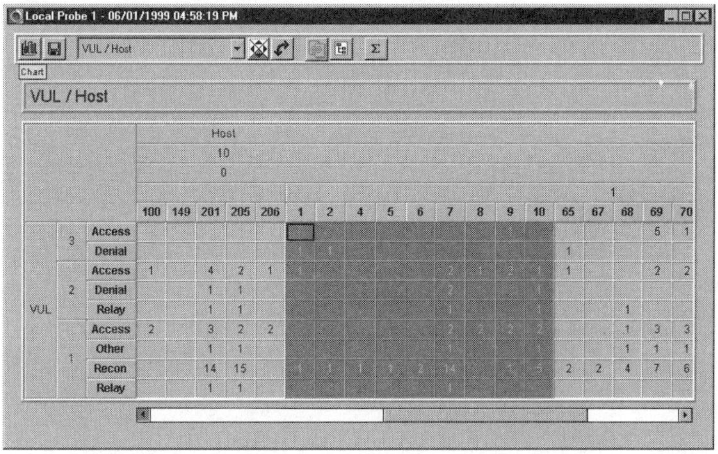

This will launch the Chart Wizard, as shown in Figure 11.21, where you can choose the type of chart you want to create. The chart types available will depend on the data you have selected. For example, a pie chart will only appear as an option if you choose a single row of data.

By selecting the first option (**3D Row**), the chart in Figure 11.22 is created.

Charts like the one shown in the previous figure are often invaluable in communicating effectively to both system managers and executive management because they can instantly communicate where mitigation or compliance efforts should be focused.

The chart is easily manipulated by right-clicking it and choosing the appropriate option, as shown in Figure 11.22. You can show/hide/manipulate the legend, change the chart type, change the background color, and tilt or pan the view. In the preceding example, the height of the bars represents the number of vulnerability types exhibited by a host. Once you save a graph, it can be incorporated into a NetSonar report or used externally as a .bmp or .gif file.

Figure 11.21 The Chart Wizard

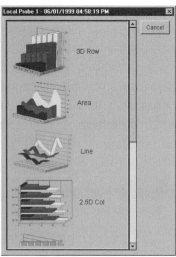

Figure 11.22 3D Row Chart

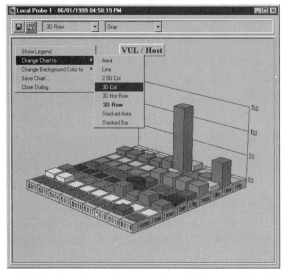

Saving Grid Views and Charts

After you have created grid views and charts, you can save them for later reference or inclusion in a report by simply right-clicking anywhere on the view or
chart and clicking **Save** or **Save Chart** options, respectively. When prompted,
enter a title and click **OK**. The grid view or chart will now appear in the **Grids**

or **Charts** subfolder (respectively) of the **Session** folder on the main screen of the Cisco Secure Scanner.

> **NOTE**
>
> You can also save any portion of a grid view by highlighting the desired data, right-clicking it, and selecting **Save**.

Reports and Wizards

Cisco Secure Scanner includes a flexible reporting and analysis tool that can generate three types of HTML reports: executive, brief technical, and full technical. As the names suggest, each type of report is aimed at different groups of people as identified in Table 11.1.

Table 11.1 Scanner Report Types

Report Type	Target Audience	Description
Executive	Executive Management	High-level overview of security vulnerabilities
Brief Technical	Corporate Security Management	Technical summary of security vulnerabilities
Full Technical	System/Network Management	Detailed technical information about security vulnerabilities

To generate a report via the Scanner Report Wizard, simply right-click the desired **Result Set** and select **Create New Report** as shown in Figure 11.23.

Figure 11.23 Creating a Scanner Report

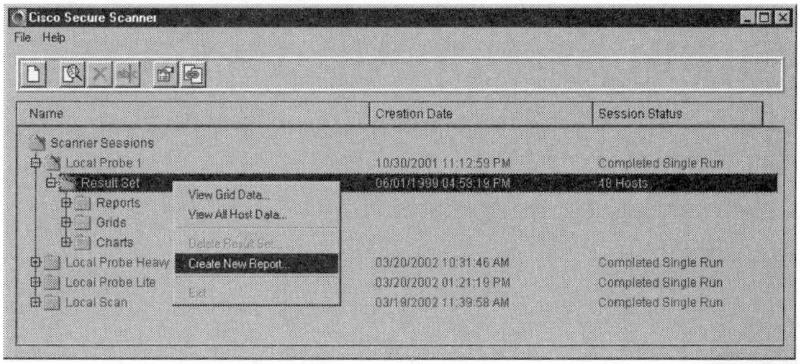

This will launch the Scanner Report Wizard shown in Figure 11.24. The wizard is easy to use to generate a report, and allows you to: Customize report types by changing the set of report components included in a report type (Executive, Brief Technical, Full Technical), change the order of report components, and include grids and charts you created and saved previously. The generated report is in HTML format, but can be manually converged into one Microsoft Word file.

Figure 11.24 The Scanner Report Wizard

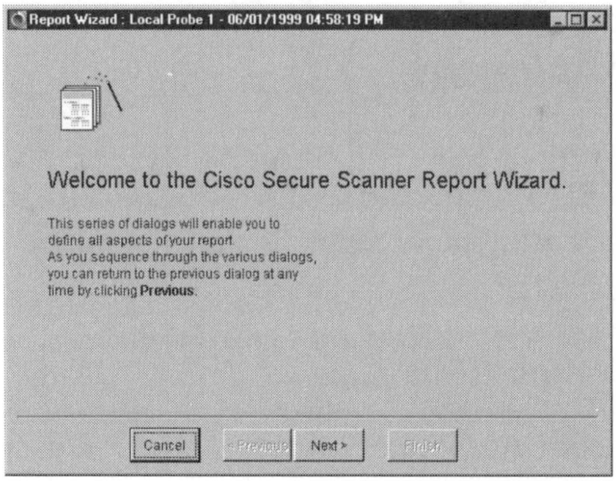

NOTE

You can customize both reports and report templates. The advantage of customizing report templates is that you can customize it once and apply it to all reports you subsequently generate using the scanner. You can find detailed guidance on customizing reports and templates at www.cisco.com/univercd/cc/td/doc/product/iaabu/csscan/csscan2/csscug/custrep.htm.

Keeping the System Up-to-Date

As Cisco Secure Scanner vulnerability exploits are updated and added, a new list will appear on the Cisco Web site. You should check the following location for new updates: www.cisco.com/kobayashi/sw-center/ciscosecure/scanner-updates.shtml.

When vulnerability exploits are updated or added, Cisco makes the appropriate updates in its Network Security Database (NSDB), which is an online HTML reference guide that provides information on the vulnerabilities detected by the Cisco Secure Scanner. The NSDB main screen is shown in Figure 11.25.

Figure 11.25 The NSDB Main Screen

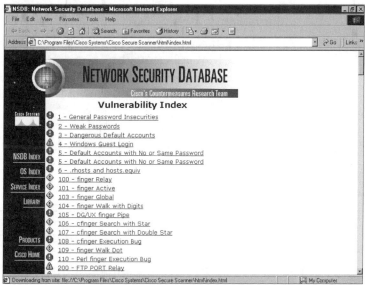

For each vulnerability, the NSDB provides the information identified in Table 11.2.

Table 11.2 NSDB Vulnerability Information

Information	Description
Vulnerability Name	The name by which the vulnerability is known in the Scanner and the NSDB.
Alias	Other names by which the vulnerability may be known.
ID Number	A number assigned to the vulnerability in the NSDB.
Severity Level	A level of 1, 2, or 3 (refer to Table 11.3).
Vulnerability Type	The type of damage the vulnerability causes.
Exploit Type	The network service the vulnerability affects.
Affected Systems	The operating systems affected by the vulnerability.
Affected Programs	The programs affected by the vulnerability.
Description	A description of the vulnerability.

Continued

Table 11.2 Continued

Information	Description
Consequences	A discussion of the vulnerability's consequences.
Countermeasures	The recommended countermeasure for the vulnerability.
Related Links	Any other sites that offer more information on the vulnerability.
User Notes	An HTML page where you can add any information you find about that vulnerability.

The severity levels that are assigned to vulnerabilities in the NSDB are identified and described in Table 11.3.

Table 11.3 NSDB Vulnerability Severity Levels

NSDB Severity Level	Description
Level 1	Generally, most Level 1 vulnerabilities permit reconnaissance activities that allow attackers to collect information that can be used to stage an attack. Examples include network topology and configuration information, including active IP addresses, active network services, operating system type and version, and valid usernames. These vulnerabilities do not directly lead to unauthorized access, but they should be corrected to make it difficult for intruders to become knowledgeable about your network and systems.
Level 2	Generally, most Level 2 vulnerabilities permit some level of unprivileged unauthorized access or denial of service. These vulnerabilities can frequently be leveraged to allow attackers to eventually gain more privileged and complete control of your network or systems. Level 2 vulnerabilities should be corrected as soon as possible.
Level 3	Generally, most Level 3 vulnerabilities permit an attacker to execute arbitrary commands on systems. The ability to execute commands on a system implies the ability either to cause denial of service or to gain unauthorized data access. These vulnerability types frequently allow attackers to establish a base of operations within your network from which they compromise other systems. Level 3 vulnerabilities should be corrected immediately.

Figure 11.26 shows the typical information provided by the NSDB for a given vulnerability.

Figure 11.26 NSDB Vulnerability Information Display

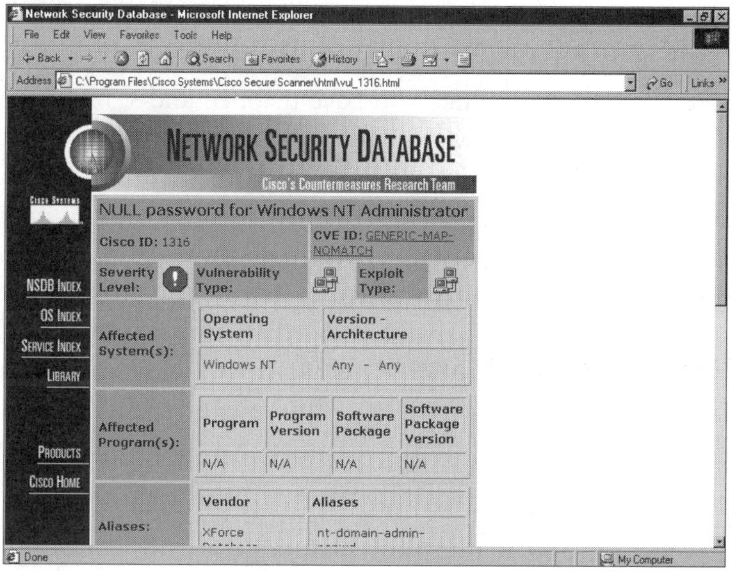

The NSDB can be accessed from within Cisco Secure Scanner in the following ways:

- From the scanner main window by selecting **File | Show NSDB**.

- From within the Grid Browser by selecting a vulnerability, service, or data cell, right-clicking it, and selecting **NSDB**.

- While data pivoting, by selecting a service or vulnerability, right-clicking it, and selecting **Vulnerabilities | NSDB**.

- From within the **Vulnerabilities** tab in the **Session Configuration** window by selecting **Enable active probes**, right-clicking any vulnerability in the **Vulnerability Confirmation** group box, and selecting **Help**.

Summary

Cisco Secure Scanner is a vulnerability scanner that maps network devices, identifies device operating systems and versions, identifies open ports and applications listening on them, and identifies vulnerabilities associated with those applications.

It can actively probe the open ports and attempt to confirm vulnerabilities in order to reduce false positives. Once you have mapped and scanned your network, the unique Grid Browser enables you to view the results of your scan from many different perspectives and at varying levels of detail. This not only provides you with the capability to identify and drill into the data that you need to implement corrective actions, but also provides you with the flexibility to generate management charts and reports that will communicate the necessary information to focus management attention and resources where it is needed. Unlike other vulnerability scanners, Cisco Secure Scanner is licensed without any ties or restrictions based on IP address; there is no requirement to modify your license as your network changes. Nor is its license based on the platform types to be scanned; all network devices are mapped and scanned, including UNIX servers, Windows servers, firewalls, routers, switches, and printers.

Solutions Fast Track

Minimum System Specifications for Secure Scanner

- ☑ Windows NT or Solaris
- ☑ 64MB RAM (96MB RAM recommended)
- ☑ Disk Space: 20MB (application), 100MB (session data), 400MB (paging file)
- ☑ TCP/IP network interface
- ☑ Microsoft Internet Explorer 4.0 or later (or Netscape Navigator 2.0 or later)

Searching the Network for Vulnerabilities

- ☑ Specify IP address ranges and details through the Network Addresses tab of the Session Configuration window.

☑ Specify the TCP/UDP ports to scan, and the vulnerabilities to attempt to confirm through the Vulnerabilities tab of the Session Configuration window.

☑ Schedule the scan session through the Scheduling tab of the Session Configuration window.

Viewing the Results

☑ The Grid Browser can manipulate the data display by changing axis views, drilling into data, pivoting on data, zooming in and out, and saving grid views.

☑ Using the Chart Wizard, you can create and save charts that graphically illustrate a particular grid view.

☑ Using the Report Wizard, you can create different report types (executive, brief technical, full technical) that are targeted at different audiences, including previously saved grid views and charts.

Keeping the System Up-to-Date

☑ Check the Cisco Web site for Cisco Secure Scanner updates that include new or updated vulnerability exploits.

☑ Use the NSDB as a resource to become knowledgeable about particular vulnerabilities.

Frequently Asked Questions

The following Frequently Asked Questions, answered by the authors of this book, are designed to both measure your understanding of the concepts presented in this chapter and to assist you with real-life implementation of these concepts. To have your questions about this chapter answered by the author, browse to **www.syngress.com/solutions** and click on the **"Ask the Author"** form.

Q: What is vulnerability scanning and how can it be leveraged?

A: Security scanning is the process of identifying security vulnerabilities associated with network devices and hosts. It can be leveraged within a company's system lifecycle process, change management process, and comprehensive risk management process. Scanning can be used in a proactive manner to identify vulnerabilities before a system is deployed, or after a significant change has occurred. In addition, it can be used as part of the vulnerability assessment phase of a continual risk management process.

Q: Do Cisco Secure Scanner users need to be experts in security in order to use it?

A: No. The graphical user interface makes it easy to initiate scan sessions, and the Grid Browser, Chart Wizard, and Report Wizard enable you to view the information needed to take corrective action. In addition, the Network Security Database provides you with comprehensive information for identified vulnerabilities so you can develop and implement effective action plans.

Q: Is Cisco Secure Scanner customizable?

A: Yes. You can define custom vulnerability rules, and customize reports and report templates.

Q: How do firewalls effect the operation of Cisco Secure Scanner?

A: If some of the target addresses you are attempting to scan are located behind a firewall or packet filtering router, you may not obtain a complete scan of the addresses. Because Secure Scanner uses ping sweeps to discover network hosts, if the packet filtering device blocks incoming pings, you will not discover the target hosts on the other side of the device if you use the default scan session configuration. The good news is that you still may be able to discover hosts behind a packet filtering device by configuring your scan session appropriately. However, your scan and probe results will be limited by the policy being enforced by the packet filter. In other words, you will only be able to identify ports and related vulnerabilities if the packet filter allows that particular traffic to reach the target host.

Q: What impact will Scanner scans have on my traffic load?

A: In general, users should be unaware that a session is in progress; however, a performance drop may occur, especially if a probe has been selected with a heavy active probe profile. The network impact will be a function of the duration of the scan and the depth of penetration. In addition, because it is possible to render a service or device unavailable by initiating an active and intrusive probe, you should conduct probe sessions outside peak network usage hours, or you should omit sensitive devices to prevent loss of service.

Chapter 12

Cisco Secure Policy Manager

Solutions in this chapter:

- **Overview of the Cisco Secure Policy Manager**

- **Features of the Cisco Secure Policy Manager**

- **Using the Cisco Secure Policy Manager**

☑ **Summary**

☑ **Solutions Fast Track**

☑ **Frequently Asked Questions**

Introduction

Network security has become more critical to organizations than ever before. The associated security risks have become very high, with most organizations configuring and deploying firewalls to improve network boundary security and virtual private networks (VPNs) to protect the integrity of the network and establish secure business-to-business communications.

As you will see, the Cisco Secure Policy Manager (CSPM) is an excellent tool that allows you to minimize costs and ensure a consistent security policy on your network. It also allows you to manage your network and associated services with a consolidated management system. It supports the different network requirements of your organization that are used to establish a secure connection for your intranets with multiple firewalls and VPN routers, and allows real-time monitoring of alerts from Intrusion Detection sensors.

In this chapter, we will take a look at the CSPM as a whole, the features that come with it, and then take some time to examine exactly how it should be used.

Overview of the Cisco Secure Policy Manager

The CSPM is a powerful policy-driven management system for Cisco PIX firewalls, IP Security (IPSec) routers, and Cisco Intrusion Detection System (Cisco IDS) sensors. With CSPM, you can define, distribute, enforce, and audit your entire network security policies from a central location. You can use CSPM to configure your PIX firewalls on the boundary of your enterprise network as well as configure Network Address Translation (NAT) and IPSec based VPNs. This allows for easy and simple deployment of your security policy to your PIX firewalls and your VPN, which should be the cornerstone of your security policy. CSPM is also capable of configuring IDS sensors and monitoring the security alerts produced by them, so you are able to see the status of your security measures at any given time.

CSPM's distributed architecture, combined with its secure remote management features, allows you to deploy the security policy in various environments by using more than one policy enforcement point. If you are administrating a large enterprise network, you can install the policy administrator, the graphical user interface (GUI) used for policy administration, in different locations across your network for distributed management of your network security policy.

The CSPM software is an immense product and could be the subject of an entire book, so this will only be a brief summary of the benefits, features, and sample configurations included in this application.

The Benefits of Using Cisco Secure Policy Manager

Using CSPM on your network gives you a great number of products to use for creating, deploying, and changing your enterprise network security policy. Some benefits of using CSPM and all the related products include:

- Scalability enables you to meet large-scale security policy requirements and network growth. It provides the capability to manage up to several hundred PIX firewall and VPN routers on your network plus corresponding number of IDS sensors.

- The built-in auditing and reporting provides up-to-date information on network and system events. It allows you to configure notifications according to your needs—from real-time alerting of urgent events to generation of scheduled reports on other events of interest.

- It allows you to define networkwide security policies based on your organization's business objectives. You can accurately define your security policies for different devices on your network and can reduce the time needed to deploy the security configurations.

- It also allows you to define networkwide monitoring for possible security policy violations by integrating IDS management features.

- You can either use a centralized standalone policy management environment, or a distributed architecture policy management environment to support your needs on the Internet, intranet, and extranet environments.

- Now you can configure and test your security policies without connecting to your live network. You can do your configurations offline and verify that your security policies are working correctly, as attended, and then deploy the policy to your live network.

- A Windows NT-based system provides you with an easy-to-use GUI to manage your security policy.

The version discussed in this chapter is CSPM 2.3.2.

Since version 2.3, the functionality of CSPM has been split into two branches. The bulk of firewall and VPN management features are implemented in the "f" series of the product. For example, 2.3f is a CSPM version with enhanced firewall/VPN management. Installation images of this series also contain basic IDS management (setup and monitoring), although another version ("i" series) contains the full range of IDS capabilities plus basic firewall/VPN features. Most of the time, this chapter will discuss the "f" series since intrusion detection is dealt with in Chapter 13. In any case, both series share the same interface and internals.

The newest version of the "f" series is 3.0f, which is offered exclusively as a part of the VPN Management Solution (VMS) for Cisco Works 2000. This version (which is very recent and still a bit "raw") continues the integration of CSPM with Cisco Works, which was started in 2.3. The most interesting feature of 3.0 that is not offered in 2.3 is a policy import from already configured devices, which allows (to some extent) automatic creation of network topology and the importing of existing device configurations into the CSPM database.

Installation Requirements for the Cisco Secure Policy Manager

Before installing CSPM on your target server, you should ensure that all the devices on the network you intend to manage are configured properly and are active on your network. You should have IP communication between the device and the target CSPM server on your network for Telnet sessions. CSPM can only be installed on Windows NT computers. Only Intel architecture is supported, a version for DEC Alpha is not available.

Next, you should insure that your target CSPM server meets the following hardware requirements:

- Pentium-compatible processor, 600MHz or better
- 256MB RAM
- System must be partitioned using NTFS, not FAT
- 8GB free hard drive space available
- One or more properly configured network adapters
- Video Display—1024×768, with 64K color support
- CD-ROM and 3.5-inch diskette drive

If you are installing the stand-alone or client-server system option on your target CSPM server, these minimum requirements would be sufficient, but would not be optimal for a distributed system. The Policy Server component is a multi-threaded application that can benefit from multiple processors and available memory.

You can install the GUI client for CSPM on a computer that runs Windows NT 4.0, Windows 95, Windows 98, or Windows 2000. This allows you to manage the network security policy from any host on your network.

The following minimum software requirements should be met before attempting the CSPM installation:

- Windows NT 4.0 with Service Pack 6a or Windows 2000 with Service Pack 1 (the latter for GUI only)

- Microsoft Internet Explorer 5.5

- TCP/IP protocol stack installed and working properly

- Static IP address with DHCP disabled

- TAPI for pager notifications

- MAPI for e-mail notifications

Configuring & Implementing...

Upgrading CSPM

If you are currently running an earlier version of CSPM (version 2.0, for example) and would like to upgrade to CSPM version 2.3f, you need to run the installation for all intermediate versions first (2.1 and 2.2). This will ensure that all data are converted properly. After this upgrade is completed successfully, you can run the installation for CSPM version 2.3f and upgrade the older version.

Upgrading to the 3.0f version is performed in the same way. Upgrade to 2.3f first and then to 3.0f. It is not possible to upgrade from 2.3i (IDS series) to 3.0f.

Before installing CSPM on your target server, you should check the Cisco Web site for the latest compatible software list with information on various softwares that have been tested for coexistence with CSPM on the same host. CSPM already supports the coexistence of Cisco Secure VPN Client 1.1, CiscoWorks 2000 with Resource Management Essentials version 3.0, and the QoS Policy Manager version 1.1 on the same computer. On the other hand, the "f" and "i" series cannot coexist on the same machine, so if you plan to use the extra IDS management features of "i" series, you will need to install it on a separate host. It is also recommended you turn off anti-virus programs while installing CSPM as they may interfere with the installation process. You can safely turn them on after CSPM has been installed.

Features of the Cisco Secure Policy Manager

The main features included in the CSPM product will be discussed in this section. Some of the features included in the CSPM product have the same function as the PIX Firewall Manager and the Access Control List (ACL) Manager. CSPM was meant to replace and improve the features provided by these products. The difference with CSPM is that you have a more centralized management approach that includes more functionality for managing your enterprise network security policy.

The main CSPM features include the following:

- **Cisco firewall management** Allows definition and management of perimeter security policies for Cisco PIX Firewalls and Cisco IOS routers running the Cisco Secure Integrated Software feature set.

- **Cisco VPN gateway management** Configuration of site-to-site IPSec VPNs based on Cisco Secure PIX Firewalls and the Cisco suite of VPN routers running Cisco IOS IPSec software.

- **Intrusion detection sensors management** Configuration and monitoring of Cisco intrusion detection sensors and Cisco Catalyst 6000 line cards.

- **Security policy management** Allows usage of enterprisewide policies for managing hundreds of Cisco security devices without dependency on the command-line interface (CLI).

- **Notification and reporting system** Provides tools to monitor, alert, and report Cisco device and policy-related activity.

Let's take a look at each of these in detail.

Cisco Firewall Management

This feature allows you to easily define the boundary security policy on PIX firewall and Cisco IOS routers running the firewall feature set. This allows for centralized configuration management of Cisco PIX firewalls and Cisco routers using the firewall feature set on your enterprise network. It will simplify your networkwide firewall and NAT management and reduce the need for management skills to manage the security policy, as well as reduce costs.

> **NOTE**
>
> A Cisco router running the firewall feature set is called a *Cisco Router/Firewall*, while a Cisco router running the IPSec VPN feature set is called a *Cisco VPN Gateway*. These feature sets are part of the *Cisco Secure Integrated Software* and *Cisco Secure Integrated VPN Software* solutions for Cisco routers.

Using this component within CSPM you can specify the outside and inside interface addresses of the specific PIX firewall. When you configure either one of the interface settings, you need to define the network the interface is connected to and specify the IP address assigned to the interface on the specific network. New versions of CSPM support multiple interfaces and failover configurations. Figure 12.1 shows what the PIX Firewall Properties panel looks like.

Figure 12.1 PIX Firewall Properties Panel

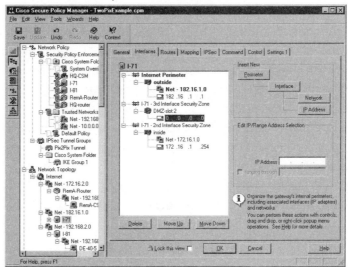

You can use the Mapping tab of the PIX Firewall Properties panel to define any NAT handled by the PIX firewall. Network routes can also be configured on the Routes tab. On the other hand, you would not use the Firewall management component to configure any of the security rules that apply to the PIX firewall on your network. For this, you should use the security policies abstractors to define any traffic filter rules that are part of your firewall security policy.

VPN and IPSec Security Management

The IPSec suite is used to seamlessly integrate security features, such as authentication, integrity, and confidentiality into IP packets. You can configure an encrypted and authenticated communication path between two clients, routers, or firewalls.

IPSec can function in two modes: tunnel and transport mode. Transport mode is used to provide end-to-end security between two nodes. Transport mode will protect all traffic between the source and destination with IPSec. In tunnel mode IPSec, the end nodes do not necessarily use or support IPSec. Instead, an IPSec-enabled security gateway or firewall functions as an IPSec peer for the communication between the end nodes. For example, a roaming user on the Internet connects to the enterprise e-mail server using an IPSec tunnel to the enterprise firewall. The traffic between the roaming user and the e-mail server is protected with IPSec up to the firewall. From there, the traffic is forwarded to the e-mail server unprotected.

IPSec uses two security protocols to provide data protection. The first one is Authentication Header (AH) protocol, which provides data integrity, data source authentication, and protection against replay attacks. When this protocol is used, the original IP packet is encapsulated into a packet that contains an extra header (AH), which contains an authentication value calculated from the contents of the packet. This value is checked when the packet arrives at its destination, ensuring the its contents were not modified on the way. The AH protocol does not provide data confidentiality, because information is not encrypted.

The second is the Encapsulation Security Payload (ESP) protocol, which provides data confidentiality, data integrity, data source authentication, and protection against replay attacks. The data confidentiality is accomplished by encrypting the original IP packet and encapsulating it into a new IP packet with the ESP header attached. The ESP header contains connection-specific encryption information in the form of reference to the Security Association (SA). This information is used on the other end of the connection to decrypt the packet after its arrival and check that the original data was not modified in any way.

The SA contains information on security protocols and encryption algorithms used to protect data for a specific connection, along with what data should be protected and which endpoints are used.

CSPM supports the configuration for IPSec SAs through the use of tunnel templates, tunnel groups, and policies. You can use the tunnel template to define the algorithms and protocols that will be used for encryption of data across the tunnel for confidentiality or authentication purposes. The tunnel group is based on one associated tunnel template and defines the tunnel peers or endpoints. This ensures that peers which are part of one tunnel group will reference the same protocols and algorithms. This will reduce risks of introducing errors when manually configuring each peer or endpoint for the tunnels. You can use the security policies to determine between services that should be routed through the tunnels, and services that should be routed using other methods.

For more information on IPSec, see Chapter 8.

CSPM allows you to create three basic types of tunnels:

- **Managed Device-to-Managed Device** Managed Device-to-Managed Device tunnels are used to securely transmit data between two managed devices (PIX firewalls or IPSec routers) across a public network, creating a VPN between two locations.

- **Policy Distribution Point-to-Managed Device** A policy distribution point is the component of CSPM that issues commands to managed devices (such as routers or Cisco Secure IDS sensors). Policy Distribution Point-to-Managed Device tunnels are used to securely transmit Managed Device configuration information to the Managed Devices over a public network. They can be used, for example, to configure and monitor remote devices over the Internet.

- **Remote User Tunnels** Remote user tunnels allow remote users secure access to internal network resources over a public network.

CSPM supports both manual and IKE tunnels. There are many preconfigured templates that can be used for creating your own tunnels. You can use them as they are or change any parameters so they suit your network setup. Figure 12.2 demonstrates one of these templates.

Figure 12.2 The IPSec Tunnel Template

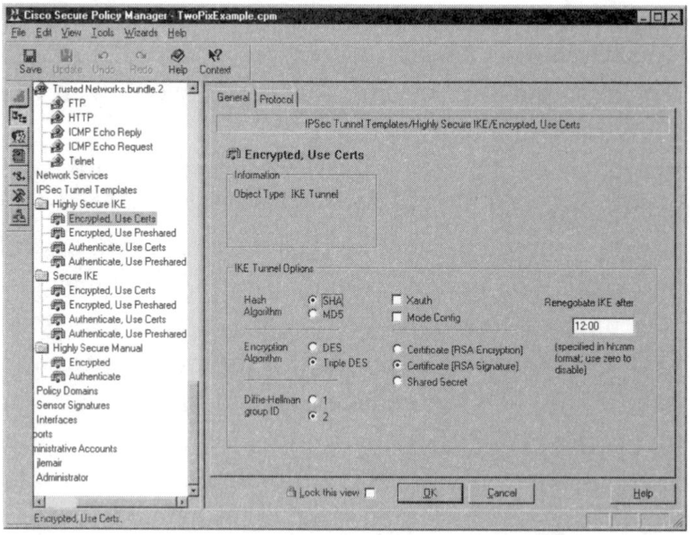

As you can see, CSPM supports all standard Cisco IPSec configuration parameters. After the template is configured, it is applied to a tunnel group to provide peers with protocol information.

Security Policy Management

CSPM is a centralized, policy-based management solution for Cisco security devices on your network. You can use CSPM to deploy a company network security policy throughout your network. The main goal of CSPM is to make the management of these policies easier. The process of policy management consists of its definition, enforcement, and auditing.

Security Policy Definition

Using CSPM, you can create high-level security policies based on the company security objectives. You can create security policy abstracts that define access and the associated level of security to specific network devices. Policy abstracts are created independently from managed devices and later assigned to them. By adjusting the parameters for the type of network service, or application, and the source and destination address of the abstracts, you can control network traffic across your enterprise network.

To simplify the creation of the policies on your network, policy abstracts can be created for a collection of services to reduce the number of policies created. When you first install the CSPM software on your server, there will be predefined abstract bundles ready for you to use in your security policies. CSPM also provides you grouping constructs for supported devices and hosts that allow you to reference multiple networks or hosts in a single policy. Figure 12.3 shows the appearance of Policy Builder—the tool used for policy creation.

Figure 12.3 Policy Builder

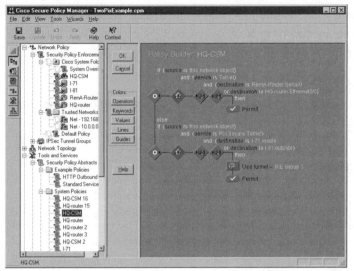

You can also use CSPM to easily define NAT policies on your PIX firewall or router on the boundary of your network. CSPM considers NAT configuration a part of device properties, not a "security policy" in the proper sense of the word. Security policies configured using Policy Builder are concerned with:

- Permitting or denying traffic for a specific user or device under certain conditions

- Use of IPSec tunnels

- Authentication, Authorization, and Accounting (AAA)

- Blocking Java in HTTP sessions

Other aspects of network traffic flow (routing, traffic shaping, general settings) are configured as the properties of corresponding devices.

Security Policy Enforcement

After you have defined the security policy, you need to apply the policy to the specific Cisco security device on your network. After the network topology is configured, you can use a simple drag-and-drop method to apply the security policies to the target network segments where they should be deployed (see Figure 12.4). The CSPM translates the policy into the device commands to apply it to the necessary PIX firewalls and VPN routers on the specified network section. You don't need to use the time-consuming CLI to configure each router for the new security policy deployed. On the other hand, if you are interested in reviewing generated commands, CSPM provides many tools for this. You can view entire sets of commands or only changes introduced by recent reconfigurations. There is also a version management utility available.

Figure 12.4 Policy Assignment

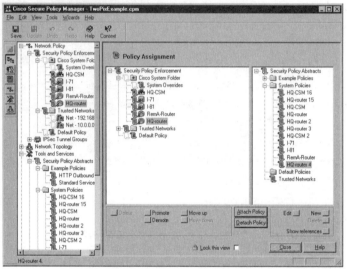

Depending on your preferences and needs, you can deploy the policy to the network automatically or manually. Manual deployment means you will need to approve each command set before it is sent to a device. Automatic approval means that commands are distributed to all devices when needed. The communication between the CSPM host and the managed devices is secure and safe to use across the network. It provides a flexible, robust mechanism to distribute configurations and enforce policies.

It allows you to have a consistent and proper policy enforcement on your network that you can easily verify and modify as required. The separate "Security Policy Enforcement" folder contains all policy enforcing devices, their hierarchy and assigned policy abstracts. You can, at any time, use the consistency check feature to ensure your network policy integrity and enforce status, or you can configure a notification if an error occurs with the policy enforcement.

Security Policy Auditing

The final part of the policy management process is the policy auditing. CSPM provides for an auditing system that enables you to log, monitor, alert, and report on the security policy events on your network where you enforced a policy. This is critical for checking the status of the policies on your network. There are two types of messages generated by Cisco security devices—firewalls and routers produce SYSLOG messages, and Cisco IDS sensors produce IDS alerts which are communicated to CSPM using Cisco proprietary protocol.

You can define filters and actions for the events related to SYSLOG messages generated on your network for the policies enforced. Any messages regarding possible network attacks and security breaches on your network can be configured for a real-time automated delivery to you using e-mail or a visual display. You can categorize the alerts based on specific events and messages for your policies to trigger only important notifications when needed. All the SYSLOG messages can be redirected to other servers on your network that could be used by third-party applications for reporting and analysis.

Cisco IDS messages are stored separately and can be viewed with the help of Event Viewer in CSPM (see Figure 12.5). This view can be manipulated by clicking plus signs (+) to open further details of the event. The special "i" series of CSPM has many extra IDS-related reports preconfigured.

Figure 12.5 Cisco IDS Sensor Events View

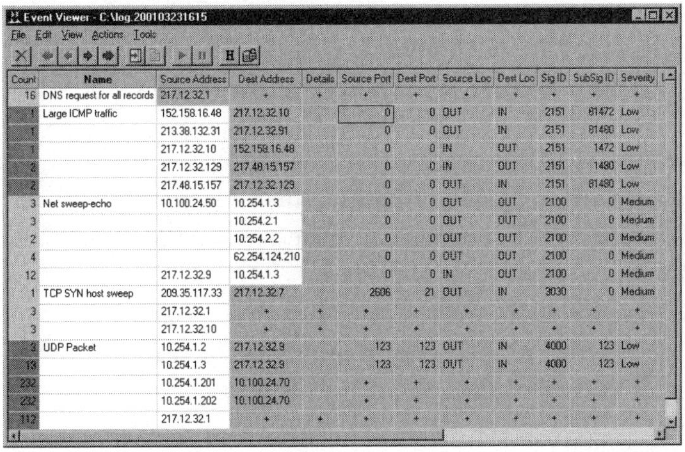

The other useful auditing and reporting CSPM tool is the Web-based reporting system that enables you to easily diagnose system security and integrity of your policies by using any host with an Internet browser. This tool allows setting access passwords and access privileges, so the reports will be open only for authorized administrators.

Network Security Deployment Options

CSPM can be used for a wide range of networks ranging from small- or medium-sized businesses that need a secure intranet connection to the Internet for networks distributed across multiple geographical locations using PIX firewalls and VPN routers for intercommunication.

When using CSPM on a large-scale enterprise network, you can deploy secure intranet connections between multiple remote sites. Using CSPM as a centralized solution for your network security management will benefit from the flexible and distributed architecture. On a large enterprise network, you could deploy CSPM in a distributed mode in which the GUI, or policy administrator, is installed on hosts in different locations on the network. The policy server includes the fundamental database, the policy translation, and the configuration distribution for CSPM. Policy server can also be installed on multiple servers in different locations on the network.

If you administer a small- to medium-sized network, you would use the perimeter, or boundary, security deployment policy available from CSPM. This gives you a simple security model and requires minimum configuration and ongoing maintenance for your security policy. Small companies usually enforce this deployment option to protect them from the Internet.

Cisco Secure Policy Manager Device and Software Support

When you use CSPM to manage your security policies in your enterprise network, you need to ensure that the managed devices comply with the list of devices and software or IOS version supported by CSPM before attempting to enforce any policies.

For all the Cisco PIX firewalls, Cisco IOS routers, and VPN routers on your network, you need to verify that they support the platform or model, as well as the software or IOS version shown in Table 12.1.

Table 12.1 Devices and Related Software Supported by CSPM 2.3.2

Device Platform	Supported Software Version
Cisco PIX Firewall	4.2(4), (5) 4.4(x) 5.1(x) 5.2.1 5.3(x) 6.0
Cisco Router/Firewall and Cisco's VPN router	IOS 12.0(5)T, XE IOS 12.0(7)T IOS 12.1(1)T, E1, XC IOS 12.1(2), T, (2) T, E, XH, (3) T, X1 IOS 12.1(4), E, T 12.1(5), 12.1(5)T

To ensure the appropriate device types are managed, CSPM includes a software version-checking mechanism that will display a warning message indicating a difference in software versions. There are also tools that allow you to manage new versions of these devices. This is called *version mapping*. Using the Version Management utility allows mapping of unsupported versions to those already known to CSPM. For example, you could create a rule that will manage Cisco PIX 6.1 using commands from the 6.0 version set.

When it comes to access control lists that need to be deployed to the specific device on the network, you would use the Policy Abstract tool to define, store, and manage your security policy abstracts that will be changed to access control lists before you enforce the policy to devices. The policy abstracts you create with this tool will support the following configuration settings:

- **Source** IP address range, specific host name, network object, policy domain, or interface defined in the network topology.

- **Destination** IP address range, specific host name, network object, policy domain or interface defined in the network topology.

- **Service type** Single or defined bundle of service types.

- **Tunnel** Uses specific IPSec tunnel groups.

- **Java** Blocks Java.

As you can see from the earlier list of allowed configuration settings to use in Policy Builder, these abstracts are mapped to standard IP ACLs and extended IP ACLs only. All other access lists have to be configured using the CLI. For example, CSPM does not support Content-Based Access-Control (CBAC) access lists. After a policy is created, you can browse the generated device commands and review to which parts of the security policy specific command sets are mapped. This is called *command to policy mapping*.

Using the Cisco Secure Policy Manager

To successfully install the CSPM on your network servers, you first need to identify the type of deployment option you will use, as discussed earlier. This will affect the number of servers you need to run the CSPM installation on, the physical location of the servers on your network, and which option you would choose during the installation based on the servers' responsibility on your enterprise network.

You have to verify that your network devices meet the necessary requirements before you can enforce any of the policies to the selected network section and related devices. In addition, you should check the minimum hardware requirements needed for your target hosts that you install the CSPM software on.

The next topics discuss the steps necessary to get CSPM installed, as well as some basic examples for configuring CSPM, and how to get CSPM up and running. Given the large amount of configuration and optional tools available in CSPM, it will be impossible to fit them all into this small section of the book. Consequently, only a few of the configurations and examples will be discussed that relate to the CSPM product. You can find additional information on the Cisco Web site at www.cisco.com. You can find almost everything you need here—from release notes for all currently supported versions of CSPM to detailed deployment guides.

Configuration

When you insert the CSPM software installation CD-ROM into the CD drive of your computer, it should autostart the Installation Wizard for CSPM. Select the **Install Product** option and then click **Next**. This will start the installation and you can follow the onscreen instructions to complete the installation. If there is no Install Product option there, this means some of the prerequisites are not fulfilled—for example, the required service pack is not installed. You will need to install it and restart installation. It is also possible to install a demo interface without installing the full product.

After installation starts, it will ask you for the location of the licence file. You can use the one supplied with the CD-ROM, which will grant you limited use of the software, and you can use the password **cisco** to continue. If you do have a licence file you purchased from Cisco, you can specify the location and enter the appropriate password.

The next option selection screen will be determined by your deployment option type on your network. You can select **Standalone CSPM** or **Client-Server CSPM,** which has two subselections to pick from, namely "Policy Server" or "Policy Client." You can also choose **Distributed CSPM** with a subselection of one of the following:

- Policy Server
- Policy Proxy-monitor
- Policy Proxy
- Policy Monitor
- Policy Admin

Designing & Planning...

Selecting between Various Deployment Types

There are many issues that affect the choice between standalone, client-server, and distributed configuration of CSPM. Some of them are:

- **Encryption of data traffic between managed devices and CSPM** This traffic will be encrypted only if the device supports IPSec and you defined IPSec tunnels for communication between the device and CSPM host. For example, if you place any part of CSPM (in a distributed configuration) on an unprotected network between the outermost managed device and your Internet provider, control traffic to that part will not be encrypted.

- **Syslog traffic** Almost all messages about the status of security policy are sent from managed devices using syslog UDP packets (the only exclusion is IDS sensors, which use their own protocol). In case of heavy attack, this UDP traffic can

Continued

> flood the network if it's busy enough, therefore it's not rec-
> ommended a standalone system or Policy Monitor compo-
> nent be placed on a busy network.
>
> ■ **IDS sensors management** CSPM does not support IDS sen-
> sors in a distributed configuration. If you plan to use Cisco
> Secure IDS sensors on the network, you will need either a
> standalone or client-server configuration. Note that only ded-
> icated sensors are supported (as standalone devices or
> Catalyst 6000 blades). There is no support for IOS IDS fea-
> tures yet.

A brief description for your selection can be found in the Installation Option box. In this window, you also specify the installation path for CSPM. The next screen allows you to enter the password for the username that will be used to install and start the relevant services on your server.

Next, you can specify the IP address on your target installation server that will be used to access and configure your CSPM. This IP address is associated with a port number, or so called service port, used for the connection to the pri-mary policy database. You can export the primary policy database key to a file in a selected path, if required. If you export the primary database key, make sure to keep it safe and secure, otherwise you might compromise the security of your network. This will start the installation of the files needed to run CSPM and configure your preferred settings.

Now that you're ready to start your CSPM, you need to get the access infor-mation for the routers and PIX firewalls you would like to manage. You will need the usernames and password to add the relevant devices to your CSPM application.

CSPM Configuration Example

The examples in this section will give you a general view of the related configu-ration screens available in CSPM. You can see some of the settings for the topics discussed previously. All the configurations can be used without connecting to your network devices and you only need to deploy your new security policy if you are satisfied with the new configuration.

Initial configuration of CSPM consists of three steps:

1. Network topology definition

2. Network policy definition and deployment

3. Generation and distribution of device commands

The first step is defining the network topology in the "Network Topology" tree in CSPM. You do not have to map your entire network to it, only devices used in security policy definition are needed here. The second step is concerned with defining security policy in terms of services permitted for different users, as well as the parameters of these services. In the last step, CSPM generates actual commands for Cisco security devices on your network based on the topology and security policies you have defined and then distributes these commands.

Network Policy Definition

Consider the following network (Figure 12.6). It is a standard example from a default installation of CSPM. It features three different remote networks connected to the Internet using Cisco routers and PIX firewalls.

Figure 12.6 Two PIX Examples

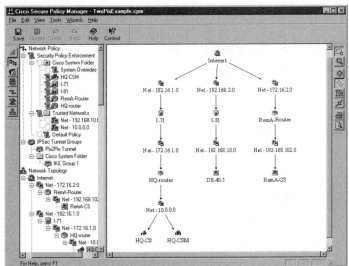

Here you will need to define hosts (servers on a network), networks, routers, and PIX firewalls in a "Network Topology" subtree. It can be done manually or by using specific wizards. For example, router configuration (probably the most complicated one judging by the amount of options available) is displayed in Figure 12.7

You can add a device by simply right-clicking the network it belongs to and clicking **New**. If you prefer to use a wizard, it is even simpler; you can select where the device has to be connected during the configuration process.

Figure 12.7 The Router Properties Panel

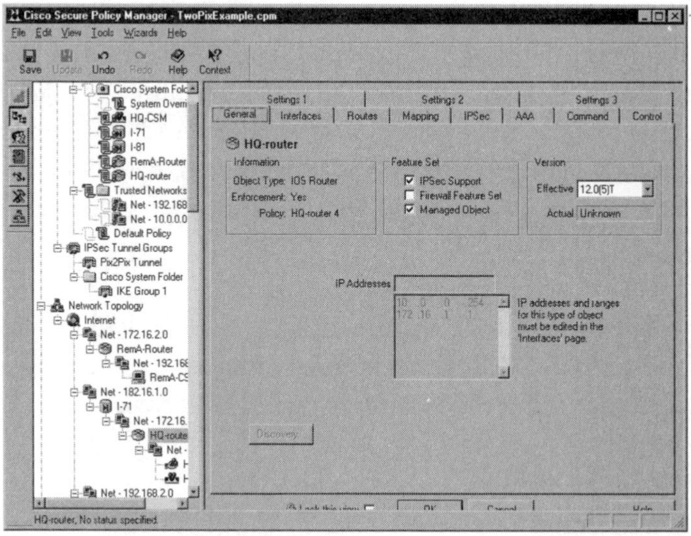

Cisco routers have many configuration options. The General tab defines general settings, such as IOS version number and feature set used. The Interfaces tab defines network perimeters, interfaces, and their IP addresses. Other panels are used to set up static routes, NAT pools, IPSec properties, authentication features, and so on. The PIX firewall configuration has fewer details (as seen in Figure 12.1). Do not forget to define your CSMP server on the network since it is a special device type (host HQ-CSM in Figure 12.6).

Network Security Policy Definition

Now that we have defined all our network assets, we need to create a security policy for the network. In order to perform this task, you will first need to place the objects, which are used to enforce the policy, in the "Security Policy Enforcement" branch of the "Network Policy" tree. The next step is to build some security policy abstracts and then assign these abstracts to the enforcement devices. If your security policy uses more complicated services than those already defined in CSPM, you will need to define them before creating policy abstracts.

Placing objects into the Security Policy Enforcement branch can be done by simply dragging-and-dropping. Policy abstracts are created using Policy Builder as in Figure 12.3. This is a context-sensitive visual tool—if you click an operator, you will be presented with a choice of possible actions, such as creating another if-then–else branch and security action selection (permit/deny/use IPSec tunnel and so on). For example, if you add another if-then branch, you are allowed to select source/destination hosts or services. Figure 12.8 shows the selection of a source of the connection.

Figure 12.8 Selecting Source Conditions for an if-then Operator

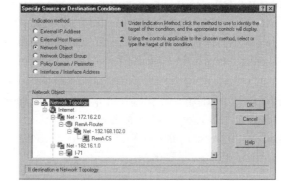

After policy abstracts are created, they need to be assigned using the policy assignment tool (as in Figure 12.4). The assignment process is very simple—just drag-and-drop policy abstracts onto corresponding enforcement points. Now everything is ready for implementation and distribution of the actual commands that will be generated by the CSPM based on your definitions. There is also a way to check some actual connections against the defined policies through use of the Policy Query tool (Figure 12.9). Using this, you can specify the source, destination, and network service of a connection and query the Policy Database on which rules actually affect this connection and what the result will be.

Figure 12.9 Policy Query

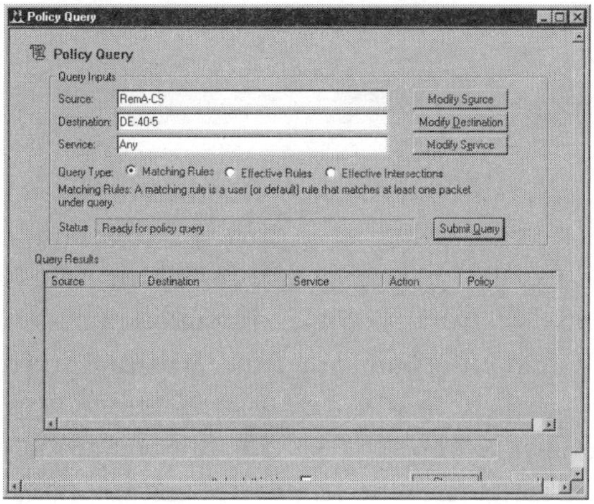

Generation and Distribution of Device Commands

The final task in the initial configuration of CSPM is generation, verification, and publishing (distribution to the actual devices) of device commands.

Device commands are generated when you select **Save and Update** from the **File** menu. The resulting command sets include all security-related commands—access lists, IPSec tunnels, and so on, plus routing and network mapping (NAT) commands, which are produced based on defined device properties. Each managed device (router or firewall) has a Command tab which allows the browsing of the resulting commands. You can also specify here any extra commands you need to send to the device (Prologue/Epilogue sections). Figure 12.10 shows the editor window for the *Epilogue* section. No commands have been generated yet, so the Command Viewer button is inactive.

Figure 12.10 Command Viewer

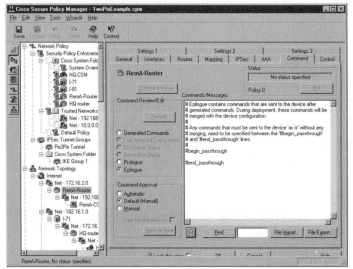

After you have reviewed the generated commands, you can distribute them to the device. This is done by clicking the **Approve Now** button. If you think you are familiar with what CSPM generates, you can change the command approval method to **Automatic** so that all commands will be published to the corresponding devices right after they are generated, meaning you aren't required to review them.

Now you are familiar with basic CSPM configuration steps from installation to the deployment of enterprisewide security policy. Of course, this was a rather sketchy description. If you plan to deploy CSPM in the real world, do not forget to consult the Cisco documentation on their Web site.

Summary

Cisco Secure Policy Manager is a scalable policy-based security management system for Cisco PIX firewalls, IPSec routers, and intrusion detection sensors. It allows network administrators to deploy their security policy from one location, or to use distributed deployment from multiple locations on the network. In addition, you can configure all the VPN tunnels using IPSec and NAT on the boundary of your network to change your private IP address range so you can communicate with outside networks.

CSPM is being distributed in two product lines: the "f" series, with enhanced support for firewalls/VPNs; and the "i" series with extended IDS reporting tools. These products cannot coexist on one host. The current version of both products is 2.3.2, with a new 3.0f version just starting to be distributed as part of CiscoWorks VMS 2.0 (VPN Management Solution) 2.0. It is also promised by Cisco that 3.0i will be released this year.

Implementation of security policies with CSPM consists of three main steps:

- Defining network topology
- Creating security policies
- Publishing generated command sets to the managed devices

All these tasks are performed inside the GUI interface. It is possible to use the various wizards or to fine-tune everything by changing the default values manually. The GUI also features many tools for checking the results of your work, such as the network graph or Policy Query tool.

CSPM can even be used for managing new, originally unsupported versions of IOS/PIX software by mapping them into supported ones with the *Version Management* utility.

Solutions Fast Track

Overview of the Cisco Secure Policy Manager

☑ CSPM is an integrated solution for management of Cisco security devices. It has distributed architecture and is policy-based. There are two product lines: The "i" series with enhanced IDS support and the "f" series with full VPN/firewall configuration capabilities.

☑ CSPM has built-in auditing and reporting tools, which provide up-to-date information on network and system events. It also supports Cisco Secure IDS sensors, which produce signature-based events, allowing you to track down network intrusions.

☑ CSPM is a Windows NT-based application. One requirement of the installation is Service Pack 6a. CSPM can coexist on the same host with Cisco Secure VPN Client 1.1, CiscoWorks 2000 with Resource Management Essentials version 3.0, and the QoS Policy Manager version 1.1. On the other hand, two different product lines, namely the "i" series and the "f" series, cannot be installed on the same computer.

Features of the Cisco Secure Policy Manager

☑ CSPM is designed to replace the PIX firewall manager and ACL manager, so it includes their functionality and enhances it with centralized management.

☑ Firewall management features of CSPM allow definition and management of perimeter security policies for Cisco PIX firewalls and Cisco IOS routers running the Cisco Secure Integrated Software feature set.

☑ Cisco IPSec VPN gateway management allows onfiguration of site-to-site IPSec VPNs based on Cisco Secure PIX firewalls and the Cisco suite of VPN routers running Cisco IOS IPSec software.

☑ Intrusion detection sensors management supports configuration and monitoring of Cisco intrusion detection sensors and Cisco Catalyst 6000 line cards. The Cisco IDS feature set of PIX firewalls and IOS routers is not supported.

☑ Another feature is security policy management. It allows usage of enterprisewide policies for managing hundreds of Cisco security devices without dependency on the command-line interface.

☑ The notification and reporting system provides tools to monitor, alert, and report Cisco device- and policy-related activity.

Using the Cisco Secure Policy Manager

☑ CSPM can be installed in standalone, client-server, or distributed mode (the latter is possible only for the "f" series). Selection between these modes depends on the size and structure of your network.

☑ Initial CSPM configuration process consists of three tasks—defining network topology, creating security policies, and distributing generated commands to managed devices.

☑ Network topology definition can be performed manually or by using wizards. There is no need to map the whole network to the CSPM database—only devices used in formulation and enforcement of security policies are important.

☑ Security policy determines user access to various services and is defined using the graphical Policy Builder. After that, it is mapped to corresponding enforcement points.

☑ The last step is command generation and distribution. There are various possibilities here—each command set may be modified (manually or automatically by adding specified prologues/epilogues) and applied to the corresponding device (again, by manually approving it or having the task performed automatically).

☑ Command differences between existing device configurations and new configurations can be viewed and checked. CSPM also supports commands to policy mapping, which allows the browsing of specific commands related to parts of security policy.

Frequently Asked Questions

The following Frequently Asked Questions, answered by the authors of this book, are designed to both measure your understanding of the concepts presented in this chapter and to assist you with real-life implementation of these concepts. To have your questions about this chapter answered by the author, browse to **www.syngress.com/solutions** and click on the **"Ask the Author"** form.

Q: Which IDS platforms are supported in CSPM?

A: Only Cisco Secure IDS sensors (former NetRanger sensors) are supported, either in standalone configuration or as Catalyst 6000 blades. Embedded IDS features of Cisco PIX firewalls and Cisco IOS routers are not supported.

Q: What network topologies are best managed by CSPM?

A: CSPM supports Cisco firewall and VPN router deployments within Internet, intranet, and extranet topologies. For VPN environments, the product supports site-to-site (router-to-router) network topologies only. RAS (client-to-router) VPN networks are not supported. The network topology discovery feature in the 3.0f version supports only "flat" networks—that is, networks without multiple layers of firewalls.

Q: Does CSPM offer user-based security policy management?

A: No, CSPM does not currently provide comprehensive management of user policies (especially user-based authentication and authorization). On the other hand, it is possible to configure AAA (authentication, authorization, and accounting) for pass-through and administrative traffic.

Q: Are there different administrator levels within CSPM?

A: Yes, the product provides three levels of administration:

- **Full access** Provides read and write access to all policy administration functions within CSPM and allows creation of other administrator accounts. Only one network security administrator can have full access rights to the system at any moment in time.

- **Read only** Provides read-only access to all policy administration functions within CSPM. This would be appropriate for help-desk personnel or network security administrators with audit/documentation responsibilities.

- **Report viewing** Provides read-only access to Web-based reports created with CSPM. This is appropriate for help-desk personnel or managers.

Q: What kind of database does CSPM use?

A: CSPM uses a proprietary object-oriented database that has been optimized for use in the policy-based management system. There are possibilities for the importing and exporting of events or topology structures into other systems, although the database itself cannot be moved to any common DBMS platform.

Q: Where can I find more information about CSPM features and requirements?

A: There is plenty of information available on the Cisco Web site at www.cisco.com/go/policymanager/.

Q: Can CSPM be integrated with third-party network management applications?

A: No, CSPM has no support for integration with any third-party applications for network management.

Intrusion Detection

Introduction

A properly configured firewall appliance is considered a first line of network defense, and controls the flow of information to your servers. Unfortunately, if the server receives information from the network, it runs a risk of compromise from the unlikely event that the firewall fails. A more likely type of failure is that the firewall does its job passing traffic but that the server itself is vulnerable to an unusual request.

Other elements of that first line of defense would include Access Control Lists (ACLs) on perimeter routers, perhaps Web caching, or load-balancing appliances. It would include operating system (OS) hardening and application configuration controls on the server, as well as ensuring that the vendor software is current according to vendor recommendations. All these things contribute to the security of the service. But because we can never be completely sure that best practices have been followed, a second line of defense is a good plan. This is known as "defense in depth." We put everything we can into the front lines, but in case that fails, we have a backup plan. A detective control is an excellent element of that second line of defense.

An intrusion detection system gives the network or security manager a tool to detect and react rapidly to an attack on the network. This chapter will investigate the various types of attacks and intrusions as well as describe the tools available from Cisco to implement an intrusion detection system.

What Is Intrusion Detection?

An intrusion detection system (IDS) is a software program, or a suite of hardware and software, that automates the investigation of unusual or potentially inappropriate activity in or around computers. It is an example of a technical security control, where the direct application of technology (as opposed to procedure or management guidance) attempts to solve security problems.

Technical controls can be classified as preventative or detective. Preventive controls attempt to avoid the occurrence of unwanted events, whereas detective controls attempt to identify unwanted events after they have occurred. An IDS is typically used as a detective control, alerting to misuse, and providing information about the frequency of the event. These detective controls typically combine signature-based approaches (similar to antivirus scanners) as well as unusual traffic analysis. This allows for more broadly based detection, but suffers from problems of false alerts.

An IDS can also be used in a preventative fashion: modern IDS can take action to interrupt a system call on a host, or interrupt network activity. In this case, the IDS must be adjusted so that this kind of activity only occurs when very clear identification of malicious activity is present.

Types of IDSs

IDSs fall into two types: network-based IDSs (NIDSs), where traffic is analyzed as it passes by a sensor on a wire; and host-based IDSs (HIDSs), where traffic is analyzed as it is accepted by the OS. The former is more readily deployed since it can be done with appliance devices rather than requiring modification of an existing server, and can provide a broader area of coverage. The latter is more precise, since it is able to understand what is occurring at the host itself: thus if an unknown form of attack attempted to cause a system to fail in a known fashion, the network-based sensor would probably miss the attack, but the host-based sensor would see the fault. This allows host-based IDS to function effectively as a preventative control, and is generally considered an appropriate use of the technology.

The Cisco Secure Network IDS product has the capability to do *shunning*. With shunning, the intrusion detection system alerts actually cause configuration changes in firewalls and routers, and block traffic from those networks.

IDS Architecture

IDSs are generally composed of a management station and one or more sensors. Because the control must see traffic to analyze it, it is generally distributed throughout a network at key locations. The management station integrates information from the distributed sensors (host and network) to provide a comprehensive and comprehensible view of the network. An operator usually interacts with the management station via a Web front-end or dedicated graphical user interface (GUI), and does not directly interact with the sensors. With the Cisco IDS, the management station can be either the IDS Director or a Cisco Secure Policy Manager (CSPM). The CSPM is documented in Chapter 12. In the fall of 2002, Cisco will be announcing a new management device to replace both the CSPM and Director consoles.

Ideally, the management station should integrate with any other operations management platforms in use. In an all-Cisco network, integration with the CSPM is helpful. In larger or nonhomogeneous networks, third-party products, such as HP OpenView, are often used to provide that integration.

Controlling the Communication between Sensor and Manager

Often people deploy the sensor and manager focusing on bandwidth issues, and don't think about the security issues. Remember, security usually revolves around CIA: confidentiality, integrity, and availability. These issues come up in spades for the sensor/manager communication:

- **Confidentiality** The output from the sensors will contain highly sensitive information, including passwords, URLs visited, and the like.

- **Integrity** If a bad guy can forge data from the sensor, he can implicate other innocent users.

- **Availability** If a bad guy can prevent the data from getting from the sensor to the manager, he can work his evil undetected.

While other IDSs may communicate using unencrypted protocols such as syslog, Cisco has thoughtfully provided for confidentiality and integrity in its Post Office protocol, used to communicate between sensor and manager. However, don't forget to protect the communication channel, and don't forget that the sensors and the managers are prime targets for the attackers!

Why Should You Have an IDS?

The security events detected by an IDS are typically of three types:

- Malicious events, such as those present at an intrusion

- Misconfigured events, such as incorrect configuration data causing system malfunction

- Ineffective events, such as ineffective network traffic

These security events are also usually classified by severity (that is, the ability of the event to harm the enterprise) and frequency (the likelihood of the occurrence). As an example of two types of malicious events, those that are severe or frequent (for example, the recent Nimda worm) are more important to identify and act upon than those that are minor or rare (for instance, a curious employee performing a port scan on his buddy's machine). Perhaps even more important is distinguishing between that curious employee port scan on an unimportant machine and a port scan on a core business asset that may signal a prelude to a determined attack.

The business drivers for each of the three types are slightly different. The driver for the first is to reduce the risk associated with a systems compromise. They may be a required part of due diligence for protection of corporate assets. The driver for the second is to identify errors in configuration so that they can be corrected. This reduces the overall cost of maintenance. The driver for the third is to optimize the use of corporate assets.

Benefits of an IDS in a Network

As stated, the tuning process can take different approaches depending upon the desired result. Usually, the desired result should follow the business driver. These are examined in turn.

Reduce the Risk of a Systems Compromise

This is the most direct driver associated with an intrusion detection system. Risk can be reduced indirectly through detection and response or through direct corrective action. As a part of the response, a forensic element can be applied. If the enterprise has the ability to document the root causes of an attack, this can reduce the frequency of occurrence, particularly among the local user community (they are put on notice that malicious activity can have severe consequences). Forensic analysis may also be of some use in recovering damages, if the activity is careful enough to survive the necessary legal proceedings.

Indirect Action

Indirect action through an incident response procedure is flexible, and can tolerate potential errors in alerting. The trade off is increased work for reduced risk. The key is to have a prepared incidence response protocol for handling events.

Direct Action

Direct corrective action can be both automated and inherent to the alert, or provide notice to a security officer so that an incident response procedure can be initiated. Examples of direct action are blocking an offending system call (for a host-based system) or reconfiguring a firewall (for a network-based system). These kinds of activity require a high degree of confidence in the alert.

Identifying Errors of Configuration

Identifying errors of configuration is an immediate benefit of an IDS. A complex environment, such as a server or a network, is usually misconfigured in several small ways. Luckily, our systems are redundant enough that the error conditions are handled by secondary systems. However, there is a risk that the secondary system may fail, causing a systemic failure; in addition, there may be improvements to service possible if the original device is correctly configured.

An IDS can usually identify this sort of invalid traffic. For example, a device may be misconfigured to have an invalid password for file access. The IDS will track this as an attempt to "break into" the file server by noting an excessive number of password failures. The detective control will allow the owner of the system to correct the password, and allow improved functionality.

Optimize Network Traffic

A third benefit of an IDS is to optimize network flows, or at least to provide insight into how networks are being used. A common component of an IDS is a statistical anomaly detection engine. Cisco calls this *profile-based detection* and notes it "involves building statistical profiles of user activity and then reacting to any activity that falls outside these established profiles." The immediate reason is to identify an intrusion through unusual behavior. However, this also permits the operator to get a feel for the behavior of the network under normal operating conditions, and that insight can provide assistance on larger network maintenance and design issues.

Documenting Existing Threat Levels for Planning or Resource Allocation

When you are drawing up a budget for network security, it often helps to substantiate claims that the network is likely to be attacked or is even currently under attack. Understanding the frequency and characteristics of attacks allows you to understand what security measures are appropriate to protect the network against those attacks.

IDSs verify, itemize, and characterize threats from both outside and inside the enterprise network, assisting security management in making sound decisions regarding the allocation of computer security resources. Using IDSs in this manner is important, as many people mistakenly deny that anyone (outsider or insider) would be interested in breaking into their networks. Furthermore, the information that IDSs give you regarding the source and nature of attacks allows you to make decisions regarding security strategy driven by demonstrated need, not guesswork or folklore.

Changing User Behavior

A fundamental goal of computer security management is to affect the behavior of individual users in a way that protects information systems from security problems. Intrusion detection systems help organizations accomplish this goal by increasing the perceived risk of discovery and punishment of attackers. This serves as a significant deterrent to those who would violate security policy.

Deploying an IDS in a Network

The placement of a NIDS requires careful planning. Cisco's Secure IDS product (NetRanger) is made up of a probe and a central management station called a Director (old style) or the CSPM (new style). Each probe has two interfaces: a *command interface*, on which configuration information is accepted and logging information is sent, and a *sensor interface*. The sensor interface has an unnumbered interface; some feel that this allows placement of the command interface on a different network than the command interface. If that is your policy, it is helpful to place the command interface on a management network. If you are concerned about the potential for a compromise through the sensor interface, then it is best to place the command interface on the same network as the sensor interface. Let's look at the best place to put the Sensor interface.

Sensor Placement

Most companies have a firewall that separates the internal network from the outside world. They typically have one or more service networks, and the internal network may also be subdivided.

Should we place the probe outside or inside? If the probe is outside, then it can monitor external traffic. This is useful against attacks from the outside but does not allow for detection of internal attacks. Of course, understanding attacks against the outside net may not be particularly valuable, since generally they would be stopped by the firewall. Also, the probe itself may become the target of an attack so it must be protected.

If you place the probe inside, it will detect internally-initiated attacks and can highlight firewall rules that are not working properly or are incorrectly configured.

Generally, the reason to put a probe outside the firewall would be to "take the temperature" of the Internet. This can be valuable to demonstrate the value of the firewall. More importantly, you should deploy sensors so they can view traffic worth sensing.

One effective strategy is to deploy probes to capture the interface of the firewall that faces the service net (or nets) so you can capture traffic from networks headed toward the service net. Other appropriate monitoring points would be near server clusters, or near router transit networks/interfaces. When you review your security policy, you may decide you need to install more probes at different points in the network according to security risks and requirements.

Here are some example locations:

- The Accounts department's Local Area Network (LAN)
- Company strategic networks (for example, the Development LAN)
- Technical department's LAN
- LANs where staff turnover is rapid or hot-desk/temp locations exist
- the Server LAN

Difficulties in Deploying an IDS

There are several difficulties associated with successful IDS deployments. One fundamental problem is that the underlying science behind intrusion detection systems is relatively new. While everyone agrees that some things can be achieved, the January 1998 paper *Insertion, Evasion, and Denial of Service: Eluding Network Intrusion Detection* by Thomas H. Ptacek and Timothy N. Newsham seemed to throw the field for a loop. They described techniques by which a properly designed IDS can be deceived, with a follow-up discussion that seemed to indicate the loftiest goal of an IDS is not achievable without a complete recreation of all network hosts. In the paper they note:

> The number of attacks against network intrusion detection systems, and the relative simplicity of the problems that were actually demonstrated to be exploitable on the commercial systems we tested, indicates to us that network intrusion detection is not a mature technology. More research and testing needs to occur before network intrusion detection can be looked to as a reliable component in a security system.

However, it should not be taken that this is seen as an unusable technology. An IDS is one of the most common security purchases today. Current (2002) Computer Security Institute (CSI)/FBI statistics show that approximately 60 percent of Fortune 500 companies deploy an IDS; in just a few years, an IDS suite will likely be as ubiquitous as firewalls. What this does point out is that this is a technology in a state of rapid change. It is also worth noting that Cisco engineering took the flaws identified to heart; today, their analysis engine is vulnerable to none of these flaws.

A second difficulty is that of expectation. Management may feel that simply purchasing an IDS will make them safe. It doesn't. It can be of assistance in identifying, imperfectly, attacks on a host or network, and can also be of use in tracking human events. But IDS tools should probably be combined with additional tools to provide a more robust detection environment.

A third difficulty is associated with the deployment phase. The network deployment is relatively straightforward but non-trivial, and coordination between multiple groups is often required. In a larger enterprise, the people who "own" the network are different from the people who "own" security, and clear communication may not always be possible. A host deployment involves interaction with a complex environment, and may involve further unknown interactions.

A fourth difficulty concerns incidence response. An incidence response procedure is a nontrivial task for most enterprises. A significant development effort is usually required. For most enterprises, such programs have not been required before. In many environments, the program is developed after the first incident, as part of a "lessons learned" analysis.

A fifth difficulty revolves around IDS tuning, described next. An IDS, out of the box, is generally not very useful. It must be adjusted to be in harmony with the local environment and the resources available to explore events. It's this level of effort associated with IDS tuning that management often underestimates.

It should be recognized that most IDS programs are at their most effective several months or even years after their initial deployment.

IDS Tuning

A detective control makes an assertion that a particular event has occurred (by flagging one or more network packets or system calls). An important aspect is to tune the tool so that the accuracy of the assertion provides maximum relevancy to the enterprise. In other words, the IDS makes a call that either something is wrong or that everything is fine. You want it to be right more often than not.

To quantify this, the language of hypothesis testing applies. Note that in the following, native errors to the tool (such as dropped packets for the NIDS or incorrect configuration of the HIDS) are not considered. An IDS makes a decision on whether a security event is taking place. Let's suppose the chance that a particular packet is an attack is "p." In most enterprises, "p" would be fairly small. This is the chance that, if you were just poking about using a sniffer, you would be able to view a malicious packet.

In hypothesis testing, a matrix is developed, as shown in Table 13.1.

Table 13.1 IDS Decision versus Truth

Truth	IDS Decision: Alert Is Generated	IDS Decision: Alert Is Not Generated
No security event is in progress (prob. 1-p)	Type I error (alpha)	Correct result
A security event is in progress (prob. p)	Correct result	Type II error (beta)

The error probability alpha represents the amount of "work" assumed by the enterprise. It is the number of stray alarms that might need to be checked out—the probability that an alert is generated even though no security event is in progress. It is often normalized by multiplying by the number of alerted events, producing the frequency of *false positives*. Thus, we say "nine out of ten of the alerts were false positives." In conventional hypothesis testing, much effort is spent to minimize alpha. The error probability beta represents the amount of "risk" assumed by the enterprise. It is also often normalized by dividing by p, the probability that a security event is occurring. This number is typically difficult to estimate, but is based upon the threat model.

With a "full bore" signature load, the error probability "alpha" is very high. By way of example, let's look at some numbers. At a recent deployment, the probes saw about 38 billion packets a day. The probes reported nearly a million events after three days. Sifting through the alerts, the security engineers found some ICMP traffic that corresponded to unauthorized test equipment; this corresponded to about ten thousand packets. They also found one server that had apparently been compromised; this probably corresponded to about a thousand packets. Therefore:

p = 11 thousand packets / 38 billion packets = 0.00000029

Without an IDS (say by using a sniffer) this would clearly be a "needle in a haystack" problem – you would have to go through about 30 million packets before finding one corresponding to a bad guy. The fact that the analysts were able to find a compromised server is a great testimonial to the power of the tool.

On the other hand, note that computing the normalized alpha, we get:

$$\text{False positive ratio} = \frac{(1 \text{ million alerts}) - (11 \text{ thousand real alerts})}{1 \text{ million alerts}} = 0.989$$

so that 99 out of 100 alerts are false positives. To be fair, with a million alerts, it is possible there were more "real" security events that were just missed. This analysis also assumes that there are no false negatives, that there were alerts on all security events, so the accuracy numbers may be lower than expected. The sheer number of packets is part of the problem with an untuned IDS deployment. It is a *lot* of work to try to classify these events. It's nice that the analyst found the compromised server, but having to explore a hundred alerts to find the smoking gun is probably not tenable over the long run.

Tuning

After the IDS is installed, a tuning phase is performed. This is to modify the performance of the tool to optimize alpha and beta. Note that it is very easy to optimize each separately: you can drop alpha to zero by never generating an alert; in this case, beta is now 100 percent. You can optimize beta by flagging every packet; unfortunately, now alpha is at nearly 100 percent error. Experience has shown that in this case, while the formal value of beta is excellent, in practice no system can respond to the high number of alarms. Managers simply turn off the system, and while the security event is detected, no action is taken, which in some respects is an even more undesirable result. This is similar to what was seen in the preceding deployment: A million alerts is too daunting.

The trick is to train the tool to provide a reasonable degree of accuracy, so the error rates of alpha and beta are both close to zero—the enterprise trades the work of investigating false positives for the risk of missing an event.

Turn It Up

There are two traditional approaches. One approach is to work through the alert information, selectively enabling only those alerts that are known to be desirable. This approach typically minimizes alpha, and is most suited to strongly controlled environments or those for which the detective control has severe consequence, such as alarms that reconfigure devices or directly notify third parties.

Tone It Down

The more common approach is to apply all possible sensitivity and slowly "tone it down," eliminating those alerts that have too high an alpha in the given environment. The best approach is to identify an acceptable false positive rate for a particular type of alert, and then enable the signature only if the observed rate is less than the desired rate. For example, if an alert indicated traffic showing a systems compromise, the acceptable false positive rate may be nine out of ten, while if the alert merely indicates traffic of a suspicious nature, the acceptable false positive rate may be one in three. The system is then allowed to run for a period, observing the environment. At the end of that time, the alerts are assessed. If more than nine out of ten of the more serious alerts prove false, the alert is disabled; if more than one out of three of the lesser severity alerts prove false, that signature is disabled.

In addition, the alerts can often be refined; the alerting procedure can selectively disable based upon known behaviors. For example, one signature may identify large numbers of User Datagram Protocol (UDP) packets in a short period as a UDP flood, often associated with malicious activity. However, large numbers of UDP packets destined to, or from, a name server is normal; thus the alert signature is revised to specify "large numbers of UDP packets in a short period EXCEPT to this host."

Network Attacks and Intrusions

An IDS provides information about network attacks and intrusions. We need to classify what these alarms are saying, which means the first step is for us to identify what an attack or intrusion is. Any action that violates the security policy of your organization should be considered a potential harm, but broadly speaking, attacks and intrusions can be summarized as an exploitation of:

- Poor network perimeter/device security
- Poor physical security
- Application and operating software weaknesses
- Human failure
- Weaknesses in the IP suite of protocols

Before we look at these threats in more detail let me suggest that you assume a devious mind, something which helps when it comes to learning about intrusion detection.

Poor Network Perimeter/Device Security

This can be described as the ease of access to devices across the network. Without access control using a firewall or a packet filtering router, the network is vulnerable.

Packet Decoders

It is very common to place packet decoders, such as Network General's Sniffer or open source products like Ethereal, onto your network to try to debug applications or diagnose network problems. The invisible becomes visible, and things on the wire are visible in text. This means that applications that send password information in the clear—Telnet, FTP, POP3 (how many users read mail), Web applications—are obvious examples.

For instance, here is a quick trace of an FTP session: This first portion is what is visible only on my private workstation.

```
C:\>ftp fred.callisma.com
Connected to fred.callisma.com.
220 ProFTPD 1.2.2 Server (ProFTPD Default Installation)
    [fred.callisma.com]
User (fred.callisma.com:(none)): luser
331 Password required for luser.
Password:
230 User luser logged in.
```

Here is what flows over the wire, visible to someone with a packet decoder—this is the "Follow TCP stream" tool from Ethereal.

```
220 ProFTPD 1.2.2 Server (ProFTPD Default Installation)
    [fred.callisma.com]
USER luser
331 Password required for luser.
PASS SeCrEt!
230 User luser logged in.
QUIT
221 Goodbye.
```

Wireless LANs suffer from the same sort of problem. It's even more sneaky, since this data can be captured without being physically present and with a much more difficult chance of being detected.

This method of intrusion is called *eavesdropping* or *packet snooping* and the type of network technology implemented directly influences its susceptibility. For instance, shared networks are easier to eavesdrop on than switched networks. Of course, confidential material should not flow across uncontrolled networks in the clear.

Scanner Programs

Certain types of software, such as Nmap, Nessus, and John the Ripper, are able to scan entire networks, produce detailed reports on what ports are in use, perform password cracking and view account details on servers. Although these are very useful tools if used for the purpose of legitimate network auditing, in the wrong hands they can be devastating. Scanning software commonly uses one or more of the following methods:

- Ping sweep
- SNMP sweep
- TCP/UDP port scans
- Scanning logon accounts

Approaching the millennium, I performed a global scan for a company using an SNMP sweep program. The objective was to ensure that all network devices were running at a compliant release of software. This was surprisingly easy and I even ended up accidentally scanning some devices outside the perimeter of our network that were inside the carrier's network. Incidentally, one device in their network was not Y2K-compliant and was upgraded on our request!

Network Topology

Shared networks are easier to eavesdrop on, as all traffic is visible from everywhere on that shared media. Switched networks, on the other hand, are more secure as, by default, there is no single viewpoint for traffic: An intruder would have to take action such as CAM table flooding, ARP cache poisoning, or route table corruption to see the packets.

Luckily, this topology does not forbid the use of IDS appliances. On Cisco Catalyst switches there is a feature where you can mirror traffic from VLANs or switch ports to a single designated switch port called the span port. Once you plug your IDS into the span port, you can easily view traffic in different VLANs by making configuration changes, allowing analysis of LAN traffic.

Configuring & Implementing…

Deploying a Cisco IDS 4230 in a LAN

The Cisco IDS 4230 is a standalone appliance used to monitor high-speed networks. In a modern switched environment, the interesting task is to see enough traffic. If you just drop the sensor interface into an unused port, you will see no traffic!

There are several approaches. One technique is to use dedicated hardware, such as a Shomiti Tap, which acts like a "mini hub" so you can monitor critical interfaces, such as areas just before a router, switch uplink, or key server.

Another technique is to use the Switched Port Analyzer (SPAN) port feature. The technique is to configure the switch with a span port combining the networks you want to monitor. The 4230 sensor interface is then plugged into the SPAN port. The problem with this is that if someone reconfigures the switch, your probe ceases to function! In that environment, it is important to verify strong change control over the LAN switch configurations, and to monitor for unexpected loss of traffic at the probe.

Unattended Modems

Installing a modem on a PC for remote access allows a quick and easy way to access the network from home. Unfortunately, this also means that the modem and PC may be prone to attack when you are not there. Detecting modems attached to PCs can be done using host auditing systems, or via network auditing systems that have direct access to the host (for instance, by inspecting the registry hive, or reviewing route tables) but this is a complex task. A better approach is to use POTS auditing software: A "war dialer" that periodically reviews all owned phone numbers to look for carriers. The problem with this approach is that the user could configure "ring back" approaches, so that the modem doesn't pick up on the first few rings. This way the war dialer would fail.

In such cases, technical controls are not the best solution: Instead use cooperation with the user community. If access is essential, you should explain the benefits of employing the (secure) corporate remote access solution instead.

Poor Physical Security

Simple measures can be taken in the physical world to ensure better security for your systems. Locking your doors is obviously a good commonsense start, but there are often a number of straightforward procedures and safeguards that companies could perform and implement that, for one reason or another, they do not.

I recently read an article in the Cisco's Packet magazine that described a theft in the Redwood City, California office of VISA of a file server that contained over 300,000 credit card numbers. The thief just unplugged the server and walked out with it. A simple tagging system would have done the trick, as alarms would have sounded when the machine was removed; even a paper authorization system would have worked. After all, it's pretty simple to bypass security on routers and switches if you can get to the console port, or in the case of servers you can remove the hard disks and reinstall them elsewhere.

Microsoft, in its Ten Immutable Laws, captures this as law number three: "If a bad guy has unrestricted physical access to your computer, it's not your computer anymore."

Application and Operating Software Weaknesses

In this context, software is a term that describes the operating system as well as the packages that run under its control. Most commercial software is, or has been, deficient at some point in its life due to poor programming compounded by commercial pressures to release software early, before it is debugged completely.

Software Bugs

Software bugs can be characterized into one of several types. The BugTraq classification scheme recognizes nine types: *boundary condition errors* (which includes buffer overflows), *access validation errors* (errors in trust), *input validation errors* (poor defensive programming), *failure to handle exceptional conditions* (more poor programming), *race conditions, serialization errors, atomicity errors* (belief that things will happen "all at once" when they might happen in stages), *environment errors*, and *configuration errors*.

Getting Passwords—Easy Ways of Cracking Programs

Most people, at some point or other, have created a simple password based on objects that are easy to remember, such as a name or favorite color. In 10 of the 15 companies I've worked for, good password management practices were rarely enforced.

It's quite simple to get someone else's password; many times, all you have to do is ask. Some other ways passwords might be obtained are:

- "Shoulder surfing," observation over the shoulder.

- Gaining access to password files.

- Using a sniffer or Trojan software to look for cleartext passwords.

- Replaying logon traffic recorded on a sniffer that contains the encrypted password.

- Dictionary-based attacks, where a software program runs through every word in a dictionary database.

- Brute force attacks, where the attacker runs a program that tries variations of letters, numbers, and common words in the hope of getting the right combination. Typical programs can try around 100,000 combinations per minute.

Human Failure

Henry Ford once said, "If there is any one secret of success, it lies in the ability to get the other person's point of view and see things from that person's angle as well as from your own."

Everyone is an individual; we all have our own thoughts, feelings, and moods. Of course, the human failure factor spans far and wide across the security spectrum and is usually a common contributing cause for security breaches. These can be caused as a result of malicious motives or innocent mistakes.

Poorly Configured Systems

The very first time I configured a Cisco router on a network I used the default password *cisco*. If anyone had decided to choose that router to attack they could have logged on, looked at the routing tables, reloaded the router (causing user disruption), or changed the password.

Many new systems when taken out of the box use default accounts or passwords that are easy to obtain. Most allow you to decide whether or not to use security features without any objections. In brief, systems are poorly configured because of:

- A lack of thought during configuration
- Insufficient time to configure the product properly
- Poor knowledge of the product

Information Leaks

Rather than a sinister individual "leaking" information to the outside, this is usually a little more straightforward. You may have seen security personal identification numbers (PINs), passwords in diaries or written on post-it notes. The list is long and an absolute feast for a nocturnal attacker wandering around the office late at night. Not shredding sensitive documents and drawings can also be a risky practice. If someone gets hold of the network diagram, they can start targeting devices and choosing points for maximum impact.

One time I was sitting in an open office one day when the LAN administrator was asked by a colleague from across the room what the supervisor account password was—he shouted it back to him. Need I say more?

Malicious Users

For various reasons, people will carry out malicious attacks or intrusions on your network—for example, downloading all customer account information onto a laptop, which can then be removed from the building. Such things are, obviously, bad for business.

Weaknesses in the IP Suite of Protocols

When most of the TCP/IP family of protocols were originally developed, the world was a nicer place; perhaps, back then, there was no need for the security we have today. Nowadays, however, it is possible for you to stroll into a bookshop and pick up a volume on how to crack a network. The success of the Internet unfortunately ensures that this type of information is readily available.

The TCP/IP stack is code written by programmers/developers, and as such, it is probable that some implementations will contain errors. If the implementation of TCP/IP is poor, then the system can be compromised in spite of the upper-layer applications being used.

Taking advantage of these weaknesses requires an in-depth knowledge of TCP/IP protocols. Flaws exploited by attackers are being countered by software developers and then recountered by attackers again.

One example of improvement is IPSec, which is an addition to the IP protocol suite. IPSec provides privacy and authentication methods creating traffic security on a network.

NOTE

Although we have discussed TCP/IP weaknesses in this section, application programs can also be poorly written or badly designed in the way that they interface with the lower-layer protocols. Bad application software can provide the attacker with a foothold to penetrate a system.

Conversely, a server running well-written applications with solid code but using a bad TCP/IP implementation can still be compromised since the application relies on the TCP/IP stack for network services.

Any member of the TCP/IP suite can be the target of an attack. Some have flaws that are easier to exploit by the cracker than others.

Layer 7 Attacks

The next sections highlight some examples of the more common attacks to date; for the purpose of our discussion, I've assumed that an Attacker (station C) can see traffic returning from its victims (stations A and B). In practice, this may not be the case, but the attack can still succeed nevertheless—it just takes a little more skill on their part. For each type of attack, I've tried to list the URL of the related CERT document for you to read.

SMTP Attacks

Simple Mail Transport Protocol (SMTP) has been used to send mail using a wide variety of mail programs, and for many years has been the e-mail standard of the Internet. A common method of attack is the buffer overrun where the attacker enters a larger number of characters in an e-mail field than expected by the e-mail server. The extra characters contain executable code that is run by the e-mail server following an error in the application. The code then facilitates further cracking. Installing the latest security patches for the e-mail system may avoid this kind of attack.

It is good practice to use digital signatures and cryptography techniques in cases where sensitive information is to be sent across shared networks. These methods can offer you excellent protection when it comes to the confidentiality and integrity of information. Digital signatures, for their part, will ensure that each message is signed and verified, while encryption techniques will make certain the mail content is viewable only by the intended receiving e-mail address. Details of these types of attack can be found at: www.cert.org/tech_tips/email_spoofing.html and www.cert.org/advisories/CA-97.05.sendmail.html

SMTP Spam

Spam is defined as unsolicited commercial e-mail (UCE). Internet service providers can restrict spamming by the implementation of rules that govern the number of destination addresses allowed for a single message. For further information, see www.cert.org/tech_tips/e-mail_bombing_spamming.html.

FTP

Anonymous connections to servers running the FTP process allow the attacking station C to download a virus, overwrite a file, or abuse trusts that the FTP server has in the same domain.

FTP attacks are best avoided by preventing anonymous logins, stopping unused services on the server, as well as creating router access lists and firewall rules. If you require the use of anonymous logons, the best course of action is to update the FTP software to the latest revision and keep an eye on related advisories. It's probably a good idea to adopt a general policy of regular checks of advisories for all software you are responsible for protecting. For further information, visit www.cert.org/advisories/CA-93.10.anonymous.FTP.activity.html.

SNMP

The Simple Network Management Protocol (SNMP) has recently been in the news for having vulnerability in ASN encoding that allowed for its compromise on essentially every implementation, including Cisco's. The basic problem is that SNMP is an unauthenticated (and because it is based upon UDP) easily spoofed service. Using *SNMP get* queries, it is possible to gain detailed information about a device. Armed with this information, the cracker can facilitate further types of attack. By using *SNMP set* queries, it is also possible to change the values of Managed Information Base (MIB) instances. In particular, one SNMP set will cause a router configuration to be written to a server, while another SNMP set will download a new configuration from a server. SNMP, and *SNMP set* in particular, are dangerous protocols, meaning access to SNMP should be carefully controlled.

Layer 3 and Layer 4 Attacks

These occur at the Network and Transport layers of the OSI model. Here are some examples of the more common attacks to date.

TCP SYN Flooding

This is best described in stages:

1. Station C sends lots of SYN packets to station B in rapid succession from nonexistent host addresses.

2. B sends back SYN/ACKs and maintains the half-opened connections in a queue as it waits for ACKs from the nonexistent hosts at the source addresses.

3. B runs out of resources waiting for ACKs back from nonexistent hosts.

4. At this point, B drops legitimate connections and is likely to hang/crash.

There is no widely accepted solution for this problem. On Cisco routers, it is possible to configure TCP Intercept that protects against SYN Floods.

TCP Intercept Configurations

This section covers the TCP Intercept feature available on Cisco routers that have Cisco Secure IS (Firewall Feature Set) installed. Here's how you configure it:

1. Make certain you have the necessary IOS Firewall Feature Set installed.

2. Create an extended access list where the source is "any" and designate internal networks to protect against SYN flooding attack.

3. In global configuration mode, enter the command:

   ```
   ip tcp intercept list <access-list number>
   ```

4. Choose what mode you want to operate in. If you don't specify it, it will be in intercept mode. In watch mode, the router "watches" TCP connection requests, if they do not become established within 30 seconds, the router sends a TCP RST to the receiving station, thus allowing it to free its resources. When operating in intercept mode, the router acts as a

"middle man" in the TCP handshake. It will keep the original SYN request, and respond back to the originator with a SYN/ACK pending the final ACK. Once this happens, the router sends the original SYN and performs a three-way handshake with the destination, it then drops out of the way allowing direct communications between source and destination. To choose the mode, enter the command:

```
ip tcp intercept mode [intercept|watch ]
```

TCP intercept will monitor for the number of incomplete connections. When this figure goes over 1100, or if a "surge" of over 1100 connections is received within 60 seconds, the router deletes the oldest connection request (like a conveyor belt) and reduces TCP retransmission time by 50 percent. This "aggressive" behavior can be adjusted to fit security policy. For further information on TCP SYN flooding, visit www.cert.org/advisories/ CA-96.21.tcp_syn_flooding.html.

Smurf Spoofing Attack

This is based on IP spoofing where multiple broadcast pings are sent out by station C with victim A's IP address as the source. A could be overwhelmed with ICMP response packets. Recommended solutions are:

- To disable IP-directed broadcasts at the router by entering the global command *no ip directed-broadcast* in the router configuration.

- If possible, to configure the operating system not to respond to broadcast pings. For more information, go to: www.cert.org/advisories/CA-98.01.smurf.html.

- Use the global command *ip verify unicast reverse-path* on the router. This will match the routing entries in the Cisco Express Forwarding (CEF) table against the source IP addresses of incoming packets. If there is no route back out of the interface, then the router drops the packet. This will only work if CEF is enabled on the router.

- Use Committed Access Rate (CAR) on the Cisco routers to limit the inbound levels of ICMP traffic. Note that CAR configurations can also reduce the amount of SYN traffic to help against SYN flooding and DDoS Attacks (discussed later in this section).

TCP/IP Sequence Number Spoofing/Session Hijacking

Let's imagine C wants to spoof B into thinking it is A.

1. Station C initiates a denial of service (DoS) attack on A and then impersonates A by spoofing its IP address. The purpose of this is to prevent the real A from interfering with the attack.

2. C initiates a connection to B and tries to guess the sequence number from frames it has sniffed.

3. If B is fooled into believing C is actually A, then data will flow freely between the two.

Older TCP/IP implementations increment SEQ numbers in a predictable manner that makes the exchange easier to intercept and spoof.

NOTE

Modern TCP/IP implementations are able to take advantage of a SYN "cookie." The idea is to eliminate the TCP_RCVD state, thus avoiding the problems of resource starvation in that state. The technique is to delay creation of the TCB until the third packet of the handshake (the final ACK) is received. This is done by responding to the initial SYN with a secure one-way hash as the sequence number, allowing for detection of bogus ACKs.

Hijack attacks from outside the network can be prevented by applying an access list to the WAN interfaces of the company router. This would prevent traffic with internal source addresses from being accepted from the outside. This type of filtering is known as input filtering and does not protect against attempts to hijack connections between hosts inside the network.

Another access list to prevent unknown source addresses from leaving the internal network should also be applied. This is to prevent attacks to outside networks from within the company. For more information on spoofing and session hijacking, visit www.cert.org/advisories/CA-95.01.IP.spoofing.attacks.and .hijacked.terminal.connections.html.

Denial of Service Type Attacks

In DoS attacks, a victim is unable to provide services due to all its resources being consumed. This is caused by a weakness in the implementation of an application, prompting its failure, or when a victim is overwhelmed by attack traffic.

Ping of Death

The ping of death attack takes advantage of the inability of poor IP implementations to cope with abnormally large IP packets. In this example, ICMP packets transmitted by the attacking station exceed 65535 bytes (the maximum IP packet size). The packet is then fragmented and the receiving station fails the reassembly process, and thereby crashes or hangs.

Several vendors have released software patches to overcome this problem. For more information, see www.cert.org/advisories/CA-1996-26.html.

Teardrop Attack

A teardrop attack targets a specific weakness in some TCP/IP implementations where the reassembly fails to work correctly because incorrect offset values are injected into IP traffic. The attack is based on the same principle as the Ping of Death attack.

The Land Attack

The land attack spoofs IP types. Here's how it works:

1. C sends a SYN packet to B using B's IP address, along with identical source and destination port numbers.

2. B is never able to complete this connection and may go into an infinite loop.

3. If B is susceptible to this type of attack, it will hang or crash.

The recommended solution is to install vendor patches. For Land attacks, it is also advisable to install input filters to combat IP spoofing. For more information, visit www.cert.org/advisories/CA-97.28.Teardrop_Land.html.

Distributed Denial of Service Attacks

Recently, distributed denial of service (DDoS) attacks have become more common. Typical tools used by attackers are Trinoo, TFN, TFN2K and Stacheldraht ("barbed wire" in German). How does a DDoS attack work? The attacker gains access to a Client PC. From there, the cracker can use tools to send commands to the nodes. These nodes then flood or send malformed packets to the victim.

Coordinated traceroutes from several sources are used to probe the same target to construct a table of routes for the network. This information is then used as the basis for further attacks.

So what makes it so nasty? In practice, there may be thousands of nodes, meaning billions of packets can be directed at the victim, taking up all available bandwidth and perhaps causing DoS.

At present, there is no solution to the problem, nor is it easy to trace the attack origin.

A list of general suggestions is as follows:

- Prevent initial compromise of the client through good security practice.

- Keep software up to date with patches and upgrades.

- Keep all antivirus software up to date.

- Run desktop firewall software where available.

- Install and activate the Cisco IDS.

Cisco also suggests the following recommendations:

- Use the *ip verify unicast reverse-path* global command (discussed earlier).

- Use ACLs to block inbound private address range traffic.

- Use input filtering (discussed earlier).

- Use CAR to limit inbound ICMP and SYN packets.

For more information, visit www.cert.org/advisories/CA-99-17-denial-of-service-tools.html and www.cert.org/reports/dsit_workshop.pdf. For more details on Cisco's recommendations, check out www.cisco.com/warp/public/707/newsflash.html#prevention.

The Cisco Secure Network Intrusion Detection System

NetRanger was originally developed by Wheelgroup, Inc. but is now owned by Cisco Systems. We will tackle this product by dividing it into five sections—overview, managing probe setup, configuration, management, and the dedicated IOS product.

What Is the Cisco Secure Network Intrusion Detection System?

This is a solution that can be added to your network to perform dynamic intrusion detection. Cisco Secure IDS will monitor for, and respond to, intrusions in real time. A simple IDS solution is made up of a distributed model with three main components: the probe, the Director, and the CSPM.

The Probe

The probe is a specialized device that uses a rule-based inference engine to process large volumes of traffic in order to identify security issues in real time. The probe is either a ready-made appliance purchased from Cisco, or it can be software-based and installed on a Windows x86 (the Catalyst 6000 IDS module) or SPARC Solaris station (the IDS 4230 and IDS 4210). The software to create your own probe can be found on the IDS CD, and can either capture traffic itself or monitor syslog traffic from a Cisco router. Once an attack or security event is detected, the probe can respond by generating alarms, logging the event, resetting TCP connections or *shunning* the attack (by reconfiguration of managed router ACLs). Probe events are forwarded to a central facility via a control/command interface.

Probes have two interfaces, one for monitoring and one for control. The monitoring interface of the probe does not have an IP address and will not respond to Layer 3 detection attempts. There are several types of monitor interfaces available from Cisco, each selected for a particular network scenario. An example is the IDS 4230 Sensor, which is capable of supporting LAN speeds of up to 100 Mbps LAN or T3 WAN speeds. Another is the Catalyst 6000 IDS module that is designed for switched networks.

The Director

The Director is a GUI software solution used to "direct" or manage Cisco IDS from a HP OpenView platform. It is installed on a HP UX or Solaris workstation. Directors are used to complete initial probe configuration, process and present information sent from sensors (in HP OpenView) and specify sensor behavior. The Director contains drivers for the Oracle RDBMS and the Remedy Trouble Ticket system. It is possible to modify these drivers to interface with Sybase or Informix systems, if required. When the Director receives information from the probes it will initially log to a flat file and then push the data to a relational database. Once stored in the database, RDBMS tools such as SQL can be used to interrogate the data. Database details such as location of files and account information have to be configured using the nrConfigure utility (discussed later in this chapter). Systems such as Oracle contain tools to generate reports containing graphical as well as numerical representation of data. To get you started, each Director ships with a sample set of SQL queries that can be easily modified and run from within your RDBMS system. It is possible to define custom actions based on events, too (this is covered in more detail later in this section). The Director also provides you with access to the NSDB for reference material on exploits.

The Cisco Secure Policy Manager

The Cisco Secure Policy Manager is a Windows-based GUI software solution that can also manage Cisco IDS. It is installed on a modern Windows NT platform. The software is very memory sensitive—specifications call for 0.5GB, but more is better. Because of the native Windows environment, it is easy for an analyst to explore the alerts generated by the platform.

Because the CSPM is documented in Chapter 12, this chapter will go over configuration and management using the Director platform.

NOTE

Cisco recommends that no more than 25 probes be configured to send information to a single Director. Cisco suggests between three and six Probes be configured per CSPM. If more probes are required for your network, you should install multiple CSPM/Directors and build a hierarchical structure of probes and Directors.

The Post Office

The Post Office is a messaging facility between management stations and sensors that uses a proprietary UDP transport protocol for communication. Rather than being unacknowledged, the protocol guarantees transmissions, maintains connection status and provides acknowledgement for packets received with lower overhead than TCP/IP. It uses an enhanced addressing structure that is ideal for building hierarchical fault-tolerant structures. Up to 255 alternate routes between each probe and its Director can be supported. The structures are comprised of multiple Directors and probes; in this way, you can support a theoretically unlimited number of probes. Probes can forward updates onto one or more Directors which can then propagate the message to other Directors in the hierarchy.

NOTE

If you need to perform any traffic filtering on routers between Directors and probes (control interfaces), you must allow traffic using UDP port 45000 to pass between the two.

Figure 13.1 shows these basic components in context.

Figure 13.1 IDS Protocols and Associated Components

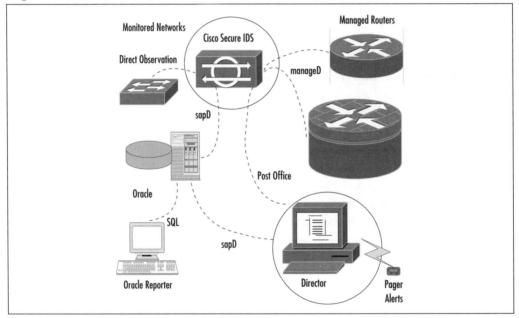

You can see the IDS components with the main daemons that are responsible for running the system. Each daemon performs a specific function, which is explained in more detail next:

- **sensord/packetd** Sensord is used to relay intrusion detection information sent from other devices capable of detecting attacks and sending data; packetd is used when the sensor itself does the intrusion detection.

- **loggerd** Used to write to log files and record events such as alarms and command instructions.

- **sapd** Provides file and data management functions, including the transfer of data to database systems such as Oracle.

- **postofficed** Manages and provides all communications between the Director and probes.

- **eventd** Performs notification management on events to pager and e-mail systems.

- **managed** Controls configuration of managed Cisco routers.

Here are some other daemons not displayed on the diagram:

- **smid** A Director daemon that converts raw information into data that ndirmap uses.

- **nrdirmap** Displays icons for NetRanger components and events such as alarms and status conditions for other daemons.

- **configd** Interprets and manages commands entered through ndirmap to interface with the other daemons.

Now we understand the components, let's discuss some of the more general features. Cisco Secure IDS is a network-based IDS system that captures packets and then performs signature analysis using an inferencing engine. The analysis involves examination of each packet's payload for content-based attacks and the examination of the header for patterns of misuse. Cisco Secure IDS classifies the types of attacks into two types: atomic (single, directed at one victim) and composite (multiple, over a period of time and involving many victims).

The Director uses an internal (upgradeable) security database (NSDB) for signature analysis, which provides information about exploits and matching countermeasures. There are two types of signatures, embedded and string matching. As the name suggests, embedded signatures are contained within the probe's system files; they cannot be modified and protect against misuse by matches against the packet header fields. String matching signatures, on the other hand, are user configurable and work by examining the payload of the packet. A description of how to do this is included later in this section.

Before You Install

It is imperative you spend time thinking out your Cisco Secure IDS design. Without this, it may end up being ineffective. You should consider all connections from your network to the outside, as well as the volumes and types of traffic in use. Also, if your network is large, perhaps multinational in nature, then you may want to consider internal boundaries. You should decide how many probes are required to monitor the network effectively.

Probes have two interfaces, one for data collection and the other, the control interface, which is used for remote communication (always Ethernet-based). The placement of the probe is important in order to protect the control port and to "sense" correctly.

Director placement is also important. It is a focal point and compromise could have serious consequences. The Director must be easily accessible for security staff yet be physically secure (in other words, protected on the network—perhaps through a firewall), and still be able to communicate with its probes.

Director and Probe Setup

Here are the minimum requirements for Director installation; the amount of RAM required varies depending on the configuration.

HP UX 10.20 (with HP OpenView 4.1) requires 125MB disk space for software directories, whereas Sun Solaris 2.5.1 or 2.6 requires 172MB. Both platforms require 1GB disk space for logging, 96MB RAM, a CD drive, a TCP/IP-enabled network card, and a current HTML browser.

Next, we will investigate how to install and configure the Director and probe. Let's start with the Director installation procedure for Unix.

Director Installation

Once you have decided on where you want to place the Director, and you have a workstation that meets the minimum system requirements, we can power up and begin the installation.

1. Log in as **root** on the chosen Director station.

2. Check that the date and time are correct.

3. Ensure /usr/sbin is in the PATH.

4. Enter **/etc/set_parms initial** and restart the machine.

5. Configure the IP address, subnet mask, default gateway, and hostname.

6. Install HP OpenView.

7. Add these lines to the root profile (watch the space between . and /)

```
.  /opt/OV/bin/ov.envvars.sh
PATH=$PATH:$OV_BIN
```

8. Modify semaphores to read:

```
semmns - 256, semmni - 128, semmnu - 90, semume - 20
```

9. Now, restart the machine.

10. Insert the Cisco Secure IDS CD into the drive and exit OpenView.

11. From the CD type **./install**. Follow the onscreen instructions and lastly restart the machine again.

Director Configuration

So, now that we have completed the basic installation of NetRanger, we must perform the following steps to configure it:

1. Log in as **netrangr**.

2. Stop all services by typing **nrstop** at the prompt.

3. Start configuration by typing **sysconfig–director**.

4. Enter all Director information, Host ID & Name, Organization ID & Name, and the IP address.

5. Exit sysconfig-director and then type **nrstart** at the prompt to restart services.

Probe Installation

Once the Director base configuration is complete, you should already know where you want to place your probe. Probe installation and configuration is done using a program called sysconfig-sensor. Here's how it works:

1. Connect all cables, and attach the probe to the network where required.

2. Sign on as **root** and enter **sysconfig-sensor** at the prompt.

3. A menu will appear where you can enter values for the IP address, subnet mask, default gateway and hostname. Figure 13.2 shows how it should look.

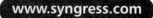

Figure 13.2 The Sysconfig-sensor Menu

```
#sysconfig-sensor

NetRanger Sensor Initial Configuration Utility

Choose a value to configure one of the following parameters:

1 - IP Address
2 - IP Netmask
3 - IP Hostname
4 - Default Route
5 - Network Access Control
6 - Netranger Communications Infrastructure
7 - System Date, Time and Timezone
8 - Passwords
x - Exit


Selection:
```

4. Connect a terminal server to the COM1 port for out of band access.

5. Using option 5, define IP addresses that are allowed to Telnet or perform file transfers to the probe.

6. Using option 6, set the Probe Host and Organization details. The corresponding Director details must also be entered.

7. Exit sysconfig-sensor and restart the Sensor device.

8. Using Unix system administration tools, modify the *netrangr* password. By default, the password is *attack*.

Completing the Probe Installation

We have almost finished. All that remains is to relate the Director and probe configurations together. Here are the steps required:

1. On the Director station, select **Security, Configure**.

2. Select **File | Add Host**, choose **Next**.

3. Enter the probe details in the next screen, select **Next**.

4. Choose **Add New Sensor Reporting To This Director**.

5. Next, enter Shunning preferences—the amount of time to wait before shun and how long to log for.

6. Enter the probe interface performing the data collection (for example, **/dev/spwr0** for Ethernet).

7. Select **Add** and then choose the IP subnets the probe is protecting.

8. The next screen is optional. Here you can enter details of a Cisco router managed by the probe.

9. Select **Next** and then **Finish.**

General Operation

The Director runs under HP OpenView. The top-level icon is **NetRanger**, which once double-clicked, shows submaps containing NetRanger nodes. As more Directors and probes are configured, these will also become visible. Each submap can represent different security regions across the company. Once you select the Director or probe icon, the application daemons running on that machine are displayed. These can be selected in turn to show alarm icons generated by each. Each type of icon describes a different classification of attack based on the signatures found in the NSDB.

From HP OpenView, selecting the **Security** option displays further NetRanger options. Some of the more significant are:

- **Show** (select icon first) Provides information on devices, configuration, alarms, the NSDB, and others.

- **Configure** (select sensor first) Starts *nrConfigure*, which is used to configure probes and Directors.

- **Network Device** (select device first) Starts the *network device configuration* utility.

- **Shun** (select alarm first) Allows you to shun devices and networks.

- **Advanced** (select probe first) Allows various options; one of the most useful is the *Statistics, Show* option.

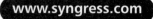

nrConfigure

When started, nrConfigure shows information regarding the device selected. You can configure communications, notification information, setup device management, log policy violations, configure shunning, and perform intrusion detection. Here are some examples of how to use nrConfigure:

Configuring Logging from a Router to a Sensor

On the router in privileged exec mode, enter global configuration mode and type these lines:

```
logging <ip address of Sensor control interface>
logging trap info
```

Modify your access list entries to include the *log* extension where required. This completes half of the configuration; the next step is to configure the probe. To do this:

1. In HP OpenView, highlight the probe.

2. From nrConfigure, select **Configure**, then select **Intrusion Detection**, **Data Sources**, and **Add**.

3. Enter the IP address of the sending router, then select **Profile**, **check the Manual box**, and **Modify Sensor**.

4. Pull down and select **Security Violations**.

5. Choose the ACL, choose the level of severity, and then select **Apply**.

Syslog traffic between the router and the probe is sent in the clear; if any networks the traffic traverses is untrusted, then this constitutes a security risk and should be avoided at all costs.

Configuring Intrusion Detection on Sensors

This can be done by using manual- or profile-based methods. The manual method allows you to configure individual signatures with complete control over configuration, whereas the profile-based one only allows selection of predefined groups of signatures. You would probably use profiles if you were integrating new signatures following a software upgrade.

Highlight the probe you wish to configure, then select one of the following methods for configuration:

1. **Profile-based** Select **Configure, Intrusion Detection, Profile,** then choose the **Profile-based** radio button, **Response.** You can then set the type of **Response,** disable Signatures, if required, or choose the **View Sensor button** to view settings. Once complete, select **OK** in the **Signatures box** and then **OK.**

2. **Manual-based** Select **Configure, Intrusion Detection, Profile** then choose the **Manual radio button.** Now choose **Modify Probe.** From the General Signatures box, configure corresponding actions. Select **OK** and choose **OK** again to exit.

By selecting **Configure | Intrusion Detection | Protected Networks tab** you can set up networks upon which you wish to perform IP packet logging using the probe.

Customizing the NSDB

This is useful for protection against vulnerabilities that are not defined in the NSDB. You can create an NSDB record that the inference engine will use as part of its analysis. Custom signatures can also be used to track host and port usage for general information. For example, you might want to look for a particular string inside the content of the packet.

Here are the steps involved in adding your own signature to the NSDB to look for the string "do not ftp" in an FTP session and then perform a session reset.

1. On the Director station, select the probe then choose **Security | Configure.**

2. Select **Intrusion Detection | Profile.**

3. Select **Manual Configuration | Modify Sensor.**

4. Choose **Matched Strings** from the **Expand** scroll box**.**

5. Select **Add,** then enter **do not ftp** in the **String** column.

6. Enter a unique ID for the signature.

7. Enter port **20** for FTP data.

8. To specify the direction, select **To & From.**

9. Enter the **Occurrences** as **1** to specify a condition to initiate an action.

10. Specify the **Action** as **Reset** and enter **5** in the destination.

11. Select **OK,** then **OK,** and finally, choose **Apply.**

The new rule will reset any FTP connections where the data contains one occurrence of the words "do not ftp" and will send out level 5 alarms to all configured logging destinations.

Upgrading the NSDB

To upgrade the NSDB, you must have a valid CCO logon. Download instructions for the NSDB file can be found at www.cisco.com by searching for "Cisco Secure IDS Update" then following instructions in the update readme file.

The Data Management Package

The Data Management Package (DMP) is contained within Cisco Secure IDS and performs two functions: 1) The collection of data in flat file logs; and 2) The manipulation of data into a relational database file format to facilitate Oracle SQL analysis (on the normalized data).

You can configure these options through *nrConfigure* and the *Data Management* options on the Director. It is possible to create triggers for execution on condition, determining log file size, and other settings. The DMP contains a basic set of SQL reports that provide detail on attack signatures with dates and times. What other components do we need to make this work? Oracle server will have to be installed either remotely or locally. It must reference the NetRanger data. Using nrConfigure, tokens must be created to allow the Oracle server access. Further details of this can be found at www.cisco.com/univercd/cc/td/doc/product/iaabu/netrangr/nr220/nr220ug/rdbms.htm#27755. Once viewable from Oracle, you can either use native scripts or third-party tools to manage the data, create graphs, and draw correlations to highlight specific areas.

An E-mail Notification Example

First of all, you must configure event notification. To do so:

1. In HP OpenView, select **Configure | Security** then **Event Processing**.

2. Select the **Application tab**.

3. Add a severity level to execute a script, and then reference the script. Enter the path to **/bin/eventd/event** in the script name field.

4. Select the **Timing option** and set the thresholds of events which will trigger the script and the interleave between sampling the event data.

5. Select **OK**, then ensure that **Daemons**, **nr.eventd** has a status of **Yes**. Select **OK**.

6. Configure the probe to send notifications to eventd. Select **Destinations** from **nrConfigure** then **Add**.

7. Enter the probe ID. Choose the application of eventd and a security level required to send the notification. Lastly, select the type of event to act upon.

8. Select **Event Processing | E-mail**.

9. Enter the Organization ID, the Type of event, and the Severity Level to trigger the mail.

10. Enter the e-mail addresses of the person(s) you wish to notify, then select **OK**.

The next time the event occurs, an e-mail notification will be sent.

NOTE

Whenever a change is made to the system using nrConfigure, it is advisable to use nrstop and nrstart to restart the services.

Cisco IOS Intrusion Detection Systems

This is one feature that puts the Cisco solution "streets ahead" of the competition because intrusion detection is integrated into the router IOS. Any traffic that passes through the router can be scrutinized for intrusions. The router acts as a probe checking for intrusions in a similar fashion to a Cisco Secure IDS Sensor device.

IOS IDS is useful to install at network perimeters, such as intranet/extranet borders or branch office routers. You may decide to deploy this method of intrusion detection where a Cisco Secure IDS Sensor is not financially viable or where a reduced set of signatures to be checked will suffice. Despite not having the same level of granularity during signature identification, and checking against a much smaller signature base than Cisco Secure IDS, it is still capable of detecting severe breaches of security, reconnaissance scans, and common network attacks. The signatures it uses constitute a broad cross section selected from the NSDB. IOS IDS will protect against 59 different types of network intrusions. It is possible to disable checking for individual signatures through modification of the router config in order to avoid false positives. The signatures can be categorized into two main types: *Info* and *Attack*. Info refers to reconnaissance scans for information gathering, and Attack refers to DoS or other intrusions. Each type can also be further divided into atomic (directed at an individual station) or compound (directed at a group of stations perhaps over an extended period of time).

IOS IDS is fully compatible with Cisco Secure IDS and can appear as an icon on the Director GUI. The router can send alarms back to a syslog server, a Cisco Secure IDS sensor, or take action by dropping unwanted packets or terminating TCP/IP sessions. Dropping packets happens transparently without the router interacting with end stations, but session termination does involve the router sending a TCP RST to source and destination devices; it is usually best to use both these actions together when configuring the router.

One important consideration is that of the impact of IOS IDS on the router. This will vary depending upon the specification of the router, the number of signatures configured, and how busy the router is. The most significant impact on the router is caused by audit rules that refer to Access Control Lists. It is probably a good idea to keep an eye on the router memory by using the *sh proc mem* command from the privileged exec prompt after configuration.

Unlike Cisco Secure IDS, IOS IDS (as the name suggests), contains the signatures within the image. For future updates to the IOS IDS signature base, the image on the router flash has to be upgraded. It is not possible to modify or add new signatures to the existing set, which is a useful feature available on Cisco Secure IDS (discussed in the previous section).

We can divide our discussion of IOS IDS into two main sections: Configuring Cisco IOS IDS features and associated commands.

Configuring Cisco IOS IDS Features

Configuration begins by initializing the IOS IDS software and then creating audit rules to specify signatures and associated actions. Rules can be applied inbound or outbound on the router interfaces. The audit rule command *ip audit* has the following extensions available:

- **smtp spam** Sets e-mail spamming restrictions.

- **po** Employed for all Post Office configurations when using a Cisco Secure IDS Director.

- **notify** Sends event information to syslog servers or a Cisco Secure IDS Director.

- **info** Specifies the action on a reconnaissance scan.

- **attack** Specifies the action to take when an attack is detected.

- **name** Specifies the name of the rule; also used to apply the rule to an interface.

- **signature** Disables individual signatures and sources of false alarms.

- **po protected** Selects which interfaces are to be protected by the router.

To investigate these commands further, we can look at an example based upon the scenario shown in Figure 13.3.

Figure13.3 The Secure IS (IOS IDS) Configuration Scenario

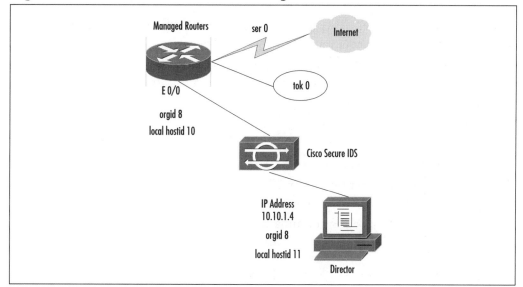

Here is the configuration for Figure 13.3:

```
ip audit smtp spam 50
ip audit po max-events 20
ip audit notify nr-director
ip audit po local hostid 10 orgid 8
ip audit po remote hostid 11 orgid 8 rmtaddress 10.10.1.4 localaddress
10.10.1.3 port-number 32000 application director
ip audit info action alarm
ip audit attack action alarm drop reset
ip audit name TEST info list 3 action alarm
```

```
ip audit name TEST attack list 3 action alarm reset drop
interface e 0/0
        ip address 10.10.1.3 255.255.0.0
        ip audit TEST in
interface tokenring 0
        ip address 11.1.3.1 255.255.255.0
        access-list 3 deny 11.1.3.1 0.0.0.255
ip audit po protected 10.10.0.0 to 10.10.255.254
```

Our objective is to protect the Ethernet network from attackers from the untrusted Internet. The example assumes that a NetRanger Director is present and that there is a trusted token ring network also attached to the router. The configuration displayed shows a subsection of commands from the router configuration.

Let's describe the commands in turn:

```
ip audit smtp spam 50
```

This sets a threshold of 50 recipients in an e-mail to denote a spam e-mail.

```
ip audit po max-events 20
```

This defines that 20 entries can be queued up for sending to the Director; above this value, events will be dropped. You need to be careful when using this command as each queue entry uses 32KB of RAM; you can monitor levels of RAM using the *show proc mem* command.

```
ip audit notify nr-director
```

This configures the Cisco Secure IDS Director as the destination for the alarms.

```
ip audit po local hostid 10 orgid 8
```

This defines the local router's Post Office details. hostid is unique, and orgid is the same as the Cisco Secure IDS Director group.

```
ip audit po remote hostid 11 orgid 8 rmtaddress 10.10.1.4 localaddress
    10.10.1.3 port-number 32000 application director
```

This is the same as the previous command but defines the Cisco Secure IDS Director hostid as 11, the Director orgid as 8, the IP address for the Director, the router's IP address, the UDP port the Director is listening on as 32000, and the type of application being used as Director (*logger* would be used in this field if logging to a syslog server).

Note that the router has to be reloaded after all Post Office config changes.

```
ip audit info action alarm
```

The default response to take on an information signature is to send an alarm.

```
ip audit attack action alarm drop reset
```

The default response to take on an attack signature is to send an alarm, drop the packet, and reset the audited session.

```
ip audit name TEST info list 3 action alarm
```

This defines an audit rule called TEST where traffic permitted by access list 3 will be processed and an alarm will be raised on an information signature match.

```
ip audit name TEST attack list 3 action alarm reset drop
```

This defines an audit rule called TEST where traffic permitted by access list 3 will be processed and an alarm will be raised, the connection reset, and the packet dropped on an attack signature match.

```
interface e 0/0
ip address 10.10.1.3 255.255.0.0
ip audit TEST in
```

This applies the audit rule to inbound traffic on the Ethernet interface.

```
interface tokenring 0
ip address 11.1.3.1 255.255.255.0
access-list 3 deny 11.1.3.1 0.0.0.255
```

This prevents Token Ring traffic from being audited since the token ring can be considered a trusted network.

```
ip audit po protected 10.10.0.0 to 10.10.255.254
```

This specifies the IP address range of the Ethernet network to be protected. Note that you can omit addresses from being protected by defining multiple ranges.

By using another command, *no ip audit signature <signature-id>* or *ip audit signature <signature-id> <disable / list ACL number>*, it is possible to omit the auditing of a particular signature globally, or for a range of addresses.

Associated Commands

These are IOS IDS commands you can enter at the Privileged EXEC prompt:

`clear ip audit configuration`

This disables IOS IDS and removes all IDS entries from the configuration.

`show ip audit interface`

Shows IOS IDS configuration from an interface perspective.

`show ip audit configuration`

Used to display the active IOS IDS configuration on the router.

`show ip audit debug`

Shows the current IDS debug flag entries.

`show ip audit statistics`

This will show you signature audited counts and TCP session statistics. You would use the *clear ip audit statistics* command to reset these figures.

Summary

An intrusion detection system (IDS) is a suite of devices, hardware and software, that automates the investigation of odd activity in or around computers. It is generally used as a detective device, highlighting unwanted events after they have occurred. The Cisco IDS can also act as a preventative device, taking steps to prevent unwanted action.

IDSs fall into two types: network-based IDSs (NIDSs), where traffic is analyzed as it passes by a sensor on a wire; and host-based IDSs (HIDSs), where traffic is analyzed as it is accepted by the operating system. Network appliances or infrastructure plug-ins are readily deployed arbitrarily into the network, while host-based solutions must be customized to the operating system of the existing server. On the other hand, host systems have better insight into how the host actually handles the event, and so the alarms are of much higher fidelity than the equivalent network solution.

The IDS architecture consists of one or more probes combined with one or more management stations. The probes have two interfaces: a sensor interface that samples traffic, and a command interface for configuration information. The sensors are generally distributed throughout the network at key locations. Sensors report back to the management station, and users will poll the management station to interpret alerts.

There are several business drivers leading to IDS deployment. The most natural one is to reduce the risk of a systems compromise. Having the detective control will reduce the frequency of events (because the vulnerabilities can be identified and addressed) and the impact of events (because root cause can be known, thus leading more rapidly to remediation). They are also good at identifying misconfigured events, such as incorrect configuration data causing system malfunction, or ineffective events, such as ineffective network traffic. Thus, in addition to traditional intrusion features, it can also help with network administration and management. Other business drivers are document existing threat levels, for planning or resource allocation purposes, and to change user behavior.

An important planning function is to determine exact placement of probes. Placing the probe outside the firewall allows you to "take the temperature" of the Internet, while placing the probe just inside the firewall allows testing of the firewall rulebase, and the possibility to identify intrusions if they pass the firewall. Other likely locations are on a service network, near server clusters, or near router transit networks/interfaces.

There are many difficulties associated with IDS deployments. One is that the underlying science behind intrusion detection systems is relatively new. Another is that management has unrealistic expectations of the capabilities of an IDS. A third is the deployment phase, since this is a security device that needs to cross organizational boundaries. A fourth is that the incidence response procedure associated with an IDS is nontrivial, and takes time to develop. A fifth is the complexity of IDS tuning, to make it a more effective product.

IDS tuning is the process of training a sensor to understand the enterprise network, so it provides a reasonable number of alerts of high fidelity. An IDS is a decision tool, and suffers from two types of errors: the Type I error, the "false positive," where it dispatches an alarm even though no event has occurred; and the Type II error, the "false negative," where it fails to send out an alarm even though an event has occurred. With a default signature load, the ratio of Type I errors to true alerts is so high that it is difficult to use on an enterprise network. In a sample data, 98.9 percent of the alerts were false positives.

There are two typical strategies for tuning. One is to "turn it up," where you review the signature database, and enable only those signatures that are of high fidelity and of interest to the site. Another (the more common of the two) is to "tone it down," where all possible sensitivity is first set, and then false positive alerts are slowly weeded out.

An IDS provides alerting for a network attack, so it's important to look at what kind of attacks occur. One type is loss of confidentiality due to packet capture on the wire. Another is reconnaissance from scanning programs. The network topology itself can help or harm you in deployments. Out-of-band communication due to unattended modems is also a risk.

Physical security of your network is always a concern. Poor physical security trumps strong technical controls.

Applications and operating systems themselves often have weaknesses, and software bugs are common in today's market. Nine types of software bugs are: boundary condition errors, access validation errors, input validation errors, failure to handle exceptional conditions, race conditions, serialization errors, atomicity errors, environment errors, and configuration errors.

Compromise of the authentication services can occur through discovery of a password. There are many ways to capture a password, from "shoulder surfing" to a brute force attack in which all possible passwords are tried in turn. Malicious code can be a source of attacks as well, and may include Trojan horses, viruses, or worms.

Errors and omissions are a major source of vulnerabilities in systems. Poorly configured systems are common as well. In addition, information leakage often occurs, simply because people don't think about what the leakage implies. Of course, malicious users are also a concern.

The IP protocols themselves can be targets of attacks. Services can be attacked, such as problems with mail bombing or spamming, together with mail impersonations. FTP is a common source of problems, particularly if anonymous ftp is permitted. SNMP has recently made news for being a source of many vulnerabilities, and unfortunately is widespread. The usual guidance of limiting access to services if they are not needed applies here.

Below the application itself, some infrastructure protocols can be vulnerable. DNS can be subject to host compromise, transparent fraudulent caching, and cache poisoning. DoS floods are also common; TCP SYN floods, an attack that sends a large number of SYN packets that never complete the handshake, in order to exhaust the TCB queue is similarly popular. A Cisco router or firewall can provide protection against this sort of flood through the use of TCP Intercept. Another common strike is the smurf attack, which depends upon forged source addresses aimed at broadcast addresses to harm hosts. TCP can also be subject to session hijacking, and various sorts of low-level packet attacks such as the Ping of Death, Teardrop, and Land attacks.

Distributed denial of service attacks are common, too, where the attacker compromises multiple computers, and installs programs like Trinoo, Tribal Flood Network, or Stacheldraht to provide an attacking agent.

As far as the equipment itself goes, the Cisco Secure IDS is either the Catalyst 6000 IDS module or a standalone Unix-based appliance. The Catalyst module is designed to be integrated natively into a switched environment, while the IDS 4230 is designed to monitor fast Ethernet links. The Director is a GUI-based plug-in for HP OpenView. The Director integrates with an Oracle relational database, and permits query of the stored information. The sensors can also report back to a Cisco Secure Policy Manager console, which provides a native Windows NT application for easy use.

In terms of the underlying communication architecture, the sensors and management console use a proprietary communication channel on UDP port 45000. This provides for native encryption, and includes reliable, acknowledged transport of the sensor data.

The IDS has several daemons responsible for successful operations. The nine daemons are sensord/packetd, loggerd, sapd, postofficed, eventd, managed, smid, nrdirmap, and configd. Signature information is stored on the sensor hard drive, and consists of a contained signature base together with a customizable string search approach.

The Director installation is an extension of HP OpenView. After that is complete, running the install script from the Cisco Secure IDS CD, and following the prompts completes the installation. The director parameter configuration is achieved with the *sysconfig-director* script; you need to specify HostID, Name, Organizational ID, Name, and IP address. Building the sensors is similar: launch an install script from the CD, and execute *sysconfig-sensor*, then follow the prompts to set up the initial communication information. Finally, the sensor is introduced to the director by selecting Add Host from the file menu, and following the prompts.

Further configuration of the sensors from inside of HP OpenView is similar to any HP OpenView plug-in. Selecting the NetRanger icon from the top-level map provides submaps containing IDS nodes. Submaps represent security zones, and various options are available from the Security menu. You can configure logging from routers to a sensor (the data is uploaded to the manager via Post Office from the sensor), and configure the IDS directly on the sensor. You can also update the network string search signatures directly from HPOV.

Other important configurations for global management are establishing the data management package (reflects flat file management and integration into Oracle) and e-mail alerting.

Cisco also has an IDS as part of the IOS firewall feature set. This is useful in integrating IDS into the infrastructure, where the expense of a dedicated probe is not justified. Its feature set is a limited subset of the probe signature-matching engine. The data will report back via a Cisco Secure IDS sensor to the management platform. Again, it is capable of alerting, and offers protective capabilities through TCP resets.

It's important to keep an eye on the performance of the router. The *sh proc mem* command is helpful in monitoring memory use. Additional commands are available under the *ip audit* menu tree; they include *smtp spam, po, notify, info, attack, name, signature,* and *po protected*. Typical Cisco IOS help systems apply. In addition, privileged commands include *clear ip audit conf, show ip audit int, show ip audit conf, show ip audit debug,* and *show ip audit stat*.

Solutions Fast Track

What Is Intrusion Detection?

☑ An IDS is a software or a suite of devices that helps investigate unusual traffic on the network. It is primarily used in a detective capability, but can also be used in a protective capability (through interrupting system calls for the host-based product, or through shunning for the network product).

☑ Usually the architecture is a typical client/server model, where the probes send data up to management consoles. Users interact with the management console to address data.

☑ The primary purposes for an IDS deployment are to reduce risk, identify error, optimize network use, provide insight into threat levels, and change user behavior. Thus, an IDS provides more than just detection of intrusion.

☑ Determining where to place the probes is not straightforward. You can place them outside the firewall if you want to gather data on attacks from the Internet, but typical locations are near critical servers, or covering interfaces between security zones.

☑ There are many difficulties associated with IDS deployment. Five important issues to overcome are: the newness of the technology, management expectation, coordination with other internal organizations, incident response procedures, and tuning IDS.

IDS Tuning

☑ What an IDS does is make a decision whether or not to alarm on a packet. The tuning process is designed to make the decision as accurate as possible.

☑ Any decision process suffers from two types of errors: the Type I error, known as the "false positive," is an alert that does not correspond to a security event. These lead to additional work as the security analyst needs to review these messages. The second is the Type II error, or the "false negative," which is a security event that isn't alarmed. This type of error leads to risk assumed by the enterprise.

☑ Untuned, an IDS deployment has a high ratio of false positives to true alerts. Based upon sample data, 99 out of 100 alerts were invalid. However, even with the high level of work, it is possible to explore the alerts to find the actual attacks.

☑ The tuning process usually follows one of two paths: "turn it up," where alerts are selectively enabled, or "tone it down," where alerts are disabled. One good approach in the "tone it down" phase is to let the appliance run, and for each alert type, disable it if the ratio of false positives exceeds the importance of the signature.

Network Attacks and Intrusions

☑ Understanding network attack and intrusion types is essential to interpreting IDS data.

☑ Five categories that correspond to network attacks are: breakdowns in perimeter/device security, harm to physical security, attacks on application/OS integrity, effects of human error and omission, and taking advantage of weaknesses in the underlying IP suite.

The Cisco Secure Network Intrusion Detection System

☑ The probe types are the Windows x86-based Catalyst 6000 IDS module, or the SPARC Solaris-based IDS 4230 and IDS 4210. Management types include the Director, a Unix-based HPOV plug-in, and the CSPM, a Windows NT-based standalone application.

☑ The Post Office is a proprietary UDP-based communication protocol between the Sensor and the management platform. It provides an encrypted channel, with reliable communications handled by the application.

☑ Nine Unix daemons handle communication between sensor and database and up to HPOV.

☑ The installation process is fairly straightforward, and is primarily prompt driven after running an install script from provided installation media. Key parameters are the IP address/routing information, host ID and Name, and Organization ID and name. Finally, the information on any new probe needs to be introduced to the management database.

☑ Probes have an atomic database, updated about every month by Cisco, and a locally customizable database. The customizable portion of the detection engine is configured from the management station and pushed out to the sensor.

☑ In addition to the conventional probes, a subset of the IDS features are available on the routers themselves. IOS IDS is useful to install at network perimeters such as branch routers. This is fully compatible with the management platform for the probes, and allows for a widespread IDS deployment.

Frequently Asked Questions

The following Frequently Asked Questions, answered by the authors of this book, are designed to both measure your understanding of the concepts presented in this chapter and to assist you with real-life implementation of these concepts. To have your questions about this chapter answered by the author, browse to **www.syngress.com/solutions** and click on the **"Ask the Author"** form.

Q: I already have a firewall. Why do I need an IDS?

A: Firewalls are gatekeepers. They allow traffic in and out of a network, and are the first line of defense. They aren't a complete solution, however. For one thing, they don't address traffic they can't see—if an internal user is playing around with a core asset and both are "internal," the firewall won't see it. For another, an IDS provides a "defense in depth." They have a different focus, and so if an attack technology penetrates the first layer of defense, there is a chance they will be picked up by the IDS. And of course, there are other advantages mentioned earlier: an IDS provides visibility into your network that can help with maintenance of applications and the network itself. An IDS is a flexible tool!

Q: I'm seeing lots of network scans on my IDS. Should I worry?

A: It depends. If your sensor covers Internet-based hosts, then port scans are a routine fact of life. Some security administrators make an effort to report the intrusion back to the owning ISP, but many do not.

On the other hand, if the scanning is going on internally, then its probably inappropriate traffic. It may be unintentional: many users install software (such as printer drivers or Visio 2000) which will attempt network scans. While harmless, eliminating this unnecessary traffic is desirable. If intentional, it could indicate someone unwilling to comply with your security policy, and a headache in development. Addressing the headache early on is the best way to keep the problem small. On the other hand, it could also indicate a compromised machine, and that is definitely worth addressing.

Q: I'm seeing an alert indicating something on my network. What should I do?

A: The first thing is to review your event management protocol; it's best to have these things thought out and documented. But essentially, if an alert comes in, you need to review the nature of the alert. For example, if the alert relates to an IIS server, and the target is a Unix host running apache, you can ignore the alert as a false positive, and perhaps tune the signature. If the event management protocol allows it, the next step might be to contact the owner of the information asset, inform them of what you are seeing, and ask them to verify the vulnerability of the device to the indicated alarm.

Q: I'm seeing an alert indicating something on my network. What does it mean?

A: Many signatures provide a context buffer; this can help you understand what it means. However, your first stop is probably the included signature database information. That provides information about the nature of the alert, and the fidelity of the signature. If you need more information, you might try the SecurityFocus database, or the ISS database. Web searches usually provide a wealth of information on the alert.

Q: How can I stay current on the various attacks?

A: CERT, the Computer Emergency Response Team at the Software Engineering Institute (SEI) of the Carnegie Mellon University (CMU), is a good source of validated information. They are online at www.cert.org. AUSCERT is the Australian CERT, available at www.auscert.org.au. Another reputable source of information on attacks is the Department of Energy's CIAC, at www.ciac.org.

While not related directly to attack information, SANS, the System Administration and Network Security Institute <http://www.sans.org>, is a good resource as well. They have a wide variety of security information, and have their own FAQ site at www.sans.org/newlook/resources/IDFAQ/ ID_FAQ.htm.

Q: Should I build a full infrastructure, or should I outsource?

A: A difficult question, as the jury is still out. On the one hand, few care as much about security on your network or have as much information about what is normal on your network as you do—and effective use of a network requires intimate knowledge of the network. On the other hand, because an IDS remains a complex and sharp tool, with skill sets that are not common, it is difficult to staff adequately. The "Managed Security Services" and "Managed Security Monitoring" companies offer services with a wide area of coverage. You need to look at your own staffing ability, your own costs and budgets, and make a decision regarding your business drivers.

Chapter 14

Network Security Management

Solutions in this chapter:

- PIX Device Manager
- CiscoWorks2000 Access Control List Manager
- Cisco Secure Policy Manager
- Cisco Secure Access Control Server

- ☑ Summary
- ☑ Solutions Fast Track
- ☑ Frequently Asked Questions

Introduction

The frequency and complexity of network security-related incidences has increased dramatically in recent years. Additionally, network infrastructure and services have grown larger and more intricate to meet continually evolving user demands for bandwidth and functionality. As a result, managing security in enterprise environments has become a challenge for administrators in companies large and small.

To overcome security management issues, Cisco has developed several security management applications including those listed next:

- PIX Device Manager (PDM)

- CiscoWorks2000 Access Control Lists Manager (ACLM)

- Cisco Secure Policy Manager (CSPM)

- Cisco Secure Access Control Server (ACS)

These applications are designed to ease the burden of security management through intuitive graphical interfaces, configuration automation, report generation, and enhanced monitoring capabilities among others. Each application is suited for a different purpose, yet the combination of these tools can represent a holistic management solution in many environments.

In addition to the applications in the preceding list, administrators can also use other tools to support and configure Cisco security devices such as the convenient command-line interface (CLI) via methods including Telnet, Secure Shell (SSH), and the out-of-band console port. Additionally, Cisco security devices can also be remotely monitored using Simple Network Management Protocol (SNMP) and syslog.

This section includes a discussion regarding the applications listed earlier. For additional information regarding more basic, CLI-based management techniques, refer to Cisco documentation.

PIX Device Manager

Companies and organizations with one or two PIX firewall devices require a tool to effectively and efficiently manage the configuration and functionality of their firewalls. PDM is an application ideally suited for such small enterprises as it enables full control over individual PIX firewalls from virtually any authorized client management platform inside an organization.

Whether it is a simple access rule change or a more advanced Network Address Translation (NAT) configuration, PDM eases administrative burdens by providing an intuitive, Web-based graphical interface to each PIX device.

With security incidents on the rise, administrators also require insight into the events and traffic patterns detected on their firewall devices. PDM provides excellent reporting and proactive IDS configuration capabilities to firewall administrators all through the Web-based interface.

PIX Device Manager Overview

The PDM is a Java-based graphical user interface used to manage the Cisco PIX firewall. It is imbedded in the PIX firewall software in all versions 6.0 and later. The PDM replaces the PIX Firewall Manager (PFM) software as of PIX Firewall software version 5.3. PDM allows firewall administrators to work from a variety of authorized workstations configured with a JDK 1.1.4-compliant browser and includes nearly all PIX command-line interface (CLI) functionalities. For example, using PDM, administrators can add, modify, and delete firewall rule sets or configure Authentication, Authorization, and Accounting (AAA). Furthermore, firewall administrators can issue command line configurations directly from the Web interface for swifter management. A more comprehensive list of capabilities is included in the sections that follow.

Using PDM for firewall management, administrators do not compromise security thanks to Secure Sockets Layer (SSL) encryption capabilities and authentication mechanisms on the PIX firewall.

PIX Device Manager Benefits

Administrators using PDM can enjoy a host of benefits over more traditional management techniques. Foremost is the ability to make configurations to PIX devices from various authorized client locations using the Web-based GUI. Doing so avoids potential configuration problems due to syntax errors and enables the administrator to swiftly alter configurations without constantly returning to a centralized management station.

Since Cisco developed PDM in Java and because the Java applets actually reside on the PIX platform, management from multiple platforms without time-consuming software installations is possible. Administrators simply need to launch a JDK 1.1.4 capable browser and connect to the PIX firewall from an authorized location.

PDM also includes helpful wizards such as the Initial Setup Wizard. The Initial Setup Wizard allows for rapid and simplified deployment of PIX firewall devices by prompting the administrator for typical information required in all firewall configurations.

With the PDM interface, administrators can also visually monitor and baseline connections, PIX system internal metrics, traffic load, IDS, and other useful information. Because PDM clients use SSL (HTTPS) to connect to the PIX, these connections are reasonably secure. However, it is recommended to further control access to PIX for administrative tasks through an Access Control List (ACL).

Finally, while PDM is designed to manage and monitor individual PIX firewalls, multiple browser windows may be opened on the management client desktop enabling the concurrent and easy management of multiple firewalls across the enterprise.

Supported PIX Firewall Versions

The PIX Device Manager application is new as of PIX Firewall software version 6.0 and replaces the PIX Firewall Management software as of PIX Firewall software version 5.3. To facilitate multiple management platforms, Cisco created the software using Java and imbedded applets directly in the OS image. All versions of the PIX Firewall software version 6.0 or later support PDM.

PIX Device Requirements

PDM is supported on all PIX 501, 506, 515, 520, 525, and 535 platforms running PIX Firewall software version 6.0 or later. Additionally, the PIX platform must meet the following requirements to run PDM:

- 8MB Flash memory
- A Data Encryption Standard (DES) or 3DES activation key

The DES or 3DES activation key supports the SSL-based communication between the remote Java management client and the Cisco PIX device. PIX devices shipped with firewall software version 6.0 and later already include DES capabilities. 3DES, which enables stronger encryption capabilities, is available from Cisco as an additional license.

Those PIX devices shipped with Firewall software versions prior to version 6.0 must be upgraded to version 6.0 or later and configured with a DES activation key before PDM will function. DES activation keys are available for free from Cisco on their Web site at www.cisco.com/kobayashi/sw-center/internet/ pix-56bit-license-request.shtml.

NOTE

Check the PIX firewall software version and DES capabilities using the *show version* console command on the selected PIX firewall.

Requirements for a Host Running the PIX Device Management Client

Because Cisco created PDM using Java technology, several client workstations are capable of running the PDM client software. However, PDM will not function on MacOS, Windows 3.1, or Windows 95 operating systems. PDM can be run from Solaris, Linux, MacOS X, and Windows 98+. The corresponding PIX Firewall IOS versions are shown in Table 14.1.

Table 14.1 PIX Device Manager Client OS Requirements

Client Operating Systems	PIX Firewall IOS Version
Solaris	Solaris 2.6 and later
Linux	Red Hat 7.0 and later
Windows	Windows 98, Windows NT 4.0 (SP4), Windows2000 (SP1), and Windows ME

When running PDM on a Solaris operating system, the following requirements apply:

- **Processor** SPARC Processor
- **Memory** 128MB RAM
- **Display** 800×600 pixel display with at least 256 colors
- **Display** CDE or OpenWindows window manager
- **Browser** Netscape Communicator 4.51 or later (4.76 recommended)

When running PDM on a Linux operating system, the following requirements apply:

- **Memory** 64MB RAM
- **Display** An 800×600 pixel display with at least 256 colors

- **Display** GNOME or KDE 2.0 desktop environment
- **Browser** Netscape Communicator 4.75 or later version

When running PDM on a Windows operating system, the following requirements apply:

- **Processor** Pentium-compatible running at 350MHz or later
- **Memory** 128MB RAM
- **Display** 800×600 pixel display with at least 256 colors
- **Browser** Either Internet Explorer 5.0 (SP1) or later (5.5 recom-
  mended), or Netscape Communicator 4.51 or later (4.76 recommended)

Regardless of the client operating system, a Web browser is required to connect to PDM on the PIX firewall. To successfully launch PDM, the Web browser
must have JavaScript and Java enabled and must support JDK 1.1.4 or later.
Finally, the browser must support SSL connectivity. All browsers listed previously
include this functionality.

Using PIX Device Manager

This section of the chapter provides insight into the logical steps and procedures
required to get PDM working and includes examples that administrators can use
to compare to their own environment. Perform the following configuration steps
to make PFM functional. Then connect to the PIX firewall via PDM and begin
changing rules for inbound and outbound connections to and from the network.
This section also includes information regarding other configuration features discussed in the previous pages.

Configuring the PIX Device Manager

Before attempting to use PDM or configure a PIX device using PDM, verify that
the PIX firewall version of the device is 6.0 or later. If the PIX firewall device
was shipped from Cisco with 6.0 or later installed, PDM is probably already
installed as part of the PIX OS. If the PIX firewall version is not 6.0 or later, the
firewall version must be upgraded and DES must be activated before PDM will
function.

To verify the PIX firewall version, log in to the command-line interface via
Telnet or a console connection and type **show version**. The first two lines of
response should display the current PIX firewall version and indicate whether

PDM is installed. Figure 14.1 shows a PIX firewall with Firewall version 6.1(1) and PDM version 1.0(2) installed.

Figure 14.1 PIX Firewall with Firewall version 6.1(1) and PDM version 1.0(2) Installed

```
Pix> show version
Cisco PIX Firewall Version 6.1(1)
Cisco PIX Device Manager Version 1.0(2)
```

If the PIX firewall version is 6.0 or later and PDM is installed, proceed to the Configuration Example Section included on the following pages. If not, perform the following steps to upgrade the PIX firewall and install the DES activation key.

Installing the PIX Device Manager

As with all upgrade and installation procedures, begin by backing up all configuration data on the existing PIX firewall devices to upgrade. If the PIX firewall is a production device, schedule the upgrade procedure during off hours and notify the users in the company of the potential service outage. Doing so helps ensure a smooth upgrade process and prevents unwarranted complaints from the user community.

NOTE

Administrators with a valid CCO login can find Cisco PIX firewall software and PDM images on the Cisco Web site at www.cisco.com/kobayashi/ sw-center/ciscosecure/pix.shtml.

Verify the PIX firewall meets all requirements listed previously in this chapter before starting with the upgrade and installation. Finally, be sure to obtain the correct version of the PIX firewall software and have a version of the PIX firewall software currently running on the PIX device in the event the new version upgrade fails. This procedure is generally trouble free, but best practice always dictates the preparation for version rollback.

The basic steps for PDM installation are:

■ Obtain a DES activation key.

■ Configure the PIX firewall for basic network connectivity.

- Install a TFTP server and make it available to the PIX firewall.

- Upgrade to a version of PIX firewall software 6.0 or later and configure the DES activation key on the PIX device.

- Install PDM on the PIX device.

These installation tasks are described in further detail next, and on the following pages.

Obtaining a DES Activation Key

The first step in configuring PDM on a PIX firewall is obtaining a new activation key to enable DES. This activation key is free from Cisco and required for PDM functionality. Because it may take some time for Cisco to issue the new key, it is best to start the request process early. Perform the following steps to request a DES activation key.

1. Establish a CLI connection to the PIX device via Telnet or the console.

2. From the command prompt, type **show version**. Note the current PIX serial number in the display. This will be required to request a new serial number and activation key.

3. From a Web browser, go to www.cisco.com/cgi-bin/Software/ FormManager/formgenerator.pl?pid=221&fid=324 and fill out the key request form. The key will be sent to you via e-mail.

Configuring the PIX Firewall for Basic Network Connectivity

To upgrade a PIX firewall and install PDM, the PIX firewall must first be capable of basic network connectivity. If the PIX firewall device is already on the network and capable of connecting to other devices, proceed to the next section and install a Trivial File Transfer Protocol (TFTP) server.

1. Establish a connection to the console port of the PIX device and log in to the CLI.

2. Enter enable mode by typing **enable** at the console prompt.

3. Type **configure terminal** to enter configuration mode on the PIX firewall.

4. Enter the setup dialog by typing **setup** after entering configure mode.

5. Follow the setup dialog prompts and enter information for the following variables:

- Enable password

- Clock variables

- IP address information

- Hostname

- Domain name

6. Save the information when prompted to write the configuration to memory.

Installing a TFTP Server and Making It Available to the PIX Firewall

After the PIX firewall is successfully placed on the network, a TFTP server must be configured to accommodate the new PIX firewall software and PDM software upload. Like other Cisco devices, using TFTP for software upload is the recommended method for performing software upgrades. If a TFTP server already exists, proceed to the next section and upgrade the PIX firewall software.

TFTP servers are usually included in all Unix and Linux distributions and can easily be configured. For information regarding TFTP configuration on a Unix or Linux platform, refer to the specific operating system documentation.

Cisco conveniently offers a TFTP server for Windows 95, Windows 98, Windows NT 4.0, and Windows2000 operating systems. The example that follows assumes the use of this software. Perform the following steps to install the Cisco TFTP server.

1. Allocate a machine to be used as the TFTP server. The Cisco software runs on the Windows 95, Windows 98, Windows NT 4.0, and Windows2000 operating systems.

2. Download the Cisco TFTP software. Administrators with a valid CCO account can find the software at www.cisco.com/cgi-bin/tablebuild.pl/tftp.

3. Run the self-extracting executable and follow the instructions included on the TFTP server download page to install the software.

Upgrading to PIX Firewall Software 6.0 and Configuring the DES Activation Key on the PIX Device

Because PDM only functions on PIX firewall software 6.0 and later, PIX devices with versions released before 6.0 must be upgraded. Furthermore, the use of PDM requires the activation of DES. To enable DES, the new key requested in previous steps must be activated during a new PIX image load using the monitor mode method on the PIX firewall. The key on the PIX firewall cannot be changed via typical copy tftp Flash upgrade procedures.

The upgrade of any operating system is a potentially difficult operation and should be thoroughly planned. Always back up configuration files and software versions before proceeding with the upgrade. Likewise, always verify that the PIX firewall meets the requirements specified for the PIX firewall software. There are several versions of PIX firewall software version 6.0 and later available on the Cisco Web site. Be sure to select the appropriate version for the installation.

To upgrade the PIX firewall software, follow these steps:

1. From the TFTP server, log in to Cisco Connection Online and download the appropriate version of the PIX firewall software. It can be found at www.cisco.com/cgi-bin/tablebuild.pl/pix.

2. Save the software in a location that can be accessed via TFTP. Note the name of the software image for later reference.

3. Log in to the PIX firewall CLI via a console connection.

4. Reboot the PIX device. As the PIX device is booting, issue a **BREAK** or **ESC** command when prompted to interrupt the Flash boot process. If using Windows HyperTerminal, the BREAK command is issued by pressing **Ctrl+Break**. The *monitor>* prompt should appear once in monitor mode.

NOTE

In monitor mode, use the **?** key to see a list of available options.

5. From the monitor prompt, type **interface 1**. This command instructs the PIX firewall to use the inside interface to connect to the TFTP server.

6. Type **address** *pix_interface_ip_address* where *pix_interface_ip_address* is the IP address of the PIX internal interface.

7. Type **server** *tftp_server_ip_address* where *tftp_server_ip_address* is the IP address of the TFTP server with the new PIX firewall software image.

8. Type **file** *filename* where *filename* is the name of the new PIX firewall software image on the TFTP server.

9. If the TFTP server is on a remote network, the gateway command must be issued to configure the PIX firewall with a default gateway. Type **gateway** *ip_address_of_default_gateway* where *ip_address_of_default_gateway* is the ip address of the default router.

10. Type **tftp** to initiate the TFTP download of the new PIX firewall software from the TFTP server.

11. When prompted, type **yes** to install the new PIX Firewall software.

12. When prompted, type **yes** to enter a new activation key. Enter the new activation key acquired from Cisco in previous steps.

Here is an example of a successful PIX firewall software upgrade:

```
monitor> interface 1

0: ethernet0: address is 0050.54ff.59cc, irq 10

1: ethernet1: address is 0050.54ff.59cd, irq 7


Using 1: i82557 @ PCI(bus:0 dev:13 irq:11), MAC: 0050.54ff.59cd

monitor> address 172.20.1.1

address 172.20.1.1

monitor> server 172.20.1.20

server 172.20.1.20

monitor> file pix613.bin

file pix613.bin

monitor> tftp

tftp pix613.bin@172.20.1.20.........................................

......

Received 2562368 bytes


Cisco Secure PIX Firewall admin loader (3.0) #0: Tue Dec  517:35:46

    EST2000

System Flash=E28F128J3 @ 0xfff00000
```

```
BIOS Flash=am29f400c @ 0xd8000

Flash version 6.1.3, Install version 6.1.3

Do you wish to copy the install image into flash? [n] y


Installing to flash


Serial Number: 480501351 (0x1ca20729)

Activation Key: 12345678 12345678 12345678 12345678


Do you want to enter a new activation key? [n] y

Enter new activation key: 87654321 87654321 87654321 87654321

Updating flash...Done.

Serial Number: 480501351 (0x1ca20729)


Flash Activation Key: 87654321 87654321 87654321 87654321


Writing 2562368 bytes image into flash...
```

Installing PDM on the PIX Device

The final step to enable PDM on the PIX firewall is to install PDM into Flash. As with the PIX firewall software upgrade, the installation of PDM is a potentially difficult operation. Always back up configuration files and software versions before proceeding with the installation. Always verify that the PIX firewall meets the requirements specified for PDM. To install PDM, follow these steps:

1. From the TFTP server, log in to CCO and download the PDM image. PDM can be found at www.cisco.com/cgi-bin/tablebuild.pl/pix.

2. Save the software in a location that can be accessed via TFTP. Note the name of the software image for later reference.

3. Log in to the PIX CLI via Telnet or the console.

4. Enter enable mode by typing **enable** at the command prompt.

5. Type **copy tftp flash:pdm**.

6. When prompted for the remote address of host, type the **ip address of the TFTP server**.

7. When prompted for the source filename, type the name of the PDM software on the TFTP server.

8. When prompted, type **yes** to proceed with the PDM installation.

9. After the installation is complete, type **show version** to verify that PDM is installed and that DES is enabled. Output similar to the following should appear:

```
pix# sh ver

Cisco PIX Firewall Version 6.1(3)
Cisco PIX Device Manager Version 1.0(2)

Compiled on Tue 11-Sep-01 07:45 by morlee

pix up 326 days 19 hours

Hardware:    PIX-515, 32 MB RAM, CPU Pentium 200 MHz
Flash i28F640J5 @ 0x300, 16MB
BIOS Flash AT29C257 @ 0xfffd8000, 32KB

0: ethernet0: address is 0050.54ff.59cc, irq 10
1: ethernet1: address is 0050.54ff.59cd, irq 7

Licensed Features:
Failover:          Disabled
VPN-DES:           Enabled
VPN-3DES:          Disabled
Maximum Interfaces:      3
Cut-through Proxy:       Enabled
Guards:            Enabled
Websense:          Enabled
Inside Hosts:    Unlimited
Throughput:      Unlimited
ISAKMP peers:    Unlimited

Serial Number: 480501351 (0x1ca20729)
Activation Key: 12345678 12345678 12345678 12345678
```

10. Type **configure terminal** to enter terminal configuration mode.

11. Enable the PDM http server on the PIX firewall by typing **http server enable**.

12. Configure internal PDM management clients by typing **http** *ip_address_of_client netmask* **inside** where *ip_address_of_client* is a specific client ip address or network ip address and *netmask* is the appropriate netmask of the client or network.

13. Save the new configuration by typing **write memory** and exit the CLI.

Configuration Examples

Configuring a PIX firewall, whether through PDM or the PIX CLI, should be the technical application of a well-developed and understood security policy. Moreover, the rules implemented on the PIX firewall often represent the enforcement of the security policy. Before configuring any security device, the firewall administrator should be aware of the specific security policy of the organization. A cohesive and comprehensive technical security solution is more likely with such an approach.

Designing & Planning…

Security Policy Development

A good security practice within any organization begins with a sound and well-developed security framework. It is from this framework that policies, standards, guidelines, and standard operating procedures flow. Organizations should clearly define this framework before embarking upon device configurations to ensure a uniform and predictable security stance.

After successfully installing PDM, connect to the PIX firewall via PDM and begin configuring a specific security policy appropriate for the company. This section includes configuration steps and examples typical of PIX firewall installations such as the following:

- Connecting to the PIX with PDM

- Configuring basic firewall properties

- Implementing Network Address Translation (NAT)
- Allowing inbound traffic from external sources

These examples represent a small portion of PDM's capabilities and are intended as a representative tour through some of the functionality PDM offers. For complete information regarding PDM functionality and methodical configuration details, refer to the Cisco PIX firewall and PDM software technical documentation.

The examples included next and on the following pages are based on the network architecture as shown in Figure 14.2.

Figure 14.2 Example Network Architecture

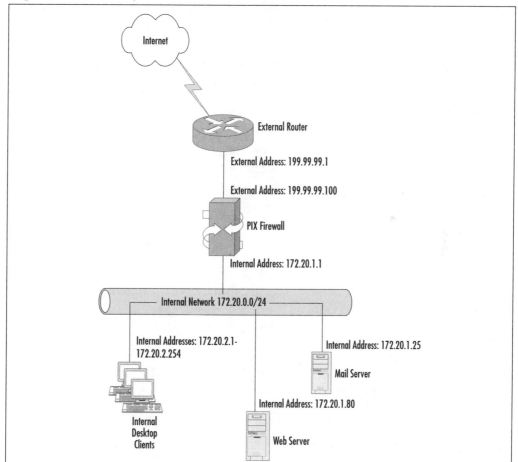

Connecting to the PIX with PDM

PDM management clients are only permitted from authorized ip addresses as specified previously using the http command. Before attempting to connect to the PIX via PDM, verify that the management workstation meets all functional requirements previously detailed. In addition, verify the PDM management client is included in the http configuration statement on the PIX firewall.

Complete the following steps to connect to the PIX firewall with PDM.

1. Launch a JDK 1.1.4 capable browser on an authorized PDM management workstation and connect to the PIX firewall internal ip address using SSL. Using the example network architecture shown previously, the URL should be entered as follows: **https://172.20.1.1**. Be sure to use https:// and not http:// in the URL string.

2. Choose to accept the SSL security certificate when prompted.

3. When prompted for authentication credentials, do not enter a username. Enter the enable password in the password field and click **OK**.

4. PDM will launch in a separate window similar to Figure 14.3.

Figure 14.3 PDM Launch Window

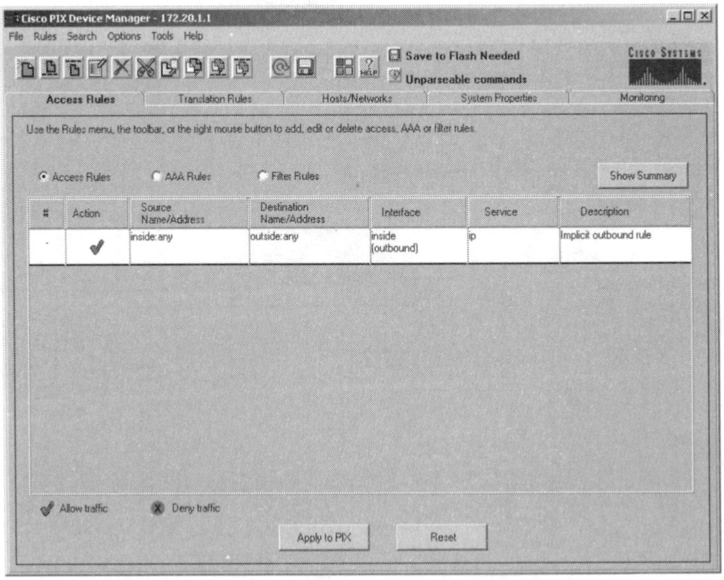

NOTE

A complete PDM troubleshooting guide is located on the Cisco Web site at www.cisco.com/univercd/cc/td/doc/product/iaabu/pix/pix_61/pdm_ig/ pdm_tsht.htm.

From the main PDM screen, notice that there are pull-down menus, toolbar buttons, and five tabbed screens to use for configuration. Click the tabs and pull-down menus to become familiar with the interface. The five tabbed screens are as follows:

- **Access Rules** The Access Rules screen is used to permit and deny specific network traffic traversing the PIX firewall. From this screen, AAA authentication and URL filters are configured as well.

- **Translation Rules** Administrators configure NAT properties from the Translation Rules screen.

- **Hosts/Networks** Entities such as networks and hosts are delineated from the Hosts/Networks screen.

- **System Properties** The basic maintenance of the PIX firewall system is performed from the System Properties screen. Properties such as DHCP client behavior, IDS configuration, interface attributes, and others are configured from this screen.

- **Monitoring** The monitoring screen is used to configure monitoring for the PIX firewall.

These screens, in addition to the pull-down menus and toolbar buttons, will be used in the following configuration examples.

Configuring Basic Firewall Properties

After connecting to the PIX firewall using PDM, click the **System Properties tab** to modify some basic firewall properties. The System Properties screen is shown in Figure 14.4.

This example includes changing the PIX firewall interface ip configuration, adding a default route, and changing the administrative password.

To alter PIX interface ip configuration information, click the **Interface Category** listed in the left portion of the System Properties screen as seen in

Figure 14.4. Highlight the specific interface to modify and click the **Edit** button. The Edit Interface screen is shown in Figure 14.5.

Figure 14.4 The System Properties Tab

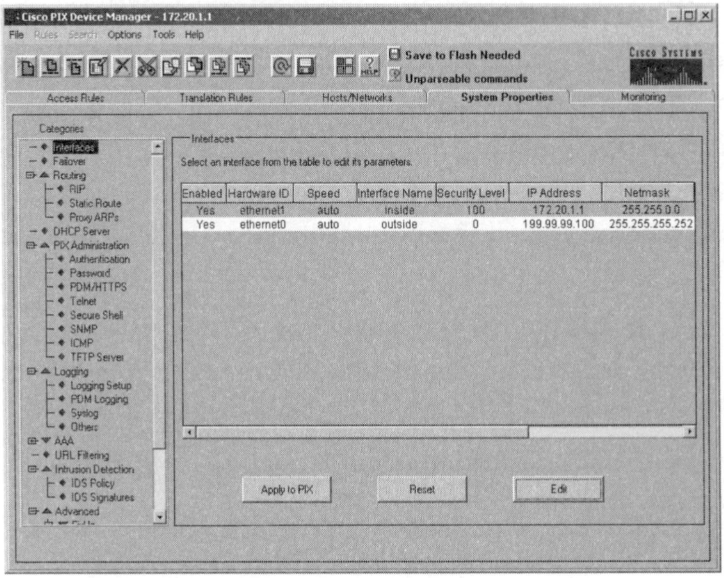

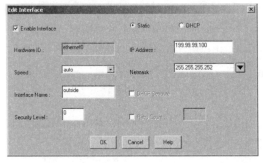

Figure 14.5 The Edit Interface Screen

Modify the attributes that require change and click **OK**. From the System Properties screen, click the **Apply To PIX button** to save changes to Flash memory on the PIX device.

To add a default route, click the **Routing Category** listed in the left portion of the System Properties screen. From the expanded category list, click **Static Routes** as shown in Figure 14.6.

Figure 14.6 Adding a Default Route

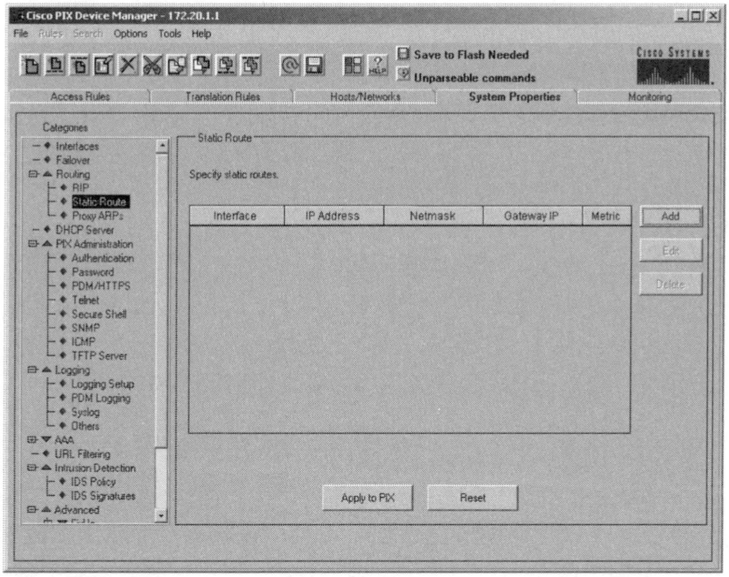

Click **Add** to add a new default route. The Add Static Route window appears, similar to the window shown in Figure 14.7. Add the required default route information as shown next and click **OK**.

Figure 14.7 The Add Static Route Window

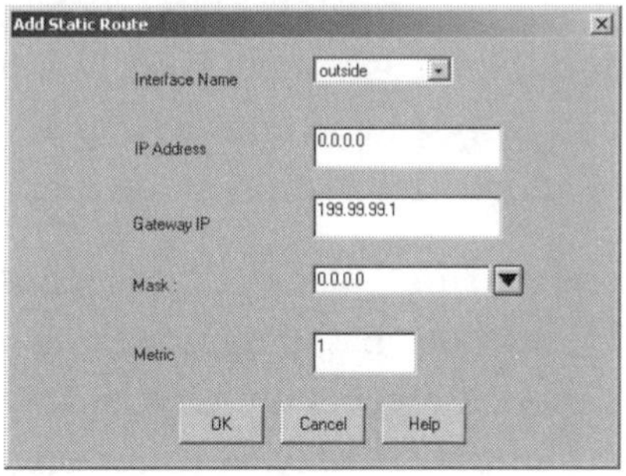

From the System Properties screen, click the **Apply To PIX button** to save changes to Flash memory on the PIX device.

To change administrative authentication variables on the PIX firewall, click the **PIX Administration** category listed in the left portion of the System Properties screen. From the expanded category list, click **authentication** as shown in Figure 14.8.

Figure 14.8 Changing the Administrative Authentication Variables

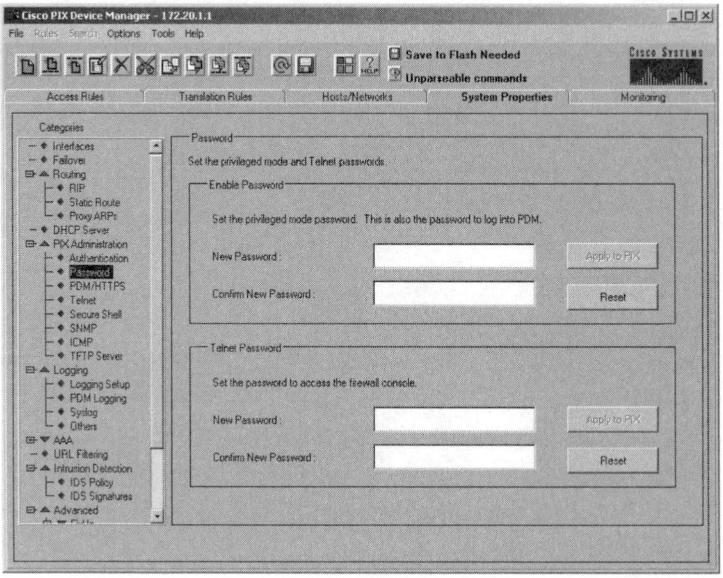

Type the new enable or Telnet (vty) password in the space provided. To confirm the password, retype the password in the space provided and click **Apply To PIX**. A dialog box will appear confirming the new password.

Implementing Network Address Translation

Network Address Translation (NAT) is widely used in networked environments to add additional layers of security and to conserve ip address space. With the PIX firewall, three types of address translation are available.

- **Static address translation** Static address translation is used to map external ip addresses to internal ip addresses on a one-to-one basis. Static mappings such as these are generally required when allowing externally originated traffic through the firewall to internal servers.

- **Dynamic address translation (PAT)** Dynamic address translation allows many internal ip addresses to be hidden behind one external IP address. Because the firewall uses ports to maintain discrete connectivity for each translated ip address, this configuration is commonly referred to as PAT. This configuration is useful for conserving external ip addresses, but cannot be used to direct externally originated traffic through the firewall to internal servers.

- **Static PAT** Static PAT is similar to dynamic address translation as described earlier. Static PAT can be used, however, to allow externally originated traffic through the firewall to internal servers. Using ports to differentiate where specific services should be sent internally, static PAT is useful in environments where only one external ip address is available for the PIX firewall. PDM does not support the configuration of static PAT.

WARNING

If static PAT is configured on the PIX device via the CLI, administrators will be unable to manage the firewall via PDM. PDM will only be able to perform monitoring on the firewall in this situation.

This configuration example includes both static address translation and dynamic address translation.

To configure NAT on the PIX firewall, click the **Translation Rules tab** as shown in Figure 14.9.

Figure 14.9 The Translation Rules Tab

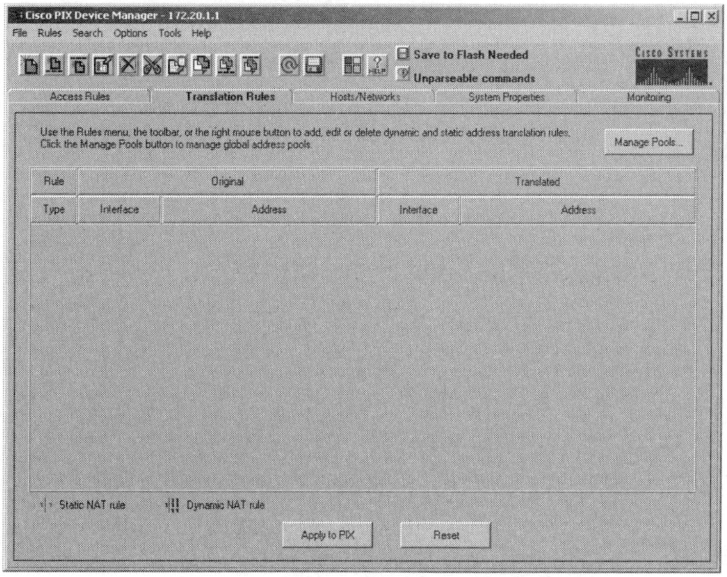

A pool must first be created on which the NAT will be based. Click the **Manage Pools...** button to add a new address pool. The Add Global Pool Item screen appears. Populate the fields with the values shown in Figure 14.10 and click **OK**.

Figure 14.10 The Add Global Pool Item Window

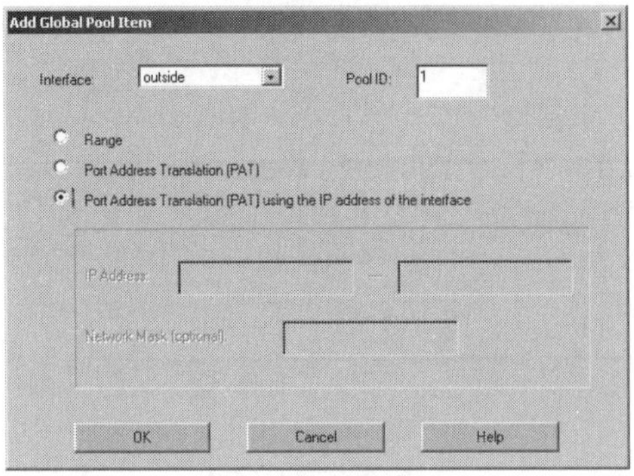

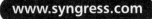

This design allows the external ip address of the firewall to be used in a dynamic NAT configuration. Next, from the Rules drop-down menu, select **Add** to create a new dynamic address translation on the firewall. Populate the Add Address Translation Rule fields with the values shown in Figure 14.11.

Figure 14.11 The Edit Address Translation Rules Window

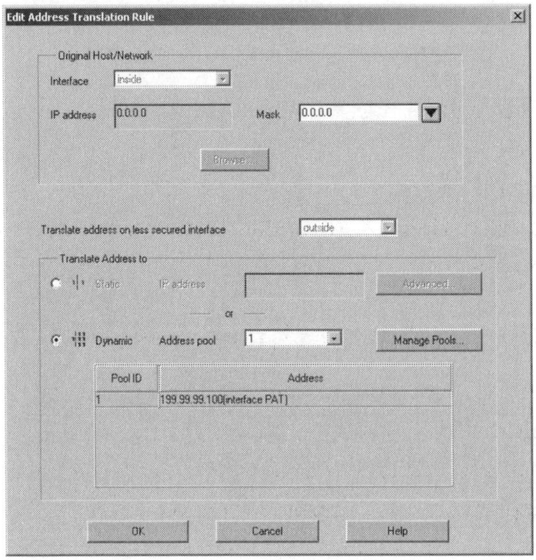

When finished, click the **OK** button. From the Translation Rules screen, click **Apply To PIX** to update Flash memory on the firewall and make the changes effective.

Now add a static NAT configuration in preparation for the next exercise of allowing inbound traffic from external sources. To do so, click the **Add From The Rules** drop-down menu again. This time, populate the Add Address Translation Rule fields with the values shown in Figure 14.12.

Figure 14.12 Adding Static NAT Configuration

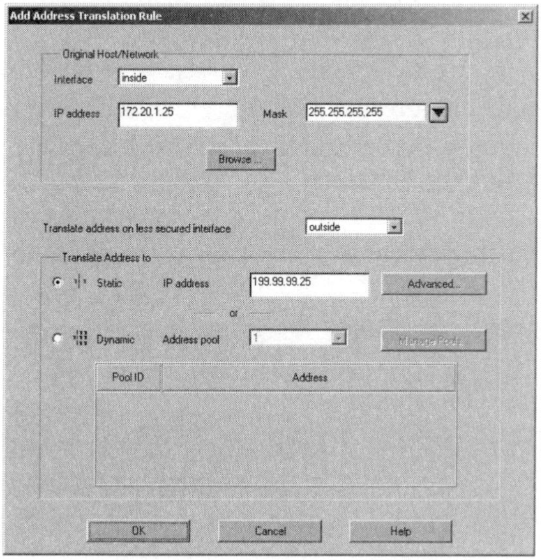

This configuration creates a static address translation mapping between the external ip address 199.99.99.25 and the internal ip address 172.20.1.25. Click **OK** to add the rule. PDM may request to add a host entity to support the rule. If so, click **OK**, then click **Add To PIX** to update the PIX firewall Flash memory. Next, add an access rule to allow traffic for this new NAT rule through the firewall.

Allowing Inbound Traffic from External Sources

Once NAT has been successfully configured, as shown in the previous exercise, internal clients should be able to access external resources. Even though a specific rule has not been manually added to allow such outbound access, it is implied through Cisco's interpretation of interface security levels.

Using Cisco parlance, traffic is always permitted from firewall interfaces with a higher security level to firewall interfaces with a lower security level. For instance, in the example network architecture previously described, the external interface of the firewall at address 199.99.99.100 has a security level of 0 and the internal interface of the firewall at address 172.20.1.1 has a security level of 100. This allows internal traffic to traverse the firewall outbound without expressly permitting it.

However, this implied rule is reversed for traffic originating on a firewall interface with a lower security level that is traversing to a higher security level. Such traffic coming from outside networks to inside networks is implicitly denied. Therefore, an access rule must be manually added to permit such traffic. The next exercise includes the configuration of such a rule and will be based on the NAT rule added previously to the mail server in the example network architecture.

To permit access to the internal mail server, click the **Access Rules tab**. Next, from the Rules drop-down menu, select **Add** to create a new access list on the firewall. The Add Rule window appears (Figure 14.13).

Figure 14.13 Permitting Access to the Internal Mail Server through the Add Rule Window

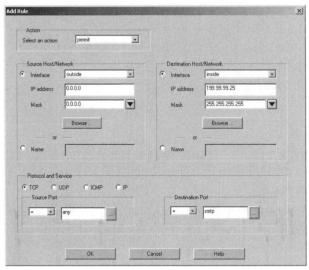

This configuration permits SMTP traffic to the external ip address 199.99.99.25. Click **OK** to add the rule. Then click **Add To PIX** to update the PIX firewall Flash memory.

The configuration of security on PIX firewall is one of many methods to protect critical network and systems resources from attack. While, PDM is oriented specifically toward the management of individual PIX firewall devices, other security devices and management applications exist in the Cisco security arsenal. The next section includes information regarding another tool, CiscoWorks2000 ACLM, and its benefits to the enterprise security suite.

CiscoWorks2000 Access Control List Manager

Another line of defense against potential intruders and malicious hackers is the configuration of Access Control Lists (ACLs) on routers, switches, and other Cisco devices. The PIX firewall is adept at providing boundary defense and other critical security functionality such as VPN termination. Moreover, the PIX firewall actually relies on ACL constructs to delineate permissible traffic from denied traffic. However, companies often require additional security throughout the network to limit access to critical resources behind boundary defenses or to simply segment certain internal network traffic. This additional security can be provided through ACLs on Cisco devices across the network.

The maintenance of ACLs on multiple devices can quickly become difficult due to complexity and quantity in a large network. To mitigate this management issue, Cisco developed a component within CiscoWorks2000 called Access Control List Manager. This section details the capabilities and functionality of the ACLM and includes examples on deployment and management within a typical network infrastructure.

ACL Manager Overview

ACLM is a component within the network management software system known as CiscoWorks2000. CiscoWorks2000 is a highly extensible application suite ideally suited for managing Cisco enterprise networks and devices. For convenience and appropriate application, CiscoWorks2000 has numerous sub-components that integrate under the CiscoWorks2000 software framework. Theses components provide management solutions for local area networks (LAN) and wide area networks (WAN) of the enterprise.

ACLM is included in the CiscoWorks2000 Routed WAN Management Solution set. In addition to ACLM, this set of applications includes the following components:

- Cisco nGenius Real-Time Monitor
- CiscoView

- Resource Manager Essentials
- Internetwork Performance Monitor

With these tools, administrators greatly increase configuration, administration, monitoring, and troubleshooting capabilities in large-scale network deployments. Furthermore, long-term performance insight and network traffic optimization are possible with the CiscoWorks2000 Routed WAN Management Solution. For additional information regarding the CiscoWorks2000 suite of productions and functionality, refer to the Cisco Web site.

As the name implies, ACLM is used to develop and maintain ACLs on Cisco devices. ACLM runs as an integrated component of Resource Manager Essentials and can manage most Cisco IOS routers, access servers, and hubs with an IOS of 10.3 through 12.1. ACLM can also manage Catalyst switches running Catalyst IOS version 5.3 through 5.5.

The Web-based Windows Explorer-like graphical interface provides powerful control of IP and IPX access lists and device access control from virtually anywhere on the network. VLAN and SNMP access control list management is also possible via ACLM. The interface eliminates the complexity and syntactical accuracy required to implement lengthy ACLs via the CLI. Furthermore, ACLM saves time and resources through batch configuration of new filters and the consistent and accurate management of existing access lists in a large-scale network.

ACLM includes several modules used to perform specific actions within the manager functionality suite. These modules are as follows:

- **Template Manager** The Template Manager module is used to construct and maintain ACL templates for the predictable and error-free security management of numerous Cisco devices. Using template manager, administrators can create appropriate templates for many devices instead of reinventing the wheel for each new network component.

- **Class Manager** This module enables the creation of service and network groups or classes. With this module, administrators can save time by designating typical groupings of rules to be quickly implemented via ACLM.

- **Template Use Wizard** Administrators use the Template Use Wizard to apply previously created packet and VLAN filtering ACLs, and line and SNMP ACLs across the network. In conjunction with Template Manager, the wizard module allows administrators to be more efficient when deploying or modifying numerous ACL configurations to devices on the network.

- **Optimizer** For additional ACL efficiency of a Cisco device, the Optimizer module can be used to inspect ACL statement ordering and syntax. Optimizer removes redundant statements and consolidates entries. Moreover, the optimizer module can automatically reorder ACL statements against hit rate utilization statistics to provide the utmost in efficiency.

- **DiffViewer** DiffViewer assists the administrator in discerning changes to ACLs of different versions. Using this module, alteration is easily identifiable making version control and version rollback simple.

- **ACL Downloader** This modules enables the scheduled or manual download of ACLs from Cisco devices in the network.

ACL Manager Device and Software Support

ACLM version 1.3 supports most Cisco IOS routers, access servers, and hubs with an IOS of 10.3 through 12.1. ACLM can also manage Catalyst switches running Catalyst OS version 5.3 through 5.5. Using ACLM, administrators can view all ACLs, regardless of type. ACLM includes full support for the following access lists:

- IP, IP_EXTENDED
- IPX, IPX_EXTENDED
- IPX_SAP, IPX_SUMMARY
- RATE_LIMIT_MAC
- RATE_LIMIT_PRECEDENCE
- VACL_Catalyst 6000

Installation Requirements for ACL Manager

Before installing ACLM, verify that the intended server meets all software and hardware requirements listed in the following. CiscoWorks2000 and Cisco Resource Manager Essentials (RME) are both prerequisites for the installation of ACLM. The software runs on either Windows NT 4.0 and Windows2000, or Solaris 2.6 and 2.7 operating systems.

When running ACLM server on a Solaris operating system, the following requirements apply:

- **System** Sun UltraSPARC 60
- **Processor** 400MHz or faster
- **Memory** 512MB RAM with 1GB swap space
- **Disk** 9GB

When running ACLM server on a Windows operating system, the following requirements apply:

- **System** Pentium-compatible
- **Processor** 500Mhz or faster
- **Memory** 512MB RAM with 1GB swap space
- **Disk** 9GB

Because the ACLM user interface is run from a browser on an authorized client machine, certain software and hardware requirements are needed on the client as well. ACLM will function on several different client platforms and operating systems as follows:

- **IBM PC-Compatible** Windows 95, Windows 98, Windows NT 4.0, and Windows2000
- **Sun Microsystems** Solaris versions 2.5.1, 2.6, or 2.7
- **IBM RS/6000** Any version of AIX supporting the required browsers listed next
- **HP-UX Workstation** Any version of HP-UX supporting the required browsers listed next

All client systems connecting to ACLM must also have either an Internet Explorer 5.0 or 5.1 browser or the Netscape Communicator 4.6 or 4.7 Internet Web browser.

ACL Manager Features

The features added when ACLM is installed concern the management of ACLs on Cisco devices in the enterprise network. ACLM is accessed through CiscoWorks2000 from any client host with an Internet browser, hardware, and that is OS-compatible with the client requirements specified earlier. All ACLM tools are found under the RME section on the left panel of CiscoWorks2000. In the following, some of the ACLM features used to manage Cisco devices are described.

Using a Structured Access Control List Security Policy

In an infrastructure consisting of multiple routers and switches, it is important to consistently manage and configure ACLs to control traffic across the network. ACLM can help ensure the uniform application of the security policy across the enterprise through Template Manager and Class Manager. These modules facilitate the creation of standardized ACL templates and classes consistent with policy on the entire network.

Decreasing Deployment Time for Access Control Lists

After creating appropriate ACL templates using Template Manager, all security policy changes and new device installations are expedited by quickly pushing the prefabricated ACL configuration to the Cisco infrastructure. In this manner, the deployment and maintenance network infrastructure is optimized for operation. When managing network security policy with ACL templates, only the initially created template must be altered to reflect policy changes. Thereafter, ACLM identifies the devices affected by the policy change and automatically generates the appropriate configurations to be deployed to the specific Cisco devices.

Using the ACL Use Wizard also decreases the deployment time for new ACLs required to enforce evolving security policy on a network. Through a methodical process, device access control or ACL filtering can be configured for devices by applying already defined templates to the device. This eases maintenance complexity and allows for quick deployment of network configuration changes across multiple devices.

Ensure Consistency of Access Control Lists

When defining ACLs on network devices, it is essential to ensure consistency of configuration throughout the enterprise. This reduces the likelihood of unauthorized network traffic by preventing unanticipated backdoor access and poorly configured ACLs. Using Template Manager with Class Manager to define network classes and services allows for the fast and consistent implementation of security policy.

ACLM always indicates the devices affected by template changes when using Template Manager, allowing administrators to confirm the new ACL configuration and fix errors before making changes to the production environment.

Furthermore, all changes to ACLs and network security policy can be reviewed with DiffViewer. DiffViewer shows a list of all affected devices and displays the current and new ACL configuration side by side. This permits the review and confirmation of ACL configuration changes before deployment to reduce the possibility of errors in the enforced security policy.

Keep Track of Changes Made on the Network

Because ACLM is installed with CiscoWorks2000 and Resource Manager Essentials (RME), it uses the RME Change Audit service. The Change Audit service is a central point from which network configuration changes can be reviewed. It displays information concerning when and what type of change was made and whether the change was made from Telnet connections, from the console port, or from a CiscoWorks2000 application like ACL Manager.

NOTE

The RME Change Audit service can filter reports using simple or complex criteria to locate specific changes in the network. Variables such as changes in time can be used to pinpoint critical infrastructure alterations.

Troubleshooting and Error Recovery

When experiencing issues on a network, it is best to first confirm that the physical network, routing, and protocols are functioning properly. After verifying such infrastructure is functional, troubleshooting ACLs on the network may be required. Using the methods previously described, investigating the nature of recent ACL changes can provide insight into whether security-related changes have negatively affected network functionality.

If issues are detected with specific ACLs, Template Manager can be used to alter the ACL template and generate appropriate configurations required to deploy new policies to network devices. In this manner, Template Manager greatly reduces the time to recovery due to unintended and erroneous ACL configurations in the enterprise.

Another error prevention feature in ACLM is the ACL Downloader, which allows administrators to select various failsafe options when deploying new ACLs to the network. One such feature forces ACL updates to abort if errors are detected in the configuration. With the "abort on error" feature enabled, ACLM will automatically revert to the original router configuration, known in Cisco ACLM parlance as *rollback*. This option prevents potentially damaging and erroneous ACL configurations from being enabled on a critical production infrastructure.

The Basic Operation of ACL Manager

With many of the useful network management features of ACLM defined, this section focuses on some of the basic operations of ACLM components. The following operational capabilities will be covered in the following sections:

- Using Templates and Defining Classes
- Using DiffViewer
- Using the Optimizer and Hits Optimizer

There are many other basic operational capabilities within the ACLM. For additional information, refer to the Cisco ACLM documentation.

Using Templates and Defining Classes

As previously discussed, templates can help ensue consistency across the network and reduce the time in deploying ACLs. Before using Template Manager however, it is important to first configure networks, network classes, services, and service classes. To do so, administrators use the Class Manager to view, add, and change classes.

The services in the Class Manager include standard services and port numbers for well-known applications like FTP, HTTP, and Telnet. New, custom services can be added to the list of services as well. To add new services, simply select the type of IP service, UDP or TCP, enter a name to identify the new service, and enter the associated port number.

Class Manager also provides the configuration of service classes, which are customized, user-defined groups of services. To add a custom service class, first specify a name to identify the service class and select the associated IP protocol type, UDP or TCP. Finally, specify the following to be part of the services class definition:

- One or more service port numbers

- A range of ports specified with a low and high port value

- One or more previously defined service classes

Additionally, the Class Manager facilitates the creation and modification of networks and network classes. Networks are created with logical names and include the IP address and corresponding subnet mask of the network. Network entities should define the smallest logical network segment on the enterprise. This allows for increased specificity when defining ACL. If necessary, network classes can be used to define larger, generalized groups of networks.

Network classes created with the Class Manager allow for the association of one or all of the following:

- One or more specific host IP addresses

- One or more ranges of IP addresses specified using a start and end IP address

- One or more networks created in the network folder

- One or more previously created network classes created in this folder

These specific service and network entities can be removed and added to new service and network classes as necessary. By defining these entities and grouping first, administrators can easily and quickly create ACL template configurations and define a standardized security policy for replication across the network.

Using DiffViewer

ACLs created and altered on the network via ACLM do not take effect immediately. Rather, changes are applied to specific routers and devices manually or at a scheduled, off-hours time with the ACL Downloader. When finished with ACL changes on the network, administrators can use the DiffViewer, as previously described, to verify all current configurations, as well as the changes made to ACLs.

The left panel of DiffViewer contains a list of all *Modified Objects*, including all network devices to which changes have been made or that are affected by other changes. This panel has subfolders under the specific devices that include detailed information concerning the altered ACLs and the affected interfaces. Using this interface, administrators can select a more specific view of changes based on an ACL or interface.

Within DiffViewer, the middle and right portion of the screen includes the original configuration and the modified configuration of the specific device selected on the right panel, respectively. Colors are used to simplify identification of changes as follows:

- Red indicates changes to access control entries (ACEs)
- Green indicates recently added ACEs in the ACL
- Blue identifies ACEs removed from the ACL

The Config and Delta buttons supply more information regarding changes to ACLs on the devices. The Config... button displays the entire new configuration for the selected device, including all changes. The Delta... button, on the other hand, shows the IOS commands to be performed on the selected device to make the necessary changes for the new security policy.

Using the Optimizer and the Hits Optimizer

The Optimizer and Hits Optimizer in ACLM help reduce processor cycles and increase packet-forwarding throughput through intelligent ACL regrouping and reordering. ACLs negatively impact the forwarding performance of a network device. When a packet is received or forwarded out an interface, it must first be compared to all ACEs in the ACL until a match is found. Once a match for the specific traffic is located in the ACL, traffic is denied or permitted according to ACE.

To prevent latency due to lengthy ACLs on network devices, the ACL Optimizer minimizes the number of ACEs used in ACLs. This is achieved by merging and removing redundant ACEs. In this manner, the Optimizer frees up processing resources and improves network performance. Table 14.2 exemplifies the positive effects of the Optimizer on some ACEs in an ACL.

Table 14.2 Beneficial Effects of the Optimizer

Original ACEs	Optimized ACEs
permit ip any host 192.168.50.8 permit ip any host 192.168.50.9 permit ip any host 192.168.50.10 permit ip any host 192.168.50.11 permit ip any host 192.168.50.12 permit ip any host 192.168.50.13 permit ip any host 192.168.50.14 permit ip any host 192.168.50.15	permit ip any 192.168.50.8 0.0.0.7

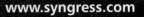
www.syngress.com

As can be seen, the Optimizer uses a process similar to that employed for route summarization on the network to improve network routing performance.

Hits Optimizer is used to improve throughput performance related to ACLs on a device. Hits Optimizer rearranges ACLs by placing the most frequently matched ACEs at the top of the ACL and moving less frequently matched ACEs to the bottom. This is achieved based on the number of matches tracked by the device IOS.

WARNING

Hits Optimizer may not always change the order of ACLs based on the number of matches for the ACEs. Hits Optimizer never alters the intent of the ACL and always preserves the security of the device since the careless reordering of access list entries can completely disable the security of an ACL.

Using ACL Manager

Before using the ACLM to manage network devices, the ACLM software must be successfully installed and the network devices configured for proper management. This section includes the procedures necessary for installation and preparation of the enterprise before ACL management can take place.

Configuring the ACL Manager

Several pieces of information must be gathered when preparing the network for ACLM. Additionally, all Cisco devices to be managed must be configured to integrate with ACLM.

Domain Name Service (DNS) entries must be configured for all devices on the network including forward and reverse resolution mapping. This information is used when adding devices to the RME inventory within CiscoWorks2000. The DNS entry should be a fully qualified domain name. When adding devices to the RME, the following information for each device on the network is required:

- Read Community String for SNMP
- Read/Write Community String for SNMP

- TACACS Username and Password, if used

- Local Device Username and Password

- Telnet Username and Password

- Enable TACACS Username and Password, if used

- Enable Password

- Enable Secret Password

Managed devices must be configured with accurate public and private SNMP community strings. All devices to be managed should be added using the Add Device tool under the Inventory folder in the RME section of CiscoWorks2000. This should be accomplished before making changes to the ACLs of the device.

NOTE

To configure the SNMP service on an ACLM managed router, use one of the following two commands in global configuration mode:

```
Rt1(config)#snmp-server community community_string ro
```

This command configures SNMP read-only access for the specified community string.

```
Rt1(config)#snmp-server community community_string rw
```

This command configures read-write access for the specific community string.

Installing the ACL Manager and Associated Software

Before beginning the ACLM installation process, ensure that the server hardware and OS meets all requirements. Also, verify that the following installation CD-ROMs or files are available:

- CiscoWorks2000 CD One

- Resource Manager Essentials

- Access Control List Manager

The software in the preceding list must be installed in sequence for the successful operation of ACL Manager on the server. Begin by installing CiscoWorks2000. If installing the software on a Windows platform, verify the server is not a primary or backup domain controller for the Windows NT domain. Furthermore, a Windows-based installation can only be performed on an NTFS file system.

After successfully installing CiscoWorks2000, install Resource Manager Essentials on the same server. Follow the onscreen wizard dialogs through the installation process, which takes approximately 30 minutes to complete.

Once RME is installed, finish by integrating ACLM on the server platform. As with the previous software installations, follow the onscreen wizards to successfully complete ACLM. This process installs the ACLM add-on to RME within CiscoWorks2000.

For detailed information regarding the installation of these software packages, refer to the appropriate Cisco documentation included with the software media.

Configuration Example: Creating ACLs with ACLM

The next example includes procedures for creating ACLs on a router. To do so, the following specific exercises are included:

- Adding a new router to the CiscoWorks2000 configuration

- Opening a new scenario to edit ACLs on the new router

- Adding an ACL and a specific ACE to the router

Additional recommended self-study exercises could include the creation of templates in the ACLM Template Editor for future security policy enforcement of the newly created ACLs.

NOTE

When using CiscoWorks2000, ensure that Java, JavaScript, and Accept all cookies are enabled in the Internet browser settings on the management client workstation. If these settings are not correct, the CiscoWorks2000 client will not function properly.

To use the CiscoWorks2000 Web-based GUI, open an HTTP connection to the specific host name or IP address of the CiscoWorks2000 server. In the URL string, include the specific TCP port number of the CiscoWorks2000 server specified during installation. The default CiscoWorks2000 port number is 1741. Use the following format in the browser: http://server_ip_address:server_port.

The initial login screen, as shown in Figure 14.14, requires a username and password to log in to the CiscoWorks2000 GUI. The default username is *admin* and the default password is *admin*.

Figure 14.14 The CiscoWorks2000 Initial Login Screen

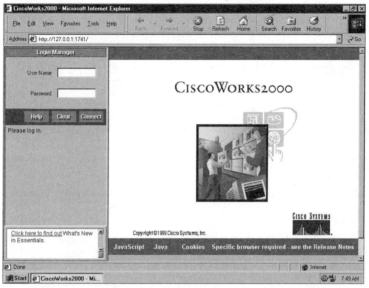

After successfully logging in to CiscoWorks2000, continue by clicking the **Resource Manager Essentials tab** on the left side of the screen. Next, click the **Administration** tree selection, followed by the Inventory subselection. Finally, click the **Add Devices** tool to add and manage the new device on the network. Figure 14.15 shows the screen used to add a device to the configuration. Enter the required information, including passwords and SNMP community strings, in the forms provided.

A scenario must be created in association with the new ACL to be configured. Figure 14.16 shows the screen on which a scenario is configured. Enter a specific name for the new scenario and select the relevant information below. Click **Next** to select the devices to be used in the scenario.

The next screen appears where the devices can be selected based on a custom view filter. Click **Add** to add the related device for the new scenario. Clicking **Next** opens a new Java applet window called "ACL Manager," which is used to configure the ACL. Apply it to the selected device. Figure 14.17 shows the ACL Manager applet window and subselections.

Figure 14.15 Adding a Device to the CiscoWorks2000 Configuration

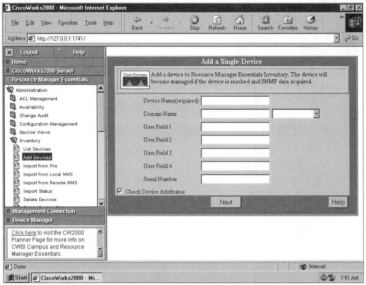

Figure 14.16 Creating a Scenario to Edit the ACL

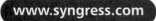

Figure 14.17 The ACL Manager Window

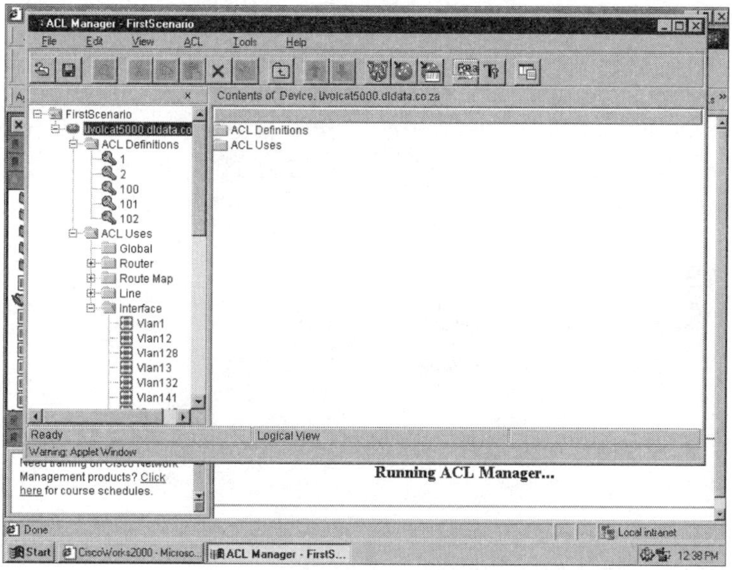

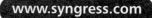

Next, add a specific ACL for the new ACE by right-clicking the **ACL Definitions folder** and selecting **New ACL**. Figure 14.18 shows the ACL Editor screen used to add an ACL to the selected router.

Figure 14.18 Adding an ACL to the Router

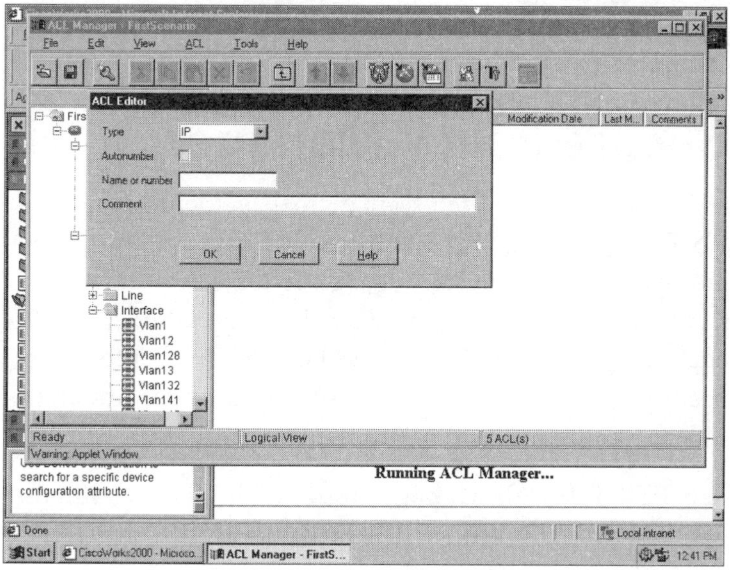

After clicking **OK**, notice the new ACL in the ACL Definition section. Right-click the new ACL to obtain a list of options related to it.

Finally, add the relevant ACEs for the specific security policy to the ACL. Figure 14.19 shows the first ACE for the new standard ACL that denies all traffic from 192.168.200.0. Click the **Expand...** button to see the list of IOS commands used to configure the selected router. To add another ACE to the ACL, click the **New** button.

Figure 14.19 Adding an ACE to the New ACL

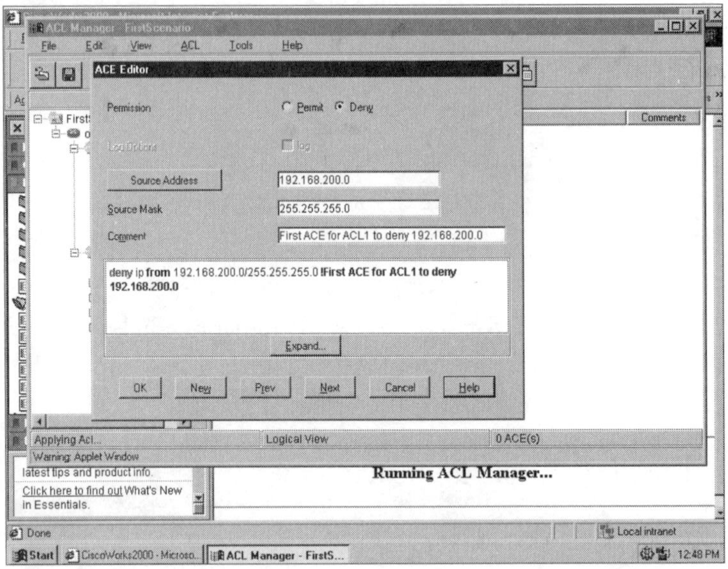

Cisco Secure Policy Manager

Another powerful tool in the Cisco security management arsenal is the CSPM. CSPM is an NT-based management tool for networks sized up to 500 devices. The application provides a complete management solution for Cisco VPN routers, IDS, and Cisco Secure PIX firewalls. Through CSPM, security administrators can effectively and securely manage the definition, enforcement and auditing of security policy from one intuitive administrative interface.

The significant features of CSPM are as follows:

- **Cisco PIX Firewall Management** With CPSM, administrators can define and maintain PIX- and IOS-based security policies via the Cisco Secure Integrated Software feature set.

- **Cisco VPN Gateway Management** VPN Gateway Management enables IPSec VPN management on PIX firewalls and Cisco VPN devices running the IOS IPSec software.

- **Config Import** Firewall administrators can import topology and security polices from PIX and IOS security network devices.

- **Security Policy Management** Up to 500 Cisco security devices can be easily managed without extensive device knowledge and dependency on the command-line interface (CLI).

- **Notification and Reporting System** CSPM includes auditing tools to monitor, alert, and report Cisco security device and policy activity.

Due to the extensive capabilities and functionality in the CSPM application, an entire chapter in this book has been devoted to the software. For additional and detailed information regarding CSPM, refer to Chapter 12.

Cisco Secure Access Control Server

In large network infrastructures, it is essential to control access to, and use of, the many diverse devices providing critical services. Without a scalable and capable management application platform to configure and monitor device access, the work of a security manager can quickly become overburdened with time-consuming and tedious administration. It is also often necessary to track specific events occurring on network devices for correlation of security breaches, configuration changes, and other access nuances.

To assist network and security administrators in these endeavors, Cisco has developed the Secure Access Control Server (Secure ACS). This application enables full control over all Cisco-based authentication, authorization, and accounting (AAA) configurations and management.

Overview of the Cisco Secure Access Control Server

Secure ACS enables centralized management of access control and accounting for dial-up access servers, VPNs and firewalls, Voice over IP (VoIP) solutions, broadband access, content networks and Cisco wireless solutions. Administrators can quickly manage user and group accounts on the entire network through security level changes and network policy alterations. Secure ACS is also designed for interoperability; administrators can leverage existing user database infrastructures such as

Lightweight Directory Access Protocol (LDAP) servers or Windows-based domain authentication mechanisms in combination with RADIUS and TACACS+ functionality to manage users. Additionally, with Secure ACS, AAA in the enterprise can be used to manage user access from disparate client mediums such as wireless networks with the Extensible Authentication Protocol (EAP) module.

Secure ACS is available on both Windows and Solaris platforms. At the time of this publication however, only the Windows release is at version 3.0, while the Solaris release remains at 2.3. All functionality described next, therefore, relates to the latest Windows release, 3.0.

Also new to Secure ACS 3.0 is a powerful new device command policy engine for TACACS+ administration control. The device command sets (DCSs) feature new, fine-grained control of administrative management, and provide for reusable policy "roles," significantly enhancing the ability to scale administrative privileges across large sets of user groups and network device groupings.

Benefits of the Cisco Secure Access Control Server

Secure ACS enables the centralized management of AAA for Cisco devices within the enterprise. The easy-to-use Web-based interface simplifies AAA configuration and permits distributed administration of Cisco device security. The capabilities of Secure ACS and AAA are described next in the following sections.

Authentication

As users require access to network resources, authentication must be used to verify the identity of the user and correlate the necessary user information. Authentication mechanisms range from simple, cleartext methods to more secure techniques such as encrypted passwords or One-Time-Password (OTP) token systems.

With Secure ACS, several methods are available for authentication between the ACS server and network components. Most simple are cleartext password mechanisms. To increase security, administrators can use encrypted methodologies such as the TACACS+ and RADIUS protocols. It should be noted, however, that this authentication connectivity is between the ACS server and the network device only. For completely secure authentication techniques, strong security measures such as OTP token systems should be implemented for user authentication to the network access device.

Finally, Secure ACS integrates with several user databases. In addition to the native Cisco Secure user database, support for the following external user databases is included:

- Windows NT/2000 User Database

- Generic LDAP

- Novell NetWare Directory Services (NDS)

- Open Database Connectivity (ODBC)-compliant relational databases

- CRYPTOCard Token Server

- SafeWord Token Server

- AXENT Token Server

- RSA SecureID Token Server

- ActivCard Token Server

- Vasco Token Server

Authorization

Authorization determines the permissible actions of a specific, authenticated user. As users access services on a network device or access server, the Secure ACS sends the users' profiles to the device to determine allowed levels of service. This enables different users and groups to possess different levels of services, access times, or security to specific devices.

Administrators can restrict users based on time of day or any one (or a combination) of the following:

- PPP

- ARA

- SLIP

- Device-based EXEC service

After the service is configured on the network, Layer 2 and 3 protocols can be restricted per user via access lists. In this manner, users or groups of users can be restricted from accessing networked devices such as FTP and HTTP servers. Additionally, authorization for Virtual Private Dial-up Networks (VPDNs) can be configured via Secure ACS to allow users and groups temporal access to secure tunnels to and from various locations. Finally, Secure ACS provides dynamic quotas for time-of-day, network usage, number of logged sessions, and day-of-week access restrictions.

An important rule to remember when configuring authentication and authorization for users on the network: those with more authorization should always require stronger authentication to access network resources.

Accounting

The final piece of AAA is accounting. With accounting enabled on network devices, Secure ACS can track user actions. Secure ACS writes accounting records to Comma Delimited (CSV) log files or to ODBC-compliant data sources for integration into third-party applications to generate items such as billing reports or security audits. For more information on AAA, see Chapter 9.

In addition to the typical AAA features listed earlier, Secure ACS also includes functionality such as IEEE 802.1x support. This permits access control for switched LANs at port-level granularity. Doing so relies on the new IETF RFC Extensible Authentication Protocol (EAP) standard. EAP is an emerging PPP authentication methodology using MD5 hashing for security and is included in Secure ACS.

Finally, ACS includes new TACACS+ management functionality known as Device Command Sets (DCS). This new administrative tool provides a central CiscoSecure ACS GUI mechanism to control the authorization of each command on each device via per-user, per-group, or per-network device group mapping.

Installation Requirements for the Cisco Access Control Server

Before installing the Secure ACS software, verify the server meets the following hardware and software requirements as shown next. Although this section focuses on the recently released Windows 3.0 functionality, specifications for the Solaris-based 2.3 version are included as well.

When running Secure ACS on a Windows operating system, the following requirements apply:

- **OS** Windows NT 4.0 SP6a or Windows 2000 SP1 or SP2
- **System** Pentium-compatible

- **Processor** 550MHz or faster

- **Memory** 256MB RAM

- **Disk** 250MB; more if the database is on the same machine

- **Browser** Microsoft Internet Explorer Versions 5.0 and 5.5 or Netscape Communicator Version 4.76

When running Secure ACS on a Solaris operating system, the following requirements apply:

- **OS** Solaris 2.5, 2.6, 7, 8

- **System** Sun SPARC 20

- **Memory** 128MB RAM with 256MB swap space

- **Disk** 500MB

- **Database** Oracle 7.33 or Sybase 11.1

- **Browser** Netscape Communicator Version 4.76

Features of Cisco Secure ACS

Secure ACS is a powerful access control server with many high-performance and scalability features such as the following:

- **Intuitive User Interface** The Web-based user interface simplifies and distributes the configuration for user profiles, group profiles, and ACS configuration.

- **Scalability** Secure ACS is built to support large networked environments with support for redundant servers, remote databases, and user database backup services.

- **Extensibility** LDAP authentication forwarding supports the authentication of user profiles stored in directories from leading directory vendors such as Netscape, Novell, and Microsoft.

- **Management** Windows 2000 Active Directory and Windows NT database support consolidates Windows username/password management and uses the Windows Performance Monitor for real-time statistics viewing.

- **Administration** Different access levels for each Secure ACS administrator and the ability to group network devices enables easier control and maximum flexibility. This facilitates enforcement and changes of security policy administration over all devices in a network.

- **Product Flexibility** Because Cisco IOS Software has embedded support for AAA, Secure ACS can be used across virtually any network access device that Cisco sells. (The Cisco IOS version must support RADIUS or TACACS+.)

- **Protocol Flexibility** Secure ACS includes simultaneous TACACS+ and RADIUS support for a flexible solution with VPN or dial support at the origin and termination of Internet Protocol Security (IPSec) and Point-to-Point Tunneling Protocol (PPTP) tunnels.

- **Integration** Tight coupling with Cisco IOS routers and VPN solutions provides features such as Multichassis Multilink Point-to-Point Protocol and Cisco IOS command authorization.

- **Third-party Support** Secure ACS offers token server support for RSA SecurID, Passgo, Secure Computing, ActiveCard, Vasco, and CryptoCard.

- **Control** Secure ACS provides dynamic quotas for time-of-day, network usage, number of logged sessions, and day-of-week access restrictions.

For more information on features available, refer to Secure ACS information on the Cisco Web site.

Placing Cisco Secure ACS in the Network

Secure ACS can control access to many devices and services on a network. Figure 14.20 depicts a typical placement of a Secure ACS server in the network.

As can be seen, Secure ACS can be used with dial-up access servers, VPNs and firewalls, voice-IP solutions, content networks and Cisco wireless solutions. Windows NT domain servers or external databases/directories, such as LDAP, can be used to manage the username database for access to network devices and dial-up user access. Centralizing control of network access simplifies access management and helps establish a constant security policy.

Between the access devices and Secure ACS, TACACS+ or RADIUS can provide authentication and authorization for network users. The ACS server checks external user databases or local accounts on the ACS server. Dial-up users from remote locations can use PPP or other methodologies to authenticate with the NAS, and the NAS can use TACACS+ or RADIUS to interact with ACS server.

Figure 14.20 A Secure ACS Server in the Network Architecture

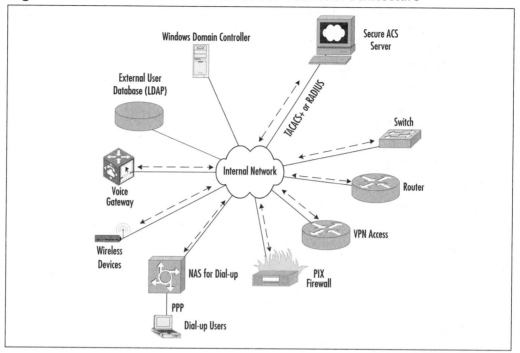

Cisco Secure ACS Device and Software Support

As previously mentioned, Secure ACS supports management of access control and accounting for dial-up access servers, VPNs and firewalls, voice-IP solutions, broadband access, content networks and Cisco wireless solutions. More specifi-cally, Secure ACS supports all devices compliant with TACACS+ or RADIUS protocol, including non-Cisco devices. For full TACACS+ and RADIUS support on Cisco IOS devices however, verify that all AAA clients are running Cisco IOS Release 11.2 or later.

When using TACACS+ and RADIUS with third-party devices via the ACS server, verify the devices conform to the following specifications:

- Cisco Systems draft 1.77: TACACS+
- IETF RADIUS RFCs: 2138, 2139, 2865, 2866, 2867, 2868

To support both the older and newer RADIUS RFCs, Secure ACS accepts authentication requests on port 1645 and port 1812. For accounting, Secure ACS accepts accounting packets on port 1646 and 1813.

In addition to supporting standard IETF RADIUS attributes, Secure ACS includes support for RADIUS vendor-specific attributes (VSAs). The following predefined RADIUS VSAs exist in Secure ACS:

- Cisco IOS/PIX
- Cisco VPN 3000
- Cisco VPN 5000
- Ascend
- Juniper
- Microsoft
- Nortel

Finally, Secure ACS supports up to ten user-defined RADIUS VSAs to be used with AAA.

Secure ACS supports several external databases for authentication in addition to the ACS internal password database as follows:

- Windows NT/2000 User Database
- Generic LDAP
- Novell NetWare Directory Services (NDS)
- Open Database Connectivity (ODBC)-compliant relational databases
- Token Card servers as follows:
  - CRYPTOCard Token Server
  - SafeWord Token Server
  - AXENT Token Server
  - RSA SecureID Token Server
  - ActivCard Token Server
  - Vasco Token Server

When dial-up users request access to a NAS server on the network, the NAS directs the dial-in user access request to the Secure ACS for authentication and authorization of privileges using TACACS+ or RADIUS. If the Secure ACS user database is not locally configured, ACS sends the authentication request to the relevant username database for authentication. The success or failure response from the Secure ACS server is relayed back to the NAS, which permits or denies user access to a network. After the user is authenticated on the network, Secure ACS sends a set of authorization attributes to the NAS and any configured accounting functions take place.

Using Cisco Secure ACS

Before using Secure ACS to manage AAA on network devices, the Secure ACS software must be successfully installed and the network devices configured for proper management. This section includes the procedures necessary for a Windows-based installation, and preparation of the enterprise before AAA management can take place. Prior to installing the software, always verify that the ACS server software and hardware meet all requirements previously specified.

Installing Cisco Secure ACS

Before initiating the installation, some information must first be gathered. Secure ACS will request the following information during the installation process:

- The AAA protocol and vendor-specific attribute to implement
- The name of the first AAA client
- The IP address of the first AAA client
- The Windows 2000/NT server IP address
- The TACACS+ or RADIUS key (shared secret)

Once you have gathered this information, begin the installation and select a location to install the server software. Next, Secure ACS requests the database format for the authentication process. Select the local Secure ACS database or the Windows NT User Database. The use of other, external authentication databases can be configured after the installation of Secure ACS.

> **WARNING**
>
> If upgrading an existing ACS installation, be sure to back up all Secure ACS system files, databases, and the Windows Registry.

Proceed with the installation through the following steps:

1. **Configure the first AAA client** Determine how to authenticate users on a specific Network Access Server on the network.

2. **Configure advanced options** Select advanced options to be enabled on the server. These options can be configured later via the Advanced Options page in the Interface Configuration section.

3. **Configure Active Service Monitoring** Determine whether active service monitoring should be enabled and how monitoring should be configured. Monitoring features can be configured later via the Active Server Management page in the System Configuration section.

4. **Configure Network Access Servers** Configure AAA in detail on network access servers, if desired.

5. **Start the ACS service and launch the Secure ACS software** Begin configuring Secure ACS via the administrative browser, if desired.

After the installation process successfully completes, access the Cisco SecureACS HTML interface using the ACS Admin desktop icon on the Windows server or open the following URL in a supported Web browser on the Windows server: http://127.0.0.1:2002.

Configuration

After installing Secure ACS, several additional administrative and configuration details must be completed. The following sequence of configuration activities is typical of most post-ACS installation processes.

- **Configure Administrators** Configure at least one administrator after installation; otherwise, remote administrative access will not be possible.

- **Configure System** Configure functions within the System Configuration section such as setting the format for the display of dates, password validation, and configuring settings for database replication and RDBMS synchronization. Set up the logs and reports to be generated by Secure ACS as well.

- **Configure Network** Establish the identity, location, and grouping of AAA clients and servers, and determine the authentication protocols each is to employ.

- **Configure External User Database** If using an external database to establish and maintain user authentication accounts, configure the database. Specify requirements for Secure ACS database replication, backup, and synchronization.

- **Configure Shared Profile Components** Before configuring user groups, configure Shared Profile Components.

- **Configure Groups** Decide how to implement unknown user processing and database group mapping. Then, configure user groups with a complete plan of how Secure ACS is to implement authorization and authentication.

- **Configure Users** Establish user accounts.

- **Configure Reports** Specify the nature and scope of logging that Secure ACS performs using the Reports and Activities section of the Secure ACS HTML interface.

Configuration Example: Adding and Configuring a AAA Client

After performing the recommended configuration tasks in the preceding list, continue to add AAA clients as necessary. This example provides information regarding the addition of new AAA clients. Begin from the Network Configuration screen shown in Figure 14.21 in order to add a device within the enterprise that requires the ACS server for AAA.

Figure 14.21 Configuring Network Devices Using Secure ACS

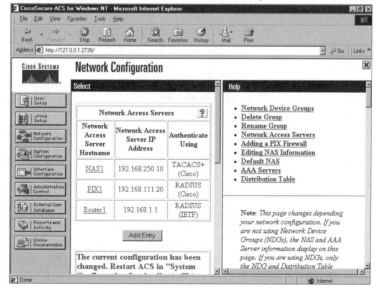

Click **Add Entry** below the AAA Clients table. The Add AAA Client page appears as shown in Figure 14.22.

Figure 14.22 Device Configuration Changes in Secure ACS

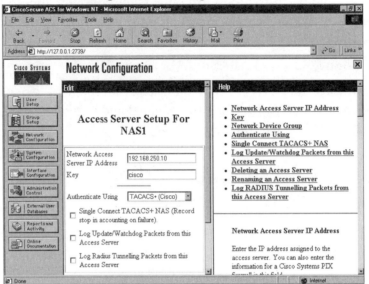

In this page, assign the following to the new AAA client:

■ Hostname

■ Client IP address

■ The shared secret that the AAA client and Secure ACS use to encrypt data

If using Network Device Groups, select the name of the Network Device Group to which the AAA client belongs from the Network Device Group list, or select **Not Assigned**. Determine the network security protocol used by the AAA client by configuring one of the following options:

■ TACACS+ (Cisco IOS)

■ RADIUS (Cisco Aironet)

■ RADIUS (Cisco BBMS)

■ RADIUS (IETF)

■ RADIUS (Cisco IOS/PIX)

- RADIUS (Cisco VPN 3000)

- RADIUS (Cisco VPN 5000)

- RADIUS (Ascend)

- RADIUS (Juniper)

- RADIUS (Nortel)

To enable a static connection for all requests from the AAA client, select the **Single Connect TACACS+ AAA Client** check box. Enable Watchdog packets by selecting the **Log Update/Watchdog Packets from this AAA Client** check box. Watchdog packets are interim packets sent periodically during a session and serve to enable an approximation of session length if the AAA client fails.

To allow RADIUS tunneling accounting packets to be logged in the RADIUS Accounting reports of Reports and Activity, select the **Log RADIUS tunneling Packets from the AAA Client** check box.

Save the changes and apply them immediately by clicking **Submit | Restart**.

NOTE

To save changes and continue working, click the **Submit** button. When finished making all changes, click **System Configuration | Service Control**. Click **Restart** to implement all changes.

Summary

Robust security management techniques are required to keep pace with the increasing complexity and frequency of security incidents. In large networks with numerous services and network ingress and egress points, the use of application tools can help administrators remain efficient and vigilant against attack while ensuring standardized security policies.

The security applications developed by Cisco (listed next) serve to enhance security management through intuitive graphical interfaces, configuration automation, report generation, and enhanced monitoring capabilities among others.

- PIX Device Manager (PDM)

- CiscoWorks2000 Access Control Lists Manager (ACLM)

- Cisco Secure Policy Manager (CSPM)

- Cisco Secure Access Control Server (ACS)

Each application is suited for different purposes, yet the combination of these applications can represent a holistic application solution in many environments. While no system or network is impervious to malicious attack, with sound management and security policy techniques, the Cisco-based solutions discussed in this chapter arm security administrators and managers with essential tools for the ongoing struggle for infrastructure security.

The Cisco-based security management solutions described in this chapter represent some of the best industry responses to the ever-evolving needs of today's security administrators and managers. Using these tools, many of the complex and tedious tasks required to manage security devices and infrastructure are simplified and automated by various application solutions.

Solutions Fast Track

PIX Device Manager

- ☑ PDM is designed to securely manage small numbers of PIX Firewalls.

- ☑ PDM has a Java-based GUI for simplified remote management.

- ☑ PDM has a powerful interface enabling nearly all CLI capabilities from a Web browser.

- ☑ PDM includes graphical reporting and monitoring capabilities.

CiscoWorks2000 Access Control Lists Manager

☑ ACLM is part of the CiscoWorks2000 Routed WAN Management Solution.

☑ ACLM enables robust control of IP and IPX access lists.

☑ ACLM automates new ACL rollout and ongoing ACL changes to multiple devices.

☑ ACLM includes version comparison tools for quick troubleshooting and change management.

Cisco Secure Policy Manager

☑ CSPM provides a complete management solution for Cisco VPN routers, IDS, and Cisco Secure PIX firewalls.

☑ CSPM is a NT-based management tool for networks sized up to 500 devices.

☑ CSPM enables the definition, enforcement, and auditing of security policy from one intuitive administrative interface.

Cisco Secure Access Control Server

☑ Secure ACS enables centralized management of access control and accounting for dial-up access servers, VPNs and firewalls, voice-IP solutions, broadband access, content networks and Cisco wireless solutions.

☑ Secure ACS provides full control over authentication, authorization, and accounting (AAA) configurations and management.

☑ Secure ACS is designed for interoperability; administrators can leverage existing user database infrastructures such as Lightweight Directory Access Protocol (LDAP) servers or Windows-based domain authentication mechanisms in combination with RADIUS and TACACS+ functionality to manage users.

Frequently Asked Questions

The following Frequently Asked Questions, answered by the authors of this book, are designed to both measure your understanding of the concepts presented in this chapter and to assist you with real-life implementation of these concepts. To have your questions about this chapter answered by the author, browse to **www.syngress.com/solutions** and click on the **"Ask the Author"** form.

Q: Is Cisco PDM compatible with other forms of management such as Cisco Secure Policy Manager (CSPM), CLI, and so forth?

A: Yes. Cisco PDM is a graphical interface to the PIX firewall, yet the resulting commands it reads and writes are CLI. PDM can read configurations that have been created via CLI or CSPM. Likewise, CLI users can view and alter configurations generated by PDM. There are some exceptions to this rule such as static PAT configurations, which cannot be interpreted by the PDM interface.

Q: Is there a limitation on the size of the configuration that Cisco PDM can handle?

A: Cisco recommends that Cisco PDM configuration files be 100KB (approximately 1500 lines) or less in size.

Q: Can Secure ACS be implemented on a platform other than Windows?

A: Yes, a Solaris version of Secure ACS exists, but is not capable of the same functionality as the Windows release at this time.

Q: Can more than one user use ACL Manager at any one time?

A: Yes, ACL Manager is designed to be a multi-user application. However, if several users are running ACL Manager and are all trying to modify ACLs on the same device, the user that downloads changes to the device first will invalidate the work of all the other users. Cisco recommends that several users use ACL Manager when the groups of devices on which they are administering ACLs do not overlap, or the user is using ACL Manager in a "read-only" manner.

Q: Will ACL Manager help reduce the time it takes to make the same changes on several devices?

A: Yes, the administrator can use the ACL Use Wizard to apply a predefined filtering policy or template to a group of devices and appropriate interfaces at one time.

## Chapter 15

Looking Ahead: Cisco Wireless Security

Solutions in this chapter:

- **Understanding Security Fundamentals and Principles of Protection**

- **MAC Filtering**

- **Reviewing the Role of Policy**

- **Implementing WEP**

- **Addressing Common Risks and Threats**

- **Sniffing, Interception, and Eavesdropping**

- **Spoofing and Unauthorized Access**

- **Network Hijacking and Modification**

- **Denial of Service and Flooding Attacks**

☑ **Summary**

☑ **Solutions Fast Track**

☑ **Frequently Asked Questions**

Introduction

There is not much indication of anything slowing down the creation and deployment of new technology to the world any time in the near future. With the constant pressure to deploy the latest generation of technology today, little time is allowed for a full and proper security review of the technology and components that make it up.

This rush to deploy, along with the insufficient security review, not only allows age-old security vulnerabilities to be reintroduced to products, but creates new and unknown security challenges as well. Wireless networking is not exempt from this, and like many other technologies, security flaws have been identified and new methods of exploiting these flaws are published regularly.

Utilizing security fundamentals developed over the last few decades, you can review and protect your wireless networks from known and unknown threats. In this chapter, we recall security fundamentals and principles that are the foundation of any good security strategy, addressing a range of issues from authentication and authorization, to controls and audit.

No primer on security would be complete without an examination of the common security standards, which are addressed in this chapter alongside the emerging privacy standards and their implications for the wireless exchange of information.

We also look at how you can maximize the features of existing security standards like Wired Equivalent Protocol (WEP). We also examine the effectiveness of Media Access Control (MAC) and protocol filtering as a way of minimizing opportunity. Lastly, we look at the security advantages of using virtual private networks (VPNs) on a wireless network, as well as discuss the importance of convincing users of the role they can play as key users of the network.

You'll also learn about the existing and anticipated threats to wireless networks, and the principles of protection that are fundamental to a wireless security strategy. And although many of the attacks are similar in nature to attacks on wired networks, you need to understand the particular tools and techniques that attackers use to take advantage of the unique way wireless networks are designed, deployed, and maintained. We explore the attacks that have exposed the vulnerabilities of wireless networks, and in particular the weaknesses inherent in the security standards. Through a detailed examination of these standards, we identify how these weaknesses have lead to the development of new tools and tricks that hackers use to exploit your wireless networks. We look at the emergence and threat of "war driving" technique and how it is usually the first step in an attack on wireless networks.

Understanding Security Fundamentals and Principles of Protection

Security protection starts with the preservation of the *confidentiality*, *integrity*, and *availability* (CIA) of data and computing resources. These three tenets of information security, often referred to as "The Big Three," are sometimes represented by the CIA triad, shown in Figure 15.1.

Figure 15.1 The CIA Triad

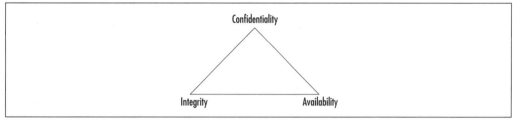

As we describe each of these tenets, you will see that in order to provide for a reliable and secure wireless environment, you will need to ensure that each tenet is properly protected. To ensure the preservation of The Big Three and protect the privacy of those whose data is stored and flows through these data and computing resources, The Big Three security tenets are implemented through tried-and-true security practices. These other practices enforce The Big Three by ensuring proper authentication for authorized access while allowing for nonrepudiation in identification and resource usage methods, and by permitting complete accountability for all activity through audit trails and logs. Some security practitioners refer to Authentication, Authorization, and Audit (accountability) as "AAA." Each of these practices provides the security implementer with tools which they can use to properly identify and mitigate any possible risks to The Big Three.

Ensuring Confidentiality

Confidentiality attempts to prevent the intentional or unintentional unauthorized disclosure of communications between a sender and recipient. In the physical world, ensuring confidentiality can be accomplished by simply securing the physical area. However, as evidenced by bank robberies and military invasions, threats exist to the security of the physical realm that can compromise security and confidentiality.

The moment electronic means of communication were introduced, many new possible avenues of disclosing the information within these communications were created. The confidentiality of early analog communication systems, such as the telegraph and telephone, were easily compromised by simply having someone connect to the wires used by a sender and receiver.

When digital communications became available, like with many technologies, it was only a matter of time until knowledgeable people were able to build devices and methods that could interpret the digital signals and convert them to whatever form needed to disclose what was communicated. And as technology grew and became less expensive, the equipment needed to monitor and disclose digital communications became available to anyone wishing to put the effort into monitoring communication.

With the advent of wireless communications, the need for physically connecting to a communication channel to listen in or capture confidential communications was removed. Although you can achieve some security by using extremely tight beam directional antennas, someone still just has to sit somewhere in between the antennas to be able to monitor and possibly connect to the communications channel without having to actually tie into any physical device.

Having knowledge that communications channels are possibly compromised allows us to properly implement our policies and procedures to mitigate the wireless risk. The solution used to ensure The Big Three and other security tenets is *encryption*.

The current implementation of encryption in today's wireless networks use the RC4 stream cipher to encrypt the transmitted network packets, and the WEP to protect authentication into wireless networks by network devices connecting to them (that is, the network adapter authentication, not the user utilizing the network resources). Both of which, due mainly to improper implementations, have introduced sufficient problems that have made it possible to determine keys used and then either falsely authenticate to the network or decrypt the traffic traveling across through the wireless network. For more information on encryption and cryptography please refer to Chapter 6.

With these apparent problems, those in charge of wireless network security should utilize other proven and properly implemented encryption solutions, such as Secure Shell (SSH), Secure Sockets Layer (SSL), or IPSec.

Ensuring Integrity

Integrity ensures the accuracy and completeness of information throughout its process methods. The first communication methods available to computers did not have much in place to ensure the integrity of the data transferred from one to another. As such, occasionally something as simple as static on a telephone line could cause the transfer of data to be corrupted.

To solve this problem, the idea of a checksum was introduced. A *checksum* is nothing more than taking the message you are sending and running it through a function that returns a simple value which is then appended to the message being sent. When the receiver gets the complete message, they would then run the message through the same function and compare the value they generate with the value that was included at the end of the message.

The functions that are generally used to generate basic checksums are usually based upon simple addition or modulus functions. These functions can sometimes have their own issues, such as the function not being detailed enough to allow for distinctly separate data that could possibly have identical checksums. It is even possible to have two errors within the data itself cause the checksum to provide a valid check because the two errors effectively cancel each other out. These problems are usually addressed through a more complex algorithm used to create the digital checksum.

Cyclic redundancy checks (CRCs) were developed as one of the more advanced methods of ensuring data integrity. CRC algorithms basically treat a message as an enormous binary number, whereupon another large fixed binary number then divides this binary number. The remainder from this division is the checksum. Using the remainder of a long division as the checksum, as opposed to the original data summation, adds a significant chaos to the checksum created, increasing the likelihood that the checksum will not be repeatable with any other separate data stream.

These more advanced checksum methods, however, have their own set of problems. As Ross Williams wrote in his 1993 paper, A Painless Guide to CRC Error Detection Algorithms (www.ross.net/crc/crcpaper.html), the goal of error detection is to protect against corruption introduced by noise in a data transfer. This is good if we are concerned only with protecting against possible transmission errors. However, the algorithm provides no means of ensuring the integrity of an intentionally corrupted data stream. If someone has knowledge of a particular data stream, altering the contents of the data and completing the transaction with a valid checksum is possible. The receiver would not have knowledge of the changes in the data because their checksum would match and it would appear as if the data was transferred with no errors.

This form of intentional integrity violation is called a "Data Injection." In such cases, the best way to protect data is to (once again) use a more advanced form of integrity protection utilizing cryptography. Today, this higher level of protection is generally provided through a stronger cryptographic algorithm such as the MD5 or RC4 ciphers.

Wireless networks today use the RC4 stream cipher to protect the data transmitted as well as provide for data integrity. It has been proven that the 802.11 implementation of the RC4 cipher with its key scheduling algorithm introduces enough information to provide a hacker with enough to be able to predict your network's secret encryption key. Once the hacker has your key, they are not only able to gain access to your wireless network, but also view it as if there was no encryption at all.

Ensuring Availability

Availability, as defined in an information security context, ensures that access data or computing resources needed by appropriate personnel is both reliable and available in a timely manner. The origins of the Internet itself come from the need to ensure the availability of network resources. In 1957, the United States Department of Defense (DoD) created the Advanced Research Projects Agency (ARPA) following the Soviet launch of Sputnik. Fearing loss of command and control over U.S. nuclear missiles and bombers due to communication channel disruption caused by nuclear or conventional attacks, the U.S. Air Force commissioned a study on how to create a network that could function with the loss of access or routing points. Out of this, packet switched networking was created, and the first four nodes of ARPANET were deployed in 1968 running at the then incredibly high speed of 50 Kbps.

The initial design of packet switched networks did not take into consideration the possibility of an actual attack on the network from one of its own nodes. As the ARPANET grew into what we now know as the Internet, many modifications have been made to the protocols and applications that make up the network, ensuring the availability of all resources provided.

Wireless networks are experiencing many similar design issues, and due to the proliferation of new wireless high-tech devices, many are finding themselves in conflict with other wireless resources. Like their wired equivalents, there was little expectation that conflicts would occur within the wireless spectrum available for use. Because of this, very few wireless equipment providers planned their implementations with features to ensure the availability of the wireless resource in case a conflict occurred.

Ensuring Privacy

Privacy is the assurance that the information a customer provides to some party will remain private and protected. This information generally contains customer personal nonpublic information that is protected by both regulation and civil liability law. Your wireless policy and procedures should contain definitions on how to ensure the privacy of customer information that might be accessed or transmitted by your wireless networks. The principles and methods here provide ways of ensuring the protection of the data that travels across your networks and computers.

Ensuring Authentication

Authentication provides for a sender and receiver of information to validate each other as the appropriate entity they are wishing to work with. If entities wishing to communicate cannot properly authenticate each other, then there can be no trust of the activities or information provided by either party. It is only through a trusted and secure method of authentication that we are able to provide for a trusted and secure communication or activity.

The simplest form of authentication is the transmission of a shared password between the entities wishing to authenticate with each other. This could be as simple as a secret handshake or a key. As with all simple forms of protection, once knowledge of the secret key or handshake was disclosed to nontrusted parties, there could be no trust in who was using the secrets anymore.

Many methods can be used to acquire a simple secret key, from something as simple as tricking someone into disclosing it, to high-tech monitoring of communications between parties to intercept the key as it is passed from one party to the other. However the code is acquired, once it is in a nontrusted party's hands, they are able to utilize it to falsely authenticate and identify themselves as a valid party, forging false communications, or utilizing the user's access to gain permissions to the available resources.

The original digital authentication systems simply shared a secret key across the network with the entity they wished to authenticate with. Applications such as Telnet, File Transfer Protocol (FTP), and POP-mail are examples of programs that simply transmit the password, in cleartext, to the party they are authenticating with. The problem with this method of authentication is that anyone who is able to monitor the network could possibly capture the secret key and then use it to authenticate themselves as you in order to access these same services. They could then access your information directly, or corrupt any information you send to other parties. They may even be able to attempt to gain higher privileged access with your stolen authentication information.

Configuring & Implementing…

Cleartext Authentication

Cleartext (non-encrypted) authentication is still widely used by many people today who receive their e-mail through the Post Office Protocol (POP), which by default sends the password unprotected in cleartext from the mail client to the server. You can protect your e-mail account password in several ways, including connection encryption as well as not transmitting the password in cleartext through the network by hashing with MD5 or some similar algorithm.

Encrypting the connection between the mail client and server is the only way of truly protecting your mail authentication password. This will prevent anyone from capturing your password or any of the mail you might transfer to your client. SSL is generally the method used to encrypt the connection stream from the mail client to the server and is supported by most mail clients today.

If you just protect the password through MD5 or a similar cryptocipher, anyone who happens to intercept your "protected" password could identify it through a brute force attack. A brute force attack is where someone generates every possible combination of characters running each version through the same algorithm used to encrypt the original password until a match is made and your password is found.

Authentication POP (APOP) is a method used to provide password-only encryption for mail authentication. It employs a challenge/response method defined in RFC1725 that uses a shared timestamp provided by the server being authenticated to. The timestamp is hashed with the username and the shared secret key through the MD5 algorithm.

There are still a few problems with this, the first of which is that all values are known in advance except the shared secret key. Because of this, there is nothing to provide protection against a brute-force attack

Continued

on the shared key. Another problem is that this security method attempts to protect your password. Nothing is done to prevent anyone who might be listening to your network from then viewing your e-mail as it is downloaded to your mail client.

You can find an example of a brute-force password dictionary generator that can produce a brute-force dictionary from specific character sets at www.dmzs.com/tools/files.

To solve the problem of authentication through sharing common secret keys across an untrusted network, the concept of Zero Knowledge Passwords was created. The idea of Zero Knowledge Passwords is that the parties who wish to authenticate each other want to prove to one another that they know the shared secret, and yet not share the secret with each other in case the other party truly doesn't have knowledge of the password, while at the same time preventing anyone who may intercept the communications between the parties from gaining knowledge as to the secret that is being used.

Public-key cryptography has been shown to be the strongest method of doing Zero Knowledge Passwords. It was originally developed by Whitfield Diffie and Martin Hellman and presented to the world at the 1976 National Computer Conference. Their concept was published a few months later in their paper, New Directions in Cryptography. Another crypto-researcher named Ralph Merkle, working independently from Diffie and Hellman, also invented a similar method for providing public-key cryptography, but his research was not published until 1978.

Public-key cryptography introduced the concept of having keys work in pairs, an encryption key and a decryption key, and having them created in such a way that generating one key from the other is infeasible. The encryption key is then made public to anyone wishing to encrypt a message to the holder of the secret decryption key. Because identifying or creating the decryption key from the encryption key is infeasible, anyone who happens to have the encrypted message and the encryption key will be unable to decrypt the message or determine the decryption key needed to decrypt the message.

Public-key encryption generally stores the keys or uses a certificate hierarchy. The certificates are rarely changed and often used just for encrypting data, not authentication. Zero Knowledge Password protocols, on the other hand, tend to use Ephemeral keys. *Ephemeral keys* are temporary keys that are randomly created for a single authentication, and then discarded once the authentication is completed.

Note that the public-key encryption is still susceptible to a chosen–ciphertext attack. This attack is where someone already knows what the decrypted message is and has knowledge of the key used to generate the encrypted message. Knowing the decrypted form of the message lets the attacker possibly deduce what the secret decryption key could be. This attack is unlikely to occur with authentication systems because the attacker will not have knowledge of the decrypted message: your password. If they had that, they would already have the ability to authenticate as you and not need to determine your secret decryption key.

Currently 802.11 network authentication is centered on the authentication of the wireless device, not on authenticating the user or station utilizing the wireless network. Public-key encryption is not used in the wireless encryption process. Although a few wireless vendors have dynamic keys that are changed with every connection, most wireless 802.11 vendors utilize shared-key authentication with static keys.

Shared key authentication is utilized by WEP functions with the following steps:

1. When a station requests service, it sends an authentication frame to the access point (AP) it wishes to communicate with.

2. The receiving AP replies to the authentication frame with its own, which contains 128 octets of challenge text.

3. The station requesting access encrypts the challenge text with the shared encryption key and returns to the AP.

4. The access decrypts the encrypted challenge using the shared key and compares it with the original challenge text. If they match, an authentication acknowledgement is sent to the station requesting access, otherwise a negative authentication notice is sent.

As you can see, this authentication method does not authenticate the user or any resource the user might need to access. It is only a verification that the wireless device has knowledge of the shared secret key that the wireless AP has. Once a user has passed the AP authentication challenge, that user will then have full access to whatever devices and networks the AP is connected to. You should still use secure authentication methods to access any of these devices and prevent unauthorized access and use by people who might be able to attach to your wireless network.

To solve this lack of external authentication, the IEEE 802.11 committee is working on 802.1x, a standard that will provide a framework for 802-based networks authenticating from centralized servers. Back in November 2000, Cisco introduced Light Extensible Authentication Protocol (LEAP) authentication to their wireless products, which adds several enhancements to the 802.11 authentication system, including the following:

- Mutual authentication utilizing Remote Access Dial-In User Service (RADIUS).

- Securing the secret key with one-way hashes that make password reply attacks impossible.

- Policies to force the user to re-authenticate more often, getting a new session key with each new session. This will help to prevent attacks where traffic is injected into the data stream.

- Changes to the initialization vector used in WEP encryption that make the current exploits of WEP ineffective.

Not all vendors support these solutions, so your best bet is to protect your network and servers with your own strong authentication and authorization rules.

Extensible Authentication Protocol (EAP)

The Extensible Authentication Protocol (EAP) was designed to provide authentication methods within the Point-to-Point-Protocol (PPP). EAP allows for the integration of third-party authentication packages that use PPP. EAP can be configured so that it can support a number of methods for authentication schemes, such as token cards, public key, certificates, PINs, and on and on.

When you install PPP/EAP, EAP will not select a specific authentication method at the Link Control Protocol (LCP) Phase, but will wait until the Authentication Phase to begin. What this does is allow the authenticator the ability to request more information, and with this information it will decide on the method of authentication to use. This delay will also allow for the implementation of a server on the backend that can control the various authentication methods while the PPP authenticator passes through the authentication exchange.

In this way, network devices like Access Points (APs) or switches do not need to understand each request type, because they will simply act as a conduit, or passthrough agent, for a server on a host. The network device will only need to see if the packet has the success or failure code in order to terminate the authentication phase.

EAP is able to define one or more requests for peer-to-peer authentication. This can happen because the request packet includes a type field, such as Generic Token, one-time password (OTP), or an MD5 challenge. The MD5 challenge is very similar to the Challenge Handshake Authentication Protocol (CHAP).

EAP is able to provide you with a flexible, link-layer security framework (see Figure 15.2), by having the following features:

- EAP mechanisms are IETF standards–based and allow for the growth of new authentication types when your security needs change:

    - Transport Layer Security (TLS)

    - Internet Key Exchange (IKE)

    - GSS_API (Kerberos)

    - Other authentication schemes (LEAP)

- There is no dependency on IP, because this is an encapsulation protocol.

- There is no windowing as this is a simple ACK/NAK protocol.

- No support for fragmentation.

- Can run over any link layer (PPP, 802.3, 802.5, 802.11, and so on).

- Does not consider a physically secure link as an authentication method to provide security.

- Assumes that there is no reordering of packets.

- Retransmission of packets is the responsibility of authenticator.

Figure 15.2 The EAP Architecture

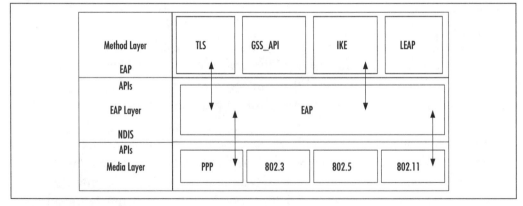

802.1x and EAP

One type of wireless security is focused on providing centralized authentication and dynamic key distribution area. By using the IEEE 802.1x standard, the EAP, and LEAP as an end-to-end solution, you can provide enhanced functionality to your wireless network. Two main elements are involved in using this standard:

- EAP/LEAP allows all wireless client adapters the capability to communicate with different authentication servers such as RADIUS and Terminal Access Controller Access Control System (TACACS+) servers that are located on the network.

- You implement the IEEE 802.1x standard for network access control that is port based for MAC filtering.

When these features are deployed together, wireless clients that are associated with APs will not be able to gain access to the network unless the user performs a network logon. The user will need to enter a username and password for network logon, after which the client and a RADIUS server will perform authentication, hopefully leading to the client being authenticated by the supplied username and password and access to the network and resources.

How this occurs is that the RADIUS server and client device will then receive a client-specific WEP key that is used by the client for that specific logon session. As an added level of security, the user's password and session key will never be transmitted in the open, over the wireless connection.

Here is how Authentication works and the WEP key is passed:

1. The wireless client will associate with an AP located on the wireless network.

2. The AP will then prevent all other attempts made by that client to gain access to network until the client logs on to the network.

3. The client will supply a username and password for network logon.

4. Using 802.1x standard and EAP/LEAP, the wireless client and a RADIUS server perform authentication through the AP. The client will then use a one-way hash of the user-supplied password as a response to the challenge, and this will be sent to the RADIUS server. The RADIUS server will then reference its user table and compare that to the response from the client. If there is a match, the RADIUS server

authenticates the client, and the process will be repeated, but in reverse. This will enable the client to authenticate the RADIUS server.

(If you are using LEAP, the RADIUS server will send an authentication challenge to the client.)

After authentication completes successfully, the following steps take place:

1. The RADIUS server and the client determine a WEP key that is unique for the client and that session.

2. The RADIUS server transmits this WEP key (also known as a session key), across the wired LAN to the AP.

3. The AP will encrypt the broadcast key and the session key so that it can then send the new encrypted key to the client. The client will then use the session key to decrypt it.

4. The client and AP then activates the WEP. The APs and clients will then use the session and broadcast WEP keys for all communications that occur during the session.

5. For enhanced security, the session key and broadcast key are regularly changed at regular periods that are configured in the RADIUS server.

A more simplified version is included in Figure 15.3.

Figure 15.3 Cisco Security Solution Using Session-Based Encryption Keys

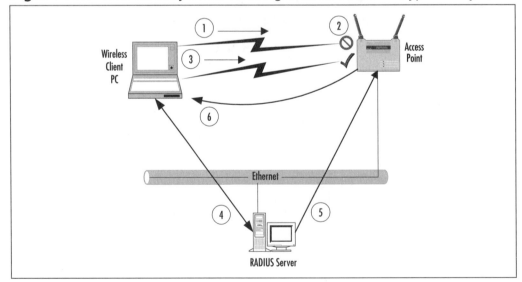

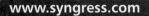

An Introduction to the 802.1x Standard

In order to better understand 802.1x, you must also understand the enhancements of current IEEE 802.11b security products and features. The current IEEE 802.11b standard is severely limited because it is available only for the current open and shared key authentication scheme, which is non-extensible.

Some of these requirements for the future security include the following:

- The creation of new 802.11 authentication methods.

- These authentication methods must be independent of the underlying 802.11 hardware.

- Authentication methods should be dynamic because hard coding it makes it difficult to fix security holes when they are found.

- It must have the ability to support Public Key Infrastructure (PKI) and certificate schemes.

Project Authorization Request (PAR) for 802.1x

Currently, no standard mechanism allows access to and from a network segment based only on the authenticated state of a port user. The problem is that network connectivity allows for the anonymous access to company data and the Internet. When 802-based networks are deployed in more accessible areas, you will need a method to authenticate and authorize basic network access. These types of projects provide for common interoperable solutions that use standards-based authentication and authorization infrastructures like those that are commonly supporting schemes such as dial-up access already.

The Objectives of the 802.1x Standard

The IEEE 802.1x Working Group was created for the purpose of providing a security framework for port-based access control that resides in the upper layers. The most common method for port-based access control is to enable new authentication and key management methods without changing current network devices.

The benefits that are the end result of this group are as follows:

- There is a significant decrease in hardware cost and complexity.

- There are more options, which allows you to pick and choose your security solution.

- You can install the latest and greatest security technology, and it should still work with your existing infrastructure.

- You are able to respond to security issues as quickly as they arise.

802.1x in a Nutshell

When a client device connects to a port on an 802.1x switch and AP, the switch port can determine the authenticity of the devices. Due to this and, according to the protocol specified by 802.1x, the services offered by the switch can be made available on that port. Only EAPOL (see the following list) frames can be sent and received on that port until the authentication is complete. When the device is properly authentication, the port switches traffic as though it were a regular port.

Here is some terminology for the 802.1x standard that you should familiarize yourself with:

- **Port** A port is a single point of connection to the network.

- **Port Access Entity (PAE)** The PAE controls the algorithms and protocols that are associated with the authentication mechanisms for a port.

- **Authenticator PAE** The authenticator PAE enforces authentication before it will allow access resources located off of that port.

- **Supplicant PAE** The supplicant PAE tries to accesses the services that are allowed by the authenticator.

- **Authentication Server** The Authentication Server is used to verify the supplicant PAE. It decides whether the supplicant is authorized to access the authenticator or not.

- **Extensible Authentication Protocol Over LAN (EAPOL)** The 802.1x defines a standard for encapsulating EAP messages so that they can be handled directly by a LAN MAC service. 802.1x tries to make authentication more encompassing, rather than enforcing specific mechanisms on the devices. Because of this, 802.1x uses Extensible Authentication Protocol to receive authentication information.

- **Extensible Authentication Protocol Over Wireless (EAPOW)** When EAPOL messages are encapsulated over 802.11 wireless frames, they are known as EAPOW.

Making it Come Together—User Identification and Strong Authentication

With the addition of the 802.1x standard, clients are identified by usernames, not the MAC address of the devices. This was designed to not only enhance security, but to streamline the process for authentication, authorization, and accountability for your network. 802.1x was designed so that it could support extended forms of authentication, using password methods (such as one-time passwords, or GSS_API mechanisms like Kerberos) and nonpassword methods (such as biometrics, IKE, and smart cards).

Key Derivation Can Be Dynamic

You can also use per-user session keys, because the 802.1x standard allows for the creation of them. Because you don't need to keep WEP keys at the client device or AP, you can dispense per-user, and/or per session–based WEP keys. These WEP keys will be dynamically created at the client for every session, thus making it more secure. The Global key, like a broadcast WEP key, can be encrypted using a unicast session key and then sent from the AP to the client in a much more secure manner.

Mutual Authentication

When using 802.1x and EAP, you should use some form of mutual authentication. This will make the client and the authentication servers mutually authenticating end-points and will assist in the mitigation of attacks from man in the middle types of devices. To enable mutual authentication, you could use any of the following EAP methods:

- **TLS** This requires that the server supply a certificate and establish that it has possession of the private key.
- **IKE** This requires that the server show possession of preshared key or private key (this can be considered certificate authentication).
- **GSS_API (Kerberos)** This requires that the server can demonstrate knowledge of the session key.

NOTE

Cisco Systems has also created a lightweight mutual authentication scheme, called LEAP (discussed later), so that your network is able to support operating systems that do not normally support EAP. LEAP also offers the capability to have alternate certificate schemes such as EAP-TLS.

Per-Packet Authentication

EAP can support per-packet authentication and integrity protection, but this authentication and integrity protection is not extended to all types of EAP messages. For example, NAK (negative acknowledgment) and notification messages are not able to use per-packet authentication and integrity. Per-packet authentication and integrity protection works for the following (packet is encrypted unless otherwise noted):

- TLS and IKE derive session key
- TLS ciphersuite negotiations (not encrypted)
- IKE ciphersuite negotiations
- Kerberos tickets
- Success and failure messages that use derived session key (through WEP)

Designing & Planning...

Preventing Dictionary Attacks Using EAP

EAP was designed to support extended authentication. When you implement EAP, you can avoid dictionary attacks by using nonpassword-based schemes such as biometrics, certificates, OTP, smart cards, and token cards.

You should be sure that if you are using password-based schemes that they use some form of mutual authentication so that they are more protected against dictionary attacks.

Possible Implementation of EAP on the WLAN

There are two main authentication methods for EAP on your wireless LAN: One is EAP-MD5, and the other is to use PKI with EAP-TLS. EAP-MD5 has a couple of issues because it does not support the capability for mutual authentication between the access server and the wireless client. The PKI schemes also has drawbacks, because it is very computation-intensive on the client systems, you need a high degree of planning and design to make sure that your network is capable of supporting PKI, and it is not cheap.

Cisco Light Extensible Authentication Protocol

LEAP is an enhancement to the EAP protocol, and as you remember, the EAP protocol was created in an effort to provide a scalable method for a PPP-based server to authenticate its clients and, hopefully allow for mutual authentication. An extensible packet exchange should allow for the passing of authentication information between the client devices and the PPP servers. The thing is that PPP servers usually rely on a centralized authentication server system that can validate the clients for them. This is where a RADIUS or a TACACS+ server usually comes into play.

This reason that the servers can work is that the servers have a protocol that will enable them to pass EAP packets between the authentication server and the PPP server. Essentially this makes the PPP server a passthrough or a relay agent, so that the authentication process happens between the client and the RADIUS server. The RADIUS server will then tell the PPP server the results of the authentication process (pass/fail) that will allow the client to access the network and its resources.

To make sure that all types of network access servers could be implemented to validate clients to network resources, the EAP protocol was created. Because we are talking about wireless connections though, the link between the AP and the client is not PPP but WLAN.

When the 802.11 specifications were standardized, it allowed for the encryption of data traffic between APs and clients through the use of a WEP encryption key. When it was first implemented, the AP would have a single key, and this key had to be configured on each client. All traffic would be encrypted using this single key. Well, this type of security has a lot of issues. In current implementations that use EAP authentication, the client and RADIUS server have a shared secret; generally this is some permutation of a username and password combination. The server will then pass certain information to the AP so that the client and AP can derive encryption keys that are unique for this client–AP pair. This is called Cisco LEAP authentication.

The previous section discussed the implementation methods of EAP (EAP-MD5, and PKI with EAP-TLS), and some of the issues that you can expect to see when you plan to implement them. LEAP may be a better option because it can offer mutual authentication, it needs only minimal support from the client's CPU, it can support embedded systems, and it can support clients whose operating system does not have the support for native EAP or allow for the use of the PKI authentication.

LEAP authentication works through three phases: the *start phase*, the *authenticate phase*, and the *finish phase*. The following sections show the process that the client and AP go through so that the client can also talk to the RADIUS server.

Start Phase for LEAP Authentication

In the start phase, information (in packet form) is transferred between the client and APs:

1. The EAPOW-Start (this is also called EAPOL-Start in 802.1x for wired networks) starts the authentication process. This packed is sent from the client to the AP.

2. The EAP-Request/Identity is sent from the AP to the client with a request for the clients Identity.

3. The EAP-Response/Identity is sent from the client to the AP with the required information.

Authentication Phase for LEAP Authentication

This sequence will change based on the mutual authentication method you choose for the client and the authentication server. If you were to use TLS for the transfer of certificates in a PKI deployment, EAP-TLS messages will be used, but because we are talking about LEAP, it would go more like this:

1. The client sends an EAP-Response/Identity message to the RADIUS server through the AP as a RADIUS-Access-Request with EAP extensions.

2. The RADIUS server then returns access-request with a RADIUS-challenge, to which the client must respond.

Cisco LEAP authentication is a mutual authentication method, and the AP is only a passthrough. The AP in the authenticate phase forwards the contents of the packets from EAP to RADIUS and from Radius to EAP.

The (Big) Finish Phase of LEAP Authentication

The steps for the finish phase are as follows:

1. If the client is considered invalid, the RADIUS server will send a RADIUS deny packet with an EAP fail packet embedded within it. If the client is considered to be valid, the server will send a RADIUS request packet with an EAP success attribute.

2. The RADIUS-Access-Accept packet contains the MS-MPPE-Send-Key attribute to the AP, where it obtains the session key that will be used by client.

The RADIUS server and client both create a session key from the user's password, when using LEAP. The encryption for the IEEE 802.11 standard can be based on a 40/64-bit or 104/128-bit key. Note that the key derivation process will create a key that is longer than is required. This is so that when the AP receives the key from the RADIUS server (using MS-MPPE-Send-Key attribute), it will send an EAPOL-KEY message to the client. This key will tell the client the key length and what key index that it should use.

The key value isn't sent because the client has already created it on its own WEP key. The data packet is then encrypted using the full-length key. The AP will also send an EAPOL-KEY message that gives information about the length, key index, and value of the multicast key. This message is encrypted using the full-length session unicast key from the AP.

Configuration and Deployment of LEAP

In this section, we talk about the installation and requirements for a LEAP solution that consists of a client, an AP and a RADIUS server for key distribution in your network.

Client Support for LEAP

You can configure your client to use LEAP mode in one of two modes:

- **Network Logon Mode** In Network logon mode, an integrated network logon provides for a single-sign on for both the wireless network as well as Microsoft Networking. This will provide users with a transparent security experience. This is probably the most common method of authenticating into the wireless network (or the wired network).

- **Device Mode** In device mode, the wireless LAN stores the username/password identification, so that you can get non-interactive authentication into the wireless LAN. You will often see this on wireless appliances where the devices that can authenticate themselves through these preconfigured credentials are enough security.

Access Point Support for LEAP

Access points can provide 802.1x for 802.11 Authenticator support. In order to make this work, you need to take the following two steps in setting up 802.1x authenticator support:

- You need to configure the AP to use 40/64- or 104/128-bit WEP mode.

- You must give the LEAP RADIUS server address and configure the shared secret key that the AP and RADIUS server use, so that they can communicate securely.

Configuring your RADIUS server for LEAP

To configure the RADIUS server for authentication and key distribution users, you will need to do the following:

- You need to create the user databases.

- You need to configure the APs as Network Access Servers (NASs). This will enable users that are configured with Cisco-Aironet RADIUS extensions on the NAS to use RADIUS. RADIUS requests from the AP with EAP extensions are passed as described earlier.

Ensuring Authorization

Authorization is the rights and permissions granted to a user or application that enables access to a network or computing resource. Once a user has been properly identified and authenticated, authorization levels determine the extent of system rights that the user has access to.

Many of the early operating systems and applications deployed had very small authorization groups. Generally, only user groups and operator groups were available for defining a user's access level. Once more formal methods for approaching various authorization levels were defined, applications and servers started offering more discrete authorization levels. You can observe this by simply looking at any standard back-office application deployed today.

Many of them provide varying levels of access for users and administrators. For example, they could have several levels of user accounts allowing some users access to just view the information, while giving others the ability to update or query that information and have administrative accounts based on the authorization levels needed (such as being able to look up only specific types of customers, or run particular reports while other accounts have the ability to edit and create new accounts).

As shown in the previous authentication example, Cisco and others have implemented RADIUS authentication for their wireless devices. Now, utilizing stronger authentication methods, you can implement your authorization policies into your wireless deployments.

However, many wireless devices do not currently support external authorization validation. Plus, most deployments just ensure authorized access to the device. They do not control access to or from specific network segments. To fully restrict authorized users to the network devices they are authorized to utilize, you will still need to deploy an adaptive firewall between the AP and your network.

This is what was done earlier this year by two researchers at NASA (for more information, see www.nas.nasa.gov/Groups/Networks/Projects/Wireless; please be aware that this URL is case sensitive). To protect their infrastructure, but still provide access through wireless, they deployed a firewall segmenting their wireless and department network. They most likely hardened their wireless interfaces to the extent of the equipments' possibilities by utilizing the strongest encryption available to them, disabling SID broadcast, and allowing only authorized MAC addresses on the wireless network.

They then utilized the Dynamic Host Configuration Protocol (DHCP) on the firewall, and disabled it on their AP. This allowed them to expressly define which MAC addresses could receive an IP address, and what the lease lifetime of the IP address would be.

The researchers then went on to turn off all routing and forwarding between the wireless interface and the internal network. If anyone happened to be able to connect to the wireless network, they would still have no access to the rest of the computing resources of the department. Anyone wishing to gain further access would have to go to an SSL protected Web site on the firewall server and authenticate as a valid user. The Web server would authenticate the user against a local

RADIUS server, but they could have easily used any other form of user authentication (NT, SecurID, and so on).

Once the user was properly authenticated, the firewall would change the firewall rules for the IP address that user was supposed to be assigned to, allowing full access to only the network resources they are authorized to access.

Finally, once the lease expired or was released for any reason from the DHCP assigned IP address, the firewall rules would be removed and that user and their IP would have to re-authenticate through the Web interface to allow access to the network resources again.

MAC Filtering

In order to fully discuss the advantages and disadvantages of MAC filtering, let's have a short review on what a MAC address is. The term *MAC* stands for Media Access Control, and forms the lower layer in the Data-Link layer of the OSI model. The purpose of the MAC sublayer is to present a uniform interface between the physical networking media (copper/fiber/radio frequency) and the Logical Link Control portion of the Data-Link layer. These two layers are found onboard a NIC, whether integrated into a device or used as an add-on (PCI card or PCMCIA card).

What Is a MAC Address?

In order to facilitate delivery of network traffic, the MAC layer is assigned a unique address, which is programmed into the NIC at the time of manufacture. The operating system will associate an IP address with this MAC address, which allows the device to participate in an IP network. Because no other NIC in the world should have the same MAC address, it is easy to see why it could be a secure way to equate a specific user with the MAC address on his or her machine.

Now, let's look at an actual MAC address. For example, my laptop has a MAC address of 00-00-86-4C-75-48. The first three octets are called the organizationally unique identifier (OUI). The Institute of Electrical and Electronic Engineers controls these OUIs and assigns them to companies as needed. If you look up the 00-00-86 OUI on the IEEE's Web site (http://standards.ieee.org/regauth/oui/index.shtml), it will state that the manufacturer of this NIC is the 3Com Corporation.

Corporations can own several OUIs, and often acquire additional OUIs when they purchase other companies. For example, when Cisco purchased Aironet

Wireless Communications in 1999, they added the 00-40-96 OUI to the many others they have.

Some other OUIs you could see on your WLAN might be the following:

- **00-02-2D** Agere Communications (previously known as ORiNOCO)
- **00-10-E7** Breezecom
- **00-E0-03** Nokia Wireless
- **00-04-5A** Linksys

The remaining three octets in a MAC address are usually burned into the NIC during manufacture, thus assuring that duplicate addresses will not exist on a network. We say "usually" because this rule has a few exceptions. For example, in some redundancy situations, one NIC on a machine is able to assume the MAC address of the other NIC if the primary NIC fails. Some early 802.11 PCMCIA cards also had the capability to change their MAC address. Although not necessarily easy to do, changing the MAC address gives a user the ability to spoof the MAC address of another PCMCIA card. This could be used to circumvent MAC filtering or be employed in a denial of service (DoS) attack against a specific user.

Where in the Authentication/Association Process Does MAC Filtering Occur?

When a wireless device wants to connect to a WLAN, it goes though a two-part process called authentication and authorization. After both have been completed, the device is allowed access to the WLAN.

As mentioned earlier, when a wireless device is attempting to connect to a WLAN, it sends an authentication request to the AP (see Figure 15.4). This request will contain the SSID of the target network, or a null value if connecting to an open system. The AP will grant or deny authentication based on this string. Following a successful authentication, the requesting device will attempt to associate with the AP. It is at this point in time that MAC filtering plays its role. Depending on the AP vendor and administrative setup of the AP, MAC filtering either allows only the specified MAC addresses—blocking the rest, or it allows all MAC addresses—blocking specifically noted MACs. If the MAC address is allowed, the requesting device is allowed to associate with the AP.

Figure 15.4 MAC Filtering

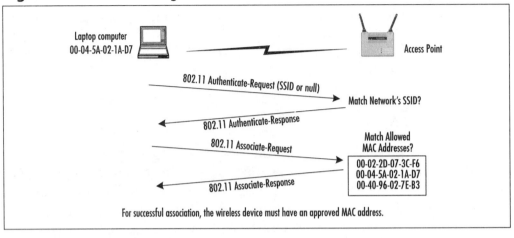

For successful association, the wireless device must have an approved MAC address.

Determining MAC Filtering Is Enabled

The easiest way to determine if a device has failed the association process due to MAC filtering is through the use of a protocol analyzer, like Sniffer Pro or AiroPeek. The difficulty here is that other factors besides MAC filtering could prevent association from occurring. RADIUS or 802.1x authentication, or an incorrect WEP key could also prevent this. These of course are costly mechanisms commonly seen in large corporate environments. Due to the costs involved with setting up the higher forms of non–AP-based authentication, most small businesses or home installations will use MAC filtering to limit access (if they use anything at all).

MAC Spoofing

If you discover that your MAC address is not allowed to associate with the AP, don't give up. There are other ways into the network besides the front door.

First off, just because you can't associate with the AP doesn't mean you can't sit there and passively watch the traffic. With 802.11b protocol analysis software, your laptop can see all the other stations' communication with any AP within range. Because the MAC addresses of the other stations are transmitted in clear text, it should be easy to start compiling a list of the MAC addresses allowed on the network.

Some early runs of 802.11 PCMCIA cards had the capability to modify their MAC addresses. Depending on the card and the level of firmware, the method to change your MAC address may vary. There are sites on the Internet that can give you more specific information on altering these parameters.

Once you have modified the MAC address, you should be able to associate it with the AP. Keep in mind however, that if the device bearing the MAC address you have stolen is still operating on the network, you will not be able to use your device. To allow the operation of two duplicate MAC addresses will break ARP tables and will attract a level of attention to your activities that is undesirable. The advanced hacker we are discussing would realize this. In attempts to subvert the security mechanisms, traffic would be monitored to sufficiently pattern the intended victim whose MAC address and identification are to be forged in order to avoid detection.

Ensuring Non-Repudiation

Repudiation is defined by West's Encyclopedia of American Law as "the rejection or refusal of a duty, relation, right or privilege." A repudiation of a transaction or contract means that one of the parties refuses to honor their obligation to the other as specified by the contract. Non-repudiation could then be defined as the ability to deny, with irrefutable evidence, a false rejection or refusal of an obligation.

In their paper "Non-Repudiation in the Digital Environment," Adrian McCullagh and William Caelli put forth an excellent review of the traditional model of non-repudiation and the current trends for crypto-technical non-repudiation. The paper was published online by First Monday—you can find it at www.firstmonday.dk/issues/issue5_8/mccullagh/index.html.

The basis for a repudiation of a traditional contract is sometimes associated with the belief that the signature binding a contract is a forgery, or that the signature is not a forgery but was obtained via unconscionable conduct by a party to the transaction, by fraud instigated by a third party, or undue influence exerted by a third party. In typical cases of fraud or repudiated contracts, the general rule of evidence is that if a person denies a particular signature, the burden of proving that the signature is valid falls upon the receiving party.

Common law trust mechanisms establish that in order to overcome false claims of non-repudiation, a trusted third party needs to act as a witness to the signature being affixed. Having a witness to the signature of a document, who is independent of the transactions taking place, reduces the likelihood that a signor is able to successfully allege that the signature is a forgery. However, there is always the possibility that the signatory will be able to deny the signature on the basis of the situations listed in the preceding paragraph.

A perfect example of a non-repudiation of submissions can be viewed by examining the process around sending and receiving registered mail. When you send a registered letter, you are given a receipt containing an identification number for the piece of mail sent. If the recipient claims that the mail was not sent, the receipt is proof that provides the non-repudiation of the submission. If a receipt is available with the recipient's signature, this provides the proof for the non-repudiation of the delivery service. The postal service provides the non-repudiation of transport service by acting as a Trusted Third Party (TTP).

Non-repudiation, in technical terms, has come to mean the following:

- In authentication, a service that provides proof of the integrity and origin of data both in an unforgeable relationship, which can be verified by any third party at any time; or

- In authentication, an authentication that with high assurance can be asserted to be genuine, and that cannot subsequently be refuted.

The Australian Federal Government's Electronic Commerce Expert group further adopted this technical meaning in their 1998 report to the Australian Federal Attorney General as:

> Non-repudiation is a property achieved through cryptographic methods which prevents an individual or entity from denying having performed a particular action related to data (such as mechanisms for non-rejection or authority (origin); for proof of obligation, intent, or commitment; or for proof of ownership.

In the digital realm, a movement is in place to shift the responsibility of proving that a digital signature is invalid to the owner of the signature, not the receiver of the signature, as is typically used in traditional common law methods.

In only a few examples does the burden of proof fall upon the alleged signer. One such example is usually found in taxation cases where the taxpayer has made specific claims and as such is in a better position to disprove the revenue collecting body's case. Another example would be in an instance of negligence. In a negligence action, if a plaintiff is able to prove that a defendant failed to meet their commitment, the burden of proof is in effect shifted to the defendant to establish that they have met their obligations.

The problem found in the new digital repudiation definitions that have been created is that they take into consideration only the validity of the signature itself. They do not allow for the possibility that the signor was tricked or forced into signing, or that their private key may be compromised, allowing the forgery of digital signatures.

With all the recent cases of Internet worms and viruses, it is not hard to imagine that one might be specifically built to steal private keys. A virus could be something as simple as a Visual Basic macro attached to a Word document, or an e-mail message that would search the targets hard drive looking for commonly named and located private key rings that could then be e-mailed or uploaded to some rogue location.

With this and other possible attacks to the private keys, it becomes difficult, under the common law position, for someone attempting to prove the identity of an alleged signatory. This common law position was established and founded in a paper-based environment where witnessing became the trusted mechanism utilized to prevent the non-repudiation of a signature. For a digital signature to be proven valid, however, it will need to be established through a fully trusted mechanism.

Thus, for a digitally signed contract to be trusted and not susceptible to repudiation, the entire document handling and signature process must take place within a secured and trusted computing environment. As we will see in some of the documentation to follow, the security policies and definitions created over the years have established a set of requirements necessary to create a secure and trusted computer system.

If we follow the definitions established in the Information Technology Security Evaluation Certification (ITSEC) to create a trusted computing environment of at least E3 to enforce functions and design of the signing process and thus prevent unauthorized access to the private key, the common law position for digitally signed documents can be maintained. E3 also ensures that the signing function is the only function able to be performed by the signing mechanism by having the source code evaluated to ensure that this is the only process available through the code. If these security features are implemented, it can be adequately assessed that under this mechanism the private key has not been stolen and as such that any digital signature created under this model has the trust established to ensure the TTP witness and validation of any signature created, preventing any possible repudiation from the signor.

One such example of a secure infrastructure designed and deployed to attempt to provide a digitally secure TTP are the PKI systems available for users of unsecure public networks such as the Internet. PKI consists of a secure computing system that acts as a certificate authority (CA) to issue and verify digital certificates. Digital certificates contain the public key and other identification information needed to verify the validity of the certificate. As long as the trust in the CA is maintained (and with it, the trust in the security of the private key), the digital certificates issued by the CA and the documents signed by them remain trusted. As long as the trust is ensured, then the CA acts as a TTP and provides for the non-repudiation of signatures created by entities with digital certificates issued through the CA.

Accounting and Audit Trails

Auditing provides methods for tracking and logging activities on networks and systems, and it links these activities to specific user accounts or sources of activity. In case of simple mistakes or software failures, audit trails can be extremely useful in restoring data integrity. They are also a requirement for trusted systems to ensure that the activity of authorized individuals on the trusted system can be traced to their specific actions, and that those actions comply with defined policy. They also allow for a method of collecting evidence to support any investigation into improper or illegal activities.

Most modern database applications support some level of transaction log detailing the activities that occurred within the database. This log could then be used to either rebuild the database if it had any errors or create a duplicate database at another location. To provide this detailed level of transactional logging, database logging tends to consume a great deal of drive space for its enormous log file. This intense logging is not needed for most applications, so you will generally have only basic informative messages utilized in system resource logging.

The logging features provided on most networks and systems involve the logging of known or partially known resource event activities. Although these logs are sometimes used for analyzing system problems, they are also useful for those whose duty it is to process the log files and check for both valid and invalid system activities.

To assist in catching mistakes and reducing the likelihood of fraudulent activities, the activities of a process should be split among several people. This segmentation of duties allows the next person in line to possibly correct problems simply because they are being viewed with fresh eyes.

From a security point of view, segmentation of duties requires the collusion of at least two people to perform any unauthorized activities. The following guidelines assist in assuring that the duties are split so as to offer no way other than collusion to perform invalid activities:

- **No access to sensitive combinations of capabilities** A classic example of this is control of inventory data and physical inventory. By separating the physical inventory control from the inventory data control, you remove the unnecessary temptation for an employee to steal from inventory and then alter the data so that the theft is left hidden.

- **Prohibit conversion and concealment** Another violation that can be prevented by segregation is ensuring that supervision is provided for people who have access to assets. An example of an activity that could be prevented if properly segmented follows a lone operator of a night shift. This operator, without supervision, could copy (or "convert") customer lists and then sell them off to interested parties. Instances have been reported of operators actually using the employer's computer to run a service bureau at night.

- **The same person cannot both originate and approve transactions** When someone is able to enter and authorize their own expenses, it introduces the possibility that they might fraudulently enter invalid expenses for their own gain.

These principles, whether manual or electronic, form the basis for why audit logs are retained. They also identify why people other than those performing the activities reported in the log should be the ones who analyze the data in the log file.

In keeping with the idea of segmentation, as you deploy your audit trails, be sure to have your logs sent to a secure, trusted, location that is separate and non-accessible from the devices you are monitoring. This will help ensure that if any inappropriate activity occurs, the person can't falsify the log to state that the actions did not take place.

Most wireless APs do not offer any method of logging activity, but if your equipment provides the feature, you should enable it and then monitor it for inappropriate activity using tools such as logcheck. Wireless AP logging should, if it's available, log any new wireless device with its MAC address upon valid WEP authentication. It should also log any attempts to access or modify the AP itself.

Using Encryption

Encryption has always played a key role in information security, and has been the center of controversy in the design of the WEP wireless standard. But despite the drawbacks, encryption will continue to play a major role in wireless security, especially with the adoption of new and better encryption algorithms and key management systems.

As we have seen in reviewing the basic concepts of security, many of the principles used to ensure the confidentiality, integrity, and availability of servers and services are through the use of some form of trusted and tested encryption. We also have seen that even with encryption, if we get tied up too much in the acceptance of the hard mathematics as evidence of validity, it is possible to be tricked into accepting invalid authorization or authentication attempts by someone who has been able to corrupt the encryption system itself by either acquiring the private key through cryptanalysis or stealing the private key from the end user directly.

Cryptography offers the obvious advantage that the material it protects cannot be used without the keys needed to unlock it. As long as those keys are protected, the material remains protected. There are a few potential disadvantages to encryption as well. For instance, if the key is lost, the data becomes unavailable, and if the key is stolen, the data becomes accessible to the thief.

The process of encryption also introduces possible performance degradation. When a message is to be sent encrypted, time must be spent to first encrypt the information, then store and transmit the encrypted data, and then later decode it. In theory, this can slow a system by as much as a factor of three.

Until recently, distribution and use of strong encryption was limited and controlled by most governments. The United States government had encryption listed as munitions, right next to cruise missiles! As such, it was very difficult to legally acquire and use strong encryption through the entire Internet. With the new changes in trade laws, however, it is now possible to use stronger encryption for internal use as well as with communications with customers and other third-parties.

Encrypting Voice Data

Voice communications have traditionally been a very simple medium to intercept and monitor. When digital cell and wireless phones arrived, there was a momentary window in which monitoring voice communications across these digital connections was difficult. Today, the only equipment needed to monitor cell phones or digital wireless telephones can be acquired at a local RadioShack for generally less than $100.

Most voice communication systems are not designed to ensure the privacy of the conversations on them, so a new industry was created to facilitate those needs. Originally designed for government and military usage, telephone encryption devices give people the option of encrypting their daily calls. A few of these devices are starting to make their way into the commercial market. Although a few are being slowed down by organizations such as the National Security Agency (NSA) and the Federal Bureau of Investigation (FBI), who argue that it will prevent their "legal" monitoring of criminal activities, consumer market needs should eventually push these devices into the mainstream.

The Internet, being a communications network, offers people the ability to communicate with anyone, anywhere. Because of this, it didn't take long for the appearance of applications enabling voice communications across the Internet. Many of the early versions, like all budding technologies, did not offer any protection methods for their users. As a result, people utilizing Internet voice communications programs could have their communications monitored by someone with access to the data stream between parties. Fortunately, encryption is making its way into some of these programs, and if you're careful, you should be able to find one that uses modern tested and secure encryption algorithms such as Twofish, a popular and publicly-available encryption algorithm created by Bruce Schneier.

Encrypting Data Systems

Data networks have traditionally been susceptible to threats from a trusted insider. However, as soon as someone connects their network to another entity, it introduces possible security compromises from outside sources. Remember, all forms of data communications, from simple modem lines to frame-relay and fiber-optic connections, can be monitored.

Reviewing the Role of Policy

Good policy is your first line of defense. A properly designed policy examines every threat (or tries to) and ensures that confidentiality, integrity, and availability are maintained (or at least cites the known and accepted risks). As we shall see, policy definition begins with a clear identification and labeling of resources being utilized that will build into specific standards that define acceptable use in what's considered an authorized and secure manner. Once a basic standard is defined, you start building specific guidelines and procedures for individual applications and services.

Many wireless manufacturers have responded to security threats hampering their initial product versions by releasing upgrades to their software and drivers. Your security policy should always require that all technology, either existing or newly deployed, have the latest security patches and upgrades installed in a timely manner. However, because the development and release of patches takes time, policy and its proper implementation tend to be the first layer of defense when confronting known and unknown threats.

A well-written policy should be more than just a list of recommended procedures. It should be an essential and fundamental element of your organization's security practices. A good policy can provide protection from liability due to an employee's actions, or can form a basis for the control of trade secrets. A policy or standard should also continue to grow and expand as new threats and technologies become available. They should be constructed with the input of an entire organization and audited both internally and externally to ensure that the assets they are protecting have the controls in place as specified in the standards, policies, and guidelines.

Designing & Planning…

The Management Commitment

Management must be aware of their needed commitment to the security of corporate assets, which includes protection of information. Measures must be taken to protect it from unauthorized modification, destruction, or disclosure (whether accidental or intentional), and ensure its authenticity, integrity, availability and confidentiality.

Fundamental to the success of any security program is senior management's commitment to the information security process and their understanding of how important security controls and protections are to the enterprise's continuity.

The senior management statement usually contains the following elements:

- An acknowledgment of the importance of computing resources to the business model

- A statement of support for information security throughout the enterprise

- A commitment to authorize and manage the definition of the lower level standards, procedures, and guidelines

Part of any policy definition includes what is required to ensure that the policy is adhered to. The prime object of policy controls is to reduce the effect of security threats and vulnerabilities to the resources being protected. The policy definition process generally entails the identification of what impact a threat would have on an organization, and what the likelihood of that threat occurring would be. Risk Analysis (RA) is the process of analyzing a threat and producing a representative value of that threat.

Figure 15.5 displays a matrix created using a small $x–y$ graph representing the threat and the corresponding likelihood of that threat. The goal of RA is to reduce the level of impact and the likelihood that it will occur. A properly implemented control should move the plotted point from the upper right to the lower left of the graph.

Figure 15.5 Threat versus Likelihood Matrix

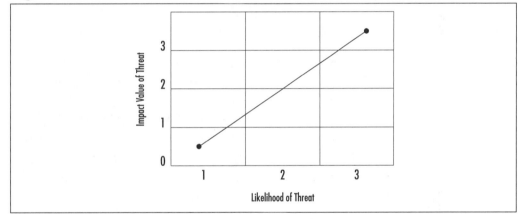

An improperly designed and implemented control will show little to no movement in the plotted point before and after the control's implementation.

Identifying Resources

To assess and protect resources, they must first be identified, classified, and labeled so that in the process of performing your risk analysis you are able to document all possible risks to each identified item and provide possible solutions to mitigate those risks.

Security classification provides the following benefits:

■ Demonstrates an organization's commitment to security procedures

- Helps identify which information is the most sensitive or vital to an organization

- Supports the tenets of confidentiality, integrity, and availability as it pertains to data

- Helps identify which protections apply to which information

- May be required for regulatory, compliance, or legal reasons

In the public sector, the common categories utilized in the classification of resources are the following:

- **Public** These are no-risk items that can be disclosed to anyone, as long as they do not violate any individual's right to privacy, and knowledge of this information does not expose an organization to financial loss or embarrassment, or jeopardize security assets. Examples of public information include marketing brochures, published annual reports, business cards, and press releases.

- **Internal Use** These are low-risk items that due to their technical or business sensitivity are limited to an organization's employees and those contractors covered by a nondisclosure agreement. Should there be unauthorized disclosure, compromise, or destruction of the documents, there would only be minimal impact on the organization, its customers, or employees. Examples of Internal Use information include employee handbooks, telephone directories, organizational charts, and policies.

- **Confidential** These are moderate-risk items whose unauthorized disclosure, compromise, or destruction would directly or indirectly impact an organization, its customers, or employees, possibly causing financial damage to an organization's reputation, a loss of business, and potential legal action. They are intended solely for use within an organization and are limited to those individuals who have a "need-to-know" security clearance. Examples of confidential items include system requirements or configurations, proprietary software, personnel records, customer records, business plans, budget information, and security plans and standards.

- **Restricted** These are high-risk critical items whose unauthorized disclosure, compromise, or destruction would result in severe damage to a company, providing significant advantages to a competitor, or causing penalties to the organization, its customers, or employees. It is intended solely for restricted use within the organization and is limited to those with an explicit, predetermined, and stringent "business-need-to-know." Examples of restricted data include strategic plans, encryption keys, authentication information (passwords, PINs, and so on), and IP addresses for security-related servers.

All information, whether in paper, spoken, or electronic form should be classified, labeled, and distributed in accordance to your information classification and handling procedures. This will assist in the determination of what items have the largest threat, and as such, should determine how you set about providing controls for those threats.

Your wireless network contains a few internal items that should be identified and classified, however the overall classification of any network device comes down the level of information that flows through its channels. While using e-mail systems or accessing external sites through your wireless network, you will likely find that your entire network contains restricted information. However, if you are able to encrypt the password, the classification of your network data will then be rated based upon the non-authentication information traveling across your wireless network.

Understanding Classification Criteria

To assist in your risk analysis, you can use a few additional criteria to determine the classification of information resources:

- **Value** Value is the most commonly used criteria for classifying data in the private sector. If something is valuable to an individual or organization, that will prompt the data to be properly identified and classified.

- **Age** Information is occasionally reclassified to a lower level as time passes. In many government organizations, some classified documents are automatically declassified after a predetermined time period has passed.

- **Useful Life** If information has become obsolete due to new information or resources, it is usually reclassified.

- **Personal Association** If information is associated with specific individuals or is covered under privacy law, it may need to be reclassified at some point.

Implementing Policy

Information classification procedures offer several steps in establishing a classification system, which provides the first step in the creation of your security standards and policies. The following are the primary procedural steps used in establishing a classification system:

1. Identify the administrator or custodian.

2. Specify the criteria of how the information will be classified and labeled.

3. Classify the data by its owner, who is subject to review by a supervisor.

4. Specify and document any exceptions to the classification policy.

5. Specify the controls that will be applied to each classification level.

6. Specify the termination procedures for declassifying the information or for transferring custody of the information to another entity.

7. Create an enterprise awareness program about the classification controls.

Once your information and resources are properly identified and classified, you will be able to define the controls necessary to ensure the privacy and security of information regarding your employees and customers. Many industries are required, either by regulation or civil law, to ensure that proper policy is in place to protect the security and privacy of nonpublic personal information. This relationship of policy, guidelines, and legal standards is shown in Figure 15.6.

Figure 15.6 The Hierarchy of Rules

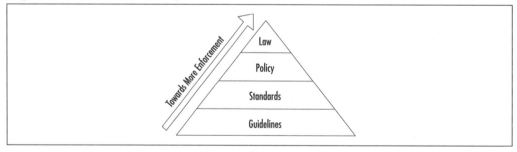

Guidelines refer to the methodologies of securing systems. Guidelines are more flexible than standards or policies and take the varying nature of information systems into consideration as they are developed and deployed, usually offering specific processes for the secure use of information resources. Many organizations have general security guidelines regarding a variety of platforms available within them: NT, SCO-UNIX, Debian Linux, Red Hat Linux, Oracle, and so on.

Standards specify the use of specific technologies in a uniform way. Although they are often not as flexible as guidelines, they do offer wider views to the technology specified. Usually, standards are in place for general computer use, encryption use, information classification, and others.

Policies are generally statements created for strategic or legal reasons, from which the standards and guidelines are defined. Some policies are based on legal requirements placed on industries such as health insurance, or they can be based upon common law requirements for organizations retaining personal nonpublic information of their customers.

Policies, standards, and guidelines must be explicit and focused, and they must effectively communicate the following subjects:

- Responsibility and authority

- Access control

- The extent to which formal verification is required

- Discretionary/mandatory control (generally relevant only in government or formal policy situations)

- Marking/labeling

- Control of media

- Import and export of data

- Security and classification levels

- Treatment of system output

The intent of policy is to delineate what an organization expects in the information security realm. Reasonable policy should also reflect any relevant laws and regulations that impact the use of information within an organization.

The System Administration, Networking, and Security Institute (SANS) offers excellent resources for implementing security standards, policies, and guidelines. You can find more information on policy implementation at the SANS Web site at www.sans.org/newlook/resources/policies/policies.htm. There you'll find example policies regarding encryption use, acceptable use, analog/ISDN lines, anti-virus software, application service providers, audits, and many others.

In this section's sidebar, "Sample Wireless Communication Policy," you will find the example wireless policy that defines the standards used for wireless communications.

Designing & Planning…

Sample Wireless Communication Policy

1.0 Purpose

This policy prohibits access to <Company Name> networks via unsecured wireless communication mechanisms. Only wireless systems that meet the criteria of this policy or have been granted an exclusive waiver by InfoSec are approved for connectivity to <Company Name>'s networks.

2.0 Scope

This policy covers all wireless data communication devices (for example, personal computers, cellular phones, PDAs, and so on) connected to any of <Company Name>'s internal networks. This includes any form of wireless communication device capable of transmitting packet data. Wireless devices and/or networks without any connectivity to <Company Name>'s networks do not fall under the purview of this policy.

3.0 Policy

To comply with this policy, wireless implementations must: maintain point-to-point hardware encryption of at least 56 bits; maintain a hardware address that can be registered and tracked (for instance, a MAC address); support strong user authentication which checks against an external database such as TACACS+, RADIUS, or something similar.

Exception: a limited-duration waiver to this policy for Aironet products has been approved if specific implementation instructions are followed for corporate and home installations.

4.0 Enforcement

Any employee found to have violated this policy may be subject to disciplinary action, up to and including termination of employment.

5.0 Definitions

Terms	Definitions
User Authentication	A method by which the user of a wireless system can be verified as a legitimate user independent of the computer or operating system being used.

6.0 Revision History

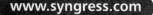

Addressing the Issues with Policy

Wireless users have unique needs that policy must address. The administrator must take diligent care in creating effective policy to protect the users, their data, and corporate assets. But just what is an effective policy for wireless users? Let's look at some common sense examples of good wireless policy.

First, wireless LANs are an "edge" technology. As such, policy should reflect a standard consistent with end users attempting to gain access to network resources from "the edge." In the case of wired LANs, typically you would set some standard physical access restrictions. This type of restriction would protect the LAN from certain types of attacks. You might also create group policy on the PC for authentication and access restrictions to corporate domains, and so long as there is no inside threat, the LAN is secured. (This scenario is unlikely in that disgruntled employees are representative of a solid portion of network hacking/misuse.) If you can't physically access the media, you cannot break in. If you do not furnish a valid username and password despite physical access, in most cases you cannot break in. Certainly some other methods of attack exist so long as you have physical access, but for all intents and purposes in this discussion, the typical, aspiring hacker is locked out. This assists in implementing the more stringent rule set as required by edge and remote access.

In a wireless environment, the rules change. How do you stop access to RF? RF travels through, around, and is reflected off objects, walls, and other physical barriers. RF doesn't have the feature-rich security support that the typical wired network has. Even though you can use the features of the wired Ethernet/IP security model after you are connected to the LAN, what about the signal from the AP to the client and vice-versa? Because of this access methodology, wireless poses some interesting policy challenges.

You can overcome one of these challenges—ease of capture of RF traffic—by preventing the broadcast of the Secure Set Identifier (SSID) to the world from the AP. Much like the Network Basic Input/Output System (NETBIOS) in the Windows world that broadcasts shares, the AP typically broadcasts the SSID to allow clients to associate. This is an advertisement for access to what you would like to be a restricted WLAN. Therefore, a good policy in the WLAN space is to prevent the AP from broadcasting this information. Instead, set up the AP to respond only to clients that already have the required details surrounding the Basic Service Set (BSS). This means that when the client attempts to associate, the AP challenges the client for the SSID and WEP encryption key information before allowing access. Of course, there are still ways to capture the traffic, but with this minor policy rule, the level of difficulty has been exponentially increased from the default implementation.

This security policy works well in the WLAN space until a technically savvy, but security ignorant, user installs a rogue AP because they wish to have their own personal AP connected to the WLAN. This poses a strong threat to the overall network security posture and must be prohibited.

What's in a name? It's imperative that you set in place a standard naming convention and WEP policy to prevent the standard defaults from being utilized. You wouldn't want your password published to the world in a set of instructions on how to access your PC, but that is exactly the case when speaking of WLAN defaults. They are published, documented, and presented as the default settings of the wireless space built from that specific hardware, and this is a *good* thing. Without this information, you would not be able to implement the hardware. However, to prevent unauthorized access, it's critical that you do not leave the default settings in place. A further consideration would be not using easily guessed names such as the company name. This should be part of your security policy for new hardware/software integration and goes toward assisting in the mitigation of capturing RF traffic.

With respect to roaming needs, these policies should not change from room to room or AP to AP. A consistent rule set (more stringent than normally internally trusted users) should be put in place across all APs where users are likely to roam while connected wirelessly. When choosing your AP, you can also add to ease of use for your wireless users by getting hardware that supports true roaming as opposed to having to lose connectivity momentarily while re-associating with another AP. The temporary loss of connectivity could lead to account lock out and the need to re-authenticate in upper layers.

Finally, strong authentication and encryption methods makes attacking the access mechanisms even more difficult, which is why the organization must include the appropriate use of authentication and encryption in its policy. Use of RADIUS or VPN solutions for authentication and tunneling sits nicely in the gap for the added protection. These authentication tools even serve as a standalone security feature for open networks where disabling the SSID is not an option.

All in all, policy should reflect these general guidelines if you intend to secure the WLAN access to corporate assets. We explore each in detail throughout this chapter to give you the information you need to secure your WLAN. Don't make the mistake of using just one of these options. Instead, look at your security policy as a tightly bound rope consisting of multiple threads. Each thread is another layer of security. In this case, your security policy will remain strong despite the failure of one or two threads. At no time do you want one solution to be the only boundary between maintaining your valuables and losing them.

Implementing WEP

Despite its critics, WEP still offers a reasonable level of security, providing that all its features are used properly. This means greater care in key management, avoiding default options, and making sure adequate encryption is enabled at every opportunity.

Proposed improvements in the standard should overcome many of the limitations of the original security options, and should make WEP more appealing as a security solution. Additionally, as WLAN technology gains popularity, and users clamor for functionality, both the standards committees as well as the hardware vendors will offer improvements. This means that you should make sure to keep abreast of vendor-related software fixes and changes that improve the overall security posture of your WLAN.

Most APs advertise that they support WEP in at least 40-bit encryption, but often the 128-bit option is also supported. For corporate networks, 128-bit encryption–capable devices should be considered as a minimum. With data security enabled in a closed network, the settings on the client for the SSID and the encryption keys have to match the AP when attempting to associate with the network, or it will fail. In the next few paragraphs, we discuss WEP as it relates to the functionality of the standard, including a standard definition of WEP, the privacy created, and the authentication.

Defining WEP

802.11, as a standard, covers the communication between WLAN components. RF poses challenges to privacy in that it travels through and around physical objects. As part of the goals of the communication, a mechanism needed to be implemented to protect the privacy of the individual transmissions that in some way mirrored the privacy found on the wired LAN. Wireless Equivalency Privacy is the mechanism created in the standard as a solution that addresses this goal. Because WEP utilizes a cryptographic security countermeasure for the fulfillment of its stated goal of privacy, it has the added benefit of becoming an authentication mechanism. This benefit is realized through a shared key authentication that allows the encryption and decryption of the wireless transmissions. Many keys can be defined on an AP or a client, and they can be rotated to add complexity for a higher security standard for your WLAN policy. This is a must!

WEP was never intended to be the absolute authority in security. Instead, the driving force was privacy. In cases that require high degrees of security, you should utilize other mechanisms, such as authentication, access control, password protection, and virtual private networks.

Creating Privacy with WEP

Let's look at how WEP creates a degree of privacy on the WLAN. WEP comes in several implementations: no encryption, and 40-bit and 128-bit encryption. Obviously, no encryption means no privacy. Transmissions are sent in the clear, and they can be viewed by any wireless sniffing application that has access to the RF propagated in the WLAN. In the case of the 40- and 128-bit varieties (just as with password length), the greater the number of characters (bits), the stronger the encryption. The initial configuration of the AP will include the setup of the shared key. This shared key can be in the form of either alphanumeric, or hexadecimal strings, and is matched on the client.

WEP uses the RC4 encryption algorithm, a stream cipher developed by noted cryptographer Ron Rivest (the "R" in RSA). Both the sender and receiver use the stream cipher to create identical pseudorandom strings from a known shared key. The process entails the sender to logically XOR the plaintext transmission with the stream cipher to produce the ciphertext. The receiver takes the shared key and identical stream and reverses the process to gain the plaintext transmission.

A 24-bit initialization vector (IV) is used to create the identical cipher streams. The IV is produced by the sender, and is included in the transmission of each frame. A new IV is used for each frame to prevent the reuse of the key weakening the encryption. This means that for each string generated, a different value for the RC4 key will be used. Although a secure policy, consideration of the components of WEP bear out one of the flaws in WEP. Because the 24-bit space is so small with respect to the potential set of IVs, in a short period of time, all keys are eventually reused. Unfortunately, this weakness is the same for both the 40- and 128-bit encryption levels.

To protect against some rudimentary attacks that insert known text into the stream to attempt to reveal the key stream, WEP incorporates a checksum in each frame. Any frame not found to be valid through the checksum is discarded. All in all this sounds secure, but WEP has well-documented flaws, which we cover in later sections. Let's review the process in a little more detail to gain a better understanding of the behind-the-scenes activities that are largely the first line of defense in WLAN security.

The WEP Authentication Process

Shared key authentication is a four-step process that begins when the AP receives the validated request for association. After the AP receives the request, a series of management frames are transmitted between the stations to produce the authentication. This includes the use of the cryptographic mechanisms employed by WEP as a validation.

Strictly with respect to WEP, in the authorization phase, the four steps break down in the following manner:

1. The requestor (the client) sends a request for association.

2. The authenticator (the AP) receives the request, and responds by producing a random challenge text and transmitting it back to the requestor.

3. The requestor receives the transmission, ciphers the challenge with the shared key stream, and returns it.

4. The authenticator decrypts the challenge text and compares the values against the original. If they match, the requestor is authenticated. On the other hand, if the requestor doesn't have the shared key, the cipher stream cannot be reproduced, therefore the plaintext cannot be discovered, and theoretically, the transmission is secured.

WEP Benefits and Advantages

WEP provides some security and privacy in transmissions to prevent curious or casual browsers from viewing the contents of the transmissions held between the AP and the clients. In order to gain access, the degree of sophistication of the intruder has to improve, and specific intent to gain access is required. Let's view some of the other benefits of implementing WEP:

- All messages are encrypted using a checksum to provide some degree of tamper resistance.

- Privacy is maintained via the encryption. If you do not have the key, you can't decrypt the message.

- WEP is extremely easy to implement. Set the encryption key on the AP, repeat the process on each client, and voilà! You're done!

- WEP provides a very basic level of security for WLAN applications.

- WEP keys are user definable and unlimited. You do not have to use pre-defined keys, and you can and should change them often.

WEP Disadvantages

As with any standard or protocol, WEP has some inherent disadvantages. The focus of security is to allow a balance of access and control while juggling the advantages and disadvantages of each implemented countermeasure for security gaps. The following are some of the disadvantages of WEP:

- The RC4 encryption algorithm is a known stream cipher. This means it takes a finite key and attempts to make an infinite pseudorandom key stream in order to generate the encryption.

- Once you alter the key—which you should do often—you have to tell everyone so they can adjust their settings. The more people you tell, the more public the information becomes.

- Used on its own, WEP does not provide adequate WLAN security.

- WEP has to be implemented on every client as well as every AP to be effective.

The Security Implications of Using WEP

From a security perspective, you have mitigated the curious hacker who lacks the means or desire to really hack your network. If you have enabled WEP as instructed in the previous pages, someone has to be actively attempting to break into your network in order to be successful. If that is the case, using the strongest form of WEP available is important. Because WEP relies on a known stream cipher, it is vulnerable to certain attacks. By no means is it the final authority and should not be the only security countermeasure in place to protect your net-work—and ultimately your job!

Implementing WEP on the Cisco Aironet AP 340

As you can see in the following, the Cisco AP340 supports 128-bit encryption. It is configured with either a HTTP connection pictured here, or a serial connec-tion. The serial interface is cryptic and in no way intuitive. If you plan on admin-istering many Cisco wireless devices, use the Web interface. In Figure 15.7, you see the Web interface for an AP340. By using the drop-down menu, you can select **Full Encryption** and then **128 bit** for the key size. Finally, select the **WEP Key** radio button for the transmission key and type the string.

Figure 15.7 WEP Configuration on the Aironet

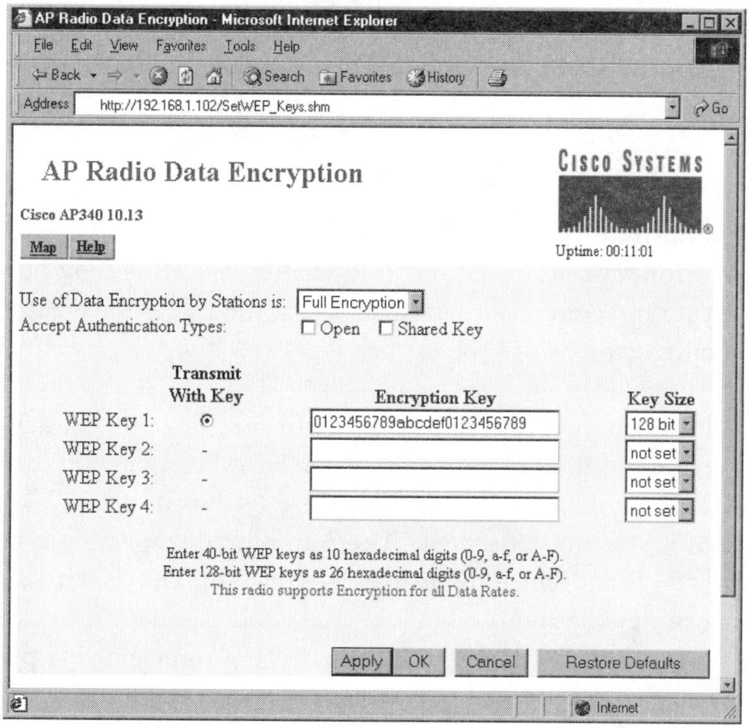

Exploiting WEP

There have been a number of well-publicized exploitations and defeats of the security mechanisms at the heart of WEP, from weaknesses in the encryption algorithm to weaknesses in key management. Although steps have been taken to overcome these weaknesses, attackers are not suffering from a lack of networks to exploit.

The first warnings regarding WEP's vulnerability to compromise came in the fall of 2000 when Jesse Walker published a document called "Unsafe at any Size: An Analysis of the WEP Encryption." In this document, Walker underscored the main weakness of WEP—the fact that it reinitializes the encrypted data stream every time an Ethernet collision occurs. Even though the 802.11 protocol attempts to avoid them with CDMA/CA, collisions are a reality that will occur. If someone is listening in on the wireless conversation, they capture the initialation vector (IV) information transmitted with each frame and in a matter of hours have all the data needed to recover the WEP key.

Although many experts have made similar discoveries regarding this and other ways to recover WEP keys, these were usually academic and only showed that the potential for vulnerability existed. This all changed with the introduction of AirSnort and WEPCrack. Both of these programs saw an initial release in the summer of 2001, and moved the recovery of WEP keys from being a theoretical to something anyone could do—if they had a wireless card based on the Prism2 chipset.

Security of 64-Bit versus 128-Bit Keys

It might seem obvious to a nontechnical person that something protected with a 128-bit encryption scheme would be more secure than something protected with a 64-bit encryption scheme. This, however, is not the case with WEP. Because the same vulnerability exists with both encryption levels, they can be equally broken within similar time limits.

With 64-bit WEP, the network administrator specifies a 40-bit key—typically ten hexadecimal digits (0–9, a–f, or A–F). A 24-bit IV is appended to this 40-bit key, and the RC4 key scheme is built from these 64-bits of data. This same process is followed in the 128-bit scheme. The Administrator specifies a 104-bit key—this time 26 hexadecimal digits (0-9, a-f, or A–F). The 24-bit IV is added to the beginning of the key, and the RC4 key schedule is built.

As you can see, because the vulnerability comes from capturing predictably weak IVs, the size of the original key would not make a significant difference in the security of the encryption. This is due to the relatively small number of total IVs possible under the current WEP specification. Currently, there are a total of 2^{24} possible IV keys. You can see that if the WEP key was not changed within a strictly-defined period of time, all possible IV combinations could be heard off of a 802.11b connection, captured, and made available for cracking within a short period of time. This is a flaw in the design of WEP, and bears no correlation to whether the wireless client is using 64-bit WEP or 128-bit WEP.

Acquiring a WEP Key

As mentioned previously, programs exist that allow an authenticated and/or unassociated device within the listening area of the AP to capture and recover the WEP key. Depending on the speed of the machine listening to the wireless conversations, the number of wireless hosts transmitting on the WLAN, and the number of IV retransmissions due to 802.11 frame collisions, the WEP key could be cracked as quickly as a couple of hours. Obviously, if an attacker attempts to listen to a WEP-protected network when there was very little network traffic, it would take much longer to be able to get the data necessary to crack WEP.

Armed with a valid WEP key, an intruder can now successfully negotiate association with an AP, and gain entry onto the target network. Unless other mechanisms like MAC filtering are in place, this intruder is now able to roam across the network and potentially break into servers or other machines on the network. If MAC filtering is occurring, another procedure must be attempted to get around this. This was covered earlier in the "MAC Filtering" section.

WARNING

Because WEP key retrieval is now possible by casual attackers, keeping the same static WEP key in a production role for an extended period of time does not make sense. If your WEP key is static, it could be published into the underground by a hacker and still be used in a production WLAN six months to a year later.

One of the easiest ways to mitigate the risk of WEP key compromise is to regularly change the WEP key your APs and clients use. Although this may be an easy task for small WLANs, the task becomes extremely daunting when you have dozens of APs and hundreds of clients to manually rekey.

Both Cisco and Funk Software have released Access Control servers that implement rapid WEP rekeying on both APs as well as the end-user client. Utilizing this form of software, even if a WEP key was to be discovered, you could rest assured that within a specified period of time, that particular key would no longer be valid.

Addressing Common Risks and Threats

The advent of wireless networks has not created new legions of attackers. Many attackers will utilize the same attacks for the same objectives they used in wired networks. If you do not protect your wireless infrastructure with proven tools and techniques, and do not have established standards and policies that identify proper deployment and security methodology, you will find that the integrity of your wireless networks may be threatened.

Finding a Target

Utilizing new tools created for wireless networks and thousands of existing identification and attack techniques and utilities, attackers of wireless networks have many avenues to your network. The first step to attacking a wireless network involves finding a network to attack. The first popular software to identify wireless networks was NetStumbler (www.netstumbler.org). NetStumbler is a Windows application that listens for information, such as the SSID, being broadcast from APs that have not disabled the broadcast feature. When it finds a network, it notifies the person running the scan and adds it to the list of found networks.

As people began to drive around their towns and cities looking for wireless networks, NetStumbler added features such as pulling coordinates from Global Positioning System (GPS) satellites and plotting that information on mapping software. This method of finding networks is very reminiscent of a way hackers would find computers when they had only modems to communicate. They would run programs designed to search through all possible phone numbers and call each one looking for a modem to answer the call. This type of scan was typically referred to as *war dialing*; driving around looking for wireless networks has come to be known as *war driving*.

NetStumbler.org created place that people can upload the output of their war drives for inclusion in a database that can graph the location of wireless networks that have been found (www.netstumbler.org/nation.php). See Figure 15.8 for output of discovered and uploaded wireless networks as of January 2002.

Similar tools soon became available for Linux and other UNIX-based operating systems, which contained many additional utilities hackers use to attack hosts and networks once access is found. A quick search on www.freshmeat.net or www.packetstormsecurity.com for "802.11" will reveal several network identification tools as well as tools to configure and monitor wireless network connections.

Finding Weaknesses in a Target

If a network is found without encryption enabled, which reports are showing to be more than half of the networks found so far, the attacker has complete access to any resource the wireless network is connected to. They can scan and attack any machines local to the network, or launch attacks on remote hosts without any fear of reprisal, as the world thinks the attack is coming from the owner of the wireless network.

If the network is found with WEP enabled, the attacker will need to identify several items to reduce the time it will take to get onto the wireless network.

First, utilizing the output of NetStumbler or one of the other network discovery tools, the attacker will identify the SSID, network, MAC address, and any other packets that might be transmitted in cleartext. Generally, NetStumbler results include vendor information, which an attacker can use to determine which default keys to attempt on the wireless network.

Figure 15.8 Networks Discovered with NetStumbler (as of January 2002)

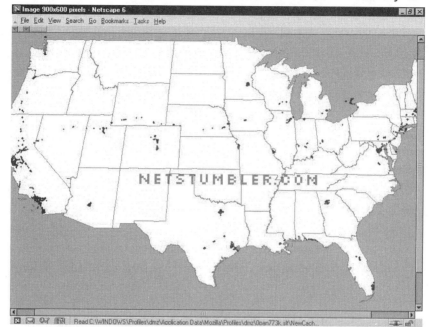

If the vendor information has been changed or is unavailable, the attacker can still use the SSID and network name and address to identify the vendor or owner of the equipment (many people use the same network name as the password, or use the company initials or street address as their password). If the SSID and network name and address has been changed from the default setting, a final network-based attempt could be to use the MAC address to identify the manufacturer.

If none of these options work, there is still the possibility of a physical review. Many public areas are participating in the wireless revolution. An observant attacker will be able to use physical and wireless identification techniques—such as finding antennas, APs, and other wireless devices that are easily identified by the manufacturer's casing and logo.

Exploiting Those Weaknesses

A well-configured wireless AP will not stop a determined attacker. Even if the network name and SSID are changed and the secret key is manually reconfigured on all workstations on a somewhat regular basis, the attacker will still take other avenues to compromise the network.

If easy access is available near to the wireless network, such as a parking lot or garage next to the building being attacked, the only thing an attacker needs is patience and AirSnort or WEPCrack. When these applications have captured enough "weak" packets (IV collisions, for example) they are able to determine the secret key currently in use on the network. Quick tests have shown that an average home network can be cracked in an overnight session. This means that to ensure your network protection, you would need to change your WEP key at least two times per day, or keep your eyes open for any vehicles that look suspicious (with an antenna sticking out the window, for instance) parked outside your home or business for hours or days at a time.

If none of these network tools help in determining which default configurations to try, the next step is to scan the traffic for any cleartext information that might be available. Some manufacturers, such as Lucent, have been known to broadcast the SSID in cleartext even when WEP and closed network options are enabled. Using tools such as Ethereal (www.ethereal.com) and TCPDump (www.tcpdump.org) allow the attacker to sniff traffic and analyze it for any cleartext hints they may find.

As a last option, the attacker will go directly after your equipment or install their own. The number of laptops or accessories stolen from travelers is rising each year. At one time these thefts were perpetrated by criminals simply looking to sell the equipment, but as criminals become more savvy, they are also after the information contained within the machines. Once you have access to the equipment, you are able to determine what valid MAC addresses can access the network, what the network SSID is, and what secret keys are to be used.

An attacker does not need to become a burglar in order to acquire this information. A skilled attacker will utilize new and specially designed malware and network tricks to determine the information needed to access your wireless network. A well-scripted Visual Basic script that could arrive in e-mail (targeted spam) or through an infected Web site can extract the information from the user's machine and upload it to the attacker.

With the size of computers so small today (note the products at www.mynix .com/espace/index.html and www.citydesk.pt/produto_ezgo.htm), it wouldn't take much for the attacker to simply create a small AP of their own that could be attached to your building or office and look just like another telephone box. Such a device, if placed properly, will attract much less attention than someone camping in a car or van in your parking lot.

Sniffing, Interception, and Eavesdropping

Originally conceived as a legitimate network and traffic analysis tool, sniffing remains one of the most effective techniques in attacking a wireless network, whether it's to map the network as part of a target reconnaissance, to grab pass-words, or to capture unencrypted data.

Defining Sniffing

Sniffing is the electronic form of eavesdropping on the communications that computers have across networks. In the original networks deployed, the equip-ment tying machines together allowed every machine on the network to see the traffic of others. These repeaters and hubs, while very successful for getting machines connected, allowed an attacker easy access to all traffic on the network by only needing to connect to one point to see the entire network's traffic.

Wireless networks function very similar to the original repeaters and hubs. Every communication across the wireless network is viewable to anyone who happens to be listening to the network. In fact, the person listening does not even need to be associated with the network to sniff!

Sample Sniffing Tools

The hacker has many tools available to attack and monitor your wireless network. A few of these tools are Ethereal and AiroPeek (www.wildpackets.com/products/ airopeek) in Windows, and tcpdump or ngrep (http://ngrep.sourceforg.net) within a UNIX or Linux environment. These tools work well for sniffing both wired and wireless networks.

All of these software packages function by putting your network card in what is called *promiscuous mode*. When in this mode, every packet that goes past the interface is captured and displayed within the application window. If the attacker is able to acquire your WEP password, they can then utilize features within AiroPeek and Ethereal to decrypt either live or post-capture data.

Sniffing Case Scenario

By running NetStumbler, the hacker will be able to find possible targets. As shown in Figure 15.9, we have found several networks that we could attack.

Figure 15.9 Discovering Wireless LANS with NetStumbler

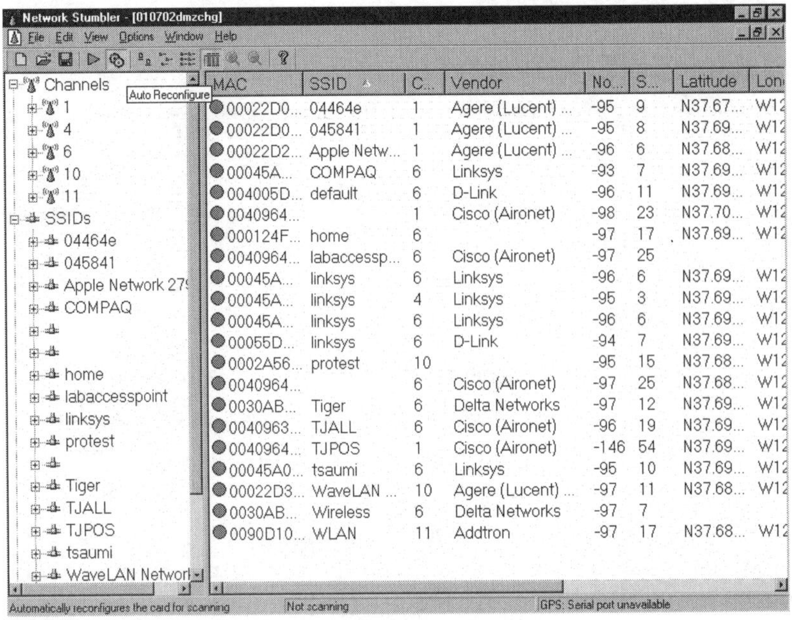

Once the hacker has found possible networks to attack, one of the first tasks is to identify who the target is. Many organizations are "nice" enough to include their name or address in the network name. For those that do not display that information, we can gather a lot from their traffic that allows us to determine who they could be.

Utilizing any of the mentioned network sniffing tools, the unencrypted network is easily monitored. Figure 15.10 shows our network sniff of the traffic on the wireless network. From this, we are able to determine who their Domain Name System (DNS) server is, and what default search domain and default Web home page they are accessing. With this information, we can easily identify who the target is and determine if they are worth attacking.

If the network is encrypted, the first place to start is locating the physical location of the target. NetStumbler has the capability to display the signal strength of the networks you have discovered (see Figure 15.11). Utilizing this information, the attacker needs to just drive around and look for where the signal strength increases and decreases to determine the home of the wireless network.

Figure 15.10 Sniffing with Ethereal

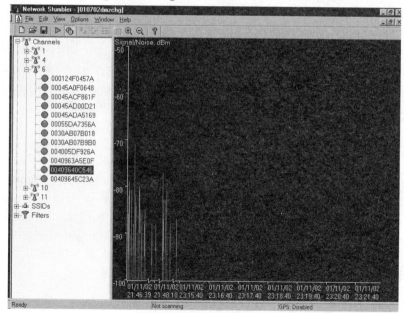

Figure 15.11 Using Signal Strength to Find Wireless Networks

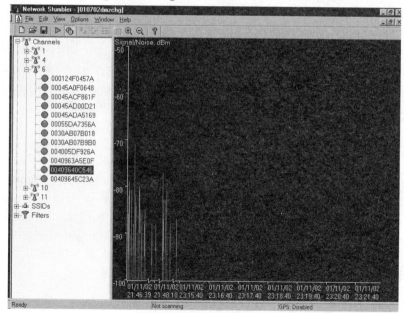

To enhance the ability to triangulate the position of the wireless network, the attacker can utilize directional antennas to focus the wireless interface in a

specific direction. An excellent source for wireless information, including information on the design of directional antennas is the Bay Area Wireless Users Group (www.bawug.org).

Protecting Against Sniffing and Eavesdropping

One protection available to wired networks was the upgrade from repeaters and hubs to a switched environment. These switches would send only the traffic intended over each individual port, making it difficult (although not impossible) to sniff the entire network's traffic. This is not an option for wireless due to the nature of wireless itself.

The only way to protect your wireless users from attackers who might be sniffing is to utilize encrypted sessions wherever possible: Use SSL for e-mail connections, SSH instead of Telnet, and Secure Copy (SCP) instead of FTP.

To protect your network from being discovered with NetStumbler, be sure to turn off any network identification broadcasts, and if possible, close down your network to any unauthorized users. This will prevent tools such as NetStumbler from finding your network to begin with. However, the knowledgeable attacker will know that just because you are not broadcasting your information does not mean that your network can't be found.

All the attacker needs to do is utilize one of the network sniffers to monitor for network activity. Although not as efficient as NetStumbler, it is still a functional way to discover and monitor networks. Even encrypted networks will show traffic to the sniffer, even if you are not broadcasting who you are. Once they have identified your traffic, the attacker will then be able to utilize the same identification techniques to begin an attack on your network.

Spoofing and Unauthorized Access

The combination of weaknesses in WEP, and the nature of wireless transmission, has highlighted the art of *spoofing* as a real threat to wireless network security. Some well publicized weaknesses in user authentication using WEP have made authentication spoofing just one of an equally well tested number of exploits by attackers.

Defining Spoofing

One definition of spoofing is where an attacker is able to trick your network equipment into thinking that the connection they are coming from is one of the valid and allowed machines from its network. Attackers can accomplish this several ways, the easiest of which is to simply redefine the MAC address of your wireless or network card to be a valid MAC address. This can be accomplished in Windows through a simple Registry edit. Several wireless providers also have an option to define the MAC address for each wireless connection from within the client manager application that is provided with the interface.

There are several reasons that an attacker would spoof your network. If you have closed out your network to only valid interfaces through MAC or IP address filtering, if an attacker is able to determine a valid MAC or IP address, he could then reprogram his interface with that information, allowing him to connect to your network impersonating a valid machine.

IEEE 802.11 networks introduce a new form of spoofing: authentication spoofing. As described in their paper "Intercepting Mobile Communications: The Insecurities of 802.11," the authors identified a way to utilize weaknesses within WEP and the authentication process to spoof authentication into a closed network. The process of authentication, as defined by IEEE 802.11, is a very simple process. In a shared-key configuration, the AP sends out a 128-byte random string in a cleartext message to the workstation wishing to authenticate. The workstation then encrypts the message with the shared key and returns the encrypted message to the AP. If the message matches what the AP is expecting, the workstation is authenticated onto the network and access is allowed.

As described in the paper, if an attacker has knowledge of both the original plaintext and ciphertext messages, it is possible to create a forged encrypted message. By sniffing the wireless network, an attacker is able to accumulate many authentication requests, each of which includes the original plaintext message and the returned ciphertext-encrypted reply. From this, the attacker can easily identify the keystream used to encrypt the response message. She could then use it to forge an authentication message that the AP will accept as a proper authentication.

Sample Spoofing Tools

The wireless hacker does not need many complex tools to succeed in spoofing a MAC address. In many cases, these changes are either features of the wireless manufacturers or easily changed through a Windows Registry modification. Once a valid MAC is identified, the attacker need only reconfigure his device to trick the AP into thinking they are a valid user.

The ability to forge authentication onto a wireless network is a complex process. There are no known "off the shelf" packages available that will provide these services. An attacker will need to either create their own tool or take the time to decrypt the secret key by using AirSnort or WEPCrack.

If the attacker is using Windows 2000, and his network card supports recon-figuring the MAC address, there is another way to reconfigure this information. If your card supports this feature, you can change it from the Control Panel by clicking the **System** icon. Once the System Properties dialog box appears, select the **Hardware** tab and choose **Device Manager**. Within the Device Manager, under the **Network Adaptors**, you should find your interface. If you open the properties to this interface, you should have an **Advanced** tab. Many network adaptors allow you to reconfigure the MAC address of the card from this area.

Now that the hacker is utilizing a valid MAC address, he is able to access any resource available from your wireless network. If you have WEP enabled, the hacker will have to either identify your secret key, or as you will see shortly, cap-ture the key through malware or stealing the user's notebook.

Protecting Against Spoofing and Unauthorized Attacks

Little can be done to prevent these attacks. The best protection involves several additional pieces to the wireless network. Using an external authentication source, such as RADIUS or SecurID, will prevent an unauthorized user from accessing the wireless network and resources it connects with.

If the attacker has reconfigured her machine to use a valid MAC address, little can be done, except the additional external authentication. The only additional protection that you can provide is if you utilize secure connections for all host services accessed by the network. If you use SSH and SSL, you can require valid client certificates to access those resources. Even if a hacker were able to access the network, this would keep her from accessing your critical systems.

However, note that even with this, and without utilizing either a dynamic firewall or RADIUS WEP authentication, an attacker could be able to get onto your network. Even if you protect your critical systems, the attacker will still have access to all workstations on the network, as well as all networks that are con-nected to the wireless network. She could then compromise those resources and acquire the valid information needed to access your systems.

Network Hijacking and Modification

Numerous techniques are available for an attacker to "hijack" a wireless network or session. And unlike some attacks, network and security administrators may be unable to tell the difference between the hijacker and a legitimate passenger.

Defining Hijacking

Many tools are available to the network hijacker. These tools are based upon basic implementation issues within almost every network device available today. As TCP/IP packets go through switches, routers, and APs, each device looks at the destination IP address and compares it with the IP addresses it knows to be local. If the address is not in the table, the device hands the packet off to its default gateway.

This table is used to coordinate the IP address with what MAC addresses are local to the device. In many situations, this list is a dynamic list that is built up from traffic that is passing through the device and through Address Resolution Protocol (ARP) notifications from new devices joining the network. There is no authentication or verification that the request received by the device is valid. So a malicious user is able to send messages to routing devices and APs stating that their MAC address is associated with a known IP address. From then on, all traffic that goes through that router destined for the hijacked IP address will be handed off to the hacker's machine.

If the attacker spoofs as the default gateway or a specific host on the network, all machines trying to get to the network or the spoofed machine will connect to the attacker's machine instead of where they had intended. If the attacker is clever, he will only use this to identify passwords and other necessary information and route the rest of the traffic to the intended recipient. This way the end user has no idea that this "man-in-the-middle" has intercepted her communications and compromised her passwords and information.

Another clever attack that is possible is through the use of rogue APs. If the attacker is able to put together an AP with enough strength, the end users may not be able to tell which AP is the real one to use. In fact, most will not even know that another is available. Using this, the attacker is able to receive authentication requests and information from the end workstation regarding the secret key and where they are attempting to connect.

These rogue APs can also be used to attempt to break into more tightly configured wireless APs. Utilizing tools such as AirSnort and WEPCrack requires a large amount of data to be able to decrypt the secret key. A hacker sitting in a car in front of your house or office is easily identified, and will generally not have enough time to finish acquiring enough information to break the key. However, if they install a tiny, easily hidden machine, this machine could sit there long enough to break the key and possibly act as an external AP into the wireless network it has hacked.

Sample Hijacking Tools

Attackers who wish to spoof more than their MAC addresses have several tools available. Most of the tools available are for use under a UNIX environment and can be found through a simple search for "ARP Spoof" at http://packetstormsecurity.com. With these tools, the hacker can easily trick all machines on your wireless network into thinking that the hacker's machine is another machine. Through simple sniffing on the network, an attacker can determine which machines are in high use by the workstations on the network. If they then spoof themselves as one of these machines, they could possibly intercept much of the legitimate traffic on the network.

AirSnort and WEPCrack are freely available. And while it would take additional resources to build a rogue AP, these tools will run from any Linux machine.

Hijacking Case Scenario

Now that we have identified the network to be attacked, and spoofed our MAC address to become a valid member of the network, we can gain further information that is not available through simple sniffing. If the network being attacked is using SSH to access their hosts, just stealing a password might be easier than attempting to break into the host using any exploit that might be available.

By just ARP spoofing their connection with the AP to be that of the host they are wishing to steal the passwords from, all wireless users who are attempting to SSH into the host will then connect to the rogue machine. When they attempt to sign on with their password, the attacker is then able to, first, receive their password, and second, pass on the connection to the real end destination. If the attacker does not do the second step, it will increase the likelihood that their attack will be noticed because users will begin to complain that they are unable to connect to the host.

Protection against Network Hijacking and Modification

You can use several different tools to protect your network from IP spoofing with invalid ARP requests. These tools, such as ArpWatch, will notify an administrator when ARP requests are seen, allowing the administrator to take appropriate action to determine if indeed someone is attempting to hack into the network.

Another option is to statically define the MAC/IP address definitions. This will prevent the attacker from being able to redefine this information. However, due to the management overhead in statically defining all network adaptors' MAC address on every router and AP, this solution is rarely implemented. In fact, many APs do not offer any options to define the ARP table, and it would depend upon the switch or firewall you are using to separate your wireless network from your wired network.

There is no way to identify or prevent any attackers from using passive attacks, such as from AirSnort or WEPCrack, to determine the secret key used in an encrypted wireless network. The best protection available is to change the secret key on a regular basis and add additional authentication mechanisms such as RADIUS or dynamic firewalls to restrict access to your wired network once a user has connected to the wireless network. However, if you have not properly secured every wireless workstation, an attacker need only go after one of the other wireless clients to be able to access the resources available to it.

Denial of Service and Flooding Attacks

The nature of wireless transmission, and especially the use of spread spectrum technology, makes a wireless network especially vulnerable to *denial of service* (DoS) attacks. The equipment needed to launch such an attack is freely available and very affordable. In fact, many homes and offices contain equipment necessary to deny service to their wireless network.

Defining DoS and Flooding

A denial of service occurs when an attacker has engaged most of the resources a host or network has available, rendering it unavailable to legitimate users. One of the original DoS attacks is known as a *ping flood*. A ping flood utilizes misconfigured equipment along with bad "features" within TCP/IP to cause a large number of hosts or devices to send an ICMP echo (ping) to a specified target. When the attack occurs it tends to use much of the resources of both the network connection and the host being attacked. This will then make it very difficult for any end users to access the host for normal business purposes.

In a wireless network, several items can cause a similar disruption of service. Probably the easiest is through a confliction within the wireless spectrum by different devices attempting to use the same frequency. Many new wireless telephones use the same frequency as 802.11 networks. Through either intentional or unintentional uses of this, a simple telephone call could prevent all wireless users from accessing the network.

Another possible attack would be through a massive amount of invalid (or valid) authentication requests. If the AP is tied up with thousands of spoofed authentication attempts, any users attempting to authenticate themselves would have major difficulties in acquiring a valid session.

As you saw earlier, the attacker has many tools available to hijack network connections. If a hacker is able to spoof the machines of a wireless network into thinking that the attackers machine is their default gateway, not only will the attacker be able to intercept all traffic destined to the wired network, but they would also be able to prevent any of the wireless network machines from accessing the wired network. To do this the hacker need only spoof the AP and not forward connections on to the end destination, preventing all wireless users from doing valid wireless activities.

Sample DoS Tools

Not much is needed to create a wireless DoS. In fact, many users create these situations with the equipment found within their homes or offices. In a small apartment building, you could find several APs as well as many wireless telephones. These users could easily create many DoS attacks on their own networks as well as on those of their neighbors.

A hacker wishing to DoS a network with a flood of authentication strings will also need to be a well skilled programmer. Not many tools are available to create this type of attack, but as we have seen in the attempts to crack WEP, much of the programming required does not take much effort or time. In fact, a skilled hacker should be able to create such a tool within a few hours. When done, this simple application, when used with standard wireless equipment, could possibly render your wireless network unusable for the duration of the attack.

Creating a hijacked AP DoS will require additional tools that can be found on many security sites. See the earlier section "Sample Hijacking Tools" for a possible starting point to acquiring some of the ARP spoofing tools needed. These tools are not very complex and are available for almost every computing platform available.

DoS and Flooding Case Scenario

Many apartments and older office buildings do not come prewired for the high-tech networks that many people are using today. To add to the problem, if many individuals are setting up their own wireless networks, without coordinating the installs, many problems can occur that will be difficult to detect.

Only so many frequencies are available to 802.11 networks. In fact, once the frequency is chosen, it does not change until someone manually reconfigures it.

With these problems, it is not hard to imagine the following situation from occurring.

A person goes out and purchases a wireless AP and several network cards for his home network. When he gets home to his apartment and configures his network he is extremely happy with how well wireless actually works. Then all of a sudden none of the machines on the wireless network are able to communicate. After waiting on hold for 45 minutes to get though to tech support for the device, the network magically starts working again so he hangs up.

Later that week the same problem occurs, only this time he decides to wait on hold. While waiting he goes onto his porch and begins discussing his frustration with his neighbor. During the conversation his neighbor's kids come out and say that their wireless network is not working.

So they begin to do a few tests (still waiting on hold, of course). First the man's neighbor turns off his AP (which is generally off unless the kids are online, to "protect" their network). Once this is done the wireless network starts working again. Then they turn on the neighbor's AP again and the network stops working again.

At this point, tech support finally answers and he describes what has happened. The tech-support representative has seen this situation several times and informs the user that he will need to change the frequency used in the device to another channel. He explains that what has happened is that the neighbor's network is utilizing the same channel, causing the two networks to conflict. Once he changes the frequency, everything starts working properly.

Protecting Against DoS and Flooding Attacks

There is little that you can do to protect against DoS attacks. In a wireless environment the attacker does not need to even be in the same building or neighborhood. With a good enough antenna, the attacker is able to send these attacks from a great distance away. There is no indication that there is any reason for the disruption.

This is one of the valid times to use NetStumbler in a nonhacking context. By using NetStumbler, you can identify any other networks that might be conflicting with your network configuration. However, NetStumbler will not identify other DoS attacks or other equipment that is causing conflicts (such as wireless telephones).

Summary

Only through a solid understanding of security fundamentals, principles, and procedures will you be able to fully identify today's security risks. From this understanding, which is built upon "The Big Three" tenets of security (confidentiality, integrity, and availability, or CIA) come the basis for all other security practices. The essential practices usually associated with security build upon the concepts of "The Big Three," which provide tools for actually implementing security into systems. The ability to properly authenticate a user or process, before allowing that user or process access to specific resources, protect the CIA directly. If you are able to clearly identify the authenticated user through electronic non-repudiation techniques usually found in encryption tools such as public-key encryption, you can ensure that the entities attempting to gain access are who they say they are. Finally, if you log the activities performed, a third party can monitor the logs and ensure that all activity happening on a system complies with the policy and standards defined, and that all inappropriate activity is identified, allowing for possible prosecution or investigation into the invalid activity.

Following these practices, through the use of tested and proven identification and evaluation standards, you can fully understand the security risks associated with any object. Once you know the risks, you can provide solutions to diminish these risks as much as possible.

The standard solution is to create a formal security policy along with detailed guidelines and procedures. These guidelines describe the actual implementation steps necessary for any platform to comply with the established security procedure.

By using these standard methods to protect your wireless network, you should be able to develop a clear and concise wireless security plan that incorporates the needs of your organization's highest levels. This plan will allow for the deployment of a wireless network that's as secure as possible and will provide clear exception listings for areas where the risks to your infrastructure cannot be fully controlled.

Through a careful examination of the design of WEP, we identified significant weaknesses in the algorithm. These weaknesses, along with implementation flaws, have lead to the creation of many new tools that can be used to attack wireless networks. These tools allow for the attacker to identify a wireless network through *war driving* and then crack the secret key by passively listening to the encrypted transmissions. Once they have access to the secret key, only those that have deployed additional security measures will have some additional protection for the rest of their infrastructure.

Even if you have a incident response plan and procedure defined in your security standards, if an attack is not known to be happening, there is little you can do to mitigate or rectify the intrusion. The entire discovery and WEP-cracking process is passive and undetectable. Only at the point of attacking other wireless hosts or spoofing their attacking machine as a valid host does the attack becomes noticeable. However, many installations do not implement system logging, nor do they have standards and practices requiring monitoring of those logs for inappropriate activity.

None of these actions will provide protection against one of the oldest attacks known—theft. There is little you can do to protect your resources if critical information, such as network passwords and access definitions, can be acquired by only gaining access to notebooks or backups. High-tech criminals are creating custom malware that can access this information through spam or disguised Web sites.

Although wireless networks are making computing easier and more accessible, understanding the design and implementation weaknesses in 802.11 will help you in preventing attacks. And at times when attacks are unavoidable, by knowing how and where the attackers will come, you may be able to identify when they are attempting to gain access and respond as defined in your standards and incident response practices.

Solutions Fast Track

Understanding Security Fundamentals and Principles of Protection

☑ "The Big Three" tenets of security are: *confidentiality*, *integrity*, and *availability*.

☑ Requirements needed to implement the principles of protection include proper authentication of authorized users through a system that provides for a clear identification of the users via tested non-repudiation techniques.

☑ Internal or external auditors can use logging or system accounting to ensure that the system is functioning and being utilized in accordance to defined standards and policies.

- ☑ Logging can also be the first place to look for evidence should an attack does occur. Ensure that logging is going to a trusted third-party site that cannot be accessed by personnel and resources being logged.

- ☑ These tools are essential to protecting the privacy of customer, partner, or trade secret information.

- ☑ Encryption has provided many tools for the implementation of these security fundamentals.

- ☑ Encryption is not the definitive solution to security problems. For example, a known secret key could be stolen, or one of the parties utilizing encryption could be tricked or forced into performing the activity, which would be seen as a valid cryptographic operation because the system has no knowledge of any collusion involved in the generation of the request.

MAC Filtering

- ☑ Media Access Control (MAC) filtering is effective against casual attackers.

- ☑ MAC filtering can be circumvented by changing the MAC address on the client device.

- ☑ It is difficult to determine if the lack of association is due to MAC filtering or other reasons like an incorrect Wired Equivalent Protocol (WEP) key.

Reviewing the Role of Policy

- ☑ Once basic fundamentals and principles are understood, through the creation of policies and standards an organization or entity is able to clearly define how to design, implement, and monitor their infrastructure securely.

- ☑ Policies must have direct support and sign-in by the executive management of any organization.

- ☑ A properly mitigated risk should reduce the impact of the threat as well as the likelihood that that threat will occur.

- ☑ A clear and well-defined classification and labeling system is key to the identification of resources being protected.

☑ Information classification techniques also provide a method by which the items being classified can then have the proper policy or standards placed around them depending on the level or importance, as well as the risk associated with each identified item.

☑ Some organizations are required by their own regulations to have clear and well defined standards and policies.

Implementing WEP

☑ To protect against some rudimentary attacks that insert known text into the stream to attempt to reveal the key stream, WEP incorporates a check sum in each frame. Any frame not found to be valid through the check sum is discarded.

☑ Used on its own, WEP does not provide adequate wireless local area network (WLAN) security.

☑ WEP has to be implemented on every client as well as every Access Point (AP) to be effective.

☑ WEP keys are user definable and unlimited. You do not have to use predefined keys, and you can and should change them often.

☑ Implement the strongest version of WEP available and keep abreast of the latest upgrades to the standards.

Addressing Common Risks and Threats

☑ By examining the common threats to both wired and wireless networks, you can see how a solid understanding in the basics of security principles allows you to fully assess the risks associated with using wireless and other technologies.

☑ Threats can come from simple design issues, where multiple devices utilize the same setup, or intentional denial of service attacks which can result in the corruption or loss of data.

☑ Not all threats are caused by malicious users. They can also be caused by a conflict of similar resources, such as with 802.11b networks and cordless telephones.

☑ With wireless networks going beyond the border of your office or home, chances are greater that your actions might be monitored by a third party.

☑ Unless your organization has clear and well-defined policies and guidelines, you might find yourself in legal or business situations where your data is either compromised, lost, or disrupted. Without a clear plan of action that identifies what is important in certain scenarios, you will not be able to address situations as they occur.

Sniffing, Interception, and Eavesdropping

☑ Electronic eavesdropping, or *sniffing*, is passive and undetectable to intrusion detection devices.

☑ Tools to sniff networks are available for Windows (such as Ethereal and AiroPeek) and UNIX (such as tcpdump and ngrep).

☑ Sniffing traffic allows attackers to identify additional resources that can be compromised.

☑ Even encrypted networks have been shown to disclose vital information in cleartext, such as the network name, that can be received by attackers sniffing the WLAN.

☑ Any authentication information that is broadcast can often be simply replayed to services requiring authentication (NT Domain, WEP authentication, and so on) to access resources.

☑ The use of virtual private networks, Secure Sockets Layer (SSL), and Secure Shell (SSH) helps protect against wireless interception.

Spoofing and Unauthorized Access

☑ Due to the design of Transmission Control Protocol/Internet Protocol (TCP/IP), there is little that you can do to prevent MAC/IP address spoofing.

☑ Only through static definition of MAC address tables can you prevent this type of attack. However, due to significant overhead in management, this is rarely implemented.

☑ Wireless network authentication can be easily spoofed by simply replaying another node's authentication back to the AP when attempting to connect to the network.

☑ Many wireless equipment providers allow for end-users to redefine the MAC address within their cards through the configuration utilities that come with the equipment.

☑ External two-factor authentication such as Remote Access Dial-In User Service (RADIUS) or SecurID should be implemented to additionally restrict access requiring strong authentication to access the wireless resources.

Network Hijacking and Modification

☑ Due to the design of TCP/IP, some spoof attacks allow for attackers to hijack or take over network connections established for other resources on the wireless network.

☑ If an attacker hijacks the AP, all traffic from the wireless network gets routed through the attacker, so they are then able to identify passwords and other information other users are attempting to use on valid network hosts.

☑ Many users are easily susceptible to these man-in-the-middle attacks, often entering their authentication information even after receiving many notifications that SSL or other keys are not what they should be.

☑ Rogue APs can assist the attacker by allowing remote access from wired or wireless networks.

☑ These attacks are often overlooked as just faults in the user's machine, allowing attackers to continue hijacking connections with little fear of being noticed.

Denial of Service and Flooding Attacks

☑ Many wireless networks within a small space can easily cause network disruptions and even denial of service (DoS) for valid network users.

☑ If an attacker hijacks the AP and does not pass traffic on to the proper destination, all users of the network will be unable to use the network.

☑ Flooding the wireless network with transmissions can also prevent other devices from utilizing the resources, making the wireless network inaccessible to valid network users.

☑ Wireless attackers can utilize strong and directional antennas to attack the wireless network from a great distance.

☑ An attacker who has access to the wired network can flood the wireless AP with more traffic than it can handle, preventing wireless users from accessing the wired network.

☑ Many new wireless products utilize the same wireless frequencies as 802.11 networks. A simple cordless telephone could create a DoS situation for the network more easily than any of these other techniques.

Frequently Asked Questions

The following Frequently Asked Questions, answered by the authors of this book, are designed to both measure your understanding of the concepts presented in this chapter and to assist you with real-life implementation of these concepts. To have your questions about this chapter answered by the author, browse to **www.syngress.com/solutions** and click on the **"Ask the Author"** form.

Q: Do I really need to understand the fundamentals of security in order to protect my network?

A: While you are able to utilize the configuration options available to you from your equipment provider, without a solid background in how security is accomplished you will never be able to protect your assets from the unknown threats that will come against your network through either misconfiguration, backdoors provided by the vendor, or new exploits that have not been patched by your vendor.

Q: Am I required by law to have a security policy?

A: If your organization is a video store, deals with children's records, or is associated with the health care or financial industries (and you are located in the United States), you are most likely required by federal regulation to have a defined security policy, and in some cases you are required to have complete third-party audits of your configuration and policies. If you are not required by legislation, you might still find yourself liable under civil law to provide proper protection for customer or partner information contained within your system.

Q: Is 128-bit WEP more secure than 64-bit WEP?

A: Not really. This is because the WEP vulnerability has more to do with the 24-bit initialization vector than the actual size of the WEP key.

Q: If I am a home user, can I assume that if I use MAC filtering and WEP, that my network is secure?

A: You can make the assumption that your home network is more secure than if it did not utilize these safeguards. However, as shown in this chapter, these methods can be circumvented to allow for intrusion.

Q: Where can I find more information on WEP vulnerabilities?

A: Besides being one of the sources who brought WEP vulnerabilities to light, www.isaac.cs.berkeley.edu has links to other Web sites that cover WEP insecurities.

Q: Can my customers really sue me or my company for being hacked and having their information leaked or misused?

A: In any situation, if you have an established trust with a customer to maintain their information securely and someone breaks into the building or into their corporate servers, a a customer can possibly pursue litigation against you if you did not have any policies or procedures in place to address the risk associated with this and other threats to the customer's information.

Q: If someone can be forced into performing an activity, why should I bother setting up complex security applications?

A: Without those applications in place, you would find that it does not take direct force to attack you or your information. There has always been the possibility that threats could force individuals in key positions to reveal damaging information and secrets, but there is a greater chance that someone will trick a user into disclosing their password or some other security key. Proper training and education are the best defenses in these situations.

Q: I added a firewall to my design. Why should I also need both a policy and external auditing?

A: Again, a firewall may protect you initially, but what do you do as technology changes, or your staff is replaced? Policies and standards ensure that current and future implementations are built in accordance to the definitions laid out by the organization. Adding logging, as well as internal and third-party auditing of the implemented resources helps ensure that the implementations are built in accordance to policy, and that all activity occurring within the environment is in compliance with your standards, guidelines, and policies.

Q: If I have enabled WEP, am I now protected?

A: No. Certain tools can break all WEP keys by simply monitoring the network traffic for generally less than 24 hours.

Q: Is there any solution available besides RADIUS to perform external user and key management?

A: No, plans are available from manufacturers to identify other ways of performing the user/key management, but to date nothing is available.

Index

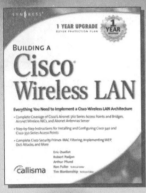
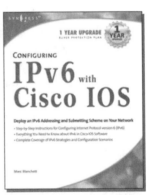
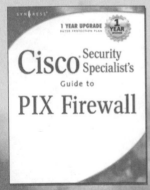
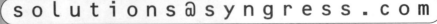